The Ship's Medicine Chest and Medical Aid at Sea

The Ship's Medicine Chest and Medical Aid at Sea

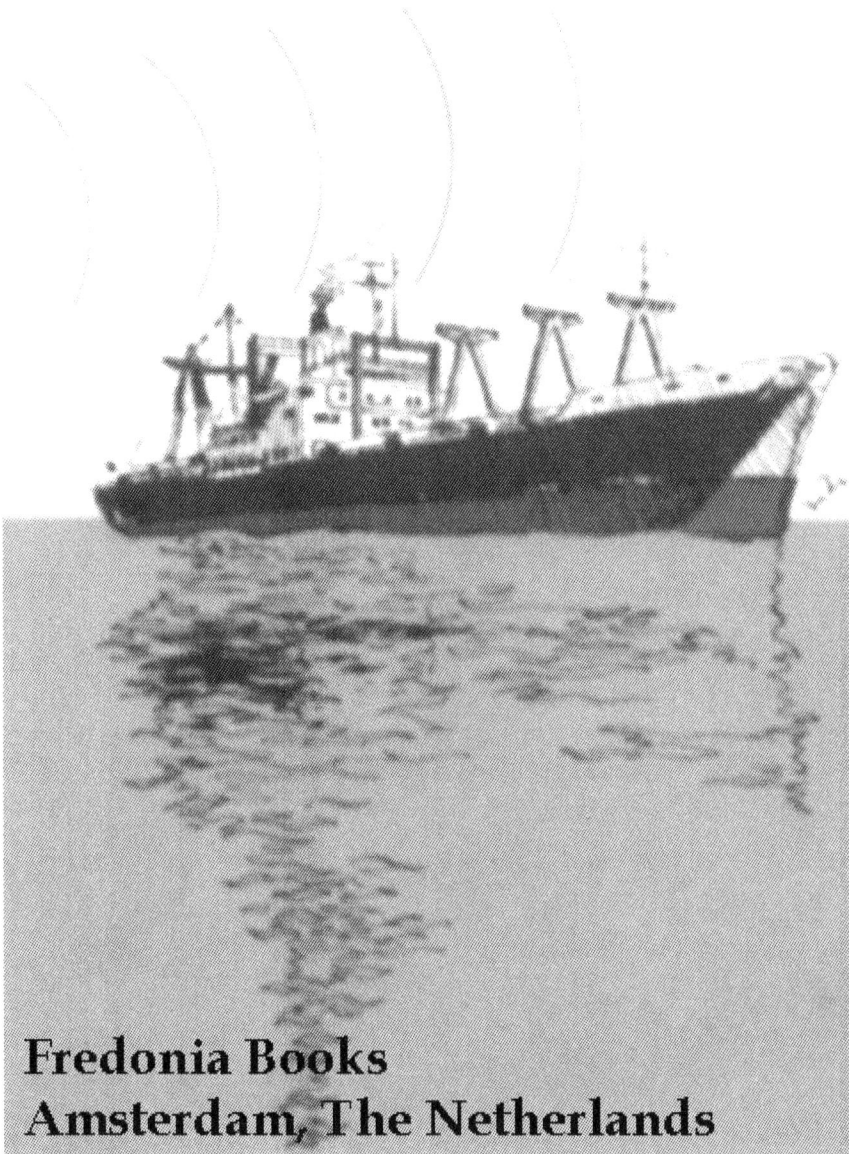

Fredonia Books
Amsterdam, The Netherlands

The Ship's Medicine Chest and Medical Aid at Sea

by
U.S. Public Health Service

ISBN: 1-58963-629-5

Reprinted from the 1978 edition

Fredonia Books
Amsterdam, the Netherlands
http://www.fredoniabooks.com

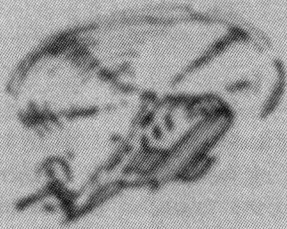

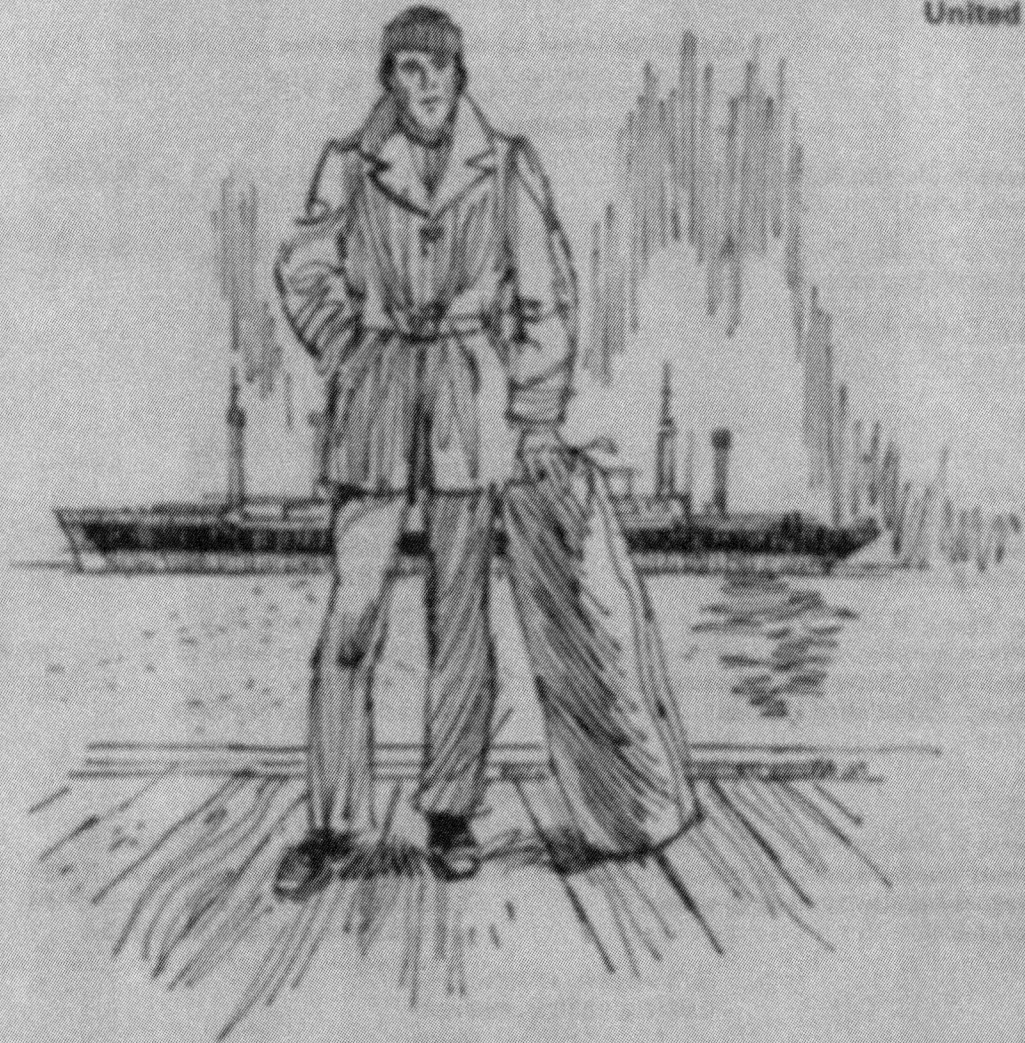

Review and Consultation

THE SHIP'S MEDICINE CHEST AND MEDICAL AID AT SEA was prepared in the Bureau of Medical Services, U.S. Public Health Service (PHS). Members of the Bureau staff are indicated below. Four senior PHS officers provided medical review and three special consultants assisted in the preparation of some of the material.

Technical-Editorial Advisory Committee

Chairman: Truman L. McCasland, Dr.P.H.
Commander (PHS)

Richard J. Bertin, R.Ph., Ph.D.
Captain (PHS)

Arthur W. Dodds, Ph.G., Ph.C.
Captain (PHS), *retired*

Jean E. Lazar, R.N.

Sanford S. Leffingwell, M.D., M.P.H.
Commander (PHS)

Pietrina Siciliano, R.N., M.S., M.P.H.
Captain (PHS)

Charles P. White, D.D.S.
Captain (PHS)

Medical Review

William A. Cherry, M.D.
Assistant Surgeon General (PHS)
Former Chief Medical Officer
U.S. Coast Guard

Roger Black, M.D.
Assistant Surgeon General (PHS), *retired*
Former Acting Director, Clinical Center
National Institutes of Health

Robert L. Brutsche, M.D.
Assistant Surgeon General (PHS)
Medical Director
Bureau of Prisons

Robert E. Streicher, M.D.
Assistant Surgeon General (PHS), *retired*
Former Director
Bureau of Medical Services

Special Consultants

Richard V. Phillipson, F.R.C. Psych., M.D.
National Institute on Drug Abuse (PHS)
  Prepared material on *drug abuse,*
  Chapter V.

James F. Beddow, Vessel Consultant
Food and Drug Administration (PHS)
  Prepared material on *environmental control aboard ship,* Chapter XI.

H. Vaughan Belcher, M.D.
Captain (PHS), *retired*

Editor: George T. Furlong, M.A., M.P.H.
Art Director: Harry J. Wiener
Typing and Review: Elizabeth Barrett

Foreword

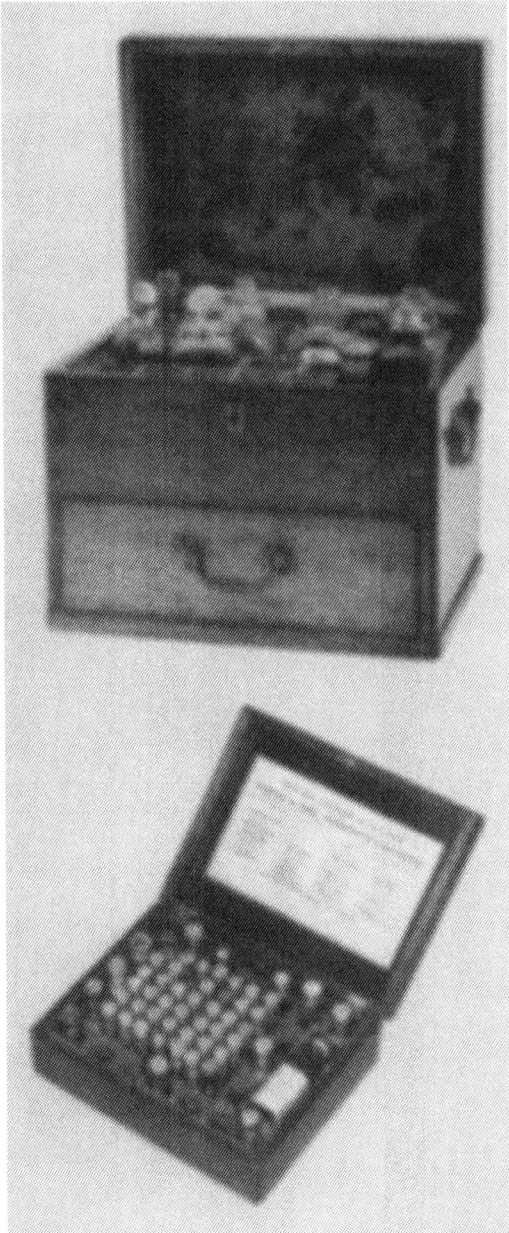

THE FEDERAL GOVERNMENT has furnished medical care to sick and disabled American merchant seamen since 1798. In 1790, eight years before the establishment of the U.S. Marine Hospital Service, legislation provided for the placement of a medicine chest on each American flag vessel over 150 tons navigated by 10 or more persons. It was not until 1881, however, that the first medical handbook was prepared for use aboard ships.

The initial edition of our present volume was published under the title, HANDBOOK FOR THE SHIP'S MEDICINE CHEST. Revised editions have been produced from time to time that incorporated new medical procedures and therapies to meet the changing needs of seamen and the conditions under which they worked.

This edition represents a major effort by many professionals to bring together in one volume the very latest principles of medical diagnosis and treatment. It is intended primarily for the information and guidance of the Master and other licensed and certificated crew members who directly or indirectly may be responsible for medical care on merchant ships at sea.

I urge all who may act as medical attendants aboard merchant vessels to study this volume carefully, and to seek professional advice by radio as soon as possible, whenever it may be necessary. The successful accomplishment of a ship's mission is directly related to the health and welfare of its crew.

As always, the U.S. Public Health Service stands ready to assist in every way possible.

James H. Erickson, M.D., M.P.H.
Assistant Surgeon General
Director, Bureau of Medical Services
U.S. Public Health Service

Early ships' medicine chests.
Courtesy of Mystic Seaport, Inc., Mystic Conn.

Preface

THE SHIP'S MEDICINE CHEST AND MEDICAL AID AT SEA is published primarily for the information and guidance of the Master and other licensed and certified crew members who may be directly or indirectly responsible for the administration of medical treatment at sea on vessels which do not carry a physician. This book attempts to describe in nontechnical language, the diseases and medical emergencies most commonly encountered while at sea and the "first aid" and "follow-up" care required until the patient can be evaluated and treated by a physician. Since the first edition of the medical handbook THE SHIP'S MEDICINE CHEST AND FIRST AID AT SEA, the book has been revised and rewritten from time to time as medical science advanced and the uses of the book expanded. The present edition, like its predecessors, is intended for ships having no physician. It cannot cover all emergencies arising on shipboard. It must be emphasized that the care and treatment of a patient at sea is much different than while ashore. The medications and treatments suggested in this book are based on the fact that a physician is not physically available and that such treatment must be carried out by intelligent seamen and ship's officers who have received training in the delivery of health care. Crew members while ashore should seek medical attention through the facilities of the Public Health Service or from other professional medical resources.

The information contained in this book is presented in a format which outlines the best approach to treatment available to the patient. When in doubt, radio communication is encouraged. Preventive medicine and environmental health principals are presented to convey the concept of reducing the incidence of disease and injury.

Previous editions of this book have been used as a textbook for the instruction of merchant marine cadets, other officer candidates, and officers and crews of American merchant vessels. It is used on fishing vessels, by outdoorsmen, explorers, and backwoodsmen as a guide when professional medical care is not available. While it may be helpful in a variety of situations, it is written with the sole intent of providing the background and procedures necessary to deliver health services to the American seaman afloat.

The principal topics or chapters have been arranged in the following order.

The first chapter describes the anatomy and major systems of the body. A basic understanding of how the body functions is necessary before the initiation of treatment.

Chapter II describes the procedures in examining a patient. This is important! It is very easy to jump to conclusions and try to form a diagnosis based on one or two impressions. Finding the right diagnosis is similar to detective work. Facts must be gathered and analyzed in a logical manner. The information obtained through the patient's history of illness, his symptoms and complaints and the physical examination must be accurately examined in order to reach a proper conclusion. Treating the wrong illness wastes time and could seriously affect the patient's prognosis.

Chapter III concentrates on the emergency treatment of injuries. The procedures described require practice and knowledge of the material before an injury occurs. The poison section presents a general explanation of the chemicals most likely found aboard ship. The variety of chemicals on the market—especially as cargo, presents a real problem to the seaman. Additional references to aid in the treatment of specific poisonings are listed in this book.

A brief description of cardiopulmonary resuscitation (CPR) is presented in Chapter IV. Cardiopulmonary resuscitation, if performed correctly, saves lives. CPR training should be required for any officer or crewman responsible for the medical care of the crew. Training courses are available through the American Red Cross as well as refresher courses to provide supervised practice. You cannot learn CPR from this book; it is only intended to provide a review of techniques.

Chapter V presents the diagnosis and treatment of common diseases. It does not list all diseases, of course, but it does provide a description of the prominent illnesses that are likely to be found aboard ship.

Chapter VI provides more detailed information on the drugs aboard. It also suggests the amount of supplies to be carried, based on the size of the crew and the accessibility of professional medical treatment. Trade names of the generic drugs suggested in Chapter IV and V are also listed.

The general nursing chapter (VII) explains the procedures that must be known in order to treat the patient. It includes instructions on how to take a temperature and blood pressure; how to catheterize and how to perform a variety of other tasks which will improve the comfort and prognosis of the patient.

Chapter VIII discusses the specific medical problems associated with castaways; both on the survival craft and after recovery. It also recommends additional medications and supplies to be added to the lifeboat first aid kits.

Birth and death at sea (Chapter IX) includes a section on the steps required to protect the mother and child during a delivery. The vast majority of births are joyful, uncomplicated deliveries, however, prior knowledge of the processes and the procedures to be taken by the attendant will avoid confusion and reduce the potential of postpartum complications. Signs of death and the procedures necessary in the care of the body are also discussed in this chapter.

Chapters X and XI discuss the prevention and control of communicable disease and environmental control aboard ship. Knowledge of these subjects can have a significant affect on the spread of communicable illnesses among the ship's company.

Chapters XII and XIII outline the procedures for obtaining medical advice by radio and patient evacuation by helicopter. THE MEDICAL SIGNAL CODE—INTERNATIONAL CODE OF SIGNALS is reproduced in this book to provide a ready reference when it is necessary to communicate with non-English speaking medical resources. We have also included a comparison list of medications found in THE MEDICAL SIGNAL CODE with equivalent drugs recommended in this book. Helicopter evacuation at sea provides a vital medical resource during certain emergencies. There are times when the medical capability aboard ship is inadequate and the patient must be transported to a hospital. There are also hazards involved in such an evacuation and it is important to understand when a helicopter can be used and the procedures required to evacuate a patient as rapidly and safely as possible.

The appendices provide specific regulations and other information concerning the medical care and protection of seamen. A list of the Public Health Service facilities and eligibility requirements are contained in Appendices A and B. The last two appendices include the Foreign Quarantine Regulations, the use of controlled substances such as depressants and stimulants aboard merchant vessels and samples of forms that are required to comply with the regulations.

There has been a conscious attempt for this book to provide guidance to the officers and crew responsible for medical care aboard our merchant ships. To some, it may prove too elementary but to most, it will be a useful guide. This book and the other suggested references should be studied and reviewed on a periodic basis. Many illnesses and traumatic injuries require a rapid assessment of the condition and immediate action. Any delay or error in judgment could cause serious complications.

It is highly desirable that the officers and crew who have the medical responsibility receive periodic refresher courses in medical care and the emergency treatment of injuries. Current certification in cardiopulmonary resuscitation should be required. This book like all others can only provide information; its success will be measured by its responsiveness to the needs of the user.

Truman L. McCasland, Dr. P.H.
Commander, U.S. Public Health Service

Acknowledgments and Copyrights

IN THE PARAGRAPHS that follow, acknowledgment is made of the several sources used by our artists to produce some of the illustrations shown. We appreciate the willingness of all concerned to allow us to adapt their copyrighted material to meet our needs.

Also acknowledged is Merck & Company's permission to use textmatter on nonbacterial food poisoning.

Sources of Illustrations

American Heart Association

JAMA SUPPLEMENT, Vol. 27, No. 7, Feb. 18, 1974: *Standards for Cardiopulmonary Resuscitation (CPR) and Emergency Cardiac Care (ECC)*, © 1974, the American Medical Association. Next two figures listed, modified with permission of the American Heart Association.

Fig. 4–6, p. 121 & Fig. 4–8, p. 122 were redrawn from JAMA figures on p. 846.

Robert J. Brady Co.

Grant, H. & Murray, R.: EMERGENCY CARE, 344 pp., © 1971 by Robert J. Brady Co., a subsidiary of Prentice-Hall, Inc., Rt. 197, Bowie, Md. 20715. The four figures listed below were redrawn from this source.

Fig. 3–34, p. 82, redrawn from p. 201 of Grant & Murray.
Fig. 3–37, p. 85, redrawn from pp. 193 & 202, Ibid.
Fig. 9–1, p. 349, redrawn from pp. 266–267 & 271–274, Ibid.
Fig. 9–2, p. 351, redrawn from p. 272, Ibid.

Fischer Medical Publications, Inc.

EMERGENCY MEDICINE, Vol. 6, No. 4, pp. 216–221, April 1974. © by Fischer Medical Publications, Inc., 280 Madison Ave., New York, N.Y. 10016. Article by Alan Dimick, M.D., entitled, *Be Aggressive with Burns*.

Figs. 3–20, 3–21, 3–22, & 3–23, pp. 67–68, were redrawn from figures on p. 219.

EMERGENCY MEDICINE, Vol. 6, No. 6, pp. 154–155, June 1974. Copyright as above. Article by Henry J. Heimlich, M.D., entitled, *Pop Goes the Cafe Coronary*.

Figs. 4–13 & 4–14, p. 132, were redrawn from figures on pages indicated.

Emergency Product News

EMERGENCY PRODUCT NEWS, Vol. 10, No. 5, Sept./Oct. 1974. Address: 6200 Yarrow Drive, Carlsbad, Calif. 92008. Copyrighted figures on unnumbered pages 24–27 of DYNA-MED advertisement.

Figs. 3–32, p. 81; Figs. 3–40 & 3–41, p. 87; and Fig. 3–42, p. 89 were redrawn from above source.

Glencoe Press

Erven, Lawrence W.: FIRST AID AND EMERGENCY RESCUE, 408 pp., © 1970 by L. W. Erven. Publisher, Glencoe Press, a Division of Macmillan Publishing Co., Inc., New York, N.Y. 10022. Twelve figures were adapted from this source.

Fig. 3–13, p. 63, adapted from fig. 8–3 of Erven.
Figs. 3–14 & 3–15, p. 64, adapted from fig. 8–4 of Erven.
Fig. 3/19, p. 66, adapted from fig. 8–24 of Erven.
Fig. 3–28b, p. 78, adapted from fig. 10–2 of Erven.
Fig. 3–33, p. 82, adapted from fig. 10–5 of Erven.
Figs. 3–35a, c, & d, p. 83, adapted from figs. 10–4 & 10–5 of Erven.
Fig. 3–43, p. 89, adapted from fig. 10–8 of Erven.
Fig. 3–46, p. 92, adapted from fig. 10–9 of Erven.
Fig. 3–49, p. 95, adapted from fig. 7–4 of Erven.
Fig. 4–1, p. 117, adapted from fig. 6–3 of Erven.
Fig. 4–7, p. 122, adapted from fig. 6–10 of Erven.

Hospital Research and Educational Trust

Hospital Research and Educational Trust: BEING A NURSING AIDE, © 1969 by the Trust, 840 N. Lake Shore Drive, Chicago, Ill. 60611.

Figs. 7–3a, 7–3b, & 7–4, pp. 306–307, adapted from illustrations on pp. 10–22, 10–23, & 10–24 of this source.

Macmillan Publishing Co., Inc.

Miller, M.A.; Drakontides, A.B.; & Leavell, L.C.: Kimber-Gray-Stackpole's ANATOMY AND PHYSIOLOGY, 17th edition, 656 pp., © 1977 by the Macmillan Publishing Co., Inc., New York, N.Y. 10022. Four figures listed below were redrawn from this source.

Fig. 1–1, p. 2, redrawn from fig. 1–1 of Kimber.
Figs. 1–11a & 1–11b, p. 10, redrawn from fig. 4–23 of Kimber.
Fig. 1–14, p. 13, redrawn from figs. 4–32 & 4–33 of Kimber.

Kimber-Gray-Stackpole's 15th edition, by Leavell, Miller, & Chapin: ANATOMY AND PHYSIOLOGY, 804 pp., © 1966, by Macmillan Publishing Co., Inc. Next three figures listed were redrawn from this source.

Fig. 1–12, p. 11 & Fig. 1–13, p. 12, redrawn from fig. 5–37 of Kimber.
Fig. 1–18, p. 18, redrawn from fig. 14–1 of Kimber.

C. V. Mosby Co.

Fig. 1–2, p. 3, redrawn after Tuttle, W.W. & Schottelius, Byron A.: TEXTBOOK OF PHYSIOLOGY, ed. 15, St. Louis, The C.V. Mosby Co.; modified from Cunningham.

Figs. 1–3 & 1–4, p. 4, redrawn after Anthony, Catherine Parker: TEXTBOOK OF ANATOMY AND PHYSIOLOGY, ed. 7, The C.V. Mosby Co.

Fig. 1–23, p. 25, redrawn after Francis, Carl C. & Farrell, Gordon L.: INTEGRATED ANATOMY AND PHYSIOLOGY, ed. 3, The C.V. Mosby Co.

Ohio State Dept. of Education

EMERGENCY VICTIM CARE, 354 pp., © 1971. Edited and distributed by the Instructional Materials Laboratory, Trade and Industrial Education, The Ohio State University, College of Education, Columbus, Ohio 43210. The four figures listed below were adapted from this source.

Fig. 1–22, p. 22, modified from fig. 23, p. 78 of EMERGENCY VICTIM CARE.
Fig. 1–28, p. 32, modified from fig. 27, p. 83, Ibid.
Fig. 3–45, p. 91, modified from fig. 13, p. 195, Ibid.
Fig. 3–48a, p. 92, modified from fig. 22, p. 202, Ibid.

W. B. Saunders Co.

Leake, Mary J.: A MANUAL OF SAMPLE NURSING PROCEDURES, 5th ed., 233 pp., © 1971, by W. B. Saunders Co., Philadelphia, Pa. 19105. Twelve figures were redrawn from this source.

Fig. 7–15, p. 310, adapted from figs. 9–14 of Leake.
Fig. 7–16, p. 320, adapted from 111–116 of Leake.

Federal Government

National Aeronautics and Space Administration: BIO-ASTRONAUTICS DATA BOOK. 2nd edition. NASA Sp—3006. U.S. Government Printing Office, Washington, D.C. 20004. 930 pp. 1973.
Fig. 8–1, p. 337, redrawn from fig. 3–31, p. 121 of above source.
U.S. Coast Guard
Fig. 13–1. Print (b&w) furnished.
U.S. Public Health Service, Food and Drug Administration
Figs. 11–1, 11–2, and 11–3. Prints (b&w) furnished.
U.S. Public Health Service, Bureau of Medical Services Colorplates in Chapter V. *Figs. 5–1, 5–2, 5–3, 5–4, 5–5, 5–6, 5–7, and 5–8.* Produced from 35 mm slides, courtesy of Herschel C. Gore, M.D., M.P.H.

Text Source

Merck & Co.

Text on *Nonbacterial Food Poisoning*, pp. 160–161, was adapted from pp. 714–716, THE MERCK MANUAL, 12th ed., International Copyright and Universal Copyright 1972, by Merck & Co., Rahway, N.J.

References for Readers

Anatomy—Physiology

Anthony, C.P. & Kolthoff, N.J.: TEXTBOOK OF ANATOMY AND PHYSIOLOGY. 9th edition. 598 pp. © 1975 by The C. V. Mosby Co., St. Louis, Mo. 63141.

Miller, M.A.; Drakontides, A.B.; & Leavell, L.C.: Kimber-Gray-Stackpole's ANATOMY AND PHYSIOLOGY. 17th edition. 656 pp. © 1977 by Macmillan Publishing Co., New York, N.Y. 10022.

Communicable Diseases

American Public Health Association (APHA): CONTROL OF COMMUNICABLE DISEASES IN MAN. Abram S. Beneson, editor, 12th edition, 413 pp. © 1975 by APHA, 1015—18 St., N.W., Washington, D.C. 20036.

Diagnosis—Therapy

THE MERCK MANUAL OF DIAGNOSIS AND THERAPY. 13th edition. 2100 pp. Copyright 1977. Publisher: Merck, Sharp & Dohme, Rahway, N.J. 07065.

Emergency Medical Care

American Academy of Orthopaedic Surgeons (AAOS): EMERGENCY CARE AND TRANSPORTATION OF THE SICK AND INJURED. 2nd edition, revised 1976. 481 pp. Publisher: AAOS, Chicago, Ill. 60680.

EMERGENCY MEDICINE: Monthly journal, edited by Irving J. Cohen. Publisher: Fischer Medical Publications, Inc., 280 Madison Ave., New York, N.Y. 10016.

Erven, Lawrence W.: FIRST AID AND EMERGENCY RESCUE. 408 pp. © 1970, Glencoe Press, a Division of Macmillan Publishing Co., New York, N.Y. 10022.

Flint, Thomas, Jr., M.D. and Cain, Harvey D., M.D.: EMERGENCY TREATMENT AND MANAGEMENT. 5th edition. 794 pp. © 1975 by W. B. Saunders Company, Philadelphia, London, Toronto.

Grant, Harvey & Murray, Robert: EMERGENCY CARE. 334 pp. © 1971. Robert J. Brady Co., Publisher, Bowie, Md. 20715.

Ohio Trade and Industrial Education Service: EMERGENCY VICTIM CARE. 471 pp. © 1976, Ohio State Dept. of Education, Columbus, Ohio 43210.

The American National Red Cross: ADVANCED FIRST AID AND EMERGENCY CARE, 1st edition. 318 pp. © 1973 by ANRC, 17th & D Sts., N.W., Washington, D.C. 20006.

CARDIOPULMONARY RESUSCITATION. 41 pp. © 1974 by ANRC (Address above).

FIRST AID FOR FOREIGN BODY OBSTRUCTION OF THE AIRWAY. 24 pp. © 1974 by ANRC (Address above).

International Health Regulations

World Health Organization: INTERNATIONAL HEALTH REGULATIONS (1969), 2nd annotated edition. 102 pp. © 1974 by the World Health Organization, Geneva, Switzerland. (Buy copies from WHO, 49 Sheridan Ave., Albany, N.Y. 12210.)

Medical Care for Eligible Seamen

U.S. Department of Health, Education, and Welfare, Public Health Service, Bureau of Medical Services: MEDICAL CARE FOR SEAMEN, 14 pp. 1976. Publication No. HEW (HSA) 76-2016. U.S. Government Printing Office, Washington, D.C. 20402. (Copies available from PHS facilities listed in Appendix A, pp. 428-9, or Bureau of Medical Services, U.S. Public Health Service, 6525 Belcrest Road, W. Hyattsville, Md. 20782.)

Prevention

U.S. Department of Transportation, Coast Guard:

A CONDENSED GUIDE TO CHEMICAL HAZARDS. January 1974. Publication Nos. CG-446-1 & 2. U.S. Government Printing Office, Washington, D.C. 20402. (A revised edition will be available in 1978 from the U.S. Coast Guard.)

A MANUAL FOR THE SAFE HANDLING OF FLAMMABLE AND COMBUSTIBLE LIQUIDS AND OTHER HAZARDOUS PRODUCTS. 150 pp. Sept. 1976. Publication No. CG-174. U.S. Government Printing Office, Washington, D.C. 20402.

A POCKET GUIDE TO COLD WATER SURVIVAL. 21 pp. Sept. 1975. Publication No. CG-473. U.S. Government Printing Office, Washington, D.C. 20402. (Available from U.S. Coast Guard.)

CHEMICAL DATA GUIDE FOR BULK SHIPMENT BY WATER. 318 pp. 1976. Publication No. CG-388. U.S. Government Printing Office, Washington, D.C. 20402.

WHEN YOU ENTER THAT CARGO TANK . . . , 17 pp. March 1976. Publication No. CG-474. U.S. Government Printing Office, Washington, D.C. 20402. (Available from U.S. Coast Guard.)

Sanitation

Lamoureux, Vincent B.: GUIDE TO SHIP SANITATION. 119 pp. Copyright 1967 by the World Health Organization, Geneva, Switzerland. (Copies may be bought from WHO, 49 Sheridan Ave., Albany, N.Y. 12210.)

U.S. Department of Health, Education, and Welfare, Public Health Service, Food and Drug Administration: HANDBOOK ON SANITATION OF VESSEL CONSTRUCTION. Standards for sanitation and ratproofing. 90 pp. Revised 1965. PHS Publication No. 393. U.S. Government Printing Office, Washington, D.C. 20402.

Contents

List of Illustrations

List of Tables

Chapter I
Human Body

Structure
and
Function

To ADMINISTER EMERGENCY TREATMENT successfully, it is essential that the person responsible for medical care at sea be able to recognize diseases and injuries. Therefore, one should have a basic knowledge of the structure of the human body as well as of the functions of its parts. A general knowledge of anatomy and physiology, similar to that given in the following pages, should help one to understand the other chapters in this book.

Anatomy is the science which deals with the structure of the body and the relationship of its parts to each other. *Physiology* is the science which deals with the *functions* of the living body and its parts. Anatomy is the science of how the machine is made (structure); physiology, the science of how it works (functions). The term *body* as used hereafter means the body as a whole, including the head, neck, trunk, and limbs *(extremities)*. The term *trunk* is limited to the chest *(thorax)* and abdomen, not including the head, neck, or limbs.

THE BODY AS A WHOLE

The human body is a complex single organism made up of several hundred trillion microscopically small cells. These basic units of life are arranged into groups that differ in size and shape to perform highly specialized functions. Such groups of cells are called tissues, organs, or organ-systems. There are muscular tissues composed of long, thin cells which have a special ability to contract and expand, permitting muscles to move the different parts of the body. There are bone cells, skin cells, and many varieties of digestive, nerve, and other kinds of cells which enable the extremely complicated human body to carry on its numerous functions.

Almost all of these different groups of cells are closely interrelated. Thus nerve cells reach into muscular tissue to stimulate the muscles into motion. Muscular motion, however, would not accomplish much were it not for the bones of the supporting skeleton and the bone cells which keep them in repair. Bone cells, together with other coordinating groups of cells, form the bone and joint *(osseo-articular)* system. Similarly, groups of different kinds of digestive cells, assembled in the mouth, stomach, liver, and elsewhere in the digestive tract contribute to different stages in the digestion of food; their different functions being closely related and their work coordinated to make up the digestive system. Other cells, tissues, and organs in the body are organized to function as the *cardio-vascular, respiratory, urinary, reproductive, nervous* and *endocrine* systems. Still others form a protective *skin* for the body or make up the special sensory organs, as the *eyes* and *ears.*

1

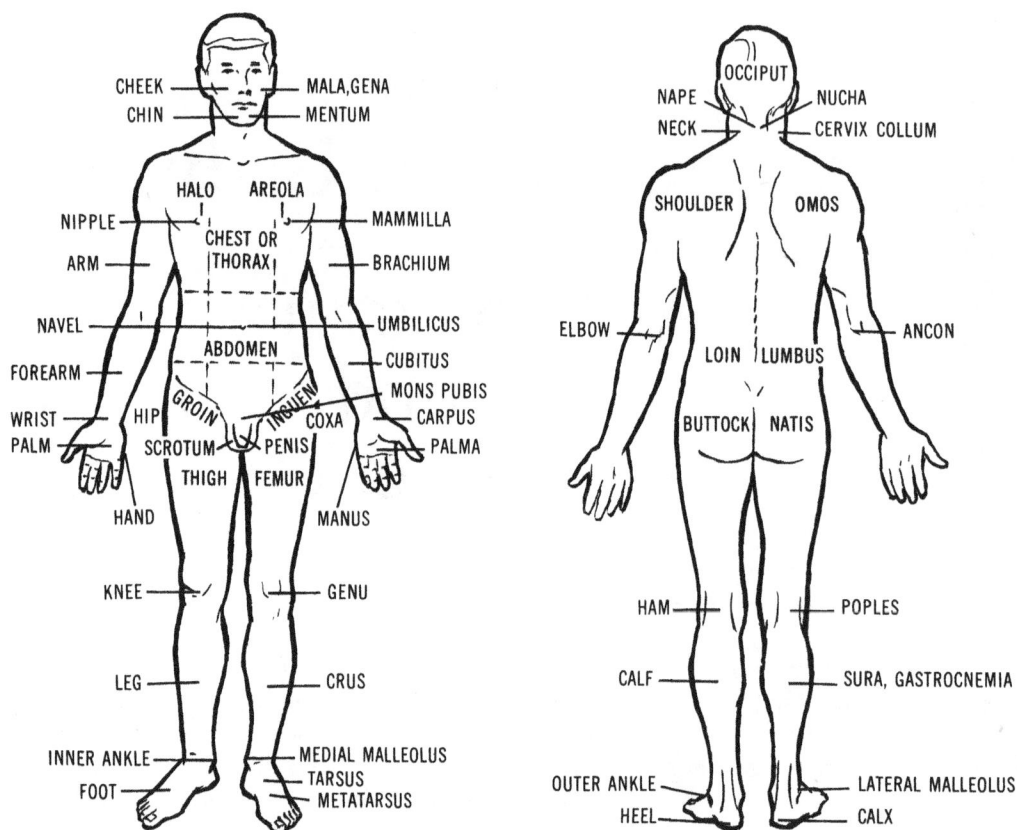

Fig. 1–1. Anatomical position and regional names of the human body.
Medical terms on right side and common terms on left side.

ANATOMICAL REGIONS

In evaluating a patient's condition, it is important to know certain external and internal landmarks; that is, the anatomical regions of the body and their related parts. Reference to these landmarks makes the description of the patient's complaint or problem more understandable to others, particularly when medical advice is sought by radio. Prominent parts of the body are shown in Fig. 1–1.

THE SKIN

The human body, composed of various tissues, organs, and systems, is separated from the outside world by the skin (integument), just as a ship is isolated by its hull plates from the surrounding ocean. The skin covers the whole body, protecting its deep tissues from injury, drying out, and invasion by bacteria and other foreign bodies. The skin helps to regulate body temperature, aids in the elimina-

tion of water and various salts, and acts as the receptor organ for touch, pain, heat, and cold.

The skin consists of two layers: the outer layer, the *epidermis*, and the inner layer, the *dermis* or *corium*. (See Fig. 1–2.)

The *epidermis*, which has no blood vessels or nerves, consists of four layers that from the surface inward, are: the *stratum corneum, stratum lucidum, stratum granulosum,* and *stratum germinativum*. The top layer of the epidermis, the stratum corneum, or horny layer, is made up of dead skin cells which gradually flake off or soak off when wet and are constantly renewed from cells formed in the stratum germinativum. The epidermis varies in thickness in different parts, being thickest on the palms and soles.

The corium or "true skin" is located beneath the epidermis and is composed of two layers. The upper *papillary layer* has small conelike elevations (papillae) which project into the epidermis. The papillae contain blood vessels and, in many cases, special nerve endings for the sense of touch. The deeper *reticular layer,* composed of a mesh of white fibers and elastic tissue, gives elasticity to the skin. In the tiny spaces within this mesh are the sweat *(sudoriferous)* glands and the oil *(sebaceous)* glands.

Beneath the corium and fused to it is the *subcutaneous layer* which contains many fat cells, blood vessels, and nerves. The subcutaneous layer links the corium with tissue covering the muscles and bones.

Sweat or perspiration glands occur in nearly all parts of the skin. Sweat contains essentially the same minerals as blood plasma and urine, but more diluted. Normally, only traces of the waste products excreted in urine are in sweat. But when sweating is profuse, or when the kidneys are diseased, the amounts of such wastes excreted in the sweat may be considerable. Several mineral salts are removed from the body in sweat. Chief among these in quantity is sodium chloride (common table salt).

The *four accessory structures of the skin* are the nails, hair, sweat glands, and oil *(sebaceous)* glands. (See Fig. 1–2.) The nails, the only external skeleton of the human body, are a

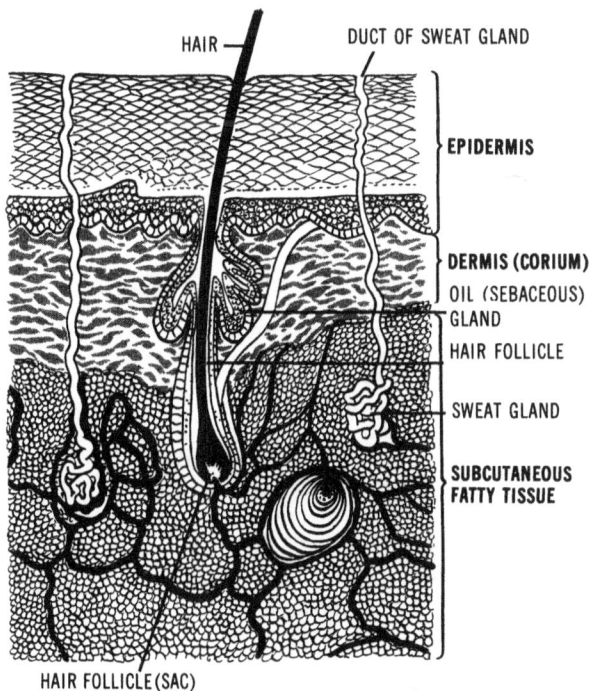

HAIR —   DUCT OF SWEAT GLAND

EPIDERMIS

DERMIS (CORIUM)

OIL (SEBACEOUS) GLAND

HAIR FOLLICLE

SWEAT GLAND

SUBCUTANEOUS FATTY TISSUE

HAIR FOLLICLE (SAC)

Fig. 1–2. Structure of the skin.

horny, elastic material growing from a root and extending beyond the tips of the fingers and toes. Hair fibers are round, oval or flat, thin or thick, and have a root and a shaft growing from a sac *(follicle).* Each hair is kept soft and pliable by two or more sebaceous glands which secrete varying amounts of a fatty substance *(sebum)* into the follicle near the surface of the skin. Between the hair follicles, coiled sweat glands open onto the skin's surface.

SKELETAL SYSTEM
(Bones and Joints)

Bones

The human body is shaped by its bony framework. Without its bones, the body would collapse.

Bone is composed of living cells and nonliving intercellular matter. The nonliving material contains calcium compounds that help to make bone hard and rigid. The body's bony framework is held together by *ligaments* which connect bone to bone; layers of *muscles; tendons* which connect muscles to bone or other structures; and various connective tissues. Bones and their adjacent tissues help to move, support, and protect the body's vital organs.

The structural framework *(skeleton)* must be strong to provide support and protection, jointed to permit motion, and flexible to withstand stress.

The skeleton in the adult has 206 bones, classified by size and shape as long, short, flat, or irregular. These may be divided into two main categories: (a) the *axial* and (b) *appendicular.* The axial skeleton consists of the bones of the head, neck, and trunk. The appendicular skeleton consists of the bones of the extremities—the arms and legs. (See Figures 1–3 and 1–4.)

Good structural design combines strength with lightness, a condition best obtained by internal bracing in a lattice arrangement. Bone has a dense, ivory-like outer shell supported by a strong inner lattice structure. Because the inner portion of the bone looks somewhat like dried sponge, it is called *spongy bone.* The crisscrossing struts of this area give support and house the *bone marrow.* Bone marrow is a

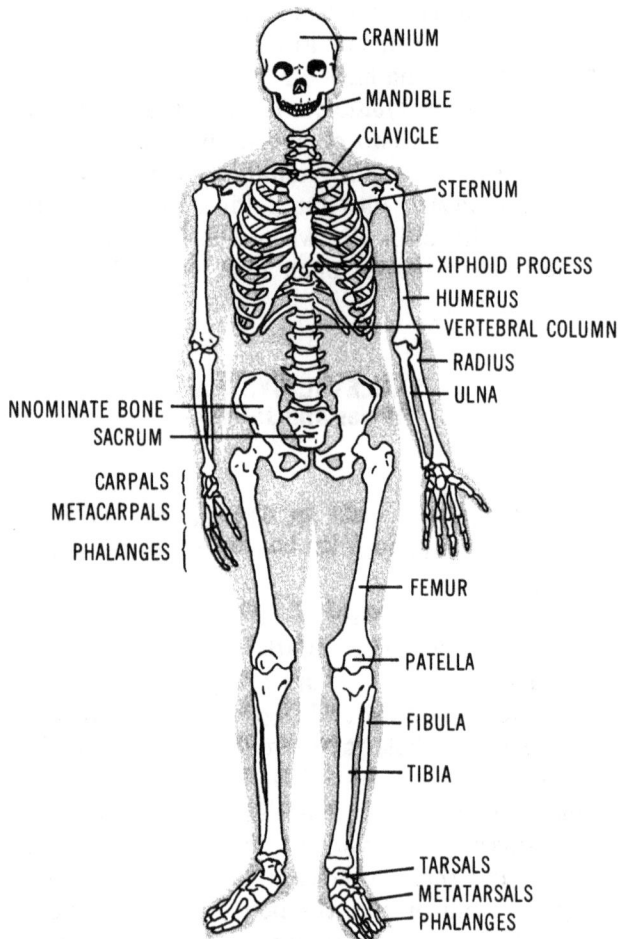

Fig. 1–3. Skeleton (front view).

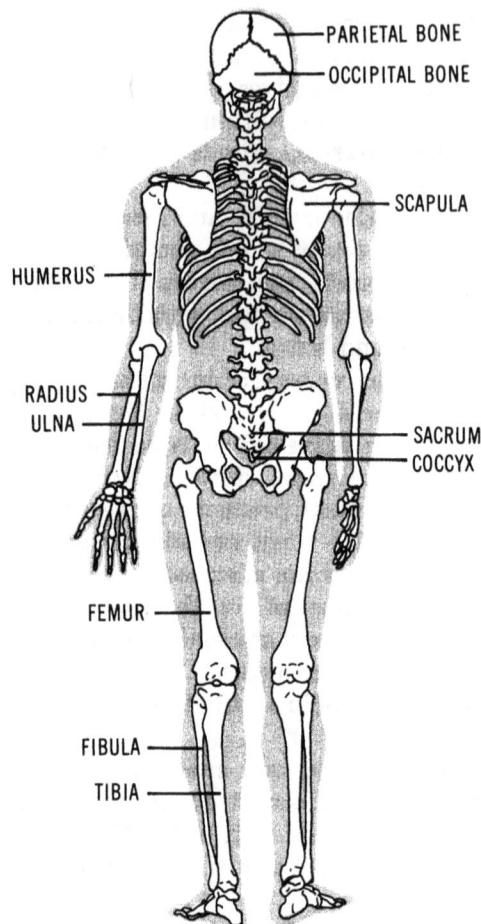

Fig. 1–4. Skeleton (back view).

principal producer of *blood cells*. Because blood cells deteriorate with use in a few weeks, an unceasing supply of new cells must be poured into the bloodstream. The *long bones* are the principal site of blood cell production.

Bone is a living tissue with numerous blood vessels and specialized bone cells (*osteoblasts*). Broken bones are repaired by bone-building cells lying in the bone and its covering sheath, the *periosteum*. New bone is formed at the site of the break, much as two pieces of steel are welded together aboard a ship.

The shapes of bones are adapted to their function. If protection is the essential function, the bone is likely to be flat, like the shoulder blade, breastbone, and bones of the skull (*cranium*). If a bone acts principally as a lever, it usually is long, such as bones of the arms, legs, and fingers. If flexibility in a group of

bones is a principal requirement, individual bones will tend to be short and irregular, as those of the wrist or ankle.

Table 1–1

THE 206 BONES OF THE SKELETON

Category	Skeleton Divisions	No. of Bones	
Axial Skeleton	Skull _____	28	
	Cranium (8 bones)		
	Face (14 bones)		
	Ear Bones (6 bones)		
	Hyoid Bone _____	1	
	Vertebral (spinal) column __	26	
	Ribs and Sternum _____	25	
Subtotal	_____		80
Appendicular Skeleton	Upper Extremities _____	64	
	Lower Extremities _____	62	
Subtotal	_____		126
GRAND TOTAL	_____		206

Joints

To allow for spatial adjustments, permit flexibility, or improve strength, the bones of the body are bound into functional units. The unit may be highly mobile (a joint), slightly movable (an articulation), or totally immobile (a fixed junction). In a typical joint the layer of cartilage or gristle, which is softer than bone, acts as a pad or buffer. The bones of such a joint are held in place by firmly attached ligaments, which are the bands of very dense, tough, but flexible connective tissue.

Joints are enclosed in a capsule, a layer of thin tough material, strengthened by the ligaments. The inner side of the capsule (synovial membrane) secretes a thick fluid (synovial fluid) which lubricates and protects the joint.

Skull

The skull rests at the top of the spinal column. It contains the brain, certain special-purpose glands (such as the pituitary and pineal), and the centers of special senses—sight, hearing, taste, and smell. The brain and the spinal cord (extending downward from the brain through the spinal column) constitute the central nervous system. Cranial nerves originate in the brain and pass through openings

Table 1–2

THE 8 BONES OF THE CRANIUM

Name	No.	Location
Occipital	1	Back of the head just above the nape of neck
Parietal	2	Sides and crown of head
Frontal	1	Forehead
Temporal	2	Ear region
Sphenoid	1	Base of skull to back of eye sockets (very irregular in shape)
Ethmoid	1	Base of skull to nose region (not visible without opening skull)

in the skull, thus differing from spinal nerves which branch from the spinal cord. (See Fig. 1–5.)

The skull has two parts, the brain case (cranium) and the face. The eight interlocking bones of the cranium form a firm cover for the brain. Four of these bones—the occipital, two parietal, and the frontal—are typical flat bones. Their outer layer is thick and tough; the inner layer is thinner and more brittle. This arrangement gives maximum strength, lightness, and elasticity.

Blood vessels and nerve trunks pass to and from the brain through openings in the

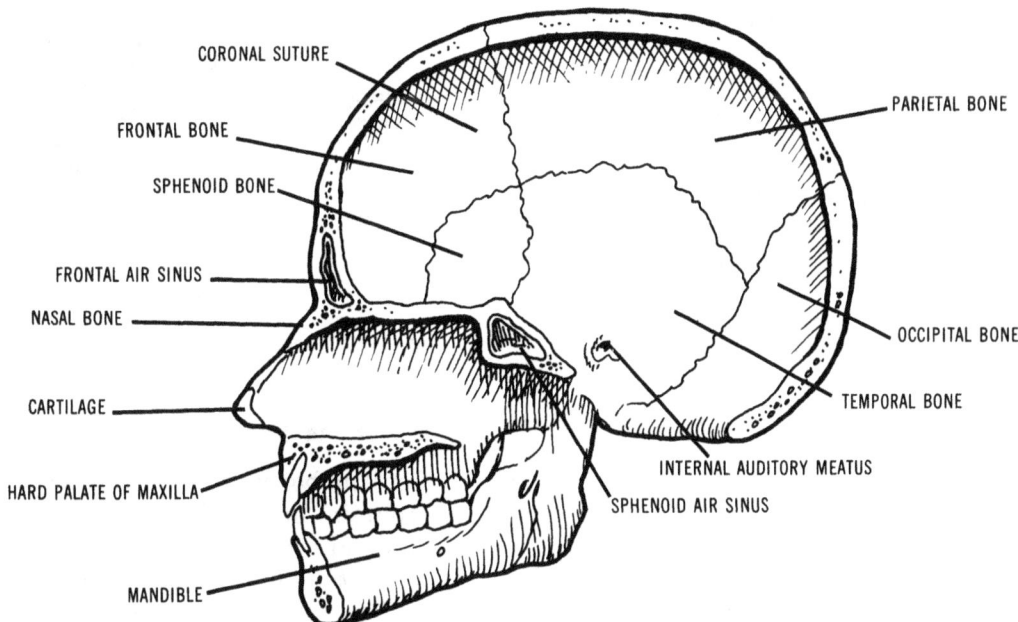

Fig. 1–5. Skull (side view).

skull, mostly at the base. The largest opening, through which the brain and spinal cord are joined, is called the *foramen magnum.*

The brain, which fits snugly into the cranium, is covered by three layers or membranes (the *meninges*). The very narrow spaces between these membranes are filled with *cerebrospinal fluid* (CSF), which is formed by a network of blood vessels in the central vesicles of the brain. It is a clear watery solution similar to blood plasma. The total quantity of CSF in the cerebrospinal system ranges from 100 to 150 ml, and the amount produced daily may range up to several liters. The CSF is constantly being produced and reabsorbed. It circulates over the surface of the brain and spinal cord, acting as a protective cushion and a means of exchange of food and waste materials. A small amount of this fluid may be removed by spinal tap *(lumbar puncture)* for study in suspected cases of brain fever *(cerebrospinal meningitis)*, syphilis of the central nervous system, and other diseases caused by infection and inflammation of the meninges.

Although the skull is very tough, a blow may fracture it. Even if there is no fracture, a sudden impact may tear or bruise the brain and cause it to swell, as any soft tissue will swell following an injury or bruise. Because the skull cannot "give," injury to the brain is magnified by the contained pressure. Unconsciousness or even death may result from swelling *(edema)*, a tearing wound *(laceration)*, bleeding, or other damage of the brain within the skull.

When recording a head injury in the ship's log, or when seeking assistance or advice by radio, the location of a visible injury should be indicated accurately by using the proper term for the area of the skull. (See Chapter XII.) Such *landmarks* as *occipital region*, right (or left) *temporal region*, right (or left) *parietal region*, or *frontal region* should be used. (See Fig. 1–5.)

Six Bones of the Ear (Ossicles)

The *temporal bones*, one on each side of the cranium, have a hollowed area with a series of small cavities. These house the *inner ear* and the *middle ear*. (See Ears, p. 33.)

Bones of the Face

The face, extending from the eyebrows to the chin, has 14 bones, 13 of which are immovable and interlocking. The immovable bones form the bony settings of the eyes, nose, cheeks, and mouth. The fourteenth bone, the lower jaw *(mandible)*, moves freely on hinge joints.

Table 1–3

THE 14 BONES OF THE FACE

Name	No.	Location
Nasal	2	Bridge of nose (upper part)
Vomer	1	Bony part of septum (dividing wall) of nose
Inferior turbinate	2	Outer walls of nostrils (scroll-like in shape)
Lacrimal	2	Inner walls of eye sockets
Zygomatic (malar)	2	Cheeks
Palatine	2	Back part of roof of mouth
Maxilla	2	Upper jaw and front part of roof of mouth
Mandible	1	Lower jaw

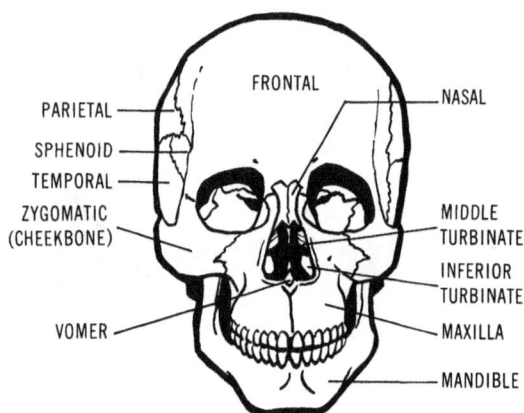

Fig. 1–6. Bones of the face and skull (front view).

Sinuses of the Head

Certain bones about the nose and inner ears contain hollows *(sinuses)*. Those about the nose are called *paranasal* or *accessory sinuses of the nose;* those about the inner ear are called *mastoid sinuses.* The paranasal sinuses communicate with the nasal passage. They are above each eye in the frontal bone

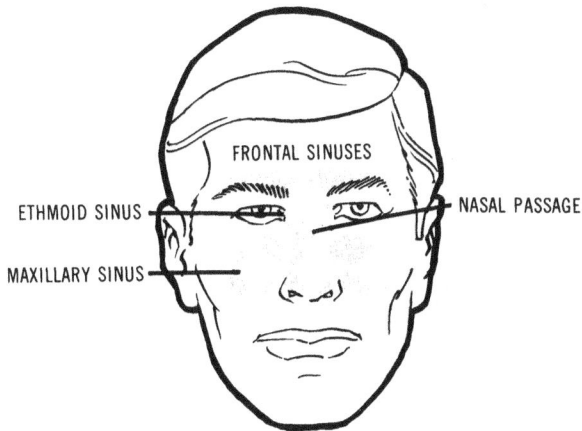

Fig. 1–7. Head showing paranasal sinuses.

(*frontal sinuses*), on each side of the nose in the upper jaw bones (*maxillary sinuses*), behind the nose in the sphenoid bone (*sphenoid sinuses*), and in the ethmoid bone (*ethmoidal sinuses*). These spaces, which contain air, reach the nose through very narrow bony openings lined by *mucous membrane*.

When a person has a head cold, infection may travel from the nose into the sinuses. The sinus membrane becomes inflamed, swollen, and produces heavy secretions and pain over the affected sinus area in the cheeks or above the eyes. The condition is called *sinusitis*. (See Fig. 1–7.)

Eye Orbits

The eye sockets, or *orbits*, are bony cavities that house and protect the eyeballs. The eyes are further protected by the bony prominences of the cheeks, the upper part of the nose, and the heavy *supraorbital ridges* just below the eyebrows.

Nose

The *nasal bones* are two small oblong bones joined together at their inner edges to form the upper, rigid part of the bridge of the nose. The lower part of the bridge is made of cartilage. The nasal bones are easily broken on impact.

Beneath the nasal bones lies the nasal cavity, which is divided into two parts or chambers by a central wall (*septum*) of bone and cartilage. Sometimes the septum is bent, misshapen or displaced to one side, making the nasal chambers unequal in size.

Turbinates are thin, scroll-shaped bones on the outer wall of each nasal chamber. (See Fig. 1–6.) They help to increase the surface area over which air passes as it flows through the nose. Thus, they assist in warming and moistening inhaled air and freeing it of dust. Deviation of the septum following fracture, with enlargement of the turbinates, may cause interference with nasal ventilation and drainage. The reduction in air-flow due to the decreased size of the nasal passage often is seen in allergy and following trauma.

Jaws

The upper jaw is formed by two *maxillary bones* which meet in the midline of the face. Together with the *palatine bones* they form part of the palate or roof of the mouth, the floor of the eye sockets, and the floor and sides of the nasal cavities.

The lower jaw (*mandible*) is shaped like a horseshoe. It is the largest and strongest bone of the face. The curved portion forms the chin. Two perpendicular portions form hinge joints with the temporal bones located on each side of the cranium just in front of the ears. Fractures and dislocations of the lower jaw are common. (See Fig. 1–6.)

Teeth

The part of a tooth normally seen above the gum tissue (*gingiva*) is called the *crown*. The rest of the tooth (about two-thirds) below the gumline is the *root*. Front teeth have one

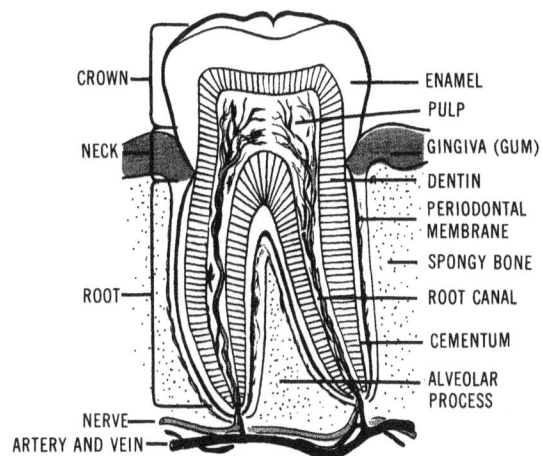

Fig. 1–8. Molar tooth and its supporting structure in the jaw.

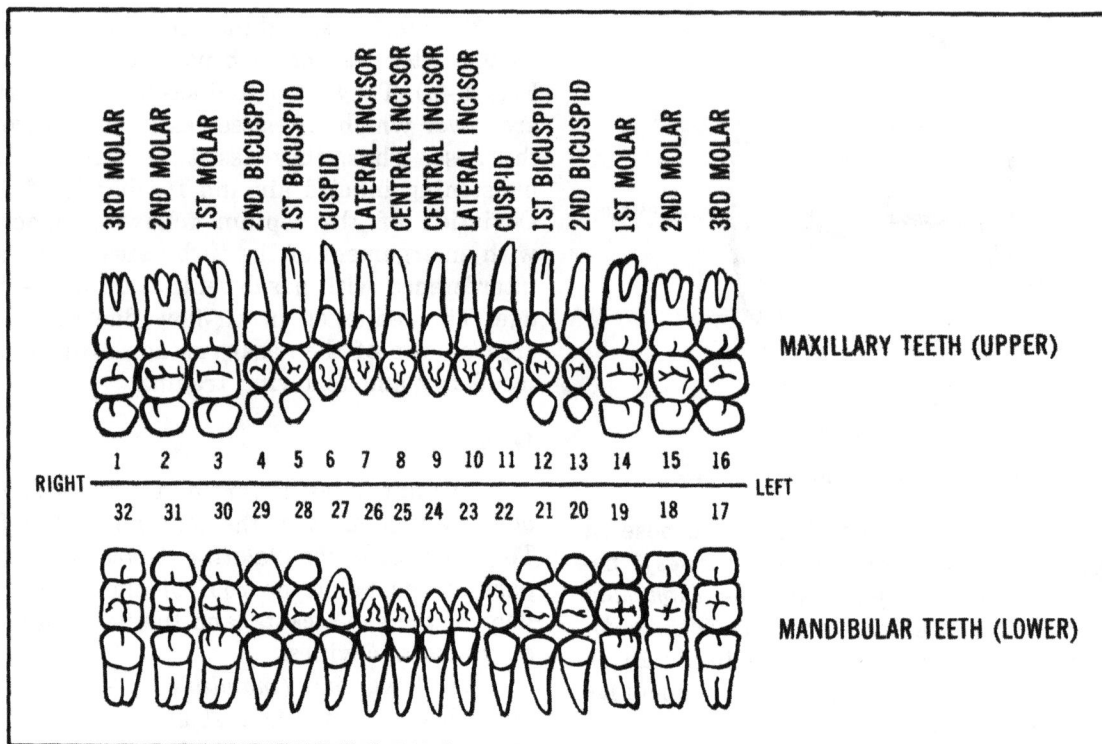

Fig. 1–9. Classification of teeth (Armed Forces System).

root while the others have two or three roots. The junction of the crown with the root is called the *neck* of the tooth. Normally the neck is at the margin of the gum tissue. (See Fig. 1–8.)

The crown is covered by a layer of *enamel,* which is the hardest substance in the human body. The root is covered with a bone-like substance called *cementum.* Beneath the covering of the enamel and cementum is the *dentin,* which is the main body of the tooth. Within the dentin is the *dental pulp,* a soft sensitive tissue composed of nerves, blood capillaries, and lymph vessels. Most of the pulp is in the crown of the tooth. The pulp in the roots extends into small canals through which the nerves and vessels pass after they enter the tooth from the jaw. The root of a healthy tooth is supported and attached to the bony socket *(alveolar bone)* in the jaw by the *periodontal membrane,* which provides both elasticity and great strength in withstanding the force required to masticate food.

Of the 32 teeth in a normal, permanent dentition, 16 are in each jaw or arch: 4 incisors, 2 cuspids, 4 bicuspids, and 6 molars. (Fig. 1–9).

In the *Armed Forces System of Classification,* the teeth are numbered from 1 to 32, beginning with the upper right third molar or wisdom tooth, and proceeding around the maxillary arch to the upper left third molar, which is No. 16. The lower left third molar is No. 17, and the numbering continues around the lower arch, ending on the lower right third molar, which is No. 32. Familiarity with the names of the teeth and the *Armed Forces System of Classification* will enable the attendant to record the site of emergency treatment.

Trunk

The trunk of the body is made up of the backbone or spine at the rear *(spinal column);* the *ribs,* which extend around the sides and meet at the breastbone *(sternum)* in front, and the heavy circular *pelvis* below. The cavity of the trunk is divided into an upper and a lower portion by a dome-shaped muscular partition *(diaphragm).* Above the diaphragm is the chest *(thorax)* ; below the diaphragm is the *abdomen.* The thorax contains the lower portions of the breathing apparatus *(bronchi* and *lungs)* and the *heart.* The abdomen contains the *stomach, intestines, liver, gallbladder, pancreas, spleen, kidneys, bladder,* and the internal organs of the *reproductive system.*

Spinal Column

The spinal column is the "principal timber" of the body. Ribs spring from it much as the ribs of a ship spring from the keel. The rest of the skeleton is directly or indirectly attached to the spine.

The spinal column has a good deal more mobility than the keel of a ship. It is made up of irregularly-shaped bones called *vertebrae* (singular-*vertebra*). Lying one on top of the other to form a strong flexible column, the vertebrae are bound firmly together by strong ligaments. Between each two vertebrae is a

Table 1–4

Cervical vertebrae	7	Neck
Thoracic vertebrae	12	Thorax, or chest
Lumbar vertebrae	5	Loins
Sacrum (5 fused vertebrae)	1	Back wall of pelvis
Coccyx (4 fused vertebrae)	1	Back wall of pelvis

pad of tough elastic cartilage (the *intervertebral disc*), a shock absorber.

The vertebrae are similar in size and shape, except for the top two. Seen from above, a typical vertebra consists of a *central body,* an *arch,* and three projections, one *spinous* and two *transverse processes* or outgrowths. The spinous process extends backward and the other two extend laterally from the *arch.* Except in the fused vertebrae (*sacrum* and *coccyx*) at the base of the spinal column, all within the vertebral arch have a central opening *(vertebral foramen)* which houses the spinal cord.

The first or top vertebra is called the *atlas* because it supports the head, as in Greek mythology, the giant Atlas was thought to have supported the universe on his back. Unlike the other vertebrae, the atlas has no body, only an

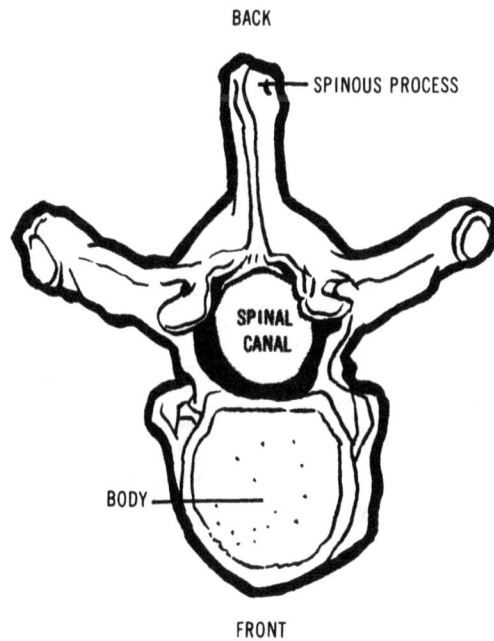

7 CERVICAL VERTEBRAE

12 THORACIC VERTEBRAE

5 LUMBAR VERTEBRAE

SACRUM

COCCYX

Fig. 1–10a. The spinal column.

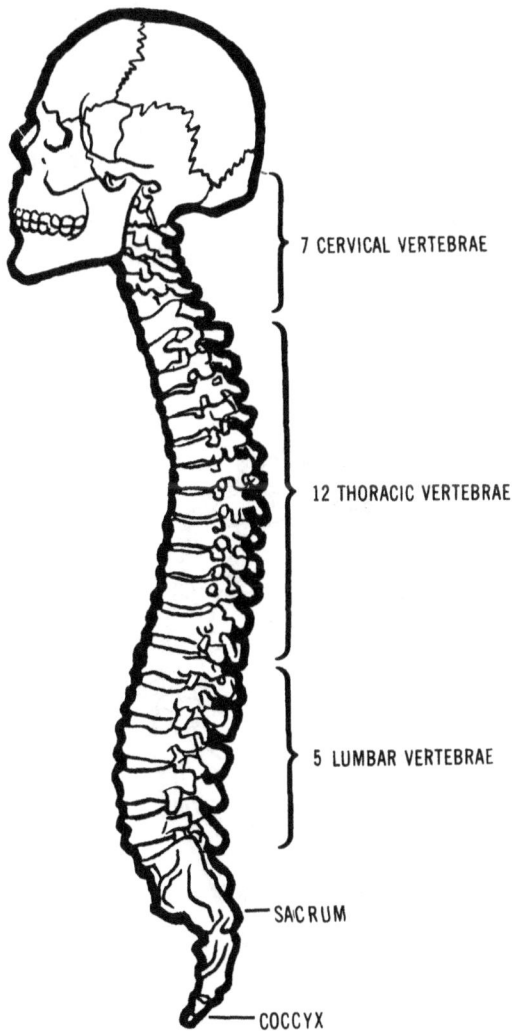

BACK

SPINOUS PROCESS

SPINAL CANAL

BODY

FRONT

Fig. 1–10b. A typical vertebra.

arch or bony ring. There are cups on the top surface into which knobs of the occipital bone of the skull fit, making possible the backward and forward movements of the head. A bony projection rising from the second neck vertebra (the *axis*) forms a pivot around which the atlas rotates when the head is turned from side to side.

In general, the spinal column viewed from the side looks like a string of spools with wing-like projections behind. The spinal column is shaped (curved) and flexible in order to carry body weight, absorb shocks, and make possible the bending of the body forward, backward, and sideways. The spinal column protects the vital spinal cord and still permits relatively free movement of the spine.

The spinal column may be damaged by disease or by injury. If any of the vertebrae are crushed or displaced, the spinal cord at that point may be squeezed, stretched, torn, or severed. Movement of the disabled part by the injured person, or careless handling by well-meaning but uninformed persons, may result in displacement of sections of the spinal column, causing further injury to the cord and possibly resulting in permanent paralysis. For this reason, a person with a back or neck injury must be handled with extreme care.

Breastbone (Sternum) and Ribs

The *sternum* is a flat, narrow bone in the middle of the front wall of the chest (*thorax*). The collar bones and certain ribs are attached to the sternum.

The 24 *ribs* are semiflexible arches of bone. There are 12 on each side of the chest. The back ends of the 12 pairs of ribs are attached to the 12 *thoracic vertebrae*. Strong ligaments bind the back ends of the ribs to the backbone but allow slight gliding or tilting movements. The front ends of the top seven pairs of ribs are attached to the breastbone by means of cartilage. They are the *true ribs*. The remaining five pairs are the *false ribs*; each of the upper three pairs is attached in front by cartilage to the pair of ribs above, and thus indirectly to the breastbone. The front ends of the last two pairs hang free; they are called *floating ribs*. (See Fig. 11a and 11b.)

The cage-like arrangement of the ribs is an admirable compromise between stability and mobility. The heart and lungs contained within this cage are indispensable organs and must be protected as much as possible. Yet, they cannot be tightly enclosed in a rigid box because the lungs must expand in breathing and the heart must change size when it beats. When a person breathes in (*inspiration*),

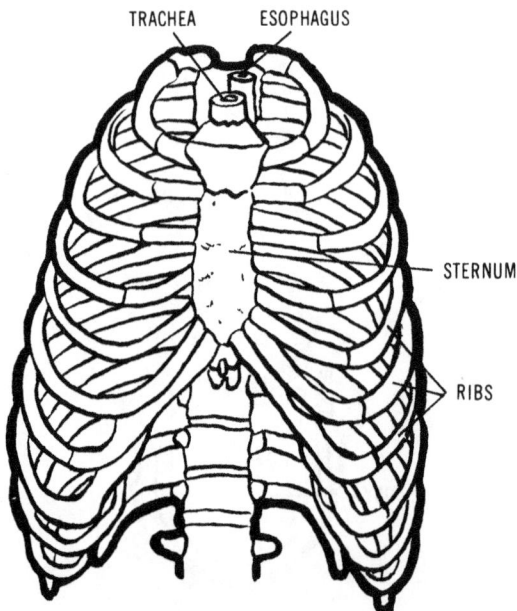

Fig. 1–11a. Ribs and sternum (front view).

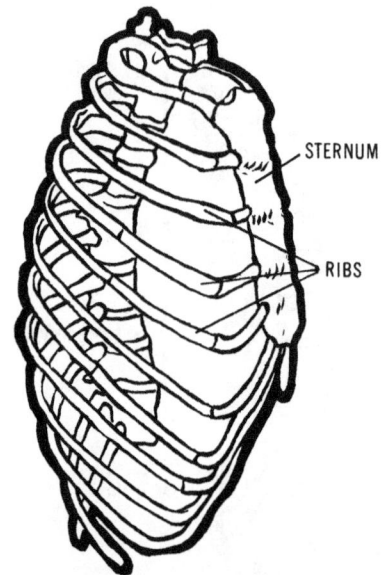

Fig. 1–11b. Ribs and sternum (side view).

muscles lift the ribs and sternum upward and outward, and the big muscle *(diaphragm)* forming the floor of the chest cavity sinks downward, creating a kind of vacuum. This permits the lungs to expand as air rushes in through the nose, mouth, and windpipe *(trachea)*.

Fracture of the sternum or the ribs usually results from crushing or squeezing the chest. A fall, blow, or penetration of the chest wall by a weapon may have the same effect. The chief danger from such injuries is that the lungs or heart may be punctured by the sharp ends of broken ribs.

Appendicular Skeleton

The arms and legs contain no vital organs. A fracture or other injury to them is not likely to cause death, except by a complication such as uncontrolled bleeding, shock, or infection. Permanent crippling can result from an injury to an arm or leg. However, this is less likely today than it was in the days before effective surgery and rehabilitative education. Nonetheless, disfigurement and disability can result from improper handling in first aid. Emergency treatment, if properly given, can minimize this possibility.

The upper and lower extremities are much alike. Each has one long strong bone nearest to the trunk; two long bones lying parallel to each other; and several small bones forming the wrist and hand, or ankle and foot. However, legs and feet, which are for locomotion, are not nearly so flexible as arms and hands, which are for manipulation. Sturdy support for the body's weight, with a reasonable degree of mobility, is all that is required of the legs and feet.

Shoulder Girdle

The collarbone *(clavicle)* and the shoulder blade *(scapula)* form each shoulder girdle. With the muscles which extend from it to the arms, thorax, neck, and head, the shoulder girdle helps attach the arms to the trunk.

Each *clavicle*—a long, slightly double-curved bone—is attached to the breastbone at its inner end and to the shoulder blade at its outer end. Fracture is common because the clavicle lies close to the surface and must absorb blows without protective padding.

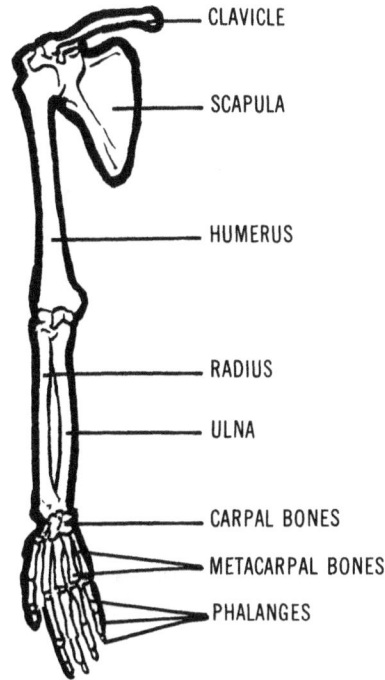

Fig. 1–12. Upper extremity, left (back view).

Each *scapula*—a large, flat, triangular bone—is located over the upper ribs at the back of the thorax. Folded back across its upper portion is a prominent ridge of bone *(the spine of the scapula)*. The ridge ends at the tip of the shoulder, to which the outer end of the collarbone is attached.

Arms

The bone of the upper arm, the *humerus,* is the arm's largest bone. Its shaft is roughly cylindrical; its upper end (the head of the

Table 1–5

Clavicle (Collarbone)	2	Shoulder girdle
Scapula (Shoulder blade)	2	Upper back
Humerus	2	Upper arm
Ulna	2	Elbow and little finger side of forearm
Radius	2	Thumb side of forearm
Carpals	16	Wrists
Metacarpals	10	Palm of hands
Phalanges	28	Two in each thumb Three in each finger.

*(See Fig. 1–12.)

humerus) is round; its lower end, flat. The round head fits into a shallow cup in the shoulder blade, forming a ball-and-socket joint. This is the most freely movable joint in the body and is easily dislocated. Dislocation may tear the capsule of the joint *(synovial membrane)* and cause irreparable damage. Improper manipulation during attempts to reduce or "set" the dislocation may add to the damage. Therefore, it is well to treat dislocation of the shoulder with gentle care.

The two bones of the forearm *(ulna* and *radius)* lie side by side. The larger ulna is on the little finger side and part of it forms the "elbow bone." The flat, curved lower end of the humerus fits into a big notch at the upper end of the ulna to form the elbow joint. This hinge joint permits movement in one direction only. The radius, shorter and smaller than the ulna, is attached to it near both ends. The wide, lower end of the radius forms a joint with the small bones of the wrist. The ulna is excluded from the wrist joint by the articular disk.

The wrist is composed of eight small, irregularly shaped bones *(carpals)* united by ligaments. Arranged in two rows of four bones each, the carpals articulate with one another as well as with the bones of the forearm and hand. This permits a wide range of motion. Tendons extending from the muscles of the forearm to the bones of the hand and fingers pass down the front and back of the wrist close to the surface. Wrist lacerations may result in cutting these tendons, yielding total or partial immobility of the fingers.

The palm of the hand has five long bones *(metacarpals)*. They articulate at their bases with the lower row of wristbones and with each other. Their heads articulate with the bases of the first row of bones of the fingers.

The 14 bones of the fingers *(phalanges)* give the hand its great flexibility. The first row of bones articulates with the heads of the metacarpals at one end and with the second row of phalanges at the other end. The second row articulates with both the first and third rows. The third, or terminal row, articulates with the second row. (The thumb is an exception; it has only two phalanges.) The thumb is the most important digit. A good thumb and one or two fingers make a far more useful hand than four fingers minus the thumb.

Pelvis and Hips

The two *hipbones*, the *sacrum*, and the *coccyx* form the pelvic girdle *(pelvis)*. Muscles help attach the pelvic bones, the trunk, thighs, and the legs. The pelvis forms the floor of the

Table 1–6
THE 62 BONES OF THE LOWER EXTREMITIES

Innominate (Hipbone)	2	Sides and front of pelvis
Femur (Thighbone)	2	Thigh
Patella (Kneecap)	2	Front of knee joint
Tibia (Shinbone)	2	Front and inner side of leg
Fibula	2	Outer side of leg
Tarsals	14	Ankle and heel of foot
Metatarsals	10	Sole and instep of foot
Phalanges	28	Two in each great toe, three in other toes

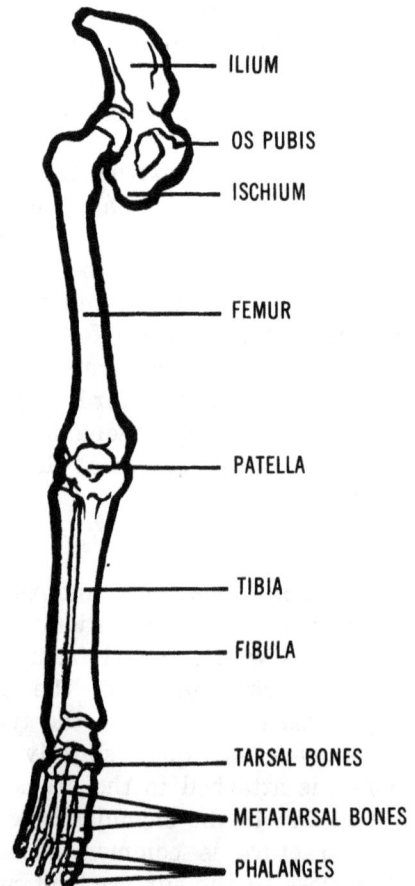

ILIUM

OS PUBIS

ISCHIUM

FEMUR

PATELLA

TIBIA

FIBULA

TARSAL BONES

METATARSAL BONES

PHALANGES

Fig. 1–13. Lower extremity, right (front view).

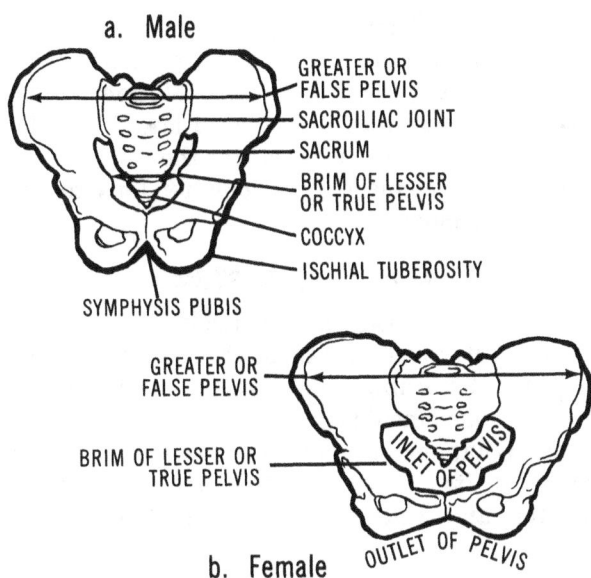

Fig. 1–14. Pelvis and hips.

abdominal cavity. The lower part of the cavity —sometimes called the *pelvic cavity*—holds the bladder, rectum, and internal parts of the reproductive organs. The floor of the pelvic cavity helps to support the intestines.

The *sacrum* and *coccyx*, parts of the spinal column, help form the pelvis. The sacrum is five vertebrae fused together; this wedge-shaped bone is united below with a smaller wedge, the coccyx. This is the "tail" of the vertebral column. (See Fig. 1–14.)

Each hipbone has three parts *(ilium, ischium, pubis)*. The ilium forms the upper prominence of the hip. It joins tightly at the back of the sacrum to form the strong *sacroiliac joint*. The sacroiliac joint does not permit much motion in the lower back region and is subjected to great pressure from the weight of the trunk. This burden is increased when one lifts objects or jumps from a height and lands on his feet. Because of its great strength and stability, the sacroiliac joint is rarely the site of back pain. The joints and muscles of the lower back *(lumbar region)* are much more susceptible to strain. Fracture of the pubis often is associated with injury to the urinary bladder or to the urethra, the tube which drains the bladder.

Thighs and Knees

At the outer side of each hipbone is a deep socket into which the round head of the thigh-

bone *(femur)* fits, forming a ball-and-socket joint. The head of the femur, not as easily dislocated as the less firmly fixed head of the humerus (upper arm bone), is likely to be more difficult to put back into its socket (reduction). The lower end of the femur, like the humerus in the upper arm, is flat and has two knobs *(condyles)*. These articulate with the shinbone *(tibia)* at the knee joint. Although the femur is the longest and strongest bone in the skeleton, its fracture is common. This is always serious because of the difficulties in getting a good position for union between the broken or splintered ends of this large, strong bone. Because of the force required to break the femur, laceration of the surrounding tissues, pain, and blood loss may be unusually extensive.

The knee joint is a strong hinge joint and like the elbow allows angular movement only. The joint is protected and stabilized in the front by the kneecap *(patella)*. The patella is a small triangular-shaped bone in front of the knee joint and within the tendon of the large muscle of the front of the thigh. Because the patella usually receives the force of falls or blows upon the knee, it frequently is bruised and sometimes fractured.

Legs

Anatomically speaking, the word "leg" is used only for that portion of the lower extremity between the knee and the ankle. Its two bones are the *tibia* and the *fibula*. The tibia is at the front and inner side of the leg. Its broad upper surface receives the condyles of the femur to form the knee joint. The lower end, much smaller than the upper end, forms the inner rounded knob of the ankle. The fibula, more slender than the tibia, is at the outer side of the leg parallel to the shinbone. The fibula, not a part of the true knee joint, is attached at the top to the tibia. The fibula is more often fractured alone than is the tibia. (Fig. 1–13.)

Ankles, Feet, and Toes

The ankle joint is the junction of the lower ends of the tibia and fibula with one of the small bones (the *talus*) of the ankle. The seven anklebones *(tarsals)* are bound firmly together by tough ligaments. They are larger and more irregular than the carpal bones in the wrist. The heel bone *(calcaneus)*, largest and strongest of the tarsal bones, transmits the weight of the body to the ground and in walking forms a base for the muscles of the calf of the leg. The heel bone forms the back anchor for the long bony arch or bridge of metatarsals that extends to the base of the toes. The arched formation of the foot gives it the power to absorb shocks and enables it to carry the weight of the body. A person with weak or broken-down arches is said to be flat-footed.

The shape of the foot is roughly a triangle with the apex pointing upward and located at the juncture of the leg and ankle bones. The sole and instep of the foot are formed by the five long *metatarsals*. These articulate with the tarsals and with the front row of toe bones

(phalanges). The phalanges forming the toes are similar in number and arrangement to the phalanges forming the fingers. Motion of the ankle, foot, and toes is produced largely by the action of muscles located in the leg. These muscles are connected by long tendons to the bones they move.

MUSCULAR SYSTEM

When the body moves itself, it is due to work performed by muscles. Examples are walking, breathing, the beating of the heart, and the movements of the stomach and intestines. What enables muscle tissue to perform work is its ability to contract—to become shorter and thicker—when stimulated by a

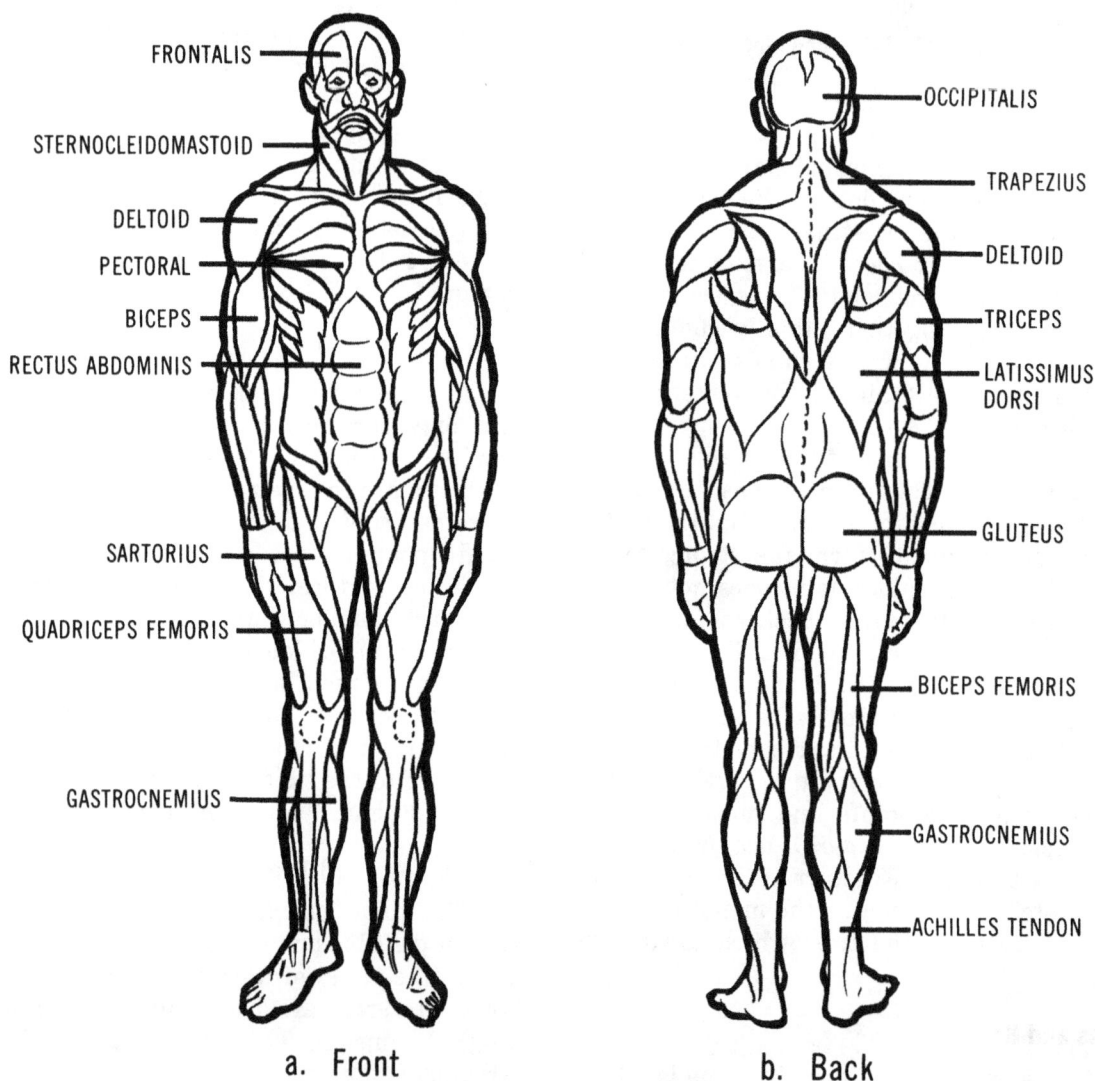

a. Front   b. Back

Fig. 1–15. Major muscles of the body.

nerve impulse. The cells of a muscle, usually long and thread-like, are called *fibers*. Each muscle has countless bundles of closely packed, overlapping fibers bound together by connective tissue. The three different kinds of muscles are (1) striated or skeletal muscle *(voluntary)*, (2) smooth muscle *(involuntary)*, and (3) heart muscle *(cardiac)*. They differ in appearance and the specific job they do.

Voluntary Muscle

Voluntary muscles, under the control of a person's will, make possible all deliberate acts: walking, chewing, swallowing, smiling, frowning, talking, or moving the eyeballs. Most voluntary muscles are attached by one or both ends to the skeleton by tendons. However, some muscles are attached to skin, cartilage, and special organs such as the eyeball, or to other muscles as the tongue. (See Fig. 1–15.)

Muscles help to shape the body and to form its walls. In the trunk, they are broad, flat, and expanded, to help form the walls of the cavities they enclose—the abdomen and the chest. In the extremities, the voluntary muscles are long and much more rounded, somewhat resembling spindles. Most voluntary muscles end in tough whitish cords *(tendons* or *leaders)* by which they are attached to the bones they move. Tendons run through sleeves of dense, strong tissue *(fascia)*. These are lined with a *synovial membrane* that secretes a lubricating substance, the *synovial fluid*. This makes it easier for the tendon to move when the muscle contracts or relaxes. If the synovial membrane becomes inflamed, stiffness and limitation of motion occur.

When not working, muscles become comparatively slack. But they are never completely relaxed; some fibers are contracting all the time. They always have some tension *(muscle tone)*. Muscle tone, which makes muscles springy and ready for instant action, also has a steadying effect, much as a steady hold on the steering wheel helps to keep a moving vehicle true to its course. When there is no muscle tone, the muscle has *flaccid paralysis*. When in continuous contraction, the muscle has a *spasm* or cramp. When a muscle cannot stop contracting, there is *spastic paralysis*.

Almost all voluntary muscles are arranged in *antagonistic* groups: one group opposes the other. For example, muscles on the front surface of the arm and forearm *(flexors)* bend the arm and hand, while *extensors* on the back surface straighten or extend the arm and hand. When a flexor group contracts to do work, the opposing extensor group automatically relaxes most of its fibers. Muscle groups, operative about a joint, act in much the same way the lines from a deck engine relax or contract in sequence to move a boom in any direction.

Muscular contraction will pull the bone in the direction permitted by the joint. The degree of movement will be limited by the countercontraction of the antagonist muscle groups attached to the same parts. Working with or against each other in different combinations, muscles produce movements of infinite variety. A simple act like smiling requires the work of many different voluntary muscles.

Muscles can be injured in many ways. Overexerting a muscle may break fibers. Muscles may be bruised, crushed, cut, torn, or otherwise injured, with or without breaking the skin. Muscles injured in any of these ways are quite likely to become swollen, tender, painful, or weak.

Involuntary Muscle

Involuntary muscles are made up of fibers that are larger than most striated fibers. A person has little or no control over these muscles and usually is not conscious of them. Involuntary muscles are in the walls of tubelike organs, ducts, and blood vessels. In the intestines they form much of the walls. Some muscles are in two principal layers *(circular* and *longitudinal)*. This arrangement strengthens the tubes and makes possible their rhythmic wavelike movements. The *peristaltic waves* in the intestines propel food through the alimentary canal.

Cardiac Muscle

The walls of the heart have a special kind of muscle. Cardiac muscle is particularly suited for the work the heart must do. It is smooth like involuntary muscle, but is striated like voluntary muscle. Unlike either, it is made up of a cellular meshwork. Heart muscle is able to stimulate itself into contraction, even when disconnected from the central nervous system.

CARDIOVASCULAR SYSTEM

Most cells of the body are anchored in one place. They cannot leave in search of food nor can they get rid of their wastes without help. These services are performed by the *cardiovascular* or *circulatory system.*

Blood is the great common carrier of the body. It carries nutrients and other products from the digestive tract in its *plasma,* and oxygen from the lungs in its *hemoglobin* to cells throughout the body. Also, it transports wastes produced by the cells to the lungs, kidneys, and other *excretory organs* for removal from the body.

Heart

The circulatory system in man is a completely closed circuit of tubelike vessels through which blood flows. The *heart,* by contracting and relaxing, pumps blood through the vessels. It is a powerful, hollow, muscular organ about as big as a man's clenched fist and shaped like a pear. It is in the left center of the chest, just behind the sternum with the apex pointing down and to the left. (See Fig. 1–16.) The heart is divided by a perpendicular wall in the middle. Right and left compartments (*right heart* and *left heart*) are divided into two chambers, *atrium* above, *ventricle* below. A check-valve is located between each atrium and its corresponding ventricle, and at the exit of the major arteries leading out of each ventricle. The opening and shutting of these valves at just the right time in the heartbeat keeps the blood from backing up. (See Fig. 1–17.)

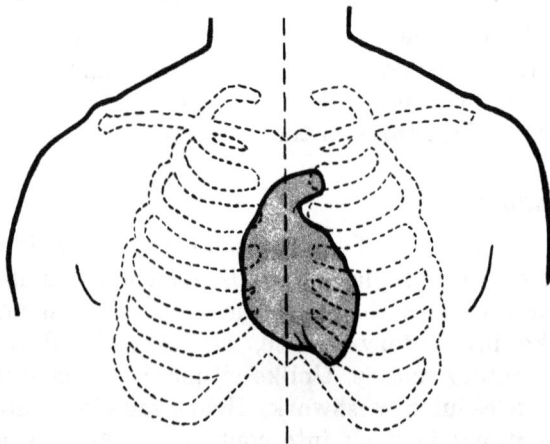

Fig. 1–16. Position of heart in chest cavity.

Blood circulates in two main systems: (a) the *pulmonary circulation* between the lungs and the heart exchanges carbon dioxide and other gas impurities for oxygen; and (b) the *corporeal systemic circulation* that distributes oxygen and food to the body while collecting carbon dioxide and other waste products. At each beat or contraction, the heart pumps blood rich in carbon dioxide and low in oxygen from the right ventricle to the lungs and back to the left atrium of the heart. Blood rich in oxygen freshly obtained from the lungs is pumped from the left ventricle to the rest of the body and back to the right atrium. At each *relaxation* of the heart, blood flows into the left atrium from the lungs and into the right atrium from the rest of the body. To hear the heart, one should put a stethoscope to the patient's chest wall, slightly to the left of the midline and just below the nipple.

Blood Vessels

The *arteries* are elastic, muscular tubes which carry blood away from the heart. They begin at the heart as two large tubes: (a) the *aorta* carries blood to all the body; and (b) the *pulmonary artery* carries blood to the lungs for *carbon dioxide-oxygen exchange.* The aorta divides and subdivides until it ends in networks of extremely fine vessels (*capillaries*) smaller than hairs. Through the thin walls of the capillaries, oxygen and food pass out of the bloodstream into the stationary cells of the body. Into the capillaries the body cells discharge their waste products. In the capillaries of the lungs, carbon dioxide is released and oxygen is absorbed. Capillaries, having reached their limit of subdivision, begin to join together again into veins. These become larger and larger, and finally form major trunks emptying into the right atrium with blood returning from the body, and into the left atrium with blood from the lungs.

It is impossible to prick the normal skin anywhere without puncturing capillaries. Because the flow of blood through the capillaries is relatively very slow and under little pressure, blood merely oozes from a punctured capillary and usually has time to clot, promptly plugging the leak.

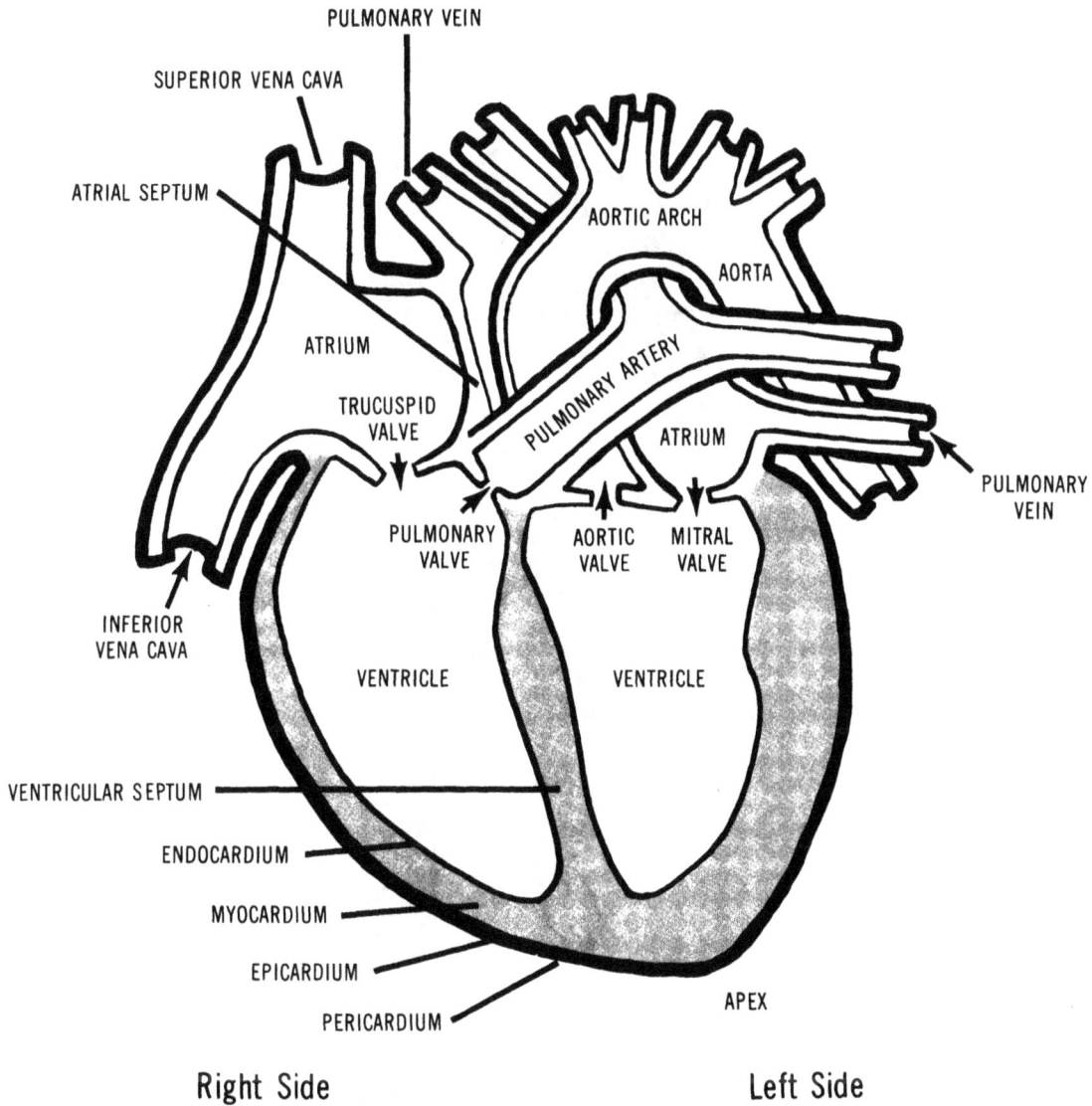

Fig. 1–17. Human heart (diagrammatic).

Right Side   **Left Side**

Pulses

Each time the heart contracts or beats, the surge of blood causes the arteries to expand or stretch. When the heartbeat is completed, the pressure is reduced and the arteries contract or recoil. This expansion and contraction, assisted by the elastic muscle tissue of the arterial walls, can be felt as a *pulse* at points where an artery lies close to the surface of the body. (See Fig. 1–18.)

Because arterial blood moves in waves, blood spurts out when an artery is cut. The spurts become weaker as the arteries grow smaller and smaller. In the capillaries, the pulse disappears. There is no pulse in a vein because the pulse is lost by the time the blood has passed through the capillaries. Hence, blood from a cut vein flows out in a steady stream. It has much less pressure behind it than blood from a cut artery.

Blood Pressure

Blood pressure is a measure of the pressure exerted by the blood on the walls of the flexible arteries. As blood is pumped by the heart into the arteries, the arterial pressure rises; as the heart relaxes between beats, the pressure falls.

The pressure may be high or low according to the resistance offered by the walls to the

17

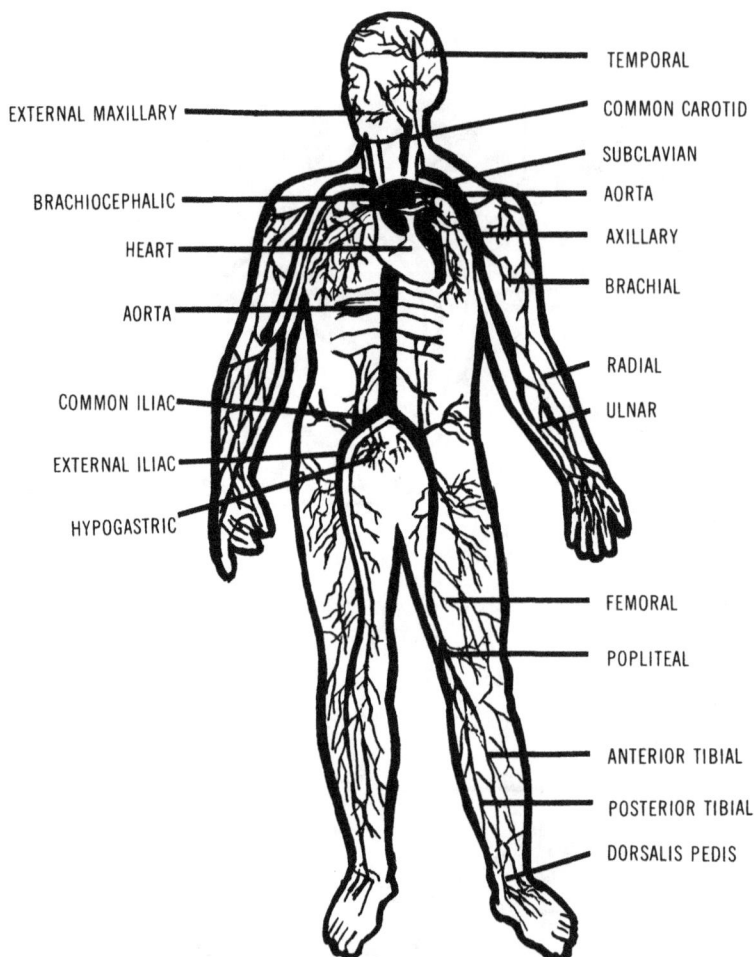

Fig. 1–18. Circulatory system (diagrammatic)—Important arteries named.

passage of blood. This difference in resistance may be due to several causes. For instance, if blood in the system does not fill it, as following hemorrhage, the pressure will be low *(hypotension)*. But if the walls of the arteries have become hard and cannot expand readily, the pressure will be higher than normal. High blood pressure *(hypertension)* may be a symptom of a serious disease.

Blood

Blood makes up about 8 percent of the body's weight. A man weighing 150 pounds, for example, has about 12 pounds of blood. A pound of blood equals about 500 ml or a *unit* of blood, as it is measured for transfusion. Blood, extremely complex, has liquid and solid portions. The liquid portion is called plasma. The solid portion, which is transported by the

plasma, includes microscopic, disk-like red blood cells (erythrocytes); slightly larger, irregularly-shaped, white blood cells (leukocytes); and an immense number of smaller bodies called blood platelets (thrombocytes). The ratio of red blood cells to white blood cells in normal blood is about 700:1.

Plasma, the liquid part of the blood, is a viscous fluid about 90 percent water, in which minerals, sugar, and other materials are dissolved. Plasma carries food materials picked up from the digestive tract and transports them to the body cells. Also, it carries waste materials produced by cells to the kidneys, digestive tract, sweat glands, and lungs for elimination *(excretion)* in urine, feces, sweat, and expired breath.

The *red blood cells*, 4½ to 5½ million per cubic millimeter of blood, contain an iron compound (*hemoglobin*) which absorbs oxygen from the lungs and unloads it in the tissues. Oxygen turns hemoglobin bright red, which is why arterial blood—blood on the way from the lungs to the tissues—is bright red. Venous blood, full of carbon dioxide, is a darker brownish-red.

The *white blood cells,* 5,000 to 9,000 per cubic millimeter, form the body's first line of defense against invading bacteria. The cells can go wherever needed within the body, as for example a wound in the skin, or to any other tissue that is diseased or injured. *Pus,* a sign of wound infection, gets its yellowish-white color from the innumerable white blood cells that fight the invading bacteria.

Blood platelets, 250,000 to 450,000 per cubic millimeter of blood, play an important role in clot formation. If blood plasma did not clot at the site of a wound, the slightest cut or abrasion would produce death from bleeding. A clot plugs the openings through which blood escapes from punctured blood vessels. Bleeding from large blood vessels may be too rapid to permit the formation of a clot. Various emergency measures must be taken to control such severe bleeding. *Hemorrhage* is the term for profuse bleeding.

LYMPHATIC SYSTEM

The human body is fed and defended from bacterial infection by the *lymphatic system.*

All substances exchanged between blood and body cells are transported in a fluid called *lymph.* Part of blood plasma, lymph seeps through the capillary walls, constantly feeding and bathing the tissues. The lymph returns to the bloodstream through the walls of the capillaries, by way of a system of thin-walled vessels *(lymphatics).* Clusters of lymph glands *(lymph nodes)* act as traps in the lymphatics for bacteria and other tiny particles. In the lymph nodes, these particles are attacked and destroyed by white blood cells. Infected lymph glands become enlarged, and can be felt as tender lumps in the neck, armpits, groin, and bend of the elbow. The *bubo* (inflammatory swelling) that may follow venereal diseases is a cluster of infected lymph glands in the groin. (See Fig. 1–19.)

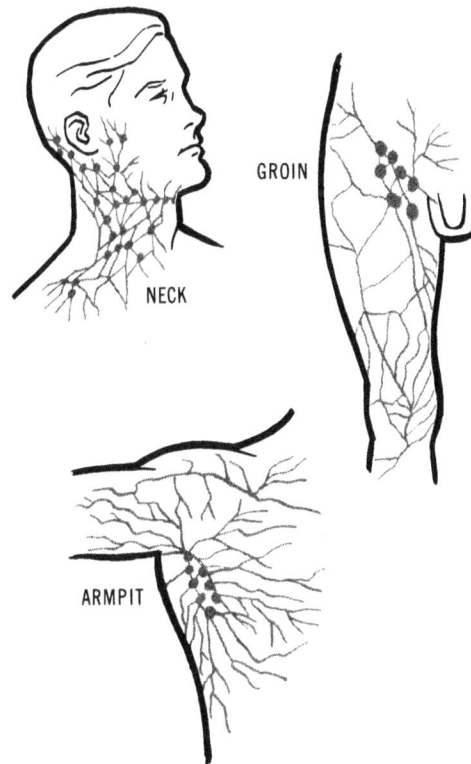

Fig. 1–19. Lymph nodes (main groups).

The lymphatic system includes:
1. A *system of tiny ducts* with walls one-cell thick (a capillary network).
2. *Larger vessels* which funnel lymph into the cardiovascular system.
3. *Lymph nodes* which act as filters and produce certain germ-fighting white blood cells (lymphocytes).
4. *Tonsils and adenoids:* tissues that strain out foreign particles.
5. *Spleen:* Over the years various functions have been attributed to the spleen, which is the largest lymphatic organ in the body. Now it is thought to enter into blood formation—especially red cells during fetal life and later in certain emergencies; and the production of some types of white blood cells throughout life. It acts as a reservoir of blood and enters into the destruction of worn-out red blood cells. There is some evidence that it may control the production of cells by the bone marrow. Other functions have been ascribed to it.

The spleen is located beneath the diaphragm, behind and to the left of the stomach, in the upper left quadrant of the abdomen. Because it lies close to the lower left ribs, fracturing them sometimes injures the spleen. Also, it may be ruptured by a severe blow, without fracture. A ruptured spleen will produce internal hemorrhage which may lead to death. A spleen can be removed surgically without seriously interfering with normal living. (See Fig. 1–22.)

RESPIRATORY SYSTEM

The body may store food to last for several weeks and water to last for several days, but it can store only enough oxygen for a few minutes. Ordinarily this does not matter because we have only to inhale air to get the oxygen we need. If the oxygen supply of the body is cut off, as in drowning, choking, or smothering, death will come in about five minutes unless oxygen intake is restored. Oxygen from air is made available to the blood through the respiratory system and then to the body cells by the circulatory system. (Fig. 1–20.)

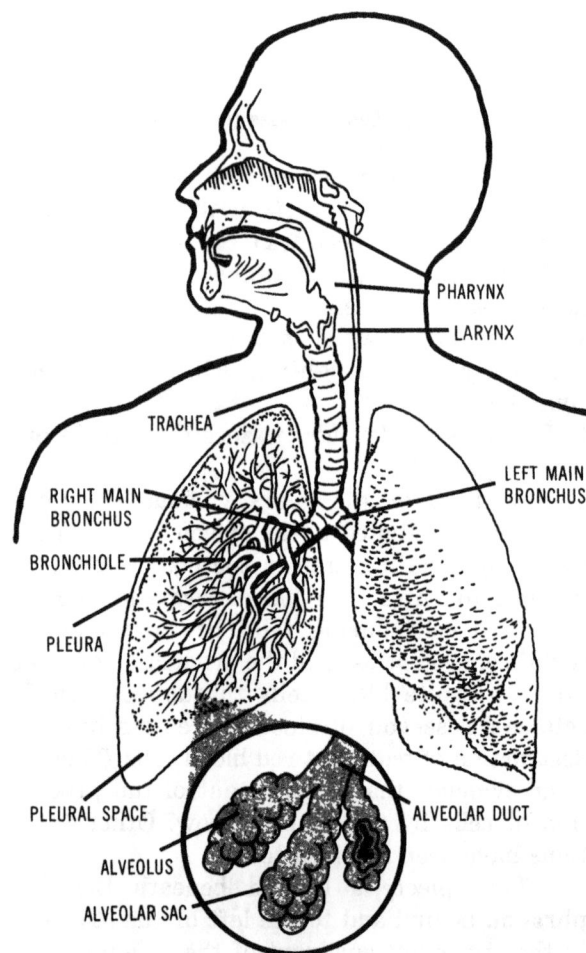

Fig. 1–20. Respiratory system.

Nasal Passages

Air normally enters the body through the nostrils. It is warmed, moistened, and filtered as it flows over the damp, sticky lining (*mucous membrane*) of the nose. When a person breathes through the mouth instead of the nose, there is less filtration and warming.

The nose is divided into two crooked passages by a wall (*septum*) of bone and cartilage. Each side of the nose has bones shaped like two inverted cones (*turbinates*). These protect the lungs from foreign body contamination, while warming and moistening the air. Breath passing through the nasal passages enters the nasal portion of the pharynx (*nasopharynx*).

Pharynx and Trachea

From the back of the nose or mouth, the air enters the throat (*pharynx*). The pharynx is a common passageway for food and air. (See Fig. 1–21.) At its lower end it divides into two passageways, one for food and the other for air. Food is routed by muscular control in the back of the throat to the food tube (*esophagus*) which leads to the stomach, and air from the pharynx to the windpipe (*trachea*) which leads to the lungs. The trachea and the esophagus are separated by a small cartilagenous flap of tissue (the *epiglottis*) which acts as a kind of valve that closes the trachea while food is being swallowed. At other times the trachea remains open to permit breathing. Usually this controlled diversion works automatically to keep food out of the trachea and air from going into the esophagus. However, when the epiglottis fails to close, food or liquids can enter the larynx instead of the esophagus.

During unconsciousness normal swallowing controls do not operate. *If liquid is poured into the mouth of an unconscious person to try to revive him, it may get into his windpipe and cause suffocation.* Foreign objects, as false teeth or a piece of food, may lodge in the throat or windpipe and cut off the passage of air.

In the upper two inches of the trachea, just below the epiglottis, is the voice box (*larynx*) which contains the vocal cords. In the front of the throat the larynx (*Adam's apple*) can be felt.

Lungs

The trachea branches into two main tubes (*bronchial tubes* or *bronchi*), one for each lung. Each *bronchus* divides and subdivides somewhat like the branches of a tree. Finally, the smallest ones end in thousands of tiny pouches (*air sacs*), just as the twigs of a tree end in leaves. Each air sac is enclosed in a network of capillaries. The adjoining walls of the air sacs and the walls of the capillaries are very thin. Through these walls, the oxygen combines with hemoglobin in red blood cells to form *oxyhemoglobin*, which is carried to all parts of the body. Carbon dioxide and certain other waste gases in the blood move across the capillary walls into the air sacs and are exhaled from the body. Tobacco smoke and certain other inhaled irritants cause the partitions between the air sacs to be destroyed, resulting in shortness of breath and eventually a disease called *emphysema*.

The lungs are very light—somewhat like large sponges. With the heart they occupy most of the chest cavity (*thoracic cavity*), which is divided into three sections, all separated from each other by a pleural membrane. The lungs are enclosed in a double-layered sac (*pleural sac*); the inner layer (*visceral pleura*) covers the lungs; the outer layer (*parietal pleura*) lines all of the chest cavity. The space between the pleural membranes contains fluid (*pleural fluid*) which acts as a lubricant to reduce friction. Inflammation of the pleurae (pleurisy) may cause friction, fever, and a stabbing pain with each breath. The lungs are open to attack by viruses and other microorganisms, notably those causing *bronchitis*, *pneumonia*, and *tuberculosis*.

Mechanics of Breathing

The passage of air into and out of the lungs is called *respiration*. Breathing in is called *inspiration* or inhalation; breathing out is *expiration* or exhalation.

Respiration is a mechanical process brought about by alternately increasing and decreasing the size of the chest cavity. During inspiration, the diaphragm is drawn downward, and the up-and-down dimension of the chest cavity is increased. At the same time, muscles attached to the chest wall tighten and lift the

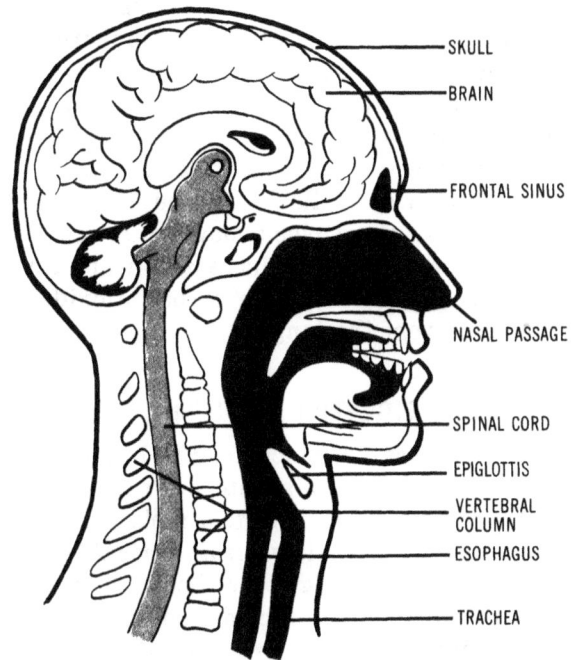

Fig. 1–21. Head and neck (sagittal plane section).

ribs and sternum upward and outward, increasing the front-to-back and side-to-side diameters of the chest. A relative vacuum in the respiratory system occurs. By way of the nose, mouth, trachea, and bronchi, air enters the lungs, which expand to fill the enlarged chest cavity and the air sacs receive fresh air. Muscles can close the larynx to hold the breath. During expiration, the muscles of the chest relax; the larynx opens to release the air trapped in the "pulmonary tree." Atmospheric pressure on the chest wall forces the ribs to fall, decreasing the size of the chest cavity. At the same time, the abdominal muscles contract, the abdominal contents press upward on the relaxed diaphragm and it domes. This further decreases the size of the chest cavity, forcing out the same volume of air that just had been taken in.

The average rate of breathing in an adult at rest is from 16 to 18 complete respirations (inspiration-expiration) per minute. Normally the rate is less when a person is lying down; faster when he is exercising vigorously.

Normally, the rate of breathing is controlled by a nerve center in the brain (the *respiratory center*). When a person does hard muscular work, the lungs cannot get rid of carbon dioxide or take in oxygen fast enough at the normal rate. As carbon dioxide increases in the blood and tissues, the respiratory center sends impulses along its nerves to cause deeper and more rapid respirations. At the same time, the heart rate increases. A greater supply of oxygen becomes available to the blood and lungs, because more blood moves through the lungs as a result of the increased heart rate. For the same reason, more carbon dioxide is discharged from the lungs.

DIGESTIVE SYSTEM

The process by which food is broken mechanically and chemically into a form the cells can use is *digestion*. This takes place mainly in the alimentary canal *(gastrointestinal tract)*, which extends through the body from the mouth to the anus and includes the esophagus, stomach, intestines, and rectum. (See Fig. 1–22.)

Abdominal Cavity

Except for the mouth and esophagus, the abdomen contains the major organs of the gastrointestinal tract. (See Fig. 1–22.) The abdominal cavity is well protected above by the thorax, below by the heavy ring of pelvic bones, and at the sides and in the back by thick tough muscles, the lower ribs, and the spinal column. It is protected in front by flat muscular layers, which for greater strength run in different directions in the abdominal wall.

Contraction of the abdominal muscles and diaphragm puts pressure on the abdominal contents from the sides, front, and above. This pressure helps defecation, urination, and vomiting. Occasionally, there are weaknesses in the abdominal wall which may "give" under pressure. These weaknesses are at points of some anatomic peculiarity, such as where two bundles of muscles cross at an angle to each other. Under sufficient pressure, the abdominal contents may bulge into or through the muscle wall but not through the skin. This is a rupture *(hernia)*. Most hernias occur in the groins *(inguinal hernias)*. A rupture at the navel *(umbilicus)* is called an *umbilical hernia*. Hernias also may occur in many other places, both superficially and deep in the abdominal cavity.

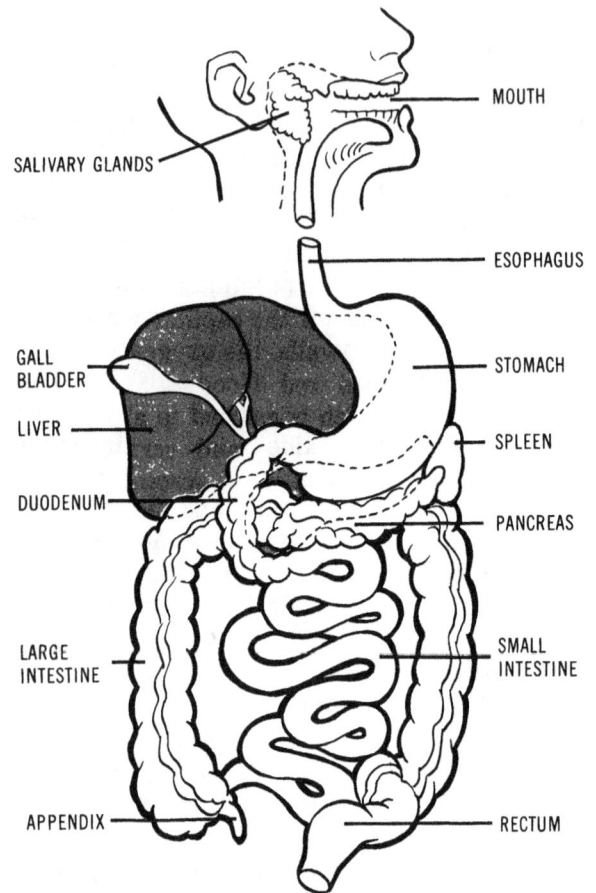

Fig. 1–22. Digestive system.

Peritoneum

The peritoneum is a sheathlike membrane in the abdominal cavity that consists of two layers. The outer layer *(parietal)* lines the walls of the abdominal cavity and the inner layer *(visceral)* surrounds and helps support some of the abdominal organs. Where the surfaces of these two layers contact each other, they secrete *peritoneal fluid*, a lubricant that prevents the layers from sticking together to form *adhesions*.

Alimentary Canal

The alimentary canal is divided into four specific parts by ringlike bands of muscles *(sphincters)*. These are at the junction of (1) the esophagus and the stomach (the *cardiac sphincter)*; (2) the stomach and small intestine *(pylorus)*; (3) the small intestine and the large intestine *(ileocecal valve)*; and (4) the end of the canal *(anal sphincter* or *anus)*. When a sphincter contracts, it closes the canal at that point so that its contents cannot pass through. The only sphincter under voluntary control is the anal sphincter, allowing control of the feces.

Food is pushed along the alimentary canal by contraction of the involuntary muscles in its wall. This *peristalsis*, besides moving food along, helps mix food with digestive juices in the stomach and small intestine. The wavelike motion of peristalsis usually is in one direction, away from the mouth; however, in vomiting, or when the bowel becomes obstructed, there may be a *reverse peristalsis* and the intestinal contents are ejected by way of the mouth.

Digestion begins in the mouth. Food is broken down and mixed with *saliva* by the action of the teeth, jaw and cheek muscles, and the tongue. Saliva, secreted by the *salivary glands*, contains an *enzyme*, a chemical which starts the digestion of starch. Later in the small intestine partly digested starch is turned into a sugar *(glucose)* which can be used by the body. Other enzymes are produced in the stomach, liver, pancreas, and small intestine for the digestion of each of the three principal components of food: *proteins* (found principally in meat, beans, and dairy products); *carbohydrates* (starches and sugars); and *fats* (both animal and vegetable).

Esophagus

Food passes from the mouth down the back of the throat *(pharynx)* and into the *esophagus*. A fairly straight, narrow, muscular tube, the esophagus passes through the chest just in front of the spinal column and into the abdomen. Through an opening in the diaphragm, it enters the stomach. Food is started down the esophagus by the action of the voluntary swallowing muscles of the mouth and pharynx. Then, peristalsis takes over. Pain sometimes occurs when the peristaltic wave presses on the food mass *(bolus)*, instead of behind it. At the lower end of the esophagus, the cardiac sphincter opens and food passes into the stomach.

Stomach

The *stomach*, a sac or pouch, is in the left, upper part of the abdomen, just below the diaphragm. (See Fig. 1–22.) It increases in size as food enters, and decreases as food passes out. The stomach holds food until it is acidified, liquified, mixed, and digested sufficiently to pass on into the small intestine. Digestion in the stomach is by gastric juices *(digestive enzymes)*. By peristalsis, the stomach mixes the food with the gastric juices. Too much hydrochloric acid causes acid indigestion *(hyperacidity)*. Haste, worry, emotional tension, tobacco, and alcohol appear to interfere with digestion. If not treated properly, hyperacidity may lead to a gastric or duodenal ulcer.

Small Intestine

From the lower end of the stomach, partially digested food *(chyme)* moves, a little at a time, through the pyloric sphincter into the small intestine. This narrow tube, about one inch in diameter and 23 feet long in the adult, extends from the stomach to the large intestine, joining the latter at the ileocecal valve in the lower right quadrant of the abdominal cavity. The upper part of the small intestine, the first 10 or 12 inches nearest the stomach, is the *duodenum*. Juices secreted by the liver and pancreas are delivered through ducts to the duodenum. These alkaline juices change the chyme from an acid to a nonacid state. The mucous membrane lining the small intestine has many tiny folds. These increase the surface in contact with the food and help in the absorption of digested food from the intestine into the blood and lymph.

Liver

The *liver*, the largest gland in the body, secretes *bile* and converts and stores sugar for use by muscles and other tissues. The liver is located in the upper right quadrant of the abdominal cavity. Its upper rounded surface fits closely into the under surface of the diaphragm, and part of its left side fits over the lower end of the stomach. Bile is concentrated and stored in a small sac *(gallbladder)*, from which it pours into the duodenum through the *bile duct* where it aids in digestion. Gallstones may form in the gallbladder by the crystallization of one or more ingredients of bile. The passage of a stone through the bile duct often causes severe pain *(gallstone* or *biliary colic)*. Gallstones may plug the bile duct, causing a back-up of bile in the liver. *Jaundice,* due to the presence of an abnormal amount of bile in the blood, gives a yellowish tinge to the skin, whites of the eyes, and membranes beneath the tongue.

There is a special system *(portal circulation)* for the transport of digested and absorbed foods from the intestines to the liver. The veins from most of the intestinal tract do not return blood directly to the heart, but convey it first to the liver. Capillaries in the liver bring this portal blood into close contact with cells that alter the partly converted food products into special materials for use by the body. These liver capillaries then funnel into a network of veins *(hepatic veins)* and the *inferior vena cava,* which delivers all the blood from the liver and the rest of the lower part of the body to the right atrium of the heart.

In certain diseases, the liver cells degenerate and are replaced by scar tissue. In this condition, *cirrhosis of the liver,* commonly seen in chronic alcoholics, blood cannot move easily through the liver. Pressure in the portal veins increases *(portal hypertension).* The portal blood may be sent on detours instead of passing normally through the liver. This may produce dilated veins *(varicose veins* or *varices)* in the stomach and esophagus, about the anus *(hemorrhoids* or *piles),* and even in the abdominal wall. The dilated veins in the stomach or esophagus are likely to rupture, with severe and often fatal hemorrhage.

Pancreas

The *pancreas* is a fish-shaped gland in the upper left quadrant of the abdominal cavity, behind the stomach and in front of the spinal column. (See Fig. 1–22.) It manufactures two important substances: (1) *pancreatic juice,* which passes from the pancreas into the duodenum through the pancreatic duct and is essential to the digestion of proteins, carbohydrates, and fats; and (2) *insulin,* which is absorbed directly from the gland into the bloodstream. An internal (or *endocrine)* secretion, insulin helps regulate the body's use and storage of sugar. The production of insufficient insulin results in *diabetes.*

Large Intestine and Rectum

Food not digested and absorbed by the small intestine passes into the *large intestine,* or *colon,* through the *ileocecal valve* in the lower right quadrant of the abdomen. The small intestine opens into the large intestine about two or three inches from the colon's beginning. This initial section of the large intestine is a kind of blind pouch called the *cecum.* At the end of the cecum is a narrow, wormlike tube (the *appendix).* Inflammation of the appendix is called *appendicitis.* The large intestine, about 2½ inches in diameter and 4 or 5 feet long, looks like a squared horseshoe. Beginning in the lower right quadrant of the abdomen, the large intestine goes up the right side *(ascending colon)* and crosses *(transverse colon)* to the left side; then goes down the left side *(descending colon).* In the lower left quadrant it makes a few turns to form the lower bowel *(sigmoid colon).* The large intestine or colon ends in the *rectum.*

The large intestine holds food residue and waste *(feces)* until some of the water is absorbed, reducing its bulk and fluidity. This absorption by the large intestine salvages large quantities of water which if lost by the body could be life-threatening.

The *rectum,* that portion of the large intestine just above the *anus,* is about five inches long. It ends in the *anal canal,* which terminates the alimentary canal. The anal canal, only about 1½ inches long, is guarded by the *anal sphincter,* which opens during a bowel movement *(defecation).*

URINARY SYSTEM

The urinary system produces urine to rid the body of certain wastes that result from cellular action. Urine normally is composed of water and salts, but in certain illnesses, sugar, albumin (a protein), cells, and cellular debris also may be present. Identifying the composition of urine helps to diagnose some illnesses. Elimination of waste matter from the body is called *excretion.*

The urinary system includes two *kidneys* (where the urine is formed); two *ureters* (tubes to carry urine from the kidneys to the bladder); the *bladder* (a reservoir for urine

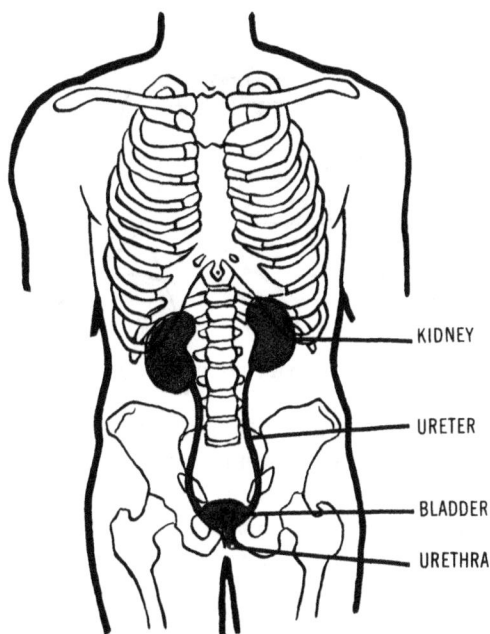

Fig. 1–23. Urinary system.

until discharged); and the *urethra* (the tube which carries the urine from the bladder to the outside of the body). (See Fig. 1–23.)

Kidneys

The *kidneys,* bean-shaped organs weighing about one-half pound each, are on either side of the spinal column in both upper quadrants of the abdominal cavity, about the level of the last lower rib. The kidneys are deeply imbedded in fatty tissue, well protected by heavy muscles of the back, and are seldom injured except by severe trauma.

The kidneys purify blood and maintain a proper fluid and chemical balance for the body. About 96 percent of urine is water. The quantity (over one liter daily) of urine excreted and the analysis of its contents *(urinalysis)* inform the physician whether the kidneys are working properly. When the kidneys fail, the body is poisoned by wastes which cannot be excreted. This *uremia,* if not treated properly, may lead to death.

Bladder and Urethra

The *bladder* is a muscular sac. When empty, it lies entirely within the pelvis behind and beneath the pubis. Because of its vulnerable location, especially when distended, the bladder

sometimes is punctured, ruptured, or otherwise injured when the abdomen is struck heavily or the pubis is broken.

The *urethra* is the canal which empties the urine from the bladder. It also carries male seminal fluid *(semen)* on ejaculation. Through the external opening of the urethra, infections from bacteria and other organisms may travel to the bladder, to the kidneys by way of the ureters, or the testicles through the seminal ducts.

REPRODUCTIVE SYSTEM

The reproductive systems in the male and female consist of complementary organs whose function is to accomplish reproduction and produce a new human being. The male, who provides the male germ cell (the *sperm*), and the female, who provides the female germ cell (the *ovum*), contribute the genes that determine the hereditary characteristics of the baby. Combination of a single sperm with a single ovum forms a fertilized ovum that can grow into an *embryo*, then into a *fetus*, and finally a newborn baby.

Male Reproductive System

The reproductive system of the male includes the two *testes* (singular, *testis*), a *duct system, accessory glands,* and the *penis.*

The *testes* are two oval glands, which produce sperm and male hormones and are enclosed within a skin-covered pouch called the *scrotum.* The structures that form the *duct system* are the *epididymides, vas deferens, ejaculatory duct,* and the *urethra.*

Each *epididymis,* located along the top and side of each testis, consists of a single tightly coiled tube which connects the testis with the

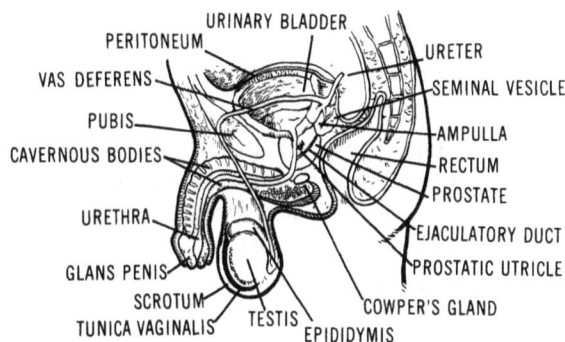

Fig. 1–24. Reproductive system (male).

vas deferens. The *vas deferens* extends upward inside the *spermatic cord,* a cylindrical casing of white fibrous tissue that also encloses blood vessels, lymphatics, and nerves, through the *inguinal canal* into the abdominal cavity. It joins the duct from the *seminal vesicle* to form the ejaculatory duct, a short tube which passes through the prostate gland and ends in the urethra.

The accessory reproductive glands of the male are the *seminal vesicles,* the *prostate gland,* and the *bulbourethral glands* or Cowper's glands.

The *seminal vesicles* are two membranous pouches lying above the prostate and behind the bladder. They secrete the viscous liquid portion of the semen.

The *prostate* is a chestnut-size, glandular body which surrounds the neck of the bladder and part of the urethra. The prostate adds a thin alkaline secretion to the seminal fluid. In older men the prostate frequently enlarges in size. As it enlarges, it compresses the urethra so that urine cannot pass readily through the tube.

The two small pea-shaped *bulbourethral glands* lie below the prostate gland on either side of the urethra. They secrete an alkaline fluid which lubricates the urethra.

The *penis* serves a double function: it contains the urethra, the terminal duct for both the urinary and reproductive systems; and is the organ of copulation by means of which sperm cells are introduced into the female vagina. The penis is composed of three cylindrical masses of erectile tissue that stiffen when engorged with blood. The head of the penis (*glans penis*), highly sensitive, is covered by a foreskin (*prepuce*). The scrotum and the penis constitute the *external genitals* of the male. (See Fig. 1–24.)

Female Reproductive System

The female reproductive system consists of two ovaries, two uterine (*fallopian*) tubes, the *uterus,* the *vagina,* and the *external genitals.* (See Fig. 1–25.) The accessory organs are the breasts (*mammary glands*).

There is an *ovary* on each side of the uterus, below and behind the fallopian tubes. The ovary, the female counterpart of the testis, is oval and covered by a special type of tissue

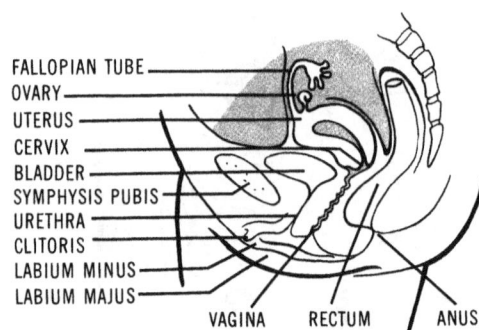

Fig. 1–25. Reproductive system (female).

(*germinal epithelium*). Beneath this tissue covering are numerous round transparent vesicles (sacs), each with an ovum in a different stage of maturation. When mature, an ovum ruptures into the abdominal cavity (*ovulation*). Ovulation usually occurs every 28 days from puberty to menopause. The ovaries also produce hormones that control the implantation of the fertilized egg in the uterus, stimulate the growth of the mammary glands, and stop ovulation during pregnancy.

The *fallopian tubes,* about four inches long, enter the uterus from the upper outer wall on the right and on the left. The tubes serve as ducts for the germ cells (*ova*) even though they are not actually connected to the ovaries. Near the ovary, each tube has a number of finger-like projections which sweep an ovum into the tube and thence to the uterus. Fertilization normally occurs in the fallopian tubes.

The *uterus,* a pear-shaped, hollow, muscular, thick-walled organ is composed of two parts: an upper portion, the *body,* and a lower, narrow section, the *cervix,* which extends into the upper vagina.

The uterus has several functions: *menstruation,* the monthly shedding of the lining of the uterus; *pregnancy,* when the embryo implants itself in the uterus a few days after fertilization and lives there throughout the fetal period; and *labor,* the powerful, rhythmic contractions which result in expulsion of the fetus from the mother at birth.

The *vagina* is a musculo-membranous collapsible tube located behind the bladder and urethra and in front of the rectum. The vagina is the site of copulation in the female. Also, it serves as the lower part of the birth canal and as the excretory duct for the menstrual flow.

The external genital structures—referred to collectively as the *vulva*—include the *mons pubis*, the *labia majora*, the *labia minora*, the *clitoris*, the *vestibule of the vagina*, and the *greater vestibular glands*, or *Bartholin's glands*.

The *mons pubis*, a fatty pad lying in front of the pubic bone, is covered with hair after puberty. Extending downward from the mons are two fleshy flaps of skin (*labia majora* and *labia minora*). Between them is the *clitoris*. Like the penis, it contains erectile tissue and is highly sensitive to stimulation. The vestibule of the vagina is in the area situated posterior to the clitoris and between the labia minora. The urethra opens into this space anteriorly and the vagina opens into it posteriorly. The Bartholin's glands open on either side of the vaginal orifice. They secrete a lubricating fluid. These glands are of clinical importance because they may become infected.

NERVOUS SYSTEM

The nervous system is a very complex collection of nerve cells (*neurons*) that coordinate the work of all parts of the human body and keep the individual in touch with the outside world. Neurons receive stimuli from the environment and transmit impulses to nerve centers in the brain and spinal cord. Then by a

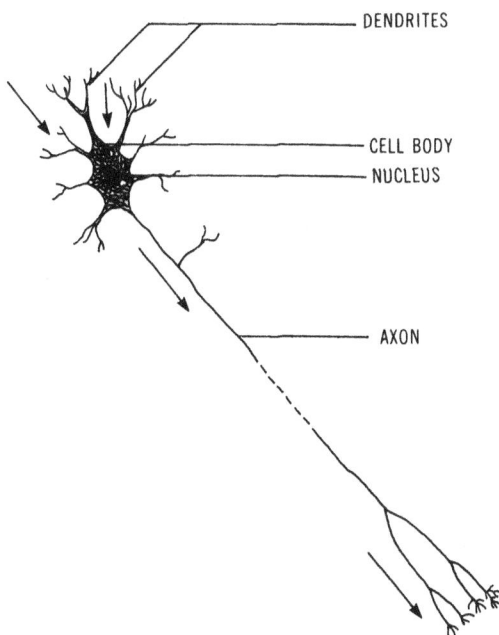

Fig. 1–26. Nerve cell (neuron). Diagrammatic. Arrows show direction of impulse.

complicated process of thinking (reasoning), plus reflex and automatic reactions, they produce nerve impulses that regulate and coordinate all bodily movements and functions, and govern behavior and consciousness.

Nerve Cells

The nervous system's basic unit, the *neuron*, transmits messages in the form of electrochemical impulses to other neurons. A neuron consists of a central cell body with threadlike extensions (processes)—an *axon* with several *dendrities*. (See Fig. 1–26.) Impulses are carried toward the cell body by dendrites. A single process called an axon transmits impulses away from the cell body. Axons and dendrites of the body's nerve cells never touch each other; there is a space or gap (a *synapse*) between them over which nerve impulses are relayed by electrochemical means. A group of nerve cells is called a *ganglion* (pl. ganglia).

In terms of function, neurons may be classed as (1) *sensory* or *afferent nerves* that carry messages toward the brain or spinal cord; (2) *motor neurons* or *efferent nerves* that carry impulses from the brain or spinal cord to *muscles* to produce various actions; and (3) *mixed nerves* that transmit impulses in both directions at once.

Once nerve cells are destroyed, the body cannot regenerate them. However, some limited nerve repair is possible as long as the vital cell body is intact. If a nerve fiber is cut or injured, the section attached to the cell body remains alive, but the part beyond the injury withers away. At times the live remnant may extend itself beyond the withered section to restore function.

Classification

The nervous system can be discussed in different ways. From a structural standpoint, there is the (1) *central or cerebrospinal nervous system* that includes the brain and spinal cord; and (2) the *peripheral nervous system*, a network of nerve cells that originates in the brain and spinal cord and extends to all parts of the body, including muscles, surface of the skin, and the special sense organs as the eye and ear. The peripheral nervous system is further subdivided into the *voluntary* and *autonomic (involuntary) nervous systems*.

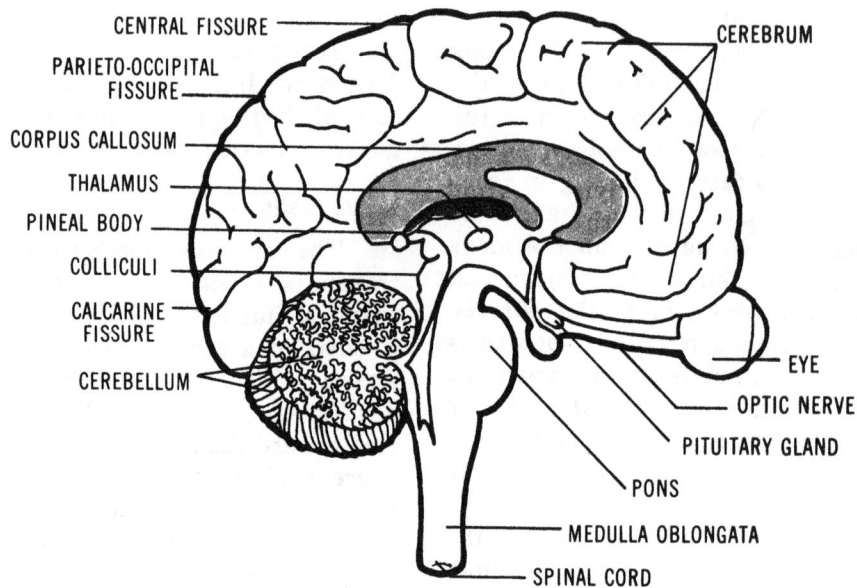

Fig. 1–27. Brain, midsection, lateral view (diagrammatic).

Another way to describe the nervous system is by *function*. Again there are two divisions: (1) the *voluntary* (cerebrospinal) system, which for the most part sets up conscious, deliberate bodily actions under the control of the will—plus reflex actions which may or may not be conscious; and (2) the *involuntary* (autonomic) system which is automatic and partly independent of the rest of the nervous system. The autonomic nervous system is subdivided into the *sympathetic* and the *parasympathetic* nervous systems.

Central Nervous System

The central nervous system is composed of two interconnected structures: the *brain* which is enclosed within the skull and protected by three membranes of connective tissue called *meninges;* and the *spinal cord* housed within a semiflexible bony column of vertebrae and composed of nerve cells that transmit impulses to and from the brain. From the brain 12 pairs of nerve trunks go out to various parts of the head and neck, and one pair goes down to the chest and the upper part of the abdominal cavity. From the spinal cord 31 pairs of nerve trunks go out to the neck, trunk, and limbs.

Brain

The brain which is the headquarters of the human nervous system is probably the most highly specialized organ in the body. It is criti-

cal to the functioning of the central and peripheral nerve networks. It weighs about three pounds in the average adult, is richly supplied with blood vessels, and requires considerable oxygen to perform effectively.

The brain has two main subdivisions: the *cerebrum* (large brain) which occupies nearly all of the cranial cavity and the *cerebellum* (small brain). The cerebrum is divided into two hemispheres by a deep cleft. The outer surface of the cerebrum, about one-eighth inch thick, is composed mainly of cell bodies of nerve cells, called "gray matter" or the *cerebral cortex.* The inner mass of cerebral tissue or "white matter" has interconnecting nerve fibers intermixed with small sections of "gray matter" that form special *ganglia* or control centers of nerve cells. These ganglia integrate and moderate the activities of nerve cells in the cortex. The surface of the brain is thrown into folds called convolutions that are separated from each other by grooves or fissures. These infoldings increase greatly the surface of the cortex.

Certain sections of the cerebrum are localized to control specific body functions as sensation, thought, and associative memory which allows us to store, recall, and make use of past experiences. Also, it initiates and manages those motions which are said to be "under the control of the will." The sight center of the brain is located in the back part called the *occipital lobe.* The *temporal lobe* at the side of the head deals with smell and hearing. The sensory and motor centers are separated by a transverse fissure at the middle of the top of the head. Centers of touch, taste, smell, and speech, among others have been recognized. An injury to any one center interferes with the specific function that it controls.

The *cerebellum* is located at the back of the cranium and below the cerebrum. Its main function is to coordinate muscular activity. Also it maintains balance in association with impulses from the eyes and the semicircular canals of the inner ears. Although the cerebellum cannot initiate a muscular contraction, it can hold muscles in a state of partial contraction which keeps a person from collapsing. It helps to coordinate the several muscular movements necessary to catch a ball.

Two smaller subdivisions of the brain that are vital to life are the *pons* and the *medulla oblongata*. The pons acts as a bridge that connects the cerebrum, cerebellum, and the medulla oblongata. The medulla oblongata protrudes from the skull slightly where it joins the spinal cord. It controls the activity of the internal organs, as the rate of respiration, heart action, muscular action of the walls of the digestive organs, and glandular secretions, among other activities.

Beneath the cerebral hemispheres of the forebrain are the *thalamus, hypothalamus,* and *pituitary* sections. The thalamus is a selective relay center for such impulses as those that relate to heat, cold, touch, and pain; also, it controls basic emotions as anger or fear. A lack of emotional control and marked changes in personality can be traced to dysfunctions of the thalamus. The hypothalamus, located next to the thalamus, has control centers that regulate the amount of fluid retained in the body, the appetite, the sex drive, the waking-sleeping cycle, and acts as a body temperature regulator. The *pituitary gland*, the master endocrine gland of the body, is attached to the hypothalamus and injury to either can upset many functions of the body's delicately balanced endocrine (glandular) system. (See Fig. 1–27.)

Within the brain are small cavities, the ventricles, which contain the *cerebrospinal fluid*. This fluid, produced by a plexus of blood vessels is a clear, watery solution similar to blood plasma. Circulating throughout the brain and spinal cord, it serves as a protective cushion and exchanges food and waste materials. The total quantity in the brain-spinal cord system is 100–150 ml, although up to several liters may be produced daily. It is constantly being produced and reabsorbed. Some diseases affect the reabsorption activity and pressure may build up within the system due to excess fluid. In the lower back between vertebrae, there is room for the insertion of a hypodermic needle to withdraw a sample of fluid for chemical examination. This spinal tap can furnish important diagnostic information on whether the volume of fluid and the pressure increased or decreased; on the fluid's composition, as content of protein or sugar; white blood cell count, and it can identify bacterial invaders.

Knowledge of nerve structure and function enables physicians to locate brain sections that are diseased. It is known that nerves from one side of the body eventually connect with the opposite side of the brain. Thus, a person whose left arm is paralyzed after a stroke is known to have suffered damage to the right side of the brain.

Spinal Cord

The spinal cord is a soft column of nerve tissue that is continuous with the lower part of the brain (*medulla oblongata*) and is enclosed in the bony vertebral column. Thirty-one pairs of spinal nerves branch from the spinal cord and are named generally for the vertebrae through which they emerge. These nerves are large trunks similar to telephone cables because they house many nerve fibers. Some fibers carry impulses into the spinal cord; others carry impulses away from it. Nerve impulses travel in one direction only along these fibers.

Spinal nerves at different levels of the cord regulate activities of various parts of the body. Eight pairs of *cervical nerves* activate muscles, bones, joints, and skin areas of the neck, shoulders, outer arm areas, wrists and hands. The next 12 pairs known as *thoracic nerves* act on parts of the trunk of the body from the shoulder level to a line about two inches below the navel; also they innervate the inner surfaces of the arm. Then come five pairs of *lumbar nerves* that emerge between lumbar vertebrae; five pairs of *sacral nerves* that emerge at the base of the spine; and one pair of *coccygeal nerves* that pass out between the sacrum and the coccyx bones. These last eleven pairs service the pelvic region of the trunk, the buttocks regions, and the legs. Also, branches of these lower spinal nerves merge to form two of the largest peripheral nerve trunks of the body: the *femoral nerve* that goes down the inner sides of the legs from groins to feet; and the *sciatic nerve* that extends along the back of the upper and lower legs to the feet.

Reflex Action

In addition to linking the brain with all the nerves of the body, the spinal cord is the center for *reflex actions.* A reflex action is the simplest form of nerve action. It is an automatic unconscious response wherein an impulse is relayed from one nerve to another without the brain being involved. The knee jerk is a good example of a simple reflex action. If the leg is allowed to swing freely and it is tapped just below the kneecap, the foot will jerk upward. The tap sets up an impulse in a sensory nerve from the lower leg. The impulse travels along a dendrite to the spinal cord where it contacts a central neuron to stimulate a motor nerve that activates leg muscles to cause a jerk. It is a split second automatic action that does not involve the brain.

When a hot object is touched, a similar reflex is experienced. The hand jerks away almost instantly. After the reflex is completed, the impulse continues to the brain and pain is registered. If the muscle response had been delayed until the pain impulse had reached the brain, and a motor impulse traveled back along the spinal cord from the cerebral motor area, there would have been a much greater burn injury. Such a reflex action not only can reduce the extent of the injury, it can be lifesaving. Other reflex actions are blinking the eyes, coughing, sneezing, and leaping when touched unexpectedly.

Peripheral Nervous System

The *peripheral nervous system* which carries both voluntary and involuntary impulses, is made up of (1) the 31 pairs of spinal nerves discussed previously that serve the spinal cord; (2) 12 pairs of cranial nerves that carry nerve messages to and from the brain; and (3) the autonomic (involuntary) nervous system.

The several divisions and subdivisions of the nervous system described herein represent an arbitrary procedure that depends upon whether we are considering its structure, function, or actions under the control of the will. No matter what specialized duties are involved, the various groups of nerves adapt to each other to form a coordinated unit.

The 12 pairs of cranial nerves innervate organs, muscles, and glands in the head. For example, the *optic nerve* innervates the eye; the *auditory nerve*, the ear; and the *olfactory nerve*, the organs of smell.

One cranial nerve—the *vagus nerve*—differs somewhat from the others in the head. It wanders out of the head to extend itself through the neck and chest to reach the abdomen. Along its path it connects with various organs to regulate rates of breathing and heartbeat, glandular secretion, and motility within the digestive tract. In this respect it acts as an *automatic nerve* to provide unbroken contact with involuntary (autonomic) control centers in the brain. This bypass of the vertebral column by the vagus nerve provides a supplemental pathway to allow the autonomic nervous system to continue its vital automatic functions unimpaired, if the spinal cord ever is injured severely or destroyed. Only when injury or disease affects the brain or brain stem will these vital involuntary body functions be disturbed.

Autonomic Nervous System

The *autonomic nervous system* is an auxiliary network of nerve tissue that regulates unconscious, involuntary body functions which must continue day and night, regardless of our desires. It excites into action the smooth muscle of the walls of blood vessels, the gastrointestinal tract, the lungs and heart, and stimulates internal secretions. The system governs automatic functions to which we normally pay no attention—including vital functions like breathing and the heartbeat.

The autonomic nerves belong to a group that is not directly under control of the brain, but usually work in harmony with those nerves that the brain controls.

The autonomic system is divided into the *sympathetic nervous system* and the *parasym-*

pathetic nervous system. Both systems act in delicate balance.

Sympathetic Nervous System

Sympathetic nerve trunks lie on both sides of the vertebral column, connect with nerve cells in the spinal cord, and extend motor fibers to the various organs that they control in the chest and the abdomen. Also, other motor fibers do not extend directly to the organs that they control; instead they unite or come together into groups of nerve cells or *ganglia* that act as interconnected control centers in the connective tissue that lines the chest and abdomen outside the spinal column on both sides. Special nerve cells in these ganglia send out fibers to form dense networks of nerves *(plexuses)* near the organs they control. The largest of these sympathetic ganglia is the *solar plexus,* located just below the diaphragm. Another is near the heart, a third is in the neck, and a fourth in the lower abdomen surrounds the testicles. The latter plexus of nerves accounts for the extreme sensitivity of the area and the excessive pain that results when struck by a blow.

The sympathetic nervous system helps to regulate heart action, arterial blood supply, secretions of ductless glands, smooth muscle action in stomach and intestine, plus action of other internal organs. An important function of the system is to increase body activity to enable it to meet danger. When challenged to meet stress, body processes are stepped up by discharge of stimulating secretions at nerve junctions. These secretions, plus adrenalin shot into the bloodstream, produce faster muscular action than could be gotten by hormonal releases from various glands. Heart and lung action increases, extra glucose is released from the liver for energy, and the body is prepared for a super effort.

Parasympathetic Nervous System

Ganglia of the *parasympathetic nervous system* are in the midportion of the brain, the medulla oblongata, and the sacral region of the spinal cord. This system opposes the sympathetic system. It prevents body processes from increasing to extremes. Secretions are discharged to slow the heartbeat, decrease lung action, and return body processes to normal after the threat of danger has been met.

Table 1–7

**FUNCTIONS OF THE
AUTONOMIC NERVOUS SYSTEM**

Sympathetic	Parasympathetic
1. Dilates pupils.	1. Contracts pupils.
2. Lessens tonus of ciliary muscles so that the eyes may accommodate to see distant objects.	2. Contracts ciliary muscles so that the eyes may accommodate to see objects near at hand.
3. Dilates bronchi.	3. Constricts bronchi.
4. Quickens and strengthens the action of the heart.	4. Slows the action of the heart.
5. Contracts blood vessels of the skin and viscera so that more blood goes to the skeletal and cardiac muscles where it is needed for "fight or flight."	5. Dilates blood vessels (except cardiac).
6. Relaxes gastrointestinal tract and bladder.	6. Increases contractions of gastrointestinal tract and muscle tone of the bladder.
7. Decreases secretions of gastrointestinal glands.	7. Increases secretions of gastrointestinal glands.
8. Increases secretion of sweat glands.	8. No action on sweat glands.
9. Causes contraction of sphincters to prevent emptying of bowels or bladder.	9. Relaxes sphincters so that waste matter can be excreted.

The principal nerve of this system is the *vagus nerve,* which has been discussed previously under the peripheral nervous system. Through surgery, impulses from the vagus nerve can be diminished to lessen excess acid secretions in the stomach of a peptic ulcer patient.

Sympathetic vs Parasympathetic Systems

The sympathetic nervous system is concerned with making rapid adjustments to meet emergencies. The parasympathetic system deals mainly with digestion and the repair of wear and tear to the body.

The opposing functions of the two systems tend to keep the body in delicate balance. For example, in times of stress or danger it is more important that the heart pump extra blood to leg muscles to have us move away quickly from danger than for blood to go to digestive organs to act on food. Sympathetic nerve impulses speed the heart and slow digestion; parasympathetic impulses oppose these. The one system constricts blood vessels, the other dilates. The parasympathetic system acts more slowly than the sympathetic system's split-second response to danger. When there is no longer a need for "flight or fight," the former system forces a gradual slowdown of heart, lungs, and other organs for a return to normal functioning of body processes.

ENDOCRINE SYSTEM

Endocrine (or *ductless*) *glands* are the body's regulators. Secretions (*hormones*) of the glands are carried by the bloodstream to all parts of the body, affecting physical strength, mental ability, build, stature, reproduction, hair growth, voice pitch, and behavior. How people think, act, and feel depends largely on these minute secretions from the endocrine glands.

Endocrine glands, having no ducts, discharge their secretions (hormones) directly into the bloodstream. Each endocrine gland produces one or more hormones, which are chemical substances that have a specific effect on the activity of certain organs. Good health depends on a well-balanced output of hormones. Endocrine imbalance yields profound changes in growth and serious changes in mental, emotional, physical, and sexual behavior.

Some endocrine glands (see Fig. 1–28) and their functions follow:

• The *thyroid* gland in the neck produces thyroxin, a catalyst for oxidative (oxygen-using) processes in tissue metabolism.

• The *parathyroid* glands, near the thyroid, produce parathormone, necessary for the metabolism of calcium and phosphorus in bones.

• The *adrenal* glands atop the kidneys produce hormones that postpone muscular fatigue, in-

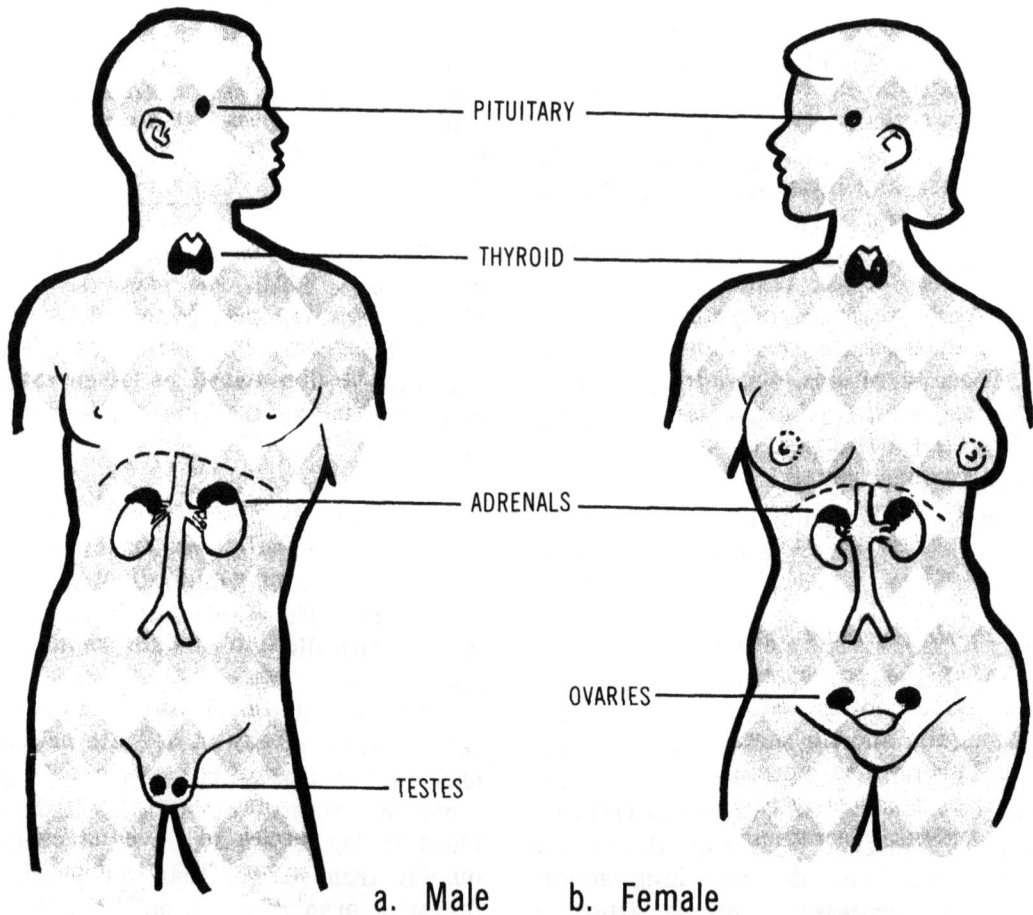

PITUITARY

THYROID

ADRENALS

OVARIES

TESTES

a. Male   b. Female

Fig. 1–28. Some endocrine glands.

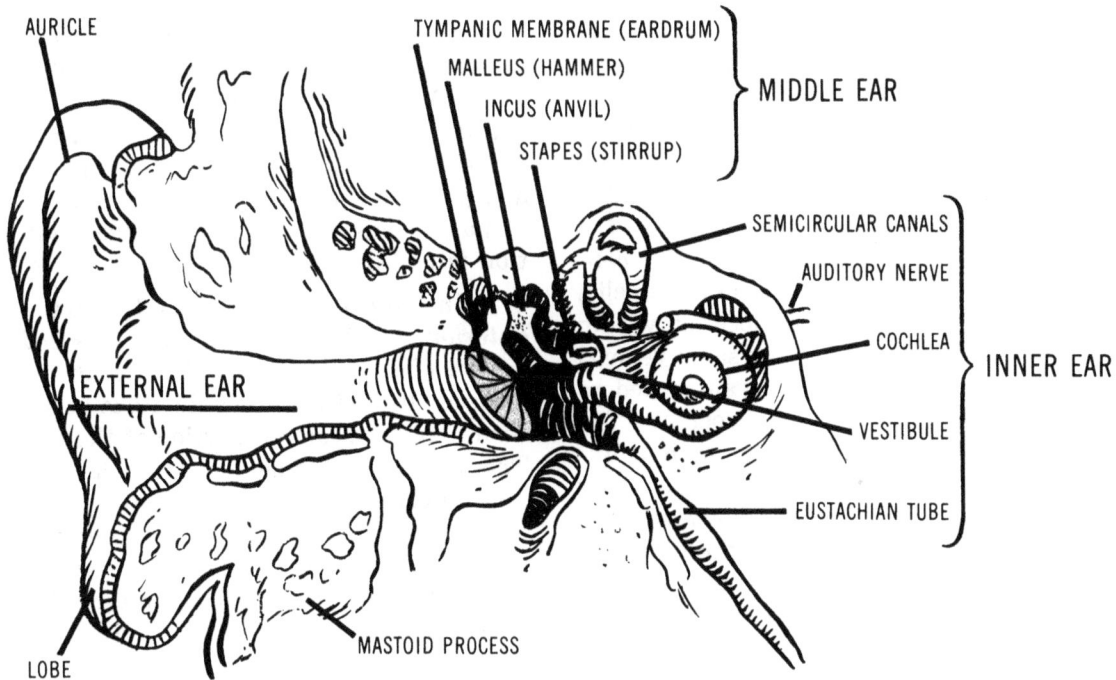

Fig. 1–29. Ear, right, diagrammatic.

crease the storing of glycogen (a sugar), control kidney function, and regulate the metabolism of salt and water.

• The *gonads* (ovaries and testes) produce the hormones governing reproduction and sex characteristics.

• The *islets of Langerhans* in the pancreas make insulin for sugar metabolism.

• The *pituitary* gland at the base of the brain behind the nose, is the "master gland" because its various hormones regulate growth, the thyroid and parathyroid glands, pancreas, gonads, metabolism of fatty acids and some basic proteins, blood sugar reactions, and urinary excretion.

EARS

The ear is concerned with the functions of hearing and equilibrium. There are three divisions of the ear: the *outer ear, middle ear,* and *inner ear.* (See Fig. 1–29.)

The outer ear is comprised of the auricle *(pinna),* a skin-covered cartilaginous framework which projects from the head and the *external auditory canal.* This canal, lined with hairs and glands that secrete earwax *(cerumen),* is S-shaped, about one inch long and extends to the middle ear.

The eardrum *(tympanic membrane* or *tympanum)* separates the external auditory canal from the middle ear. In the middle ear, three tiny movable bones (the *ossicles*) modify and conduct sound vibrations from the eardrum to the inner ear.

The eardrum and the ossicles are so delicate that violent vibrations of the air, like those caused by the explosion of a bomb or the firing of a heavy gun, may injure them. The three ossicles of each ear are called *malleus, incus,* and *stapes,* and in the order named, resemble a miniature hammer, anvil, and stirrup.

Air is let into or out of the middle ear through the *eustachian tube,* which leads to the upper part of the throat. The eustachian tube allows air pressure in the middle ear to equal that of air entering the external ear canal. A nose or throat infection can spread to the middle ear by way of the eustachian tube. Blowing the nose may force infected material into the middle ear. An infection of the middle ear may abscess (form pus), and running ears may result. Sometimes infection may extend from the middle ear to the *mastoid cells* in the temporal bone and cause mastoiditis. When this happens, a brain abscess or permanent deafness may result.

Vibrations that are carried to the inner ear by the external canal, the eardrum, and the ossicles are converted into nerve impulses and transmitted to the brain by the auditory nerve. The inner ear consists of the *osseous* (bony) labyrinth and the *membranous* labyrinth. The osseous labyrinth is composed of a series of cavities: the vestibule, three *semi-circular canals,* and the *cochlea* (snail shell). The membranous labyrinth is located within the osseous labyrinth and has the same general shape. The sense of hearing is transmitted to the auditory nerve through the cochlea. The semicircular canals are concerned with equilibrium. They are filled with fluid and any movement of the head results in a corresponding movement of the fluid in the three canals. The movement of the fluid generates nerve impulses, which cause a person to make adjustments in position to maintain balance. Motion of an airplane or of a ship can produce dizziness and nausea. This *motion sickness* may be called "sea sickness," "air sickness," or "bus sickness," depending upon the type of vehicle in which the person is riding when he experiences the symptoms.

EYES

The eye is a sphere approximately one inch in diameter formed by a tough outer coat called the *sclera* and the clear front portion known as the *cornea.* There are six muscles attached to the sclera which work in various combinations to move the eye. The ocular movements are very precise and rapid; primarily because there is more brain tissue devoted to controlling eye movements than to any other single motor function.

The cornea is the window through which light enters the eye. There are no blood vessels in the normal cornea, and it is extremely sensitive and especially susceptible to injury or infection. If scarring occurs from injury, the cornea loses its transparency at the site of the scar, which may markedly impair vision. The cornea has an extremely high concentration of nerve fibers which make it extremely sensitive to the slightest insult. A superficial scratch, abrasion, or the smallest foreign body can cause extreme pain with reflex tearing and redness (inflammation) of the eye.

The back surface of the eyelids and the exposed portion of the white part of the eye (sclera) are lined with a paper-thin covering called the *conjunctiva;* it does not cover the cornea. The conjunctiva may become infected and produce a red eye with a variable amount of pus, mucus, or water discharge. This infection is called conjunctivitis.

The internal portions of the eye are the *anterior chamber, iris, lens, vitreous body,* and *retina.* (See Fig. 1–30.) The anterior chamber, a space filled with watery fluid lies between the cornea and the colored portion of the eye (iris). The *iris* is a pigmented muscular structure which opens and closes the pupil to allow more or less light to enter the eye, depending on the level of illumination. This works much the same as the iris diaphragm on a camera which controls the amount of light that enters the camera.

Just behind the iris is a structure known as the *lens,* which can change shape to focus light rays on the back of the eye. When the lens becomes cloudy, it is called a *cataract.* In middle age the lens usually becomes somewhat less flexible, making it necessary to get reading glasses or bifocals. Behind the lens is the *vitreous body,* a cavity filled with a clear jelly known as the *vitreous humor.*

The innermost layer of the eye is the *retina* with specialized nerve cells, which are sensitive to light and color. The retina acts much the same as the film in a camera, except the retina receives the light rays and converts them into nerve impulses which are transmitted to the

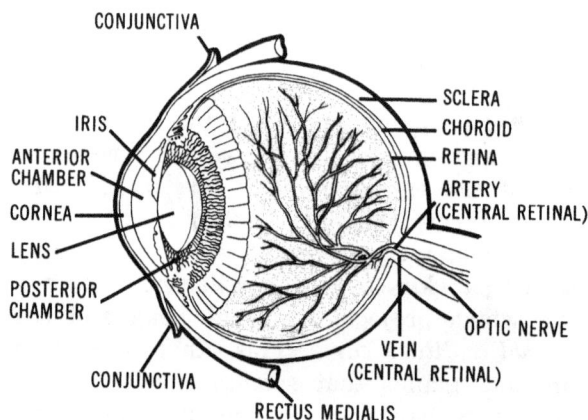

Fig. 1–30. Human eye.

brain by the *optic nerve*. In the brain the nerve impulses are interpreted as sight.

A tear gland (*lacrimal gland*), located under the outer part of the upper lid, is constantly producing tears to keep the eye moist and lubricated so the eyeball can glide smoothly under the eyelid. When the eye is irritated, tear production is increased to help wash away the irritant.

The eye is protected and cleansed by the *eyelids*. They spread the tears over the front of the eye and tend to wipe away dust and other foreign particles. Along the edges of the eyelids are openings of many small oil glands which help prevent too rapid evaporation of tears. The lashes and eyebrows tend to prevent foreign material from entering the eye. At the inner corner of each upper and lower lid is a small pinpoint opening called the *punctum*. Through this opening the tears drain into a small tube which in turn empties into a passage known as the nasolacrimal duct. This duct empties the tears into the nose.

Chapter II

Examination of the Patient

GENERAL CONSIDERATIONS

A SYSTEMATIC AND COMPLETE EXAMINATION of the patient is essential to evaluate the extent of a person's illness. An examination is composed of two basic parts: (1) the *history*, a chronological story of the patient's illness from the first symptoms to the present time; and (2) the *physical examination*, in which the patient is examined for physical evidence of disease. The findings should be recorded accurately, concisely, and completely.

Many patients reporting to sickbay may have a minor illness or injury, as a splinter or blister which often requires only a brief examination prior to treatment for the specific complaint. Patients who appear quite ill will require a thorough evaluation and a more detailed examination.

An accurate record should be made of all phases of every illness, beginning with the history and physical examination. Daily records should be kept during the course of the illness. Many times, the diagnosis will not be evident when the patient is first seen; but, as complaints and delayed physical signs appear in the next several days, the symptom complex may become clearer. Originally, many infectious diseases present themselves with only fever and general malaise, but in several days a rash may appear (as in measles); or jaundice (as in hepatitis); or a stiff neck and coma (as in menin-

gitis). These signs and symptoms help to establish a definitive diagnosis. Many times the patient's complaints will change after a period of time ranging from several hours to days; or more information will be offered. Many patients unconsciously omit important facts due to fear created by their illness. This added information may modify or change the diagnosis.

A clear, concise recording of signs and symptoms of the patient's illness is important in communication by radio, or when a patient is transferred to a physician's care. At times, the patient may be unable to speak coherently or remember exactly what has happened during the illness. If accurate and complete records have been made, they may prove lifesaving in establishing a correct diagnosis promptly.

HISTORY TAKING

Taking the history is an important part of the examination and often a diagnosis may be made from the history alone. Techniques that help to obtain a meaningful history should be studied, practiced, and reviewed. A patient may tell his history in various ways. All possible information should be obtained and organized logically to tell the story of the patient's illness. Arranging symptoms into a diagnostic pattern may seem difficult at first; however, this will become easier with experience.

37

Recording the History

The recorded history should begin with the time the patient first noted any symptoms of sickness, body changes, or a departure from good health. Symptoms and events up to the present time should be included. The dates or times that various symptoms appeared should be noted as precisely as possible. The patient should be encouraged to talk freely without interruption. Specific leading questions should be asked. Many patients cannot give a good history and it will be necessary to prod their memories with leading questions, or encourage them to be more detailed in describing the illness.

Some questions that will help the patient to give the history are:

"How did your illness start?"
"What was the first symptom you noticed?"
"How long have you had this?"
"How and where does it affect you?"
"What followed?"

Later, more detailed questions may be asked that will help to diagnose the illness. To help decide on other questions to ask, reference may be made to sections of this book, or other medical books available aboard ship. *It's important to be specific about the main symptom or symptoms*, such as pain in the abdomen (See Table 2–1) or severe headache. Time should not be wasted with vague symptoms such as tiredness, weakness, and loss of appetite. These non-specific symptoms are a part of almost every illness. The patient should be asked if ever he had experienced similar symptoms or had the condition or problem before. He should be asked for the diagnosis of any similar situation in the past, the treatment that was prescribed, and the medications he had taken. Also, any medications that the patient is taking now should be noted, because his present illness might be an aggravation or complication of a chronic illness or a reaction to the medication.

Pain

Pain is one of the most common bodily symptoms. These are questions that should be asked:

"How did the pain start?" "What were you doing at the time?"

"Where is the pain located?" (Ask the patient to point to the area of pain so you can be specific in your notes.)

"How severe is the pain?" "Does it make you double up?" "What is the pain like?" (Such as cramping, sharp, dull, or aching.) "Is it constant or intermittent?"

"Does the pain radiate to any other body area?"

"Has it ever moved from one area to another?"

"Is there a way you can bring on the pain or relieve it?"

"Is there anything that makes the pain worse?"

"Do medications help?"

Past Illnesses

Next, the patient should be asked to describe any past illnesses, injuries, or operations. This will help rule out certain conditions. For example, if he has had an appendectomy, then pain in the right lower quadrant of the abdomen can't be acute appendicitis. Or an illness may be a recurrence. If he had been hospitalized in the past for a duodenal ulcer and now comes in with burning mid–upper abdominal pain that is relieved by antacids and milk, then he probably is having pain from a recurrent ulcer. Previous diagnoses should be kept in mind, such as diabetes or high blood pressure; these conditions may get worse during an illness and cause complications. The patient should be asked if he is allergic to any drugs, or if any drugs have made him ill.

REVIEW OF BODY SYSTEMS

When the diagnosis is not obvious or complete and if time permits, a general review of the various body systems and associated symptoms may be helpful. It may help to see that different symptoms relate to one system. For example a patient may have chest pain, shortness of breath when lying in bed, swelling of his legs, and a history of high blood pressure. These symptoms can be found in a cardiac patient so the possibility of heart disease should be considered. However, too much importance should not be placed on just one symptom. For example, shortness of breath can relate to other systems, as the respiratory system (as

Table 2-1. SEVERE ABDOMINAL PAIN

Position and Type of Pain	Associated Symptoms		General Condition of Patient	Associated Signs			Probable Cause of the Pain
	Vomiting	Diarrhea		Temperature	Pulse Rate	Abdominal Tenderness	
All over abdomen, or mainly about navel and lower half; sharp, coming and going in spasms	None	Usually not at first, but sometimes coming on later	Not ill; usually walks about, even if doubled up	Normal	Normal	None; on the contrary, pressure eases the pain	Intestinal colic (see page 148)
In upper part, and under left ribs, a steady burning pain	Present, and usually repeated	Not at first; it may follow 24–48 hours later	Wretched, because of nausea, vomiting and weakness, but soon improving	Usually normal; may be raised up to 100° F (37.8° C) in severe cases	Slightly raised, up to 80-90	Sometimes, but not severe and confined to upper part of abdomen	Acute indigestion (see page 163)
Shooting from loin to groin and testicle; very severe, agonizing spasms	May be present, but only with the spasms	None	Severe distress	Normal, or below normal	Rapid, as with shock	Over the loin	Renal colic (kidney stones) (see page 170)
Shooting from the upper part of the abdomen to the back or right shoulder; agonizing spasms	May be present, but only with the spasms	None	Severe distress	Normal, or below normal	Rapid, as with shock	Just below the right ribs	Gallstones (biliary colic) (see page 162)
Around navel at first, settling later in the lower part of the right side of abdomen; usually continuous and sharp; not always severe	Soon after onset of pain, usually only once or twice	Sometimes once at commencement of attack; thereafter constipation exists	An ill patient—tends to lie still	Normal at first, but always rising later, up to 100° F (37.8° C); it may be raised more	Raised all the time (over 85), and tending to increase in rate hour by hour	Definitely present in the right side of the lower part of the abdomen	Appendicitis (see page 149)
All over the abdomen, usually severe and continuous	Present, becoming more and more frequent	Usually none	An extremely ill patient with wasted appearance, afraid to move because of pain	Present up to 103° F (39.4° C) or more, except in final stage near death	Rapid (over 110) and feeble	Very tender, usually all over; wall of abdomen tense	Peritonitis (see page 165)
Spasmodic at first, but later continuous	Increasing in frequency and amount of brown fluid	None; complete constipation exists	Very ill	Normal	Rising steadily, feeble	Slightly, all over. Wall of abdomen not hard but distended	Intestinal obstruction (see page 163)
In the groin, a continuous and severe pain	Not at first, but later as with obstruction	None; as with obstruction	Very ill	Normal	Rising steadily, feeble	Over the painful lump in the groin	Strangulated hernia (rupture) (see page 167)
Severe and continuous pain, worst in the upper part of the abdomen	Rare	None	Severe shock at first, then very ill; afraid to move because of the pain	Normal or below normal at first; rising about 24 hours later	Normal at first, rising steadily a few hours later	All over; worst over site of pain. Wall of abdomen hard	Perforated ulcer of stomach (see page 164)

Source: The Ship Captain's Medical Guide. Department of Trade and Industry, Her Majesty's Stationery Office, London, England. Twentieth Edition. Reprinted 1973. p. 171.

in pneumonia), or it can follow a bleeding episode.

The patient should be asked if he *now* has any of the following things to report:

Head—History of wounds (trauma), severe headaches.

Eyes—Blurred vision, double vision, pain, yellow color of the sclera (white part of eye), pain on looking at light.

Ears—Loss of hearing, severe dizziness, pain, or drainage.

Nose—Bleeding, runny, or stuffy.

Mouth—Sores, pain, trouble swallowing.

Neck—Stiffness, enlarged glands, tenderness.

Respiratory—Cough and character of material coughed up, coughing up blood, chest pain when breathing, shortness of breath.

Cardiac—Pain in middle of chest, swelling of both legs, shortness of breath on exercising or when sleeping flat in bed, forceful or rapid heart beat, history of high blood pressure, heart attack, history of rheumatic fever.

Gastrointestinal—Poor appetite, indigestion, nausea, vomiting, diarrhea, constipation, jaundice, pain in stomach, blood in stool or vomitus.

Genitourinary—Pain when urinating, pain in middle of back, frequent urination, straining to urinate, blood or pus in urine, discharge from penis.

Neurological—Paralysis or severe weakness of a part of the body (an arm or legs), convulsion, or seizure.

Family and Social History—The patient should be asked if diabetes, tuberculosis, heart disease, cancer, or other diseases ever appeared in other members of his family. These now may be appearing in the patient. Also ask about the amount of alcohol and tobacco the patient uses. The date of his last drink should be noted if chronic alcoholism is suspected, because delirium tremens may start five to seven days after a patient stops drinking.

Endocrine Disorders—Weight change, unusual hunger, unusual thirst, bulging eyes, intolerance to heat or cold.

PHYSICAL EXAMINATION

This is the second basic part in the evaluation of the patient. By this time, some observations of the patient will have been made, such as speech, general appearance, and mental status. Now, another system of collecting information must be used, wherein definitive signs of disease must be observed. Check the corresponding parts of the patient's body. For example, compare his right eye with the left eye, right arm with the left arm, and the right side of the chest with the left side.

To do a basic examination, a clock or watch with a second hand, blood pressure apparatus, stethoscope, thermometer, and a quiet room will be needed.

Vital Signs

• What is the blood pressure? Does it drop 15 mm or more when the patient stands for 3 minutes?

• What is the pulse rate per minute? Is it regular? Does it increase 15 beats or more per minute when the patient stands 3 minutes?

• What is the respiratory rate per minute?

• What is the patient's temperature?

General Appearance

• Note the position of the patient's body and his facial expression.

• Is he tense, restless, or in any unusual posture? Note his general ability to move and respond.

Skin

• Note location of rashes or sores.

• Is the rash red, made up of small or large spots? Are the spots separated, or do they run together? Do they itch? Are they elevated or flat?

• Is the skin hot and dry, or cold and wet?

• What is the color of the skin? Is there evidence of jaundice (yellowness)?

• Are his lips and nailbeds a dusky blue color, or are they pale and white?

Head

• Is there evidence of trauma, such as a cut, bruise, or swelling?

Eyes

- The patient should be asked if he can see. Each eye should be tested independently by having him identify certain objects or numbers.

- Is there evidence of jaundice or inflammation in the sclera (white part of the eye)? (Check for jaundice in the sunlight, if possible; in many normal people, there is a slight yellow cast of the sclerae in artificial light.)

- Can he move both eyes together up and down, and to each side? Is there an abnormal twitching to the eyes in any position?

- Are the pupils the same size? Do they get smaller when a light is shined into the eyes?

Ears

- Check for blood in the ear canal, especially if a blow to the head is known or suspected.

- Check his ability to hear by having him listen for ticking of a watch held at about the same distance from each ear. If the examiner's hearing is normal, he may compare his hearing with that of the patient.

Nose

- Look for bleeding or abnormal discharge.

Mouth and Throat

- Are the gums swollen or extremely red?

- Are the color and movement of the tongue unusual?

- Does the throat have abnormal redness, swelling or ulcerated patches?

- Observe the patient swallow. Does he have difficulty swallowing?

- Note any abnormal odor to the breath.

Neck

- The patient should be asked to lie down and the examiner's hands placed behind his head. When he is relaxed, the head should be lifted gently, bending the neck so that his chin will touch his chest. Observe for (1) an unnatural stiffness of the neck or (2) discomfort when the legs are lifted from the table with the knees straight.

- Check for any enlarged glands on the side of his neck. Note if they are tender, movable, soft, or hard.

Chest

- The patient's breathing should be observed. Note if it is painful, and if both sides of the chest move together.

- Note if he has to sit up to breathe.

- The hand should be placed flat on different parts of his chest to check for abnormal vibrations or tenderness.

- A stethoscope should be used to listen to all areas in the front and back, and compare each side. Normally, when a patient breathes, the air can be heard moving in and out, sounding like wind blowing through trees. Listen for wheezes, bubbling, or other sounds that are abnormal.

Abdomen

- Look at the contour. Is it symmetrical?

- Ask about any scars. They may indicate previous surgery and rule out certain diseases of the gallbladder or appendix, if these organs have been removed.

- Feel the abdomen noting tender areas or masses. Is the abdomen soft or rigid?

- If any organs such as the liver can be felt, note if they are tender, firm or soft. (Any time the examiner causes pain during an examination, he should ask the patient if this duplicates pain that has been described previously in the history.)

- Listen to the abdomen with the stethoscope. Low gurgling sounds should be heard about every 30 seconds. (They may be loud enough to hear without a stethoscope, as when one's stomach "growls." It is important to determine if this occurs almost constantly or not at all.)

Genitalia

- Check for sores, as in syphilis, being careful not to touch any sores.

- Is there any discharge from the penis?

- Check the testicles for swelling and tenderness.

- Check the groin for swollen glands and for hernia (rupture).

Rectum and Anus

- Look for hemorrhoids, which are usually swollen, blue, and often painful.

• Note if there is any blood around the anus.

Arms and Legs

• Check for movement and strength of all parts. Is there any weakness or paralysis? (If the patient is unable to move his leg, for example, find out if it is due to pain; or if it truly is paralysis, which usually causes no pain.) Is the grip stronger with one hand than the other?

• Check for swelling and for tenderness. Is it one leg or arm, or both?

Back

• Is there tenderness or deformity?
• The kidney area should be tapped gently with the fist to check for tenderness. This area lies in the back on either side of the spine and between the top of the pelvic bone and last rib.

Nervous System

• Does he show abnormal concern about his illness?

• Note general mental status. Is he rational? Is his behavior abnormal? Can he remember today's date and do simple arithmetic?

• Are his coordination and gait normal? As a test, have the patient take a few steps and pick up with each hand an object from a table or chair. If the patient is too ill to walk, note how he moves, turns over, and picks up objects in bed.

SYMPTOMS AND SIGNS

The preceding section of this chapter described how to obtain useful information on a patient. The approach included questions about symptoms, things that the patient feels and describes, plus an examination of the patient for signs or things that can be seen without relying on the patient's cooperation. The examiner's observation of the patient should begin at the head and proceed systematically to the feet.

After the examiner has obtained all the information, it must be sorted and rearranged in different ways in order for it to make sense. Related things must be brought together. A recommended way to organize the information when asking for medical advice by radio is described in Chapter XII. (See the outline, p. 386+.)

In general, information should be organized as it relates to body systems. From the signs and symptoms gathered, try to decide what body system(s) might be involved. Do the signs and symptoms suggest involvement of the digestive system, the excretory system, the circulatory system, or others? If possible, relate the signs and symptoms to one system. For example, pallor of the hands or feet is related to circulation—not to muscles or skeleton. So with pallor present, concern should be given primarily to blood pressure, heart rate, signs of bleeding, or evidence of injury to an artery, instead of signs of arthritis or skin rashes.

MAKING CONCLUSIONS

One way to approach the problem of diagnosis is to write down the main complaints, note the body systems that might be involved, and ask more detailed questions about these symptoms. The physical examination may be performed, again noting the body systems affected by the abnormal findings. If necessary, ask further questions or reexamine areas that will help to clarify the findings. Often by a process of elimination, the problem will be reduced to a few possible diagnoses. Next, turn to the chapters of this book that describe the diseases or conditions possibly involved, and decide which one comes closest to explaining all the signs and symptoms. The material in the chapters might suggest other special tests or additional questions that should be asked.

At this point, if a definitive diagnosis cannot be made, knowledge of the case will be sufficient for presentation by radio to a physician. Also, it will be easier to follow the course of the disease as it progresses. Some parts of the physical examination will have to be repeated daily. Changes that are observed in the patient should be recorded.

Body discharges, such as vomitus, feces, sputum, and urine should be examined carefully to note abnormal color, consistency, and above all the presence of blood. Blood in the feces may be bright red, dark brown, or have the color of tar. Blood in the urine is usually red in color; but the urine may have to settle for several hours before blood can be seen. If the patient appears jaundiced, his urine usually will have a dark yellow color. To confirm a jaundiced condition, the urine should be put into a small bottle and shaked vigorously. In jaundice the foam will have a yellow color; normally the color of the foam is white. This can be compared to a normal urine specimen. The volume of vomitus, diarrhea, and urine output should be measured and recorded.

Two important final points: *First,* when in doubt always compare the physical findings on a patient to those of a normal person; or compare corresponding left and right parts, as the eyes or ears in the same patient. *Second,* continue to observe and recheck the patient for things that may have been missed. Avoid a quick decision or diagnosis! Snap decisions might be wrong and the illness could be prolonged.

DIAGNOSING THE UNCONSCIOUS PATIENT

Signs and symptoms of several causes of unconsciousness are shown in Table 2–2. Although the specific cause of the unconsciousness may not be known at once, an orderly diagnostic routine is urgent. Immediate findings may call for first aid measures. Some general rules follow:

1. Breathing and bleeding are top priorities. First, make sure that the airway is open; if there is no breathing, begin artificial respiration at once. Make a quick overall check for serious bleeding; if found, it must be stopped.

2. Unless the patient is lying in a dangerous spot, do not move him until first aid is completed.

3. Remove spectacles or dentures and loosen tight clothing around neck, chest, and abdomen.

4. Look into the patient's wallet for a *card,* or elsewhere on his person for a *metal tag or bracelet* that shows the *Emergency Medical Identification Symbol.* The symbol identifies people with special medical problems that might be neglected in an emergency or aggravated by usual emergency treatment. (See p. 46 for additional information.)

5. If the patient is breathing, lay him on one side so vomitus will run out of the mouth and the tongue will be kept from falling back into the throat to choke him.

6. If breathing seems difficult, extend the head by pushing the jaw forward with fingers pressing behind the angle of the jaw. This will keep the tongue from falling back into the throat.

7. Put blankets or coats over and under the patient to keep him warm.

8. Give nothing by mouth until the patient regains consciousness.

9. Never give morphine sulfate; an unconscious patient does not feel pain.

10. Keep him under continuous observation, noting color of face and rates of pulse and respiration. If the face is pale, the head should be on the deck. If the face is flushed, use a pillow, rolled clothing, or towels underneath head and shoulder to raise these a few inches.

11. If the patient is restless, restrain gently any movements that might be injurious—but do not use force.

12. As consciousness returns, treat for shock (see p. 57).

13. Question observers of the incident that caused the unconsciousness before taking a history or making a more detailed examination.

14. Get medical advice by radio. When a specific diagnosis is made, refer elsewhere in the text for further treatment. (Also refer to Chapter III for more detail on the emergency treatment of injuries.)

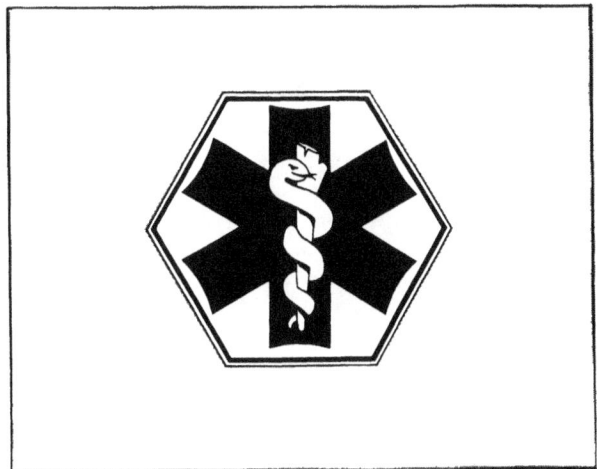

Emergency Medical Identification Symbol.

Table 2-2. **DIAGNOSING**

	1 Fainting	2 Concussion	3 Brain compression	4 Epilepsy	5 Apoplexy (stroke)	6 Alcohol	7 Opium and morphine
Onset	Usually sudden	Sudden	Usually gradual	Sudden	Sudden as a rule	Gradual	Gradual
Mental condition	Complete unconsciousness	Unconsciousness but sometimes confusion only	Unconsciousness deepening	Complete unconsciousness	Complete or partial unconsciousness	Stupor, later unconsciousness	Unconsciousness deepening
Pulse	Feeble and fast	Feeble and irregular	Gradually slower	Fast	Slow and full	Full and fast, later fast and feeble	Feeble and slow
Respiration	Quick and shallow	Shallow and irregular	Slow and noisy	Noisy, later deep and slow	Slow and noisy	Deep, slow, and noisy	Slow, may be deep
Skin	Pale, cold, and clammy	Pale and cold	Hot and flushed	Livid, later pale	Hot and flushed	Flushed, later cold and clammy	Pale, cold, and clammy
Pupils	Equal and dilated	Equal	Unequal	Equal and dilated	Unequal	Dilated, later may contract. Eyes bloodshot	Equal, very contracted
Paralysis	None	None	Present (of leg or arm)	None	Present in leg, arm, or face or all three, on one side	None	None
Convulsions	None	None	Present in some cases	Present	Present in some cases	None	None
Breath	—	—	—	—	—	Smells of alcohol	With opium, musty smell
Special points	Often giddiness and swaying before collapse	Often signs of head injury. Vomiting on recovery	Often signs of head injury. Remember delayed onset of symptoms	Tongue often bitten. Urine or feces may be voided. Sometimes injury in falling	Over middle age. Eyes may look to one side. Sometimes loss of speech	Absence of the smell of alcohol excludes it as cause, but its presence does not prove that alcohol is the cause	Look for source of supply

*Source: **International Medical Guide For Ships**. World Health Organization, Geneva, Switzerland. 1967. pp. 84-85.*

THE UNCONSCIOUS PATIENT

8 Barbiturate (sedative tablets)	9 Uremic coma	10 Sunstroke and heat-stroke	11 Electric shock	12 Cyanide (prussic acid)	13 Diabetic coma	14 Shock	
Gradual	Gradual	Gradual or sudden	Sudden	Very rapid	Gradual	Gradual	**Onset**
Stupor, later deepening unconsciousness	Very drowsy, later unconsciousness	Delirium or unconsciousness	Unconsciousness	Confusion, later unconsciousness	Drowsiness, later unconsciousness	Listlessness, later unconsciousness	**Mental condition**
Feeble and fast	Full	Fast and feeble	Fast and feeble	Fast and feeble, later stops	Fast and feeble	Fast and very feeble	**Pulse**
Slow, noisy, and irregular	Noisy and difficult	Difficult	Shallow and may cease	Slow, gasping, and spasmodic	Deep and sighing	Rapid and shallow with occasional deep sigh	**Respiration**
Cold and clammy	Shallow, cold, and dry	Very hot and dry	Pale, may be burnt	Cold	Livid, later pale	Pale, cold, and clammy	**Skin**
Equal, somewhat contracted	Equal and contracted	Equal	Eyes may squint	Equal, staring eyes	Equal	Equal, dilated	**Pupils**
None	None	None	May be present	None	None	None	**Paralysis**
None	Present in some cases	Present in some cases	Present in some cases	Present	None	None	**Convulsions**
—	Sometimes smells of urine	—	—	Smells of bitter almonds	Smells of acetone	—	**Breath**
Look for source of supply	Vomiting in some cases	Vomiting in some cases	Muscular spasm often causes tight gripping of the electrified object	Rapid deterioration. Breathing may stop	In early stages, headache restlessness, and nausea. Test urine for sugar	May vomit. In early stages shivering, thirst, defective vision, and ear noises	**Special points**

Why You Should Carry Emergency Medical Identification

An emergency medical identification card is your protection in an emergency. If you are not able to tell your medical story after an accident or sudden illness, the information entered on this card can save your life.

You may have health problems which can affect your recovery from an emergency. You may have a problem which is no emergency but often is treated as one, such as epilepsy. Even if you do not have a health problem, the information on this card can be of valuable assistance to the first aid and attendant.

Why You Should Wear an Emergency Medical Signal Device

In an emergency, you may be separated from your pocket card. Possibly you are one who has a medical problem so critical that it must be immediately known to those who help you. If so, a signal device of durable material should be worn around your neck, wrist, or ankle in such a way that it can be present at all times—even while swimming.

The device should be fastened to the person wearing it with a strong nonelastic cord or chain so designed that it does not become an accident hazard in itself.

On this device there should be

• The universal symbol of emergency medical identification
• The name of your major health problem
• For children and the aging, the name and address of a responsible relative and a telephone number, including area code

Carry Your Card and Wear Your Signal Device at All Times!

EMERGENCY MEDICAL IDENTIFICATION

Reprinted by permission of the
AMERICAN MEDICAL ASSOCIATION
U S DEPARTMENT OF HEALTH
EDUCATION AND WELFARE
Public Health Service

ATTENTION

In an emergency where I am unconscious or unable to communicate, please read the other side to know the special care I must have

PERSONAL IDENTIFICATION

Name _____
Address _____
Religion _____

NOTIFY IN EMERGENCY

Name _____
Address _____
Phone _____

Name _____
Address _____
Phone _____

My Doctor is _____
Address _____
Phone _____

Detach card here

MEDICAL INFORMATION
(with date of notation)

Present Medical Problems _____

Medicines Taken Regularly _____

Dangerous Allergies _____

Other Important Information _____

Last Immunization Date

Tetanus Toxoid _____   Polio   Salk _____
Diptheria _____   Sabin _____
Smallpox _____   Typhoid _____
Measles _____   Others _____

REMEMBER This is the minimum medical and personal information needed by those who help you in an emergency. It is not designed to be a complete medical record. Check its accuracy with your doctor

---

To put your EMERGENCY MEDICAL IDENTIFICATION CARD to work for you, fill in both sides of this card. For example, under

Present Medical Problems, include
Epilepsy   Tracheotomy (neck breather)
Diabetes   Pneumothorax
Glaucoma   Pneumoperitoneum
Hemophilia   Colostomy
Chorea

Medicines Taken Regularly
Anticoagulants   When noting drugs, ask your
Cortisone or ACTH   doctor for the name to use that
Heart drugs such as   will be easy to identify in an emer-
  digitalis or nitrites   gency.
Thyroid preparation

Dangerous Allergies
Drug allergies   Feathers (pillows)
Horse serum (as in   Common foods
  tetanus antitoxin)   Penicillin sensitivity

Other Information
Scuba diver   Speak no English (note the
Recurring unconsciousness   language you speak)
Hard of hearing   Wearing contact lenses

Immunizations
The date is important. If you note immunization over three years old, ask your doctor about a booster immunization. For tetanus toxoid, note the date of your first immunization as well as your last

Reprinted by permission of the AMERICAN MEDICAL ASSOCIATION
U S DEPARTMENT OF HEALTH EDUCATION AND WELFARE
Public Health Service

Copr ght AMERICAN MEDICAL ASSOCIATION 1965

Detach card here

Fig. 2–1. Emergency medical identification (EMI) card.

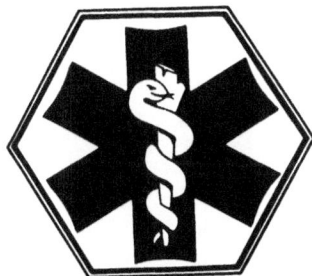

Emergency Medical Identification Symbol

Stop! Look before you treat. This is the message of the *Emergency Medical Identification (EMI) symbol* that is worn or carried by many people. The American Medical Association designed the symbol to identify people who have medical problems that might be neglected in an emergency or aggravated by usual emergency treatment.

Learn to recognize the symbol. It may save a life or lessen disability. Worn as a bracelet, necklace, or anklet, the symbol means that the person has special health needs that must not be ignored if he is injured or suddenly taken ill. A card in pocket, wallet, or purse will explain the patient's special needs. Everyone with special medical problems, or who takes medicines regularly, or has dangerous allergies, or who requires special medical attention of any kind—such as the hard-of-hearing, heart patients, contact lens wearers, epileptics, diabetics, or non-English speakers—should wear the *Emergency Medical Identification* symbol, or carry an *Emergency Medical Identification* card.

EMI Cards and Emblems

Pocket or wallet cards are available from the American Medical Association or some voluntary health agencies that deal with special health problems. (See sample card on previous page.) Bracelets and necklaces may be obtained from several sources including the Medic Alert Foundation, Turlock, California 95380.

For information about the symbol and its uses, contact the

American Medical Association
535 North Dearborn Street
Chicago, Illinois 60601.

Chapter III

Emergency Treatment of Injuries

Section A
INTRODUCTION

FIRST AID IS THE EMERGENCY TREATMENT given to the ill or injured before professional medical services can be obtained. It is given to prevent further injury or death, to counteract shock, and to relieve pain. Certain conditions, such as severe bleeding or asphyxiation, require *immediate* treatment if the patient is to survive. In such cases, seconds might mean the difference between life and death. However, the treatment of most injuries or other medical emergencies may be postponed safely for the few minutes required to locate a crew member skilled in first aid, or to locate suitable medical supplies and equipment.

All crew members should be prepared to administer first aid. They should have sufficient knowledge of first aid to be able to apply true emergency measures and decide when treatment can be delayed safely until more skilled personnel arrive. Limitations must be recognized. Procedures and techniques beyond the rescuer's ability should *not* be attempted. More harm than good might result.

The person responsible for administering first aid should think and act carefully, and not become unduly excited or emotionally upset. Unnecessary haste and the appearance of uncertainty or confusion should be avoided.

First aid must be administered *immediately* to:

- Restore breathing
- Control bleeding
- Remove poisons
- Prevent further injury to the patient, such as his removal from a room containing carbon monoxide or smoke.

A rapid, emergency evaluation of the patient should be made immediately at the scene of the injury to determine the type and extent of the trauma. Because seconds may count, only the essential pieces of the patient's clothing should be removed. The rescuer must be prepared to observe, speak to the patient, and act *all at once*.

The patient's pulse should be taken. If it cannot be felt at the wrist, it should be felt at the carotid artery at the side of the neck. If there is no pulse, cardiopulmonary resuscitation must be started (see p. 115). The patient should be treated for shock if the pulse is weak and rapid, or the skin pale, cold, and possibly moist, with an increased rate of shallow, irregular breathing. The patient should be kept in the best position that provides relief from his

49

injuries. Usually this is lying down, which increases circulation of the blood to the head. The patient should *not* be moved if injuries of the neck or spine are suspected. The patient should be covered to prevent loss of body heat.

The patient should be observed for the type of breathing and possible bleeding. If not breathing, mouth-to-mouth ventilation or mouth-to-nose ventilation must be given (see p. 117+). The opening of a sucking wound of the chest must be closed (see p. 95) to prevent air from flowing in and out of the chest cavity as the patient breathes. The fractured ribs of a flail chest should be splinted (see p. 88) because the chest wall between the breaks will collapse instead of expanding when the patient tries to inhale. Severe bleeding *must* be controlled.

During this time, the patient if conscious should be reassured and told that all possible help is being given. The rescuer should ask about the location of any painful areas. Also, talking with the patient will help the rescuer to determine the state of consciousness and any reaction to the injury. There may be the presence or absence of consciousness, mental dullness or confusion, anxiety or fear, overactivity or excitement, and complaints of abnormal sensation.

Once lifesaving measures have been started or deemed not necessary, the patient should be examined more thoroughly for other injuries.

If necessary, additional clothing of the patient may be removed, including constricting articles such as belts. The patient should be kept in a lying-down position and moved only when absolutely necessary. The general appearance of the patient should be observed, including any signs and symptoms which may indicate a specific injury or illness. Signs of a head injury should be sought, and the eyes examined for a reaction of the pupils to light. Deformities and wounds indicating a fracture are important. The patient should be asked about any lack of motion, tenderness, or pain. *Fractures should be splinted before moving a patient (see p. 81+).* No attempt should be made to set the fracture.

The rescuer should ask if the patient can move either the arms or legs. If neither arms nor legs can be moved, the neck probably has been injured. The spine probably is injured if the arms can be moved, but not the legs. *When these conditions are present, a spine board must be used to move the patient (see p. 85).* Any loss of sensation is serious and should be treated as a spinal cord injury.

Wounds and most burns should be covered to prevent infection. The treatment of specific injuries will be discussed more fully in the rest of this chapter.

Always remember that the rescuer will be expected to provide assistance to the patient, until the patient is placed in the care of qualified medical personnel.

Chapter III

Emergency Treatment of Injuries

Section B
WOUNDS

A WOUND IS AN INJURY caused by external physical forces. An *open wound* is one where the skin or mucous membranes have been broken. A *closed wound* occurs when underlying tissues are involved and the skin and mucous membranes are intact. In wounds there is an immediate risk of hemorrhage, after which the greatest danger is infection. Thus disinfection of the wound should follow first aid procedures. Other concerns will be shock, nerve injury, and the extent of tissue destruction.

from bacteria usually ground into the wound with dirt, grease, and other foreign matter.

TYPES OF WOUNDS

Abrasions

An abrasion is an open wound that is caused by rubbing or scraping the skin. (See Fig. 3–1.) The wound may be quite painful when large areas of skin are scraped off. An abrasion usually is not very deep and bleeding is limited to an oozing from damaged capillaries and small veins. There is a danger of infection

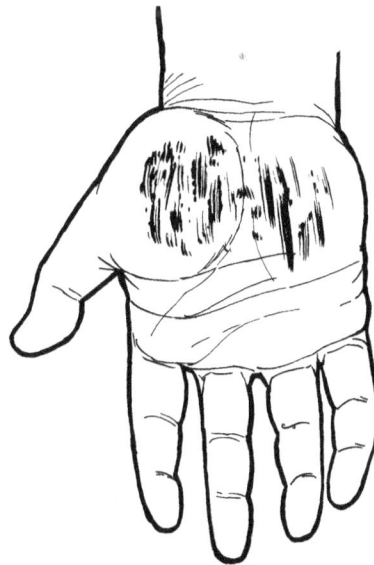

Fig. 3–1. Abrasion.

Avulsions

An avulsion is an open wound that may be caused by explosions, accidents from vehicles, heavy machinery, and animal bites. (See Fig. 3–2.) Tissue is separated forcibly or torn with loss of skin and soft tissue. Heavy bleeding usually follows immediately.

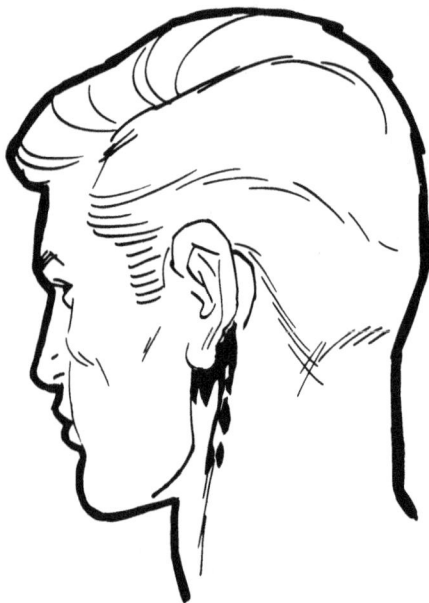

Fig. 3–2. Avulsion.

Contusions (Bruises, Blood Blisters)

A contusion is a closed, superficial wound usually caused by a blow from a blunt object, a bump against a stationary object, or a crush. Blood seeping into soft tissues from injured vessels and capillaries causes swelling and pain that may be severe at the site of the injury. If the injury is over a bone, the possibility of a fracture should be kept in mind.

Incisions

An incision is an open wound caused by sharp objects as knives, broken glass, and sharp metal edges. (See Fig. 3–3.) The wound is smooth-edged and bleeds freely. The amount of bleeding depends upon the depth, location and size of the wound. There may be severe damage to muscles, nerves, and tendons if the wound is deep.

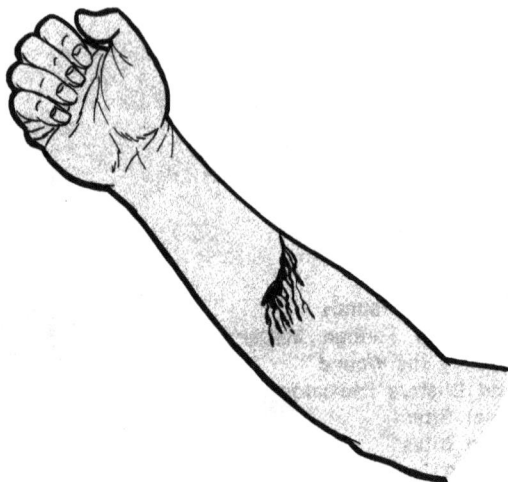

Fig. 3–3. Incision.

Lacerations

A laceration is an open wound caused by objects as dull knives, broken glass, stones, moving parts of machinery, and direct blows. (See Fig. 3–4.) The edges of the wound usually are jagged and irregular, and pieces of tissue may be partly or entirely pulled away. Bleeding may be scant or rapid and extensive. Contamination of the wound with dirt, grease, or other material increases the chance of infection.

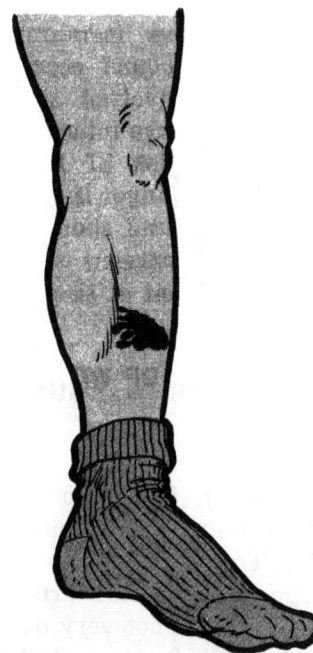

Fig. 3–4. Laceration.

Punctures

A puncture is an open wound caused by such objects as wooden or metal splinters, knives, nails, fishhooks, ice picks, and bullets. (See Fig. 3–5.) Although the opening of a puncture wound may be small with minor external bleeding, the object may penetrate far into the body to cause internal hemorrhage and injure organs. Because the wound is not cleansed by external bleeding, the chance of infection is increased, including possible tetanus (lockjaw) or gas gangrene.

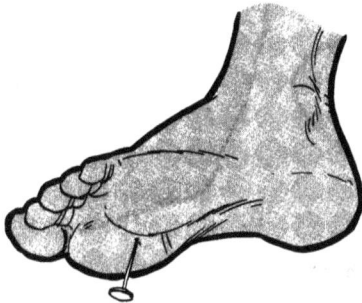

Fig. 3–5. Puncture.

CONTROL OF BLEEDING

The human body contains approximately six quarts of blood. A healthy adult can lose up to one pint of blood without developing harmful effects, but the loss of more than a quart can be life-threatening. Hemorrhage from major blood vessels of the arms, neck, and thighs may occur so rapidly and extensively that death occurs in a few minutes. Hemorrhage must be controlled immediately to prevent excessive loss of blood. In any medical emergency, only the restoration of breathing takes priority over the control of bleeding.

External bleeding may occur following an injury to the outside of the body, or internally from an injury in which blood escapes into tissue spaces or the body cavity.

External bleeding frequently is divided into arterial, venous, or capillary. However, such a classification is of little value because blood may escape at the same time from all three types of vessels when a wound is large. In capillary bleeding, blood and serum ooze to the surface as in an area of scraped skin. Blood from a vein is dark red in color and has a steady flow. Arterial blood is bright red in color and flows from the wound in spurts. In emergencies, the important consideration is the amount of bleeding and how it can be controlled, not its source.

Internal bleeding may occur as a result of a direct blow to the body, strains, sprains, and from diseases as a bleeding ulcer. When vessels are ruptured, blood leaks into tissue spaces and body cavities. Internal bleeding should be suspected in all cases that involve penetrating or crushing injuries of the chest and abdomen.

The signs and symptoms of excessive loss of blood are weakness or actual fainting; dizziness; pale, moist, and clammy skin; nausea; thirst; fast, weak, and irregular pulse; shortness of breath; dilated pupils; ringing in the ears; restlessness; and apprehension. The patient may lose consciousness and stop breathing. The number of symptoms and their severity is generally proportionate to how fast the blood is lost and the amount.

Once the bleeding has been controlled, the patient should be placed in a reclining position, encouraged to lie quietly, and treated for shock. (See p. 57.) *Fluids should not be given by mouth when internal injury is suspected.*

Bleeding may be controlled by direct pressure, elevation, and pressure at pressure points. A tourniquet should be applied *only* when every other method fails to control the excessive bleeding.

Direct Pressure

The simplest and preferred method to control severe bleeding is to place a dressing over the wound and apply pressure directly to the bleeding site with the palm of the hand. (See Fig. 3–6.) Although a sterile dressing should be applied, one may not be available at the time

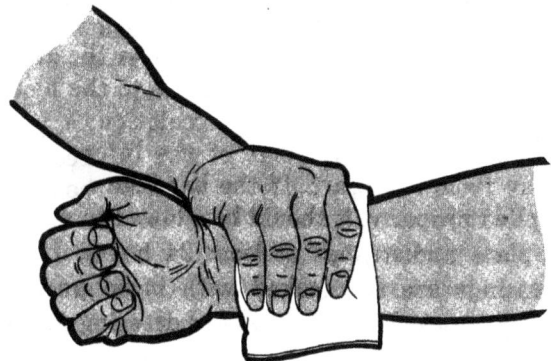

Fig. 3–6. Applying direct pressure to a wound.

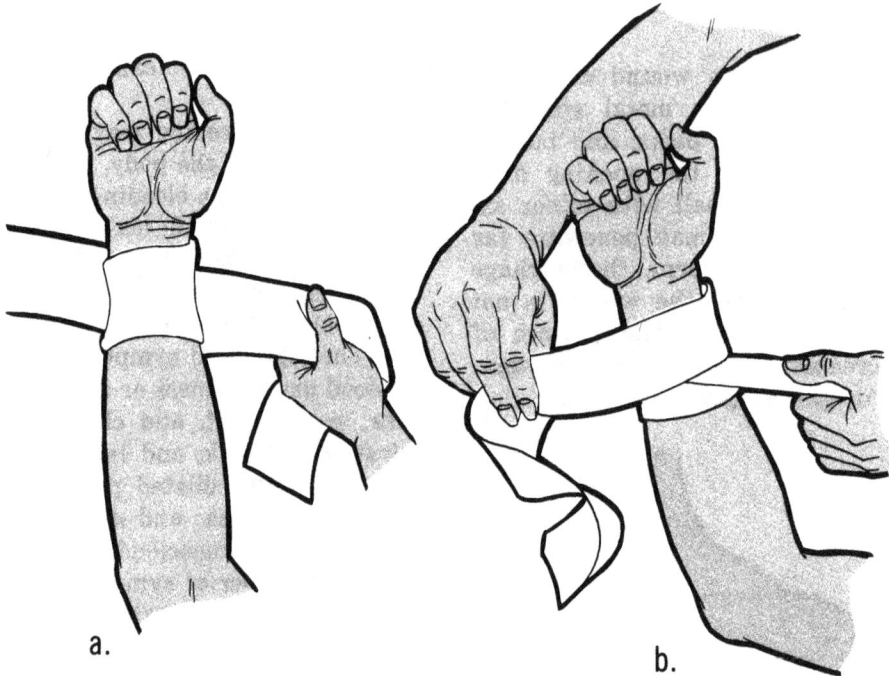

Fig. 3–7. Applying a pressure bandage.

of the emergency; so the cleanest cloth on hand may have to be used. In the absence of a dressing or cloth, the bare hand may be used until a dressing is available. If the dressing becomes soaked with blood, another dressing should be applied over the first one with firmer hand pressure. The initial dressing *never* should be removed because this will disturb the clotting process.

A pressure bandage can be applied over the dressing to hold it in place while additional emergency care is given to the patient. The center of the bandage should be placed directly over the dressing on the wound. A steady pull should be maintained as the ends of the bandage are wrapped around the injured part of the body. (See Fig. 3–7.) Unlike the normal bandaging of wounds or the splinting of fractures, the bandage should be tied over the dressing to provide additional pressure to the bleeding area. Do *not* cut off the circulation. A pulse should be felt on the side of the injured part away from the heart. If the bandage has been applied properly, it should be allowed to remain in place undisturbed at least 24 hours. If the dressings are not soaked with blood and the circulation beyond the pressure dressing is adequate, they need not be changed for several days.

Elevation

When there is a severely bleeding wound of an extremity or the head, direct pressure should be applied on a dressing over the wound with the part elevated. The force of gravity then lowers the blood pressure in the affected part and the flow of blood is lessened.

Pressure Points

When direct pressure and elevation cannot control severe bleeding, pressure should be applied to the artery that supplies the area. Because this technique reduces the circulation to the wounded part below the pressure point site, it should be applied only when absolutely necessary and only until the severe bleeding has lessened. There are a large number of pressure point sites where the fingers may be applied to help control bleeding. (See Fig. 3–8.) However, the brachial artery in the upper arm and femoral artery in the groin are the most effective pressure points.

The pressure point for the brachial artery is located midway between the elbow and the armpit on the inner arm between the large muscles. To apply pressure, one hand should be around the patient's arm with the thumb on the outside of the arm and the fingers on the inside. Pressure is applied by moving the

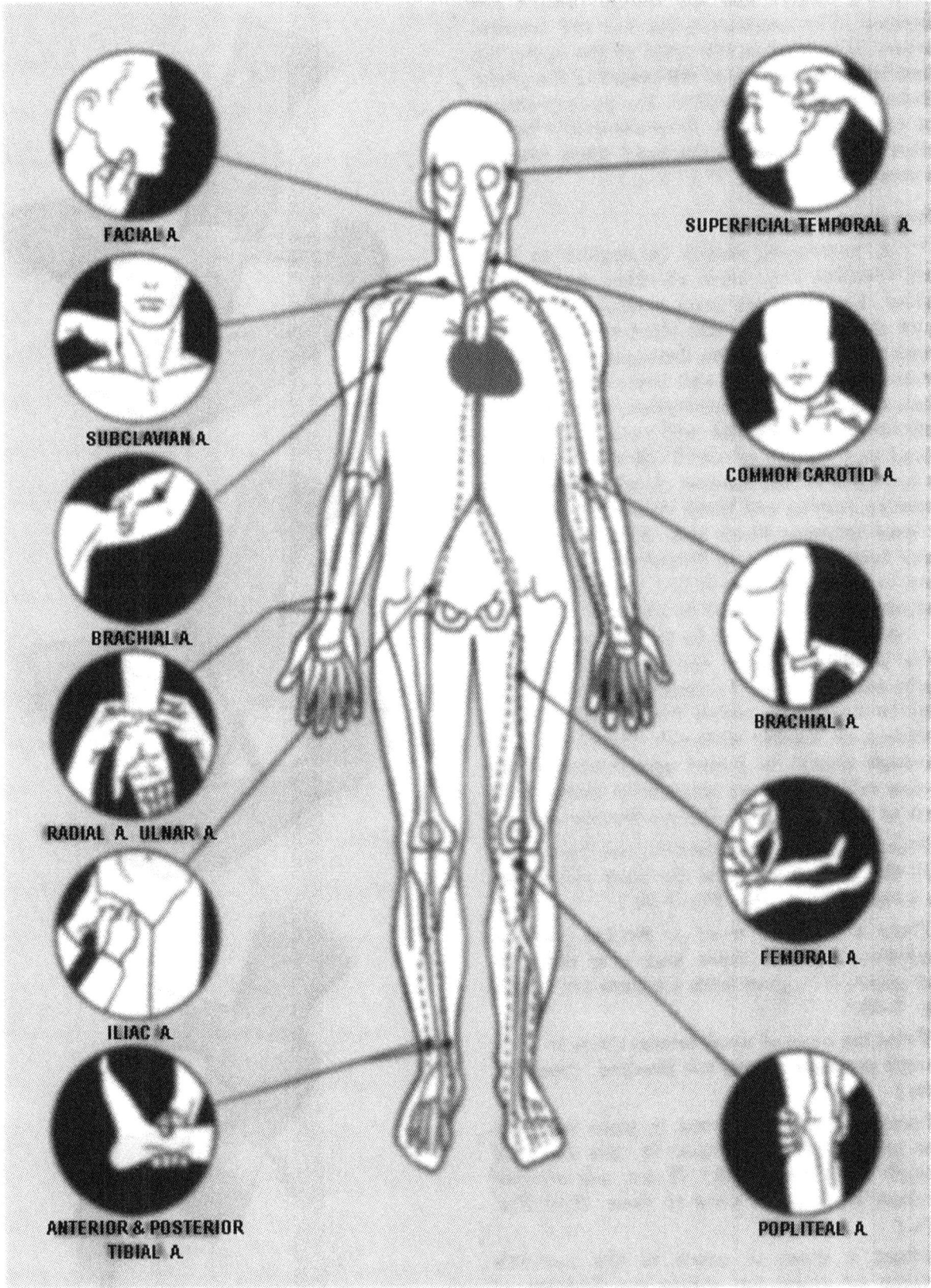

Fig. 3–8. Pressure points (arteries).

flattened fingers and the thumb toward one another. The pressure point for the femoral artery is located on the front of the upper leg just below the middle of the crease of the groin. Before pressure is applied, the patient should be turned on his back. Pressure should be applied with the heel of the hand while keeping a straightened arm.

Tourniquet

A tourniquet should be applied to control bleeding *only* when all other means have failed. Unlike direct hand pressure, a tourniquet shuts off all normal blood circulation beyond the application site. Damage to the tissues from a lack of oxygen and blood may result in limb destruction or amputation. Releasing the tourniquet periodically will result in loss of blood and danger of shock. If the tourniquet is too tight or too narrow, it will damage the muscles, nerves, and blood vessels; if too loose, it may increase blood loss. Also, tourniquets have been applied and forgotten. *If a tourniquet is applied to save a life, immediate medical advice by radio must be obtained.*

A tourniquet must be improvised from a *wide* band of cloth or one prepared commercially may be used. An improvised tourniquet may be made from folded triangular bandages, clothing, or similar material. The clothing or bandage should be folded approximately two inches wide and long enough to encircle the limb at least twice. To apply a tourniquet:

• Place the tourniquet slightly above the wound, fold the material around the limb twice, and tie a simple knot. (See Fig. 3–9a.)

• Place a piece of wood or similar material approximately six inches long over the knot and secure it in place with a square knot. (See Fig. 3–9b.)

• Twist the piece of wood several times to exert enough pressure to stop the bleeding. (See Fig. 3–9c.)

• Secure the piece of wood in place with the free ends of the tourniquet if they are long enough. (See Fig. 3–9d.) If not, use another bandage to hold the wood in place. (See Fig. 3–9e.)

• Attach a sheet of paper to the patient's clothing or extremity, giving the location of the tourniquet and the time that it was applied.

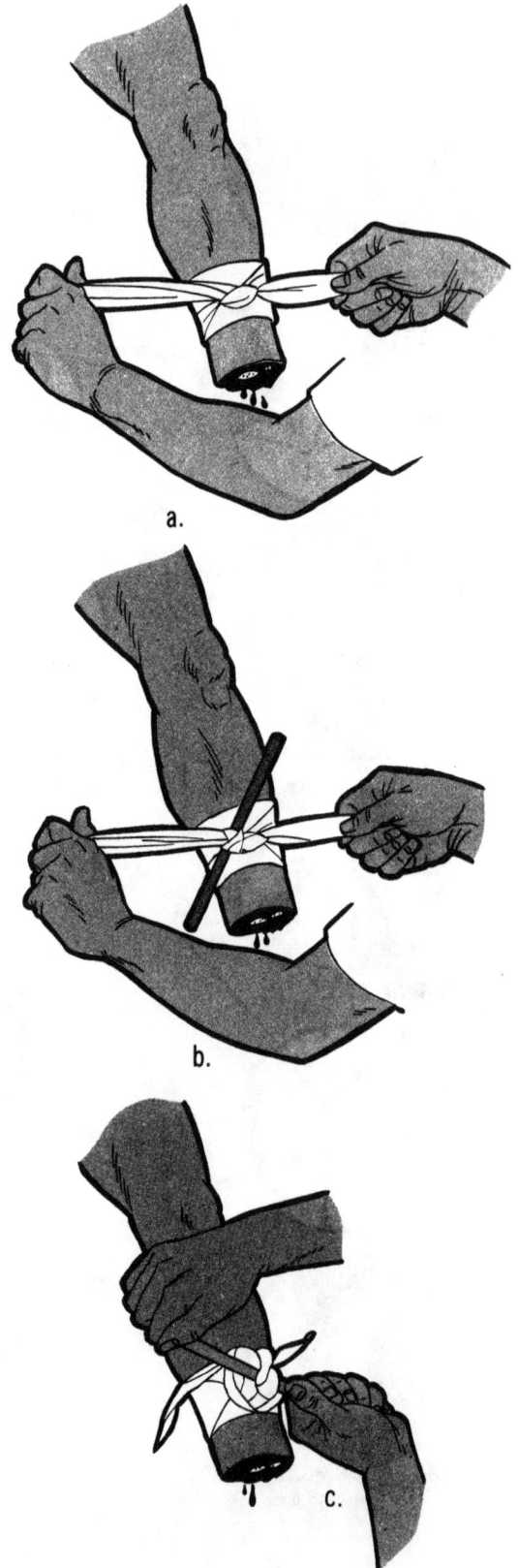

Fig. 3–9. Applying a tourniquet.

d.

e.

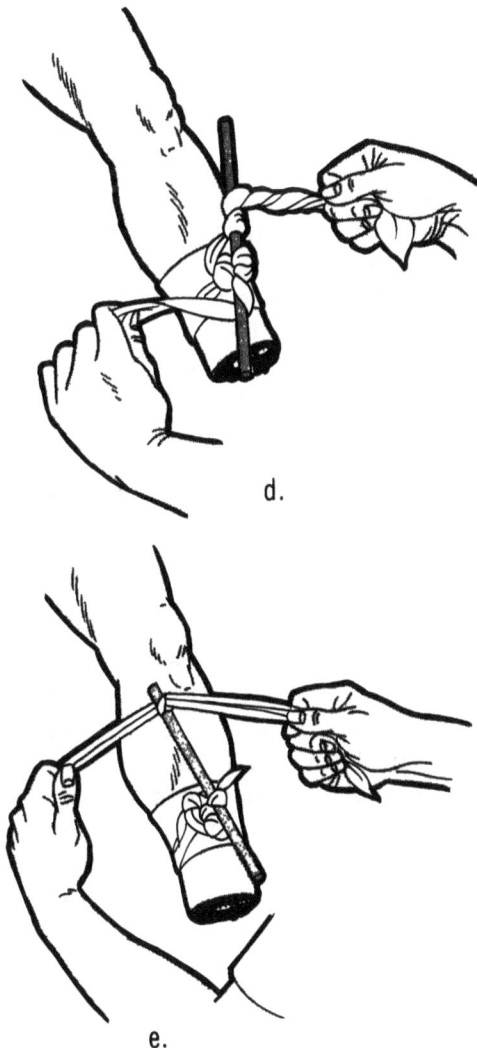

Fig. 3–9. (Continued)..Applying a tourniquet.

• *Never* cover the tourniquet with clothing, bandages, or hide it in any way.

• *Never* loosen the tourniquet, unless a physician advises it.

SHOCK

Shock following an injury is the result of a decrease in the vital functions of the various organs of the body. These functions are depressed because of inadequate circulation of blood or an oxygen deficiency. Injury-related (traumatic) shock differs from other forms, as insulin shock and electric shock, which are discussed in other sections of this book.

Shock usually follows severe injuries as extensive burns, major crushing injuries particularly of the chest and abdomen, fractures of large bones, and other extensive or extremely painful injuries. Shock follows the loss of large quantities of blood; allergic reactions; poisoning from drugs, gases, and other chemicals; alcohol intoxication and the rupture of a stomach ulcer. It also may be associated with many severe illnesses as infections, strokes, and heart attacks.

In some individuals the emotional response to trivial injuries or even to the mere sight of blood is so great that the person feels weak, nauseated, and may faint. This reaction may be considered to be an extremely mild form of shock which is not serious and will disappear quickly if the patient lies down. The signs and symptoms of the more severe degrees of shock are quite similar to those of the extremely mild form. Severe shock, however, tends to become progressively worse, does not respond readily to treatment, and seriously threatens the life of the patient.

Signs and Symptoms of Shock are:

Paleness. The skin is pale, cold, and often moist. Later it may develop a bluish, ashen color. When the patient has dark skin, the color of mucous membranes and nail beds should be examined.

Rapid and shallow respirations. The breathing possibly could be irregular and deep.

Thirst, nausea, and vomiting. These frequently occur in a hemorrhaging patient in shock.

Weak and rapid pulse. Usually the pulse rate is over 100.

Restlessness, excitement, and anxiety. These occur early, later change to mental dullness, and still later to unconsciousness. In this late stage the pupils are dilated, giving the patient a vacant, glassy stare.

Although symptoms of shock may not be evident, all seriously injured persons should be treated for it to prevent its possible development.

Treatment for Shock:

• *Eliminate the causes of shock.* This includes control of bleeding, restoration of breathing, and relief of severe pain.

• *Have the injured person lie down.* The patient should be placed in a horizontal position and covered with a blanket only heavy enough to maintain normal body temperature. However, when there is a neck or back injury, the patient should *not* be moved until he is prepared for safe transportation. Further injury must be prevented. A patient with a head injury should be positioned with the head at the same level or higher than the body. An unconscious person or one with facial injuries should be placed on the side to allow for the drainage of fluids from mouth and nose.

The patient's legs may be elevated approximately 12 inches to assist the flow of blood to the heart and head. The legs should not be elevated if there is a head or chest injury, or difficulty in breathing.

• *Keep the patient warm, but not hot.* Too much heat raises the surface temperature of the body and causes the blood supply to leave vital organs and move to the skin.

• *Relieve pain as quickly as possible.* If pain is severe, morphine sulfate 10 mg may be given by intramuscular injection. If the blood pressure is low, morphine sulfate should *not* be given because it may cause an additional drop in the pressure. Also, it should not be given to injured patients without severe pain. The dosage should be repeated only after medical advice by radio.

• *Administer fluids.* Liquids should not be given by mouth if the patient is unconscious, drowsy, convulsing, or about to have surgery or an anesthetic. Also, fluids should *not* be given if there is a puncture or crush wound to the abdomen or a brain injury. If none of the above conditions is present, lukewarm water containing one teaspoonful of salt and a half teaspoonful of baking soda to each quart of water should be given. One-half glass may be given to an adult every 15 minutes, two ounces to children, and one ounce to infants under a year. Alcohol *never* should be given.

The intravenous administration of fluids is preferable in the treatment of shock if a person trained to administer them is available. (See p. 314.) Lactated Ringer's Injection may be started intravenously.

Medical advice should be obtained by radio.

TREATMENT OF WOUNDS

Removal of Foreign Matter

Wood splinters, glass, wood and metal fragments, clothing threads, dirt, and other foreign matter that remain in a wound should be removed if they are near the surface and visible. Such materials in a wound may not cause discomfort to the patient but may result in bacterial infection if allowed to remain. However, deeply embedded material should *not* be removed for fear of causing additional damage.

A sterile forceps and hemostat may be used to remove foreign matter; also, irrigation of the wound with sterile water is helpful. The tip of a sterile needle can be used to remove small particles of matter.

Large Objects

Large penetrating objects *never* should be removed from the body. Also, the body should not be removed from a fixed object, as a ground stake. Medical advice and assistance needed to remove the object should be obtained immediately. Any movement of an impaled object should be prevented. If it cannot be broken off close to the body, dressings should be placed around the object to immobilize it. Doughnut-shaped dressings are most effective because they fit securely around the object and are less likely to come undone. The dressings should not be added until the object's position is stabilized. Then, a dressing should be placed over the area and a bandage applied to hold the object securely in place. Plans should be made to evacuate the patient to the nearest medical facility as soon as possible.

Fishhooks

A fishhook can be removed easily when only the point and not the barb penetrates the skin. If the barb of the hook enters the skin, it must be pushed until it has penetrated through the skin on the opposite side. Then, the barb should be cut off with a wire cutting instrument and the rest of the hook removed. (See Fig. 3–10.) After the wound has been cleansed, a bandage should be applied. The wound should be observed for any signs of infection and tetanus toxoid given if required. (See p. 292.)

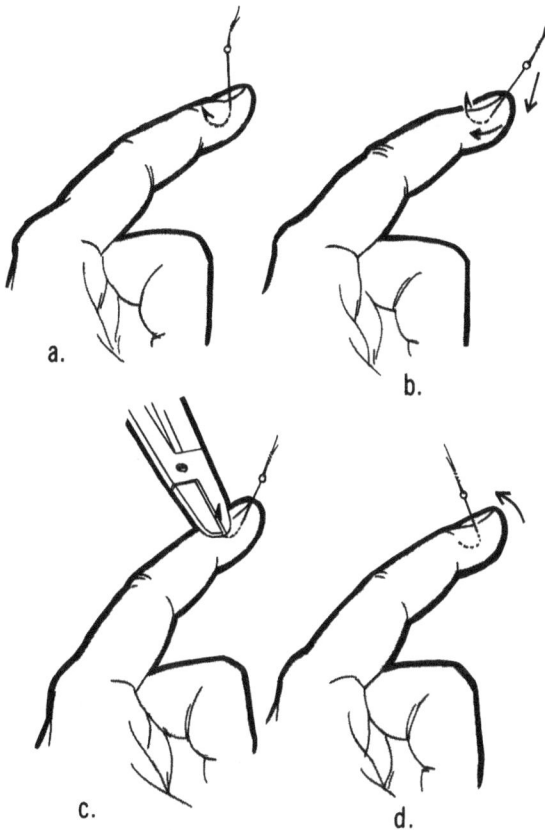

Fig. 3–10. Removing a fishhook from a finger.

Cleansing the Wound

Appropriate measures should be taken to prevent or reduce the chance of a wound infection. However, when a bandage has been applied to control severe bleeding, it *never* should be removed to cleanse a wound because additional bleeding may occur.

Before cleansing any wound, the attendant should wash both hands thoroughly with soap and water. If the wound involves tissue other than skin, it is advisable to put on sterile rubber gloves before proceeding with the treatment.

When the wound involves only the skin and no deeper tissues, it should be washed thoroughly with clean water and blotted dry with a sterile dressing. Povidone-iodine solution may be applied to the wound area. A sterile dressing should be applied over the wound and bandaged securely in place. (See Bandaging, p. 62.)

If wounds of the skin and deeper tissues are not bleeding excessively and are not band-aged to control bleeding, they should be rinsed thoroughly with sterile saline solution. Then, the wound should be blotted dry with a sterile dressing. A sterile dressing should be placed over the site and bandaged securely in place. (See Bandaging, p. 62.)

If the patient is in severe pain, morphine sulfate 10 mg may be given by intramuscular injection and may be repeated every 4 hours upon medical advice by radio. If the wound is severe, medical advice by radio should be obtained and plans made to transfer the patient to the nearest medical facility.

Blood Blisters (Hematomas)

Blood blisters that occur under fingernails and toenails as a result of a blow are very painful. If a hole is made in the nail to allow the blood to escape, the patient will obtain some relief.

Treatment

The patient's hand should be cleansed with soap and water, and povidone-iodine solution applied. The head of a straight pin should be heated until it glows—then carefully pressed through the nail into the center of the blood blister. If this is done carefully, a tiny opening will be made in the nail, and the hot pin will not penetrate into underlying tissues. The hole releases pressure, drains the blood blister, and gives the patient prompt relief from pain. A sterile dressing should be applied over the area.

Animal Bites

Open wounds as abrasions, lacerations, and punctures may be caused by animal bites. Not only is there a danger of bacterial infection including tetanus from these wounds, but rabies also is a threat. (See Rabies, p. 185.)

Insect Bites and Stings

The bite or sting of an insect produces an open wound in the skin. The venom which is injected under the patient's skin generally causes local discomfort with some swelling, itching, and redness. Allergic reactions will vary in different individuals from a minor condition to anaphylactic shock. A person extremely sensitive to the venom may not live an hour unless treatment is given immediately.

Anyone who receives a bite or sting should be observed for one or two hours for a possible reaction.

Treatment

The stinger should be removed with a forceps if it is still in place. Venom will continue to be released slowly from the stinger of a bee if left in the skin. When there are minor allergic reactions, the wound should be cleansed with soap and water, and cold applications used to reduce the swelling. If the patient is uncomfortable, diphenhydramine hydrochloride 25 mg may be given by mouth every 6 hours until the reaction subsides.

If an anaphylactic reaction occurs, 0.5 ml epinephrine 1:1,000 should be given subcutaneously. After normal breathing is restored, the patient should be kept under observation for several hours. Medical advice by radio should be obtained for additional treatment of insect bites.

Spider Bites

The *black widow spider*, identified by the red hourglass design on its bottom surface, injects a powerful venom through two puncture sites. A severe cramping muscular pain spreads within an hour to the chest, abdomen, back and leg muscles. The patient may have a headache, difficulty in speaking, and may be perspiring and restless.

Treatment

Treatment should be calcium gluconate 10% injected intravenously slowly *only* until the muscular cramps are relieved. Then, medical advice should be obtained by radio for additional treatment. The wound should be washed with soap and water, and povidone-iodine solution and a dressing applied. Adults usually recover from the bite of a black widow spider in about three days.

Tarantula bites may cause severe local reactions. Usually they do not cause generalized reactions, but they can be fatal. The wound should be cleansed as directed for bites by the black widow spider. Medical advice by radio should be obtained, especially on whether calcium gluconate may be administered.

Snakebites

The severity of local and generalized reactions to a snakebite will vary in relation to the kind and size of the snake, the amount of venom it is carrying, and the location of the bite. Venom from some snakes is more toxic than others, and some inject more venom. If some venom was discharged in a recent strike, the remaining amount will produce a milder reaction.

The location of the bite will influence the reaction. Venom in a muscle is absorbed faster than in subcutaneous tissue. A healthy adult will have a milder reaction than a child. The amount of time it takes before antivenin therapy can be started influences the severity of the reaction. Clothing such as gloves and shoes may have provided some protection.

Venom from *pit vipers such as rattlesnakes and water moccasins* affects the victim's circulatory system. The skin is discolored due to destruction of red blood cells and interference with clotting. There is pain at the site, swelling, at least one fang mark, a rapid pulse, and general weakness. The swelling tends to progress and the entire extremity may be swollen if the victim does not receive treatment for a period of time after the bite. Nausea, vomiting, breathing difficulty, and shock may occur gradually over one to two hours.

Venom from a *coral snake* affects the nervous system of the victim. Usually only a slight burning pain and slight swelling may be present at the bite. However, slurred speech, blurred vision, drowsiness, drooping eyelids, sweating, and increased salivation occur. Additional symptoms might include breathing difficulty, nausea, vomiting, convulsions, paralysis, and coma.

Symptoms from the bite of a *cobra* are similar to that of a coral snake. However, there is more intense local pain and tissue may die (undergo necrosis) at the site of the wound.

Treatment

For snakebite aim to maintain breathing, reduce the spread and absorption of the venom, and protect the wound from additional injury. The following should be done:

- Immobilize the affected extremity.

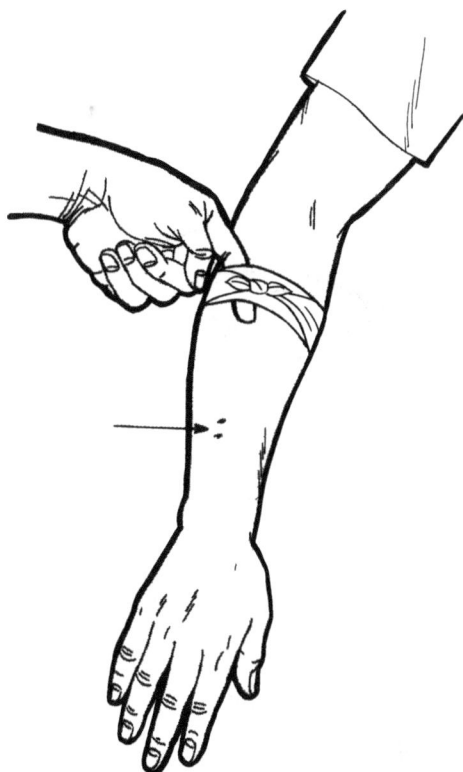

Fig. 3–11. Applying a constricting band for a snakebite.

• Apply a constricting band about two to four inches above the bite between the heart and the wound. (See Fig. 3–11.) The band should be tight enough to decrease the flow of blood in the superficial veins and lymphatic return. It should be released for 90 seconds every 15 minutes and reapplied above the advancing swelling.

• Make an incision through or near each fang mark with the blade from a snakebite kit or with one sterilized over a flame. The incision should only be one-eighth to one-fourth of an inch long and should extend only through the full thickness of the skin. If incisions are deeper, muscles and nerves might be injured.

• Apply intermittent suction to the cuts with the suction cup in the snakebite kit or with the mouth. The poison should be rinsed from the mouth, although it is not poisonous in the stomach. The poison could be dangerous to anyone with cuts, wounds, or bleeding gums in the mouth. The suction should be continued for the first hour. Suction applied after the first 30 minutes is of little value.

• Cleanse the wound with soap and water, dry, and apply a sterile dressing.

• Apply ice wrapped in waterproof material to the wound to slow down the spread of the venom.

• Treat for shock. (See p. 57+.)

• The victim may be given sips of fluid, unless nauseous or unconscious. Do *not* give alcohol. The resulting dilation of the superficial blood vessels will increase the absorption of the venom.

• Give antivenin serum for the specific type of snakebite, if known. The directions on the package should be followed when administering it. If antivenin is not available, an attempt should be made to obtain it or to transport the victim to the nearest medical facility as soon as possible.

• Obtain medical advice by radio for additional treatment, including antibiotic therapy and prevention of tetanus.

The patient should be kept quietly in bed and observed for at least two days following a snakebite. If death should occur, it usually will happen during the first two days.

Human Bites

A severe infection may develop in a wound caused by human teeth because the mouth abounds with potentially harmful bacteria. However, self-inflicted bites of the tongue and lip are tolerated well.

The bite should be treated the same as other wounds (see p. 58+) and observed carefully for any infection. Treatment for tetanus is not needed because the causative organism is not found in the human mouth.

INFECTION

All open wounds contain bacteria. The potential for an infection to develop is dependent upon the type and quantity of bacteria present, the adequacy of the blood supply to the area, and the amount of damaged tissue within the wound. Normal body tissues are capable of destroying large numbers of some bacteria. However, other bacteria resist destruction by the body's defense mechanisms. Careful cleansing of a wound and removal of foreign matter will help to prevent an infection.

Wound infections usually do not become evident until some time after the injury. During the first two or three days there may be throbbing pain, swelling, redness, and excessive warmth in the area of the wound. These are symptoms of infection; also they occur following most extensive injuries. The symptoms tend to diminish toward the end of the first 48 hours if the wound is healing satisfactorily. However, if the symptoms increase, infection may have set in. As an infection progresses, the patient will develop a rising temperature and pulse rate. Pus may develop beneath the skin or drain from an open wound. The size of the inflamed area will increase as surrounding tissues become involved. Red streaks that radiate upward from the infected area indicate the spread of infection through the lymphatic circulation. Swollen lymph glands may appear as tender nodes in the groins, armpits, or neck; this indicates that the infection has spread beyond the immediate site of the injury. A systemic infection of this type is very serious and medical advice from a physician should be obtained by radio.

Treatment

The patient should be placed in bed with the infected body part elevated, if possible. This will reduce swelling and pain. To improve the circulation warm, moist packs (see p. 323) should be applied to the wound four times daily for periods of 30 minutes. Daily redressing of the wound is necessary to remove the infected discharge from the surface of the wound.

BANDAGING

Butterfly

A butterfly strip may be applied to hold together the gapping edges of a small wound. (See Fig. 3–12.) When commercially-produced butterfly strips are not available, they can be improvised from adhesive tape. If a dressing is needed, it may be applied directly over the strips. A splint or sling may be applied to prevent reopening a wound when it is near a joint, or an area where movement might separate the edges.

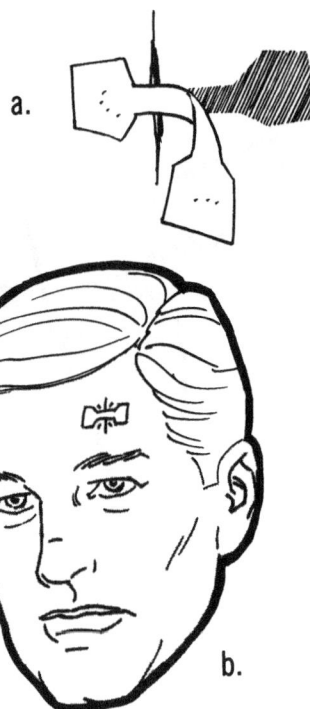

Fig. 3–12. Applying a butterfly strip.

Roller Bandage

A roller bandage is applied to hold a dressing securely in place over a wound. For this reason, it should be applied snugly, but not tightly enough to interfere with the circulation. Fingers and toes should be checked periodically for coldness, swelling, blueness, and numbness. If any of these symptoms occur, the bandage should be loosened immediately.

Anchoring a Roller Bandage

• Hold the roll of bandage in the right-hand with the loose end on the bottom. The left-hand may be used if left-handed.

• Place the outside surface of the loose end at an angle on the body part. (See Fig. 3–13a.)

• Roll the bandage around in a direction away from the body part.

• Bring the bandage from under to over the body part, and turn down the uncovered triangle on the end. (See Fig. 3–13b.)

• Roll the bandage over the end two more times to anchor it and begin circling the body part. (See Fig. 3–13c.)

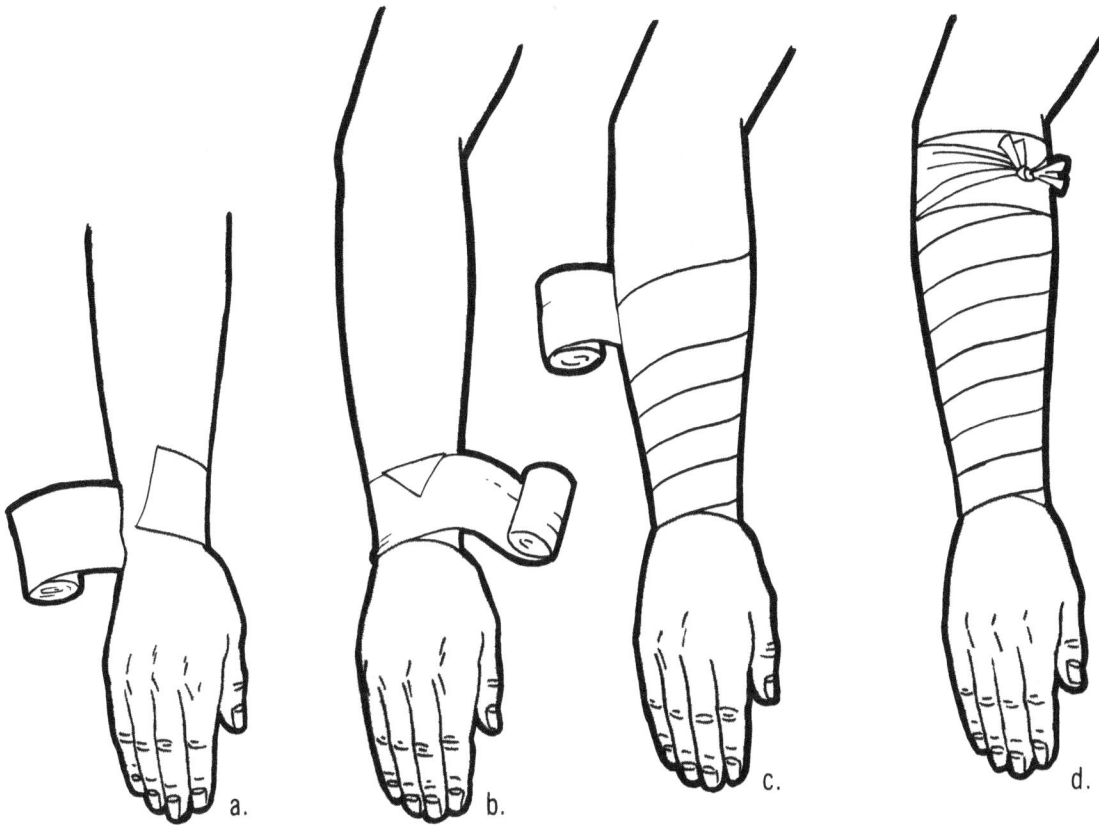

Fig. 3–13. Applying a roller bandage.

Applying a Roller Bandage

• Continue to circle the body part with the bandage using spiral turns. (See Fig. 3–13d.)

• Space the turns so they overlap and completely cover the skin.

Fastening a Roller Bandage

Roller bandages may be fastened with such items as clips, safety pins, or tape. Two methods of fastening them by tying are:

Method 1

• Fold the bandage back upon itself. (See Fig. 3–14.)

• Pass the loose end through the loop formed by folding the bandage backward and tie.

Method 2

• Split the end of the bandage lengthwise for approximately 12 inches and tie a knot to prevent further splitting. (See Fig. 3–15.)

• Pass the ends in opposite directions around the body part and tie.

Chest or Back Bandage

A triangular bandage may be used to secure large dressings on wounds and burns.

• Place the point of the bandage over the shoulder. Let the rest of the bandage drop down over the chest or back with the middle of the base under the point. (See Fig. 3–16a.)

• Fold the base of the bandage up far enough to secure the dressing and tie the ends in the back below the shoulder blade. One long and one short end will be left. (See Fig. 3–16b.)

• Bring the long end up to the shoulder and tie it to the point of the triangle. (See Fig. 3–16c.)

Chest or Abdomen Bandage

This bandage may be used to secure large, bulky dressings in place on the abdomen or chest. It may be improvised from a piece of cloth, a bedsheet, or large bath towel. The bandage should be placed under the patient and pinned securely in the front. (See Fig. 3–17.)

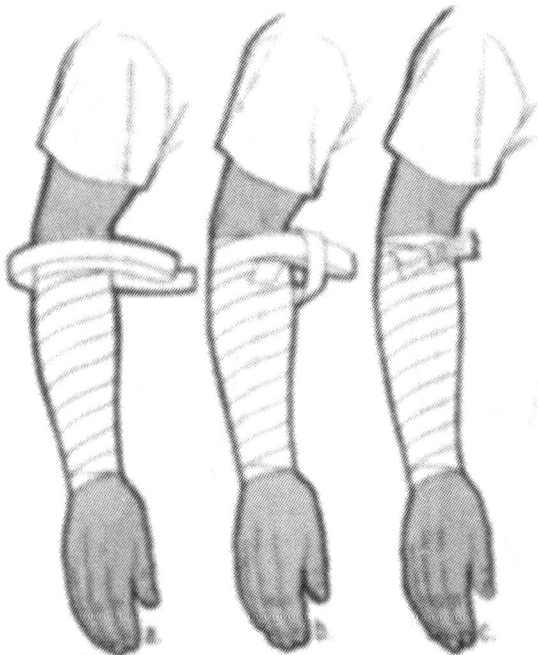

Fig. 3–14. Fastening a roller bandage, method 1.

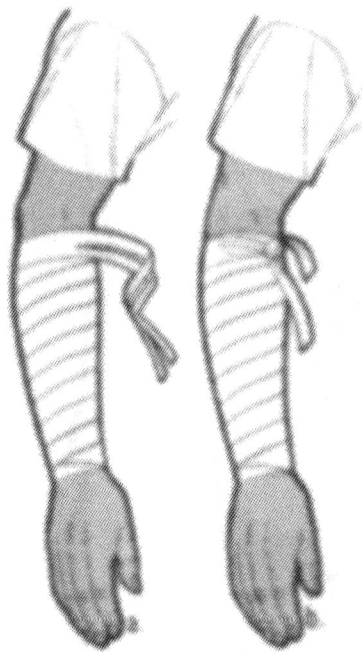

Fig. 3–15. Fastening a roller bandage, method 2.

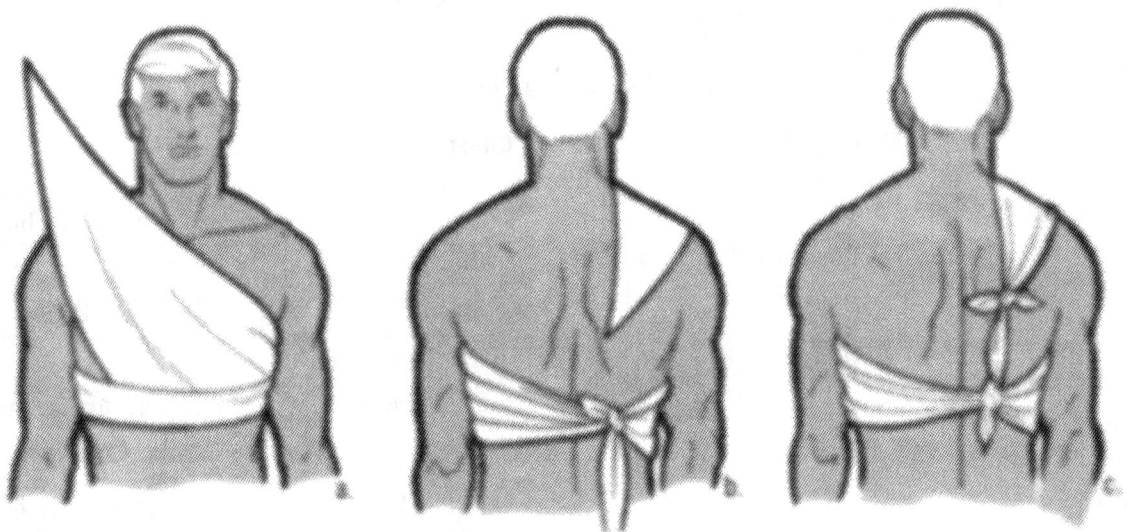

Fig. 3–16. Bandage for chest or back.

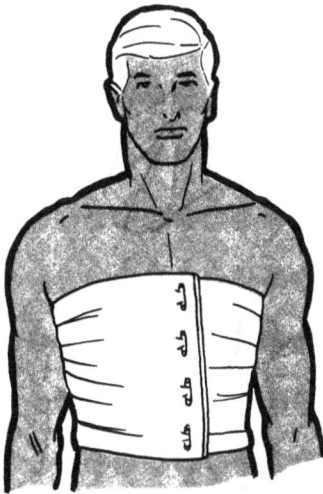

Fig. 3–17. Bandage for chest or abdomen.

angular bandage and place it on top of the cravat. (See Fig. 3–18.)

• Place the center of the cravat over the injured shoulder. Bring the back end of the cravat under the opposite armpit and tie slightly in front of it.

• Bring the base of the folded triangular bandage down and over the dressing on the shoulder.

• Fold up the base of the triangular bandage. Wrap the ends around the arm and tie in front.

• A view of the bandage applied to the hip is shown in Fig. 3–18d.

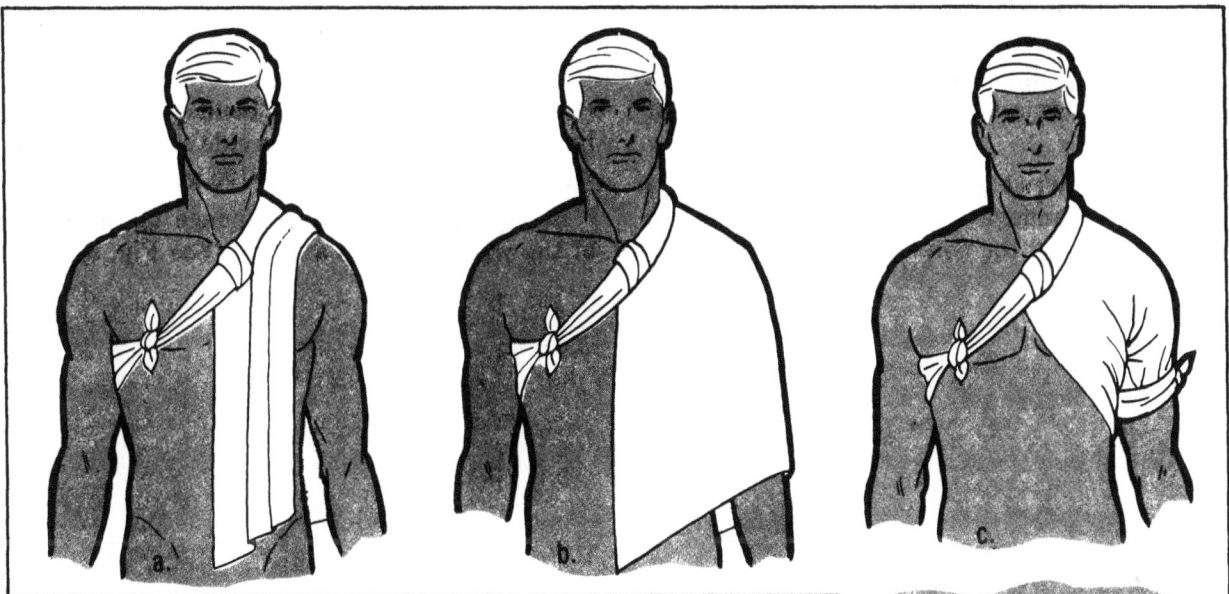

Fig. 3–18. Bandage for shoulder or hip.

Shoulder or Hip Bandage

This bandage is used to secure a dressing in place over a wound or burn on the shoulder or hip. A triangular bandage and a cravat bandage together should be used. The cravat bandage may be made by folding a triangular bandage into a narrow band; or it may be improvised from such items as a roller bandage, tie, or belt.

• Place the cravat bandage on the point of the triangular bandage and roll them together several times. Fold the remainder of the tri-

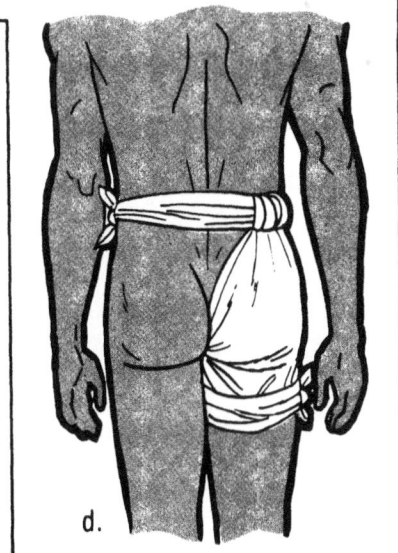

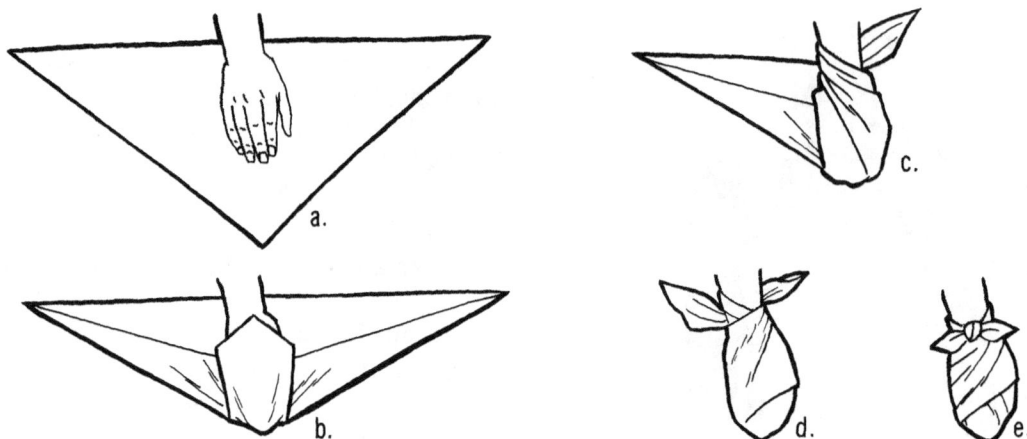

Fig. 3–19. Bandage for hand or foot.

Hand or Foot Bandage

One triangular bandage may be used to secure large dressings in place on the hand or foot.

• Place the wrist or heel in the center of a triangular bandage with the finger or toes pointing toward the point. (See Fig. 3–19a.)

• Fold the point of the bandage up and over the fingers or toes. (See Fig. 3–19b.)

• Wrap the ends of the bandage across the hand or foot to the opposite side and around the wrist or ankle. (See Fig. 3–19c and d.)

• Bring the ends of the bandage to the front of the wrist or ankle and tie. (See Fig. 3–19e.)

Chapter III

Emergency Treatment of Injuries

Section C
BURNS

SOME BURNS CAN BE VERY SEVERE, painful injuries that require many months of costly care. They are a leading cause of accidental death in the United States. These injuries are caused by heat, electricity, chemicals, and radiation.

Burns caused by excessive heat are called thermal burns. Injuries from moist heat result from contact with such things as steam and hot liquids. Injuries from dry heat result from contact with such things as lighted cigarettes, open fires, hot metal, and explosions. Faulty wiring often is the cause of electrical burns. The improper use of chemicals such as lye, strong cleaning products, and acids also may result in burns. Radiation burns result from X-rays, radioactive substances, or ultraviolet rays.

CLASSIFICATION

Burns may be classified by depth which may vary in severity in different areas of the body. Depth is spoken of in "degrees."

First-Degree Burns

Normal skin is made up of two main layers: the outer epidermis and the dermis. (See

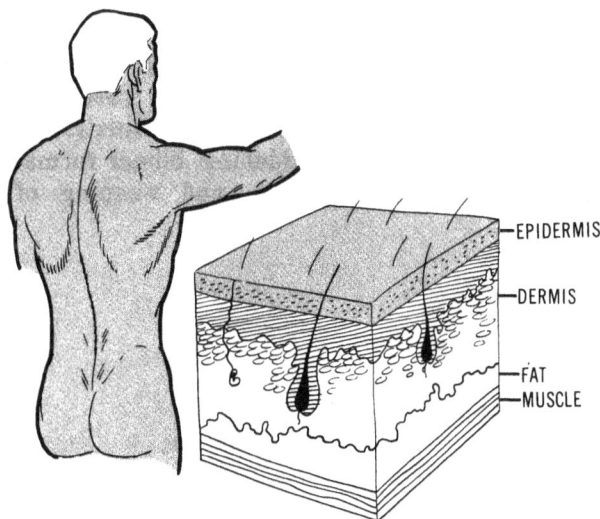

Fig. **3–20.** Normal skin.

Figs. 3–20 & 1–2.) The dermis is a deep inner layer that has sweat glands and hair follicles which are important in the regrowth of skin in first-degree and second-degree burns.

First-degree burns affect only the outer epidermal area and are characterized by redness, mild swelling, increased warmth, tenderness,

67

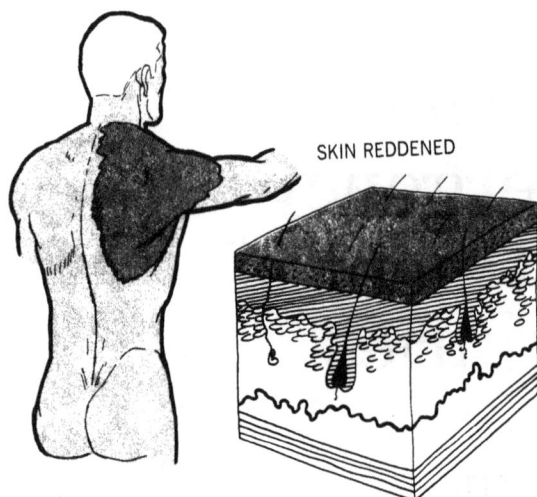

Fig. 3–21. First-degree burn.

and pain. (See Fig. 3–21.) These burns often are the result of sunburn, scalding by hot water or steam, and sudden flash burns. Although quite painful at first, first-degree burns usually heal without scarring within a week.

Second-Degree Burns

Second-degree burns involve the entire layer of the epidermis and extend into the under layer of the skin (dermis). (See Fig. 3–22.) Superficial second-degree burns are characterized by deep reddening, blister formation, considerable swelling, and weeping of

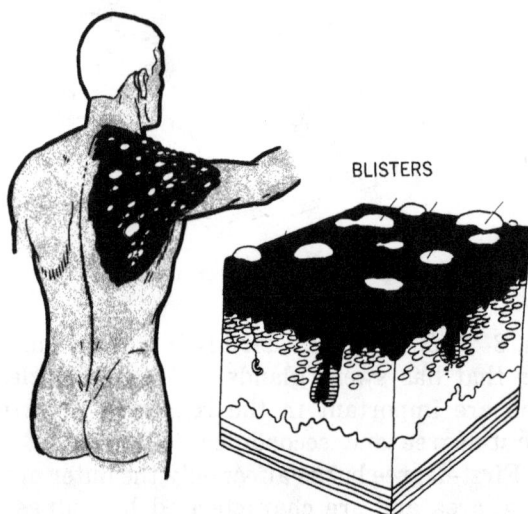

Fig. 3–22. Second-degree burn.

fluid. Deep second-degree burns may not be distinguishable from third-degree burns immediately after the injury. There is severe pain because of the irritated and overly sensitive nerve endings; and any breeze, pressure, or disturbance to the area will cause increased pain. These burns often are the result of a very deep sunburn, contact with scalding liquid, and flash burns from such things as gasoline and kerosene. If the burns do not become infected, they should heal with little scarring in about three weeks. If infection does occur, the burn may transform into a third-degree type injury.

Third-Degree Burns

Third-degree burns involve the epidermis, dermis, and may extend to the underlying fat,

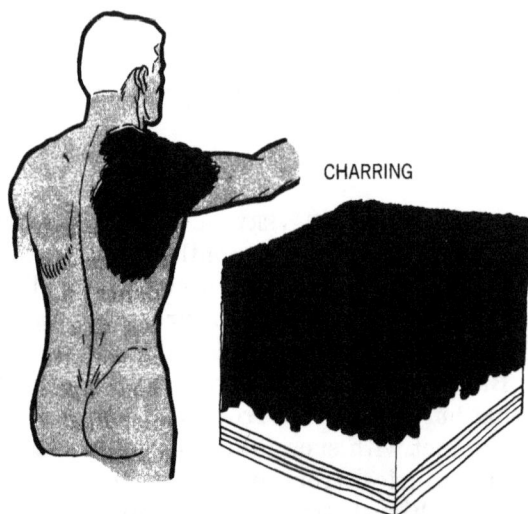

Fig. 3–23. Third-degree burn.

muscle, and bone. (See Fig. 3–23.) They usually are characterized by charring of the skin which may be black or dark brown, hard, cherry red and dry, milk white, thick, and leathery. Coagulated blood vessels frequently may be identified. Pain may be absent due to the destruction of the nerve endings. These burns may be the result of hot liquids, ignited clothing, explosions, electricity, and gasoline or oil fires. This type of burn will not heal properly by itself, except at the margins of the wound. Early skin grafting must be done to prevent contractures which may occur as scar tissue covers the damaged area.

EXTENT OF THE BURN

The amount of burned skin surface in an *adult* can be estimated by using the *rule of nines*. (See Fig. 3–24.) The head and neck represent 9% of the body surface, each arm 9%, the chest 9%, the upper back 9%, the abdomen 9%, the buttocks and lower back 9%, the front of each leg 9%, the back of each leg 9%, and the perineum and genitalia 1%. In *children,* the head is larger in relationship to the body and should be counted as 18%; otherwise, the basic rule may be used. The *rule of eights* is used to estimate the burned surface in *newborns.* Because the head and upper extremities are larger in relationship to the body, the head alone will represent 16% of the body surface, the neck 4%, each arm 16%, front of the body 16%, back of body 16%, and each leg 8%.

Generally, an adult with second-degree burns of 15% or more of the body surface, and children with second-degree burns of 10% or more of the body surface may require hospitalization. Critical burns require immediate examination and hospitalization because of their life-threatening nature.

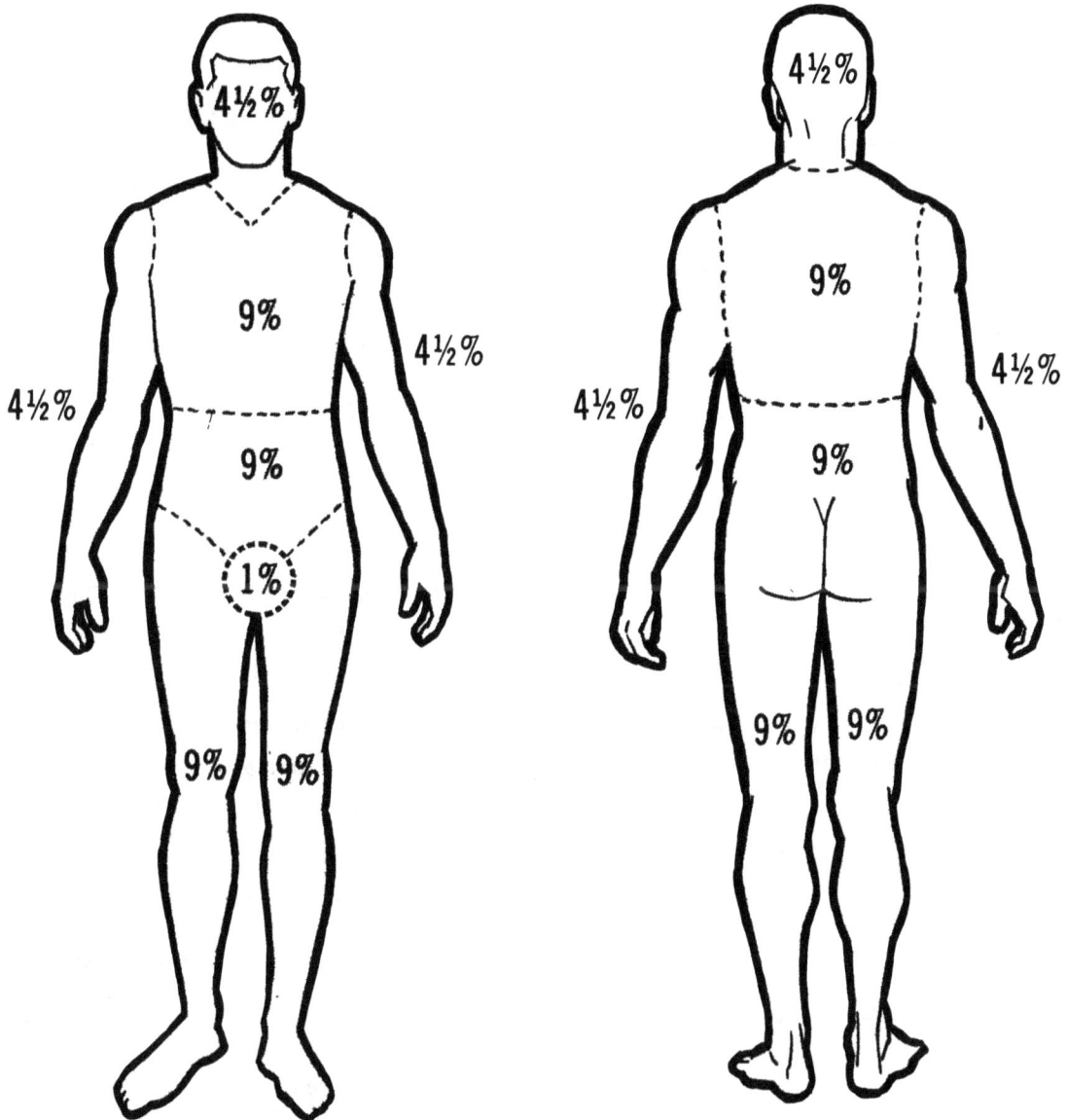

Fig. 3–24. Rule of nines to determine extent of burns.

Burns that involve the respiratory tract are considered critical because breathing may become obstructed as the swelling increases. Respiratory burns can be suspected if the patient has obvious burn injury to the face and neck. This may be identified by singed eyebrows, eyelashes, or hair. More insidious is the respiratory burn suffered by the patient caught in a closed room who inhales superheated gases and carbonaceous particles. This type of respiratory burn may be identified by hoarseness, increased respiratory rate, and carbonaceous particles in patient's sputum. (See p. 73.) Other critical burns would include third-degree burns of 10% and second-degree burns of 30% or more of the body surface; burns of the face, hands, feet, and perineum; and burns associated with soft tissue injuries and fractures.

The prognosis is poor for patients with third-degree burns that cover 50% or more of the body surface. However, the rate of recovery has increased for patients treated in modern burn centers where newer methods of treatment are used. The age and health of the patient are determining factors in the survival rate. Although a young adult may recover, the very young and elderly may not recover from burns of the same extent and degree. Patients under four and over 40 years of age should be considered more critical when burned.

TREATMENT

First-Degree

First-degree burns that involve only a small area usually require little treatment. To relieve the pain, cold water applications can be applied, or the burned area can be submerged in cold water. Unclean areas should be cleansed with soap and water and left open to air; or if desired, covered with a clean dry dressing. If sunburned areas are clean, they should not be washed.

Second-Degree (Small)

To relieve pain and reduce blister formation, cold water applications should be applied or the burned area of the skin should be immersed immediately in cold water from 1 to 2 hours. Salt lowers the temperature of ice water and *never* should be added as it may cause further injury. Following the cold treatment, the area should be cleansed with soap and water and blotted dry with either sterile gauze or a clean towel.

• Do *not* break the blisters.

• Apply sulfadiazine silver cream, 1% to the burned area and wrap with sterile dressing. Remove the sterile dressing daily and reapply the medication and a new sterile dressing.

• Do *not* try to remove pieces of body tissue that adhere to the wound.

The dressing may be changed more frequently if it develops an odor or becomes soaked with exudate. When the dressing needs to be replaced, it *never* should be pulled from adhering surfaces; the area should be soaked with large amounts of water to free the material from the wound. Before a new dressing is applied, the burned area should be washed gently with soap and water and sulfadiazine silver cream, 1% applied.

First- and Second-Degree (More Extensive)

First-and second-degree burns may require hospitalization when they cover 15% or more of the body surface of an adult. Burns which involve the hands, face, feet, and perineum should be considered serious. Plans should be made as soon as possible to evacuate these patients to the nearest medical facility.

Major Burns—Second- and Third-Degree Burns

(On More than 30% of the Body Surface of Adults and Children)

Treatment for severe burns:

Establish an Airway

The patient should be checked immediately for breathing, and an open airway established. Artificial ventilation or cardiopulmonary resuscitation should be performed, as required (see p. 115+).

Respiratory problems always should be anticipated if there are burns around the face, head, and neck; or if during a fire the patient was caught in an enclosed area. Oxygen should be administered to *all* major burn victims with breathing difficulties, because injury to the respiratory tract may have been caused by the inhalation of smoke or other products of incomplete combustion. Carbon monoxide poisoning also may accompany the burn. These problems may not be evident at the time of the burn but will occur later as the membranes swell due to inflammation.

The tongue of an unconscious patient may drop back into the throat and block the air passage. Usually resuscitation can be accomplished with proper positioning of the head and neck; however, in certain instances an oropharyngeal airway may be required. An oropharyngeal airway is a curved breathing tube which, when inserted into the patient's mouth, holds the base of the tongue forward so it does not block the air passage.

An untrained person should not attempt to insert an airway because of the possibility of damaging the soft tissues and mucous membranes in the victim's throat. Two basic guidelines should be followed to determine whether or not an airway is to be used: (1) when the patient is conscious and breathing normally, no attempt should be made to insert an airway because it will cause him to vomit; (2) when the patient is found to be unconscious with breathing obstructed, an airway should be inserted if breathing remains obstructed in spite of head tilt and attempts at artificial ventila-

tion. If the patient reacts by swallowing, retching, or coughing after an airway is in place, the airway must be removed quickly because it may make the patient vomit and increase the likelihood of an airway obstruction.

The best way to ascertain the correct size of an airway is to hold the airway to the side of the face. The lower tip should touch the angle of the jaw just below the earlobe, and the other end should extend beyond the lips. Generally, a size 4 can be used for an adult, size 2 for children, and a size 0 for infants.

To install an airway properly, the patient's mouth should be opened wide using one hand. With the other hand, insert the airway between the patient's teeth with the curve backward at first, then turned to the proper position as it is inserted deeper. This twisting maneuver prevents the tongue from being pushed further back into the throat since the airway must be inserted over the tongue. The airway should be inserted by placing its tip against the roof of the mouth, just behind the upper teeth and sliding it down the throat following the contour of the roof of the mouth until the flange comes to rest at the victim's lips. *Do not push the tongue back into the throat.* At the first sign of a gag reflex, remember to remove the airway. (See Fig. 3–25.)

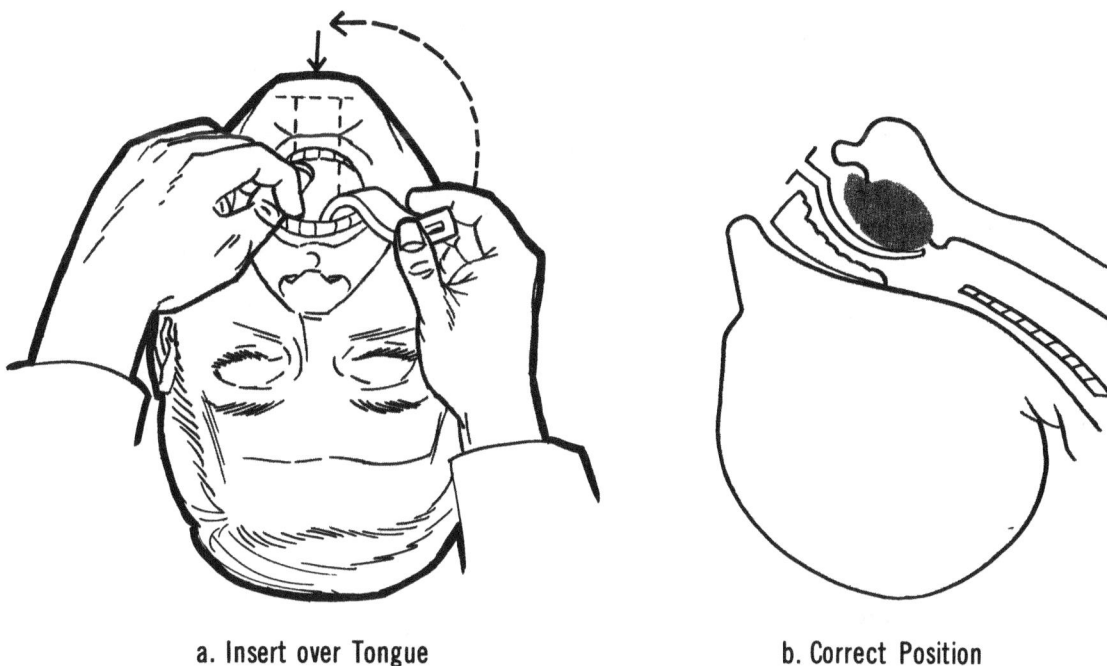

a. Insert over Tongue   b. Correct Position

Fig. 3–25. Inserting an airway.

Treat for Shock

Although there may be no immediate signs of shock, it should be anticipated and treated before local therapy of the burn wound is initiated. Loss of plasma from severely burned areas lowers the patient's blood volume and causes shock.

Replacement of fluids can be accomplished most effectively through intravenous therapy. Lactated Ringer's Solution 1,000 ml intravenously should be started immediately. Medical advice by radio should be obtained for additional treatment, and plans should be made to evacuate the patient to the nearest medical facility as soon as possible.

A person who is trained adequately to administer intravenous therapy may not be aboard ship. If so, the patient who is not vomiting and is conscious should be given weak solutions of sodium bicarbonate and sodium chloride (½ teaspoonful of baking soda and one teaspoonful of salt to a quart of water) slowly by mouth. The solution should be at room temperature. An adult should be given approximately ½ glass (120 ml) every 15 minutes; a child ¼ glass; and an infant ⅛ glass. The fluids should be discontinued immediately if vomiting occurs.

Relieve Pain

If the adult patient is *not* in shock and there is *no* head injury, morphine sulfate 10 mg may be given intramuscularly for severe pain. (Seek medical advice by radio for a child's proper dosage.) If additional doses of morphine sulfate are required, the condition warrants getting medical advice by radio before continuing the medication. When a patient is in shock, intramuscular medication is not absorbed normally. If one gives repeated doses of morphine sulfate intramuscularly, *an overdose might occur.*

Treat the Burned Area

The medical attendant's hands should be scrubbed and sterile gloves applied before the burned area is treated. (See p. 320.) The area should be cleansed gently with water and povidone-iodine solution. All debris and dirt *around* the burned areas should be removed to avoid additional contamination of the area. When cleansing the area, remember:

(1) *No attempt should be made to open blisters or to remove pieces of tissue from the burned surface.* The blisters are not harmful; they protect the underlying tissues against the entry of bacteria.

(2) *No attempt should be made to apply ice water to extensively burned surfaces.* This may increase the patient's shock reaction.

(3) Sulfadiazine silver cream, 1% should be applied in a thin layer to the burned areas and wrapped in sterile dressing. If medical aid is more than 24 hours away, the dressing should be removed, the wounds washed, and sulfadiazine silver cream and dressings reapplied every 24 hours.

After the initial treatment, a more accurate assessment of the burned area should be made. This information should be reported when medical advice by radio is obtained.

After the burned area has been cleansed and the sulfadiazine silver cream applied, multiple layers of sterile dressings should be added to absorb the large amount of fluid that is produced. Roller bandages can be used to hold the dressings in place. If adhesive tape is used to fasten the bandage, it should *not* come into contact with the skin. If the burns are extensive and sterile dressings are scarce, a freshly laundered or ironed sheet can be used.

The face, neck, genitals, and other small areas of skin may be left open to the air, and sulfadiazine silver cream applied, if the burn can be kept clean. There should be no direct contact against bed linens, clothing, or other objects. If the hands and feet are involved, sulfadiazine silver cream should be applied and sterile dressings placed between the fingers and toes to prevent them from sticking together.

Dressings should be left in place for 24 hours unless they become soaked with drainage. If this should occur before the patient can be evacuated from the ship, the dressings should be replaced under as sterile conditions as possible. (See p. 317.) If there is evidence of infection, the treatment should be the same as for an infected wound. (See p. 61.) Fever following serious burns is common, and does not necessarily indicate infection.

When treating burn injuries, *always* remember to examine the patient for other injuries. If there are fractures and lacerations, they should be treated the same as when burns are not present.

Give Tetanus Prophylaxis

Tetanus prophylaxis is recommended for all patients with major burns who have not received a booster dose or a full basic series within the past 12 months. The patient should be given a booster injection of adsorbed tetanus toxoid 0.5 ml subcutaneously, if there is knowledge of previous active immunization within the past five years. If the patient has not been immunized, or has not been immunized in the last five years, tetanus immune human globulin (250 units) should be given intramuscularly in one arm, and adsorbed tetanus toxoid 0.5 ml subcutaneously in the other arm.

RESPIRATORY BURNS

Respiratory burns (see p. 70) are caused by the inhalation of hot gases and air, particles, and smoke. They should be anticipated when burned areas are found around the mouth, nose, face, hair, and neck. However, sufficient heat from a flash fire may cause edema (swelling) of the larynx with little evidence of other burns.

The patient with a mild injury to the respiratory passages may have only a cough, hoarseness, or a sore throat. Complete obstruction of the respiratory passages may occur as a result of a severe injury. Also, partial collapse of a lung may occur. The patient first may exhibit cyanosis (blue color of the skin), dyspnea (shortness of breath), coughing, wheezing, and hoarseness.

Treatment

An airway must be maintained. An oropharyngeal airway should be inserted (see p. 70+) and oxygen administered. Medical advice by radio should be obtained. If necessary, plans should be made to evacuate the patient to the nearest medical facility.

ELECTRICAL BURNS

The severity of electrical burns often is difficult to determine because the deeper layers of the skin, muscles, and internal organs may be involved. Also, the burns may be followed by a paralysis of the respiratory center and an irregularity in the beat of the heart. Unconsciousness or instant death may occur.

Treatment

The patient must be removed from the source of the electrical current as quickly as possible, without endangering the rescuer. Electrical lines may be removed with a wooden pole, chair, or other non-metal object. Cardiopulmonary resuscitation (see p. 115+) may be required because the shock may affect the patient's heart and lungs. The treatment of the burn would be the same as for any thermal burn of the same extent and depth. This would include relief of pain, prevention and treatment of shock, care of the wound, and control of infection.

CHEMICAL BURNS

Chemical burns occur when acids, alkalis, and other corrosive chemicals come in contact with the skin and mucous membranes. These will include alkalis such as sodium hydroxide (caustic soda, soda lye), potassium hydroxide (lye), and calcium oxide (quick-lime); and such acids as nitric acid, hydrochloric acid, and sulfuric acid. Chlorine, ammonia, mustard gas, and white phosphorus may cause serious burns.

Treatment

The chemical should be washed away immediately with large amounts of water, using a hose or shower, if available. The washing should be continued for a minimum of five minutes. All of the patient's clothing which has become contaminated with the chemical should be removed. *This washing technique must be modified for dry lime and phenol (carbolic acid) burns.* Before washing, the lime should be brushed away gently. Water mixed with the lime reacts chemically to produce heat, which may further burn the skin. Phenol crystals or liquefied phenol should be washed from the skin with ethyl alcohol or isopropyl alcohol, then the skin washed with water.

After copious washing, any chemical remaining should be neutralized carefully. If the appropriate antidote is not known, medical advice by radio should be obtained. Additional treatment would be the same as for any thermal burn of the same extent and depth.

Chapter III

Emergency Treatment of Injuries

Section D
ORTHOPEDIC EMERGENCIES

GENERAL TREATMENT

Sprains

A SPRAIN IS AN INJURY to a joint in which the ligaments and other tissues are damaged by violent stretching or twisting. The ankle, wrist, back, and knee joints are the ones most often sprained. Sharp pain and marked swelling are characteristics of this type of injury. Attempts to move or use the joint increase the pain. With severe sprains the patient may be unable to use the injured hand or walk on the injured leg. The skin about the joint may be discolored due to bleeding from torn tissues.

It often is difficult to distinguish between a severe sprain and a fracture. The injury should be treated as a fracture until the advice of a physician can be obtained, or until the patient's improvement reduces the possibility of a fracture. It may be necessary to obtain an X-ray before the extent of the injury can be determined.

Serious sprains may require complete rest in bed for a period of two days to one week. The arm should be placed in a sling if the injury involves an arm or a shoulder. (See Fig. 3–26.) If the hip, thigh, or leg is involved, the leg on the injured side should be elevated by placing a pillow or folded blanket under it. A patient with a sprained back should be placed on his back with a board under the mattress. A pillow under the knees will provide further comfort. A patient with a severe sprain involving the lower back should not stand or walk for several days after the injury, or until the pain has subsided.

Ice bags and cold wet compresses should be applied to the injured area to control swelling and to relieve pain. For severe pain, the patient may be given aspirin 600 mg with

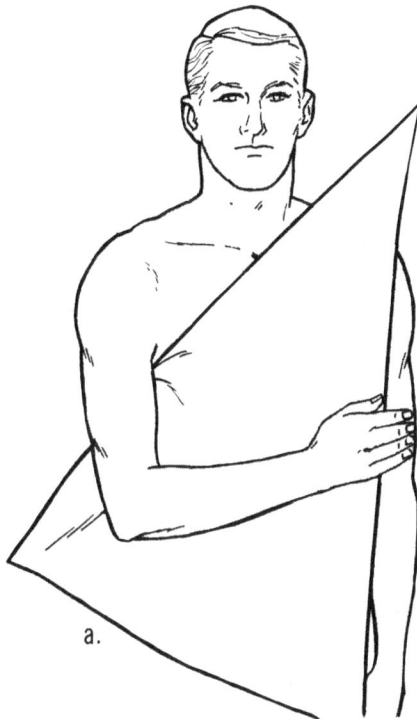

applied firmly, but not too tightly. Fingers and toes should be checked periodically for blue or white discoloration, indicating that the bandage has been applied too tightly. Pain, tingling, loss of sensation, and loss of pulses indicate impaired circulation. The bandage should be loosened if any of these signs or symptoms are present.

Strains

A *strain* is an injury to a muscle or tendon caused by sudden, forcible overstretching due to vigorous muscular effort, such as heavy lifting, running, or jumping. The muscles of the back are involved more often than the thigh and leg muscles. Strains usually occur over the midportion of a long bone, and not at the joint itself. Injuries of this type are characterized by pain, weakness, stiffness, and knotting of the muscles (charley horse). Discoloration may be present due to blood escaping from injured vessels into the tissues.

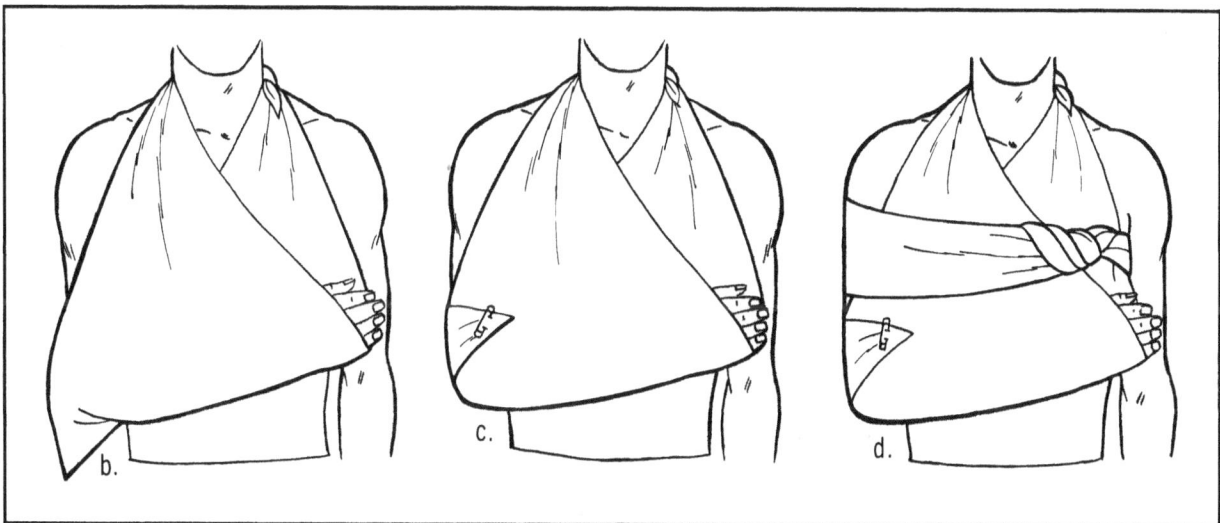

Fig. 3–26. Applying a sling and cravat bandage.

codeine sulfate 30 mg by mouth. Aspirin alone may control the pain after four or five doses. If the patient does not tolerate aspirin, acetaminophen 600 mg should be given with the same frequency. To continue the codeine sulfate, medical advice by radio should be obtained.

The injured joint should be immobilized with pillows, blankets, or bandaged with a wide elastic bandage. The bandage should be

The injured part should be kept at rest in a position that is comfortable for the patient. Heat (preferably moist heat) should be applied to the area involved to relax the muscle spasms. Pain may be relieved and circulation stimulated by rubbing. Often it is difficult to differentiate between a sprain and a strain. If so, the injury should be treated as a sprain for 24 to 48 hours.

Dislocations

A *dislocation* occurs with severe wrenching or twisting of a joint. The ligaments holding the bones in position are stretched and sometimes torn, and the bone ends are forced into an abnormal relationship. A dislocation generally is caused by a blow or a fall, or by strenuous lifting, pulling, or twisting in which a sudden, violent strain is placed on a joint.

Severe pain, rapid swelling, discoloration, and loss of ability to use the joint are characteristic symptoms of this injury. The joint has an abnormal appearance and is generally stiff and immobile. Although a fracture and dislocation can occur at the same time, fractures usually occur between joints. The joints most frequently dislocated are the shoulders and the fingers. The ankle joint often is dislocated and fractured at the same time.

Cold compresses may help to relieve the pain and to keep the swelling down. If severe pain is present, morphine sulfate 10 mg may be given by intramuscular injection. Before repeating the morphine sulfate, medical advice by radio should be obtained.

Treatment for specific dislocations will be discussed later.

Fractures

Fractures are classified as simple or compound. (See Fig. 3–27.)

A simple (closed) fracture is an injury in which the bone has been broken but does not penetrate the skin. Surrounding tissues and blood vessels may suffer damage. Simple fractures that do not produce obvious deformities may be very difficult to detect and may not be discovered without an X-ray. Fractures always should be suspected following a severe injury. The type of accident that is most likely to cause a fracture is a sudden twist, sharp blow, fall, or crushing injury. A fracture may occur even though the injury seems relatively slight. For example, a fracture of the anklebone often is confused with a sprained ankle.

A compound (open) fracture is an injury in which the bone is broken and there is an adjoining wound through the soft tissues and skin. The skin is pierced by the bone end, or from the external source which caused the fracture, such as a gunshot wound or penetrating materials. Careless handling of a patient may change a simple fracture into a compound fracture by forcing the jagged ends of bone

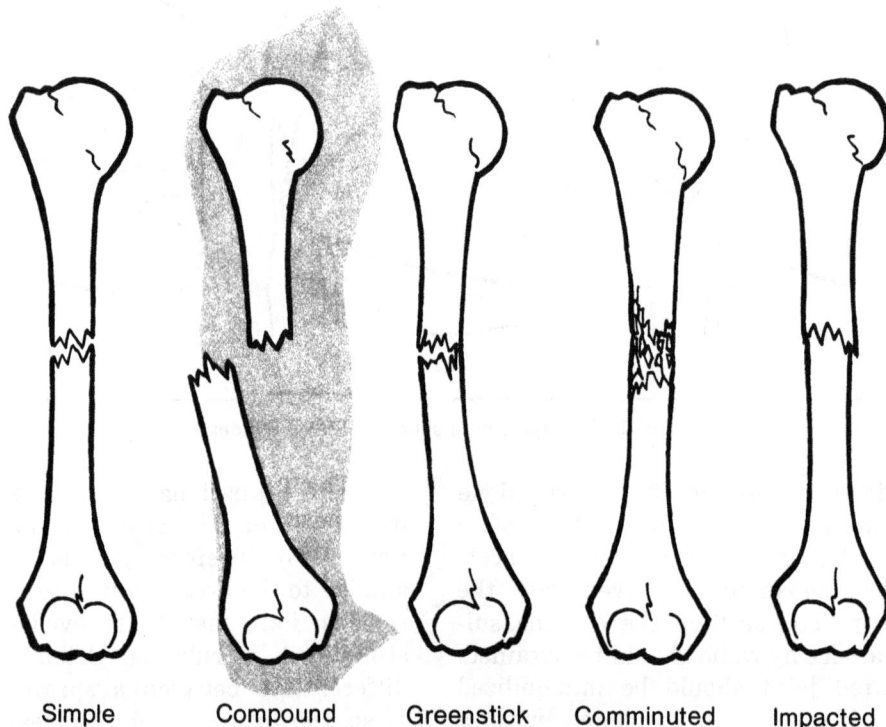

Simple   Compound   Greenstick   Comminuted   Impacted

Fig. 3–27. Types of fractures.

through intact overlying skin. A compound fracture should be considered to be present when an open wound is located at or near the site of a fracture.

There are several types of simple and compound fractures. A *greenstick fracture* occurs when a bone does not break completely through. This is common in children because of their soft and pliable bones. There is little or no separation of the bone ends in *fissure or crack fractures*. They require only adequate immobilization to heal. In an *impacted fracture*, one end of the broken bone is driven into the other end. In a *comminuted fracture*, the bone is broken into three or more pieces that may be crushed, splintered, or fragmented. (Fig. 3–27.)

Fractures, whether simple or compound, usually cause severe pain. Although pain generally is present at the fracture site, the area around the injury may be tender to the touch. Swelling almost always occurs immediately and discoloration of the skin may follow. It may be difficult or impossible for the patient to move the part beyond the injury. However, because the part can be moved, it does not rule out the possibility of a fracture. Also, he may be reluctant to move the part because of the severe tenderness and throbbing pain. Even if the bone is cracked, the part may be moved without difficulty. When the part is moved, the patient may feel a grating sensation as the ends of the bones rub together. Unnecessary movements should be avoided as the grating may increase the damage to the bone ends and soft tissue. The injured part may be deformed or may be in an unnatural position. One limb may be shorter than the other if the broken ends of the bone overlap. Compound fractures may be accompanied by serious bleeding, and shock is likely to develop, especially if a large bone is involved.

Medical advice by radio should be sought early because it might be necessary to evacuate a patient with a compound fracture.

General Treatment

Unless there is an immediate danger of further injury, the patient should not be moved until bleeding is controlled, and all fractures are immobilized by splinting. A pressure dress-

ing can be devised to control almost any bleeding from wounds in compound fractures. A tourniquet is rarely, if ever, indicated. Bulky sterile dressings can be applied and held firmly in place with an elastic bandage. If the bleeding is severe, it may bleed through this dressing. More bulky sterile dressing should be added and the elastic bandage tightened. The fingers or toes beyond the break should be examined at intervals to assure adequate circulation. If they become bluish or white, the dressing should be loosened. As soon as temporary splinting has been applied, the patient should be placed carefully into bed as quickly as possible.

If the patient is in severe pain, morphine sulfate 10 mg may be given by intramuscular injection. To repeat the dosage medical advice by radio should be obtained. Care should be taken not to aggravate pain by moving or roughly handling the injured part.

The pressure dressing, placed over the wound in compound fractures, should be removed after approximately one hour. If bleeding is well controlled, the wound can be treated. The area around the wound should be cleansed thoroughly with soap and water, after which surface washings should not be allowed to spill into the wound. *The wound itself should not be washed.* The wound should be covered with a sterile dressing. Particles of dirt, pieces of clothing, wood, and metal should be removed gently from the wound with a sterilized forceps. Blood clots should not be disturbed as this may cause fresh bleeding. One should not probe for deeply buried objects. Isopropyl alcohol or other anti-infective solutions should not be applied because they will irritate damaged tissue. The wound should not be sutured. A sterile gauze compress or pad should be placed over the wound, and gauze bandage or elastic bandage used to secure it. As a general rule, dressings should be allowed to remain in place four or five days. Changing them earlier is justified only if evidence of wound infection develops.

If a long bone in the arm or leg has been fractured, it should be straightened carefully. Traction should be applied on the hand or the foot, and the limb moved back into position. (See Fig. 3–28.) Compound fractures of joints, such as the elbow or knee, should not be manipulated. They should be placed gently into a

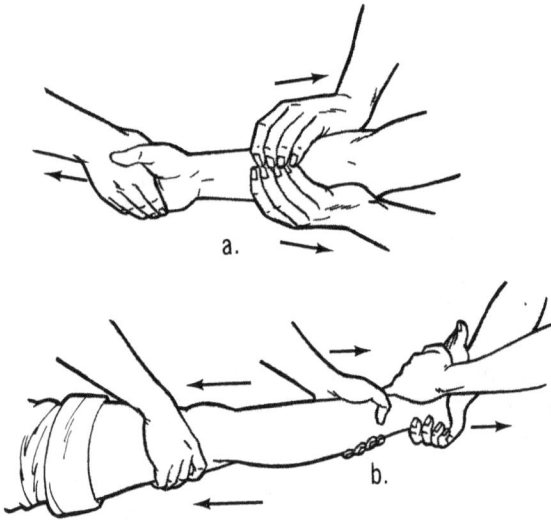

Fig. 3–28. Straightening a fractured limb.

proper position for splinting. The knee should be splinted straight. The elbow should be splinted at a right angle. Inflatable splints (see Fig. 3–32) may be used for some fractures; others will require a different type of splinting. To provide adequate stability, the splint should be long enough to extend beyond the joints at the end of the fractured bone. Splinting will be covered in more detail later in the treatment of specific fractures.

The advice of a physician on handling these injuries should be obtained by radio as soon as possible.

HEAD

Skull

A fracture of the skull may be caused by a fall, direct blow, crushing injury, or a penetrating injury such as a bullet wound. The patient may be conscious, unconscious, or dizzy, and have a headache or nausea. Bleeding from the nose, ears, or mouth may be present; and there may be paralysis and signs of shock.

Treatment

The patient with a head injury should receive immediate attention to prevent additional damage to the brain. The patient should be kept lying down. If the face is flushed, the head and shoulders should be elevated slightly. If the face is pale, the head should be kept level

with the body or slightly lower. Bleeding can be controlled by direct pressure on the temporal or carotid arteries. The patient should be moved carefully with the head supported on each side with a sandbag. *Depressant drugs, such as morphine sulfate never should be given.*

Upper Jaw

In all injuries of the face, an adequate airway must be considered first. (Refer to Cardiopulmonary Resuscitation, p. 115+.)

Treatment

If there are wounds, bleeding should be controlled. Dental consultation should be obtained after the patient has been transported to a medical facility. Loose teeth should not be removed without medical advice by radio, unless it is feared that they will be swallowed or block the airway.

Lower Jaw

A dislocation or fracture of the lower jaw may occur as a result of a direct blow or fall. The pain from the injury is likely to become severe when an effort is made to open or close the jaw. A fracture may cause a deformity of the jaw, missing or uneven teeth, bleeding from the gums, swelling, and difficulty in swallowing. Dental consultation should be obtained after the patient has been transported to a medical facility. Dislocation of the lower jaw may be associated with a fracture of the lower jaw and other facial injuries. A lower jaw dislocation may occur simply from opening the mouth too wide while yawning or eating. In the most common type of acute dislocation, the lower jaw is locked open to make eating and talking almost impossible. Medical advice by radio should be obtained on the proper course of action.

Treatment

The injured jaw may interfere with breathing. If this occurs, the jaw and tongue should be pulled forward and maintained in that position. (Refer to Cardiopulmonary Resuscitation, p. 115+.) If unconscious, the patient should be placed on his side or on his stomach, with the face tilted to one side to avoid aspiration of blood, mucus, and vomitus.

Application of cold compresses may reduce the swelling and pain. The patient's jaw must be immobilized by closing his mouth as much as possible (depending on the degree of deformity) and applying a bandage. (See Fig. 3–29 for method *a* or method *b*.) If the patient is unconscious, bleeding from the mouth, or there is danger of vomiting, an attendant must be present at all times to loosen the bandage when an emergency occurs.

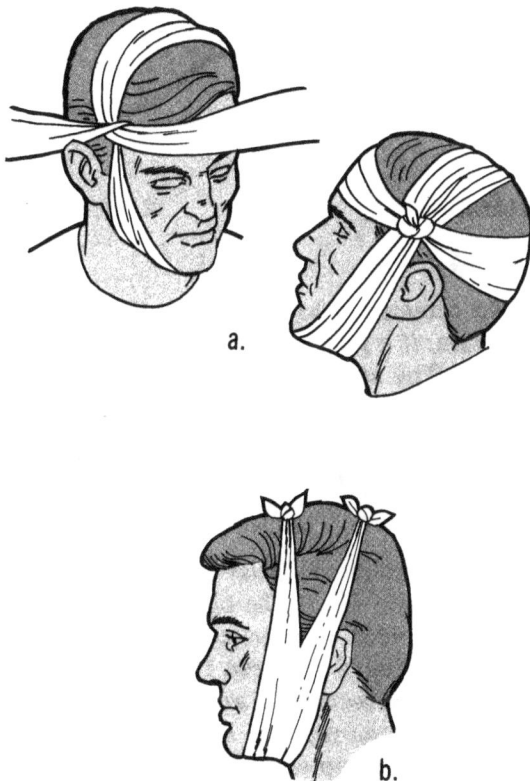

Fig. 3–29. Bandages for a fracture of the jaw: method a or method b.

Aspirin 600 mg with codeine sulfate 30 mg by mouth, or acetaminophen 600 mg with codeine sulfate 30 mg by mouth may be given for pain. To repeat the codeine sulfate, or if the patient cannot take oral medication, medical advice by radio should be obtained.

Nose

A fracture of the nose usually is caused by a direct blow. Generally, there will be pain, swelling, bleeding, and a deformity which is easy to detect.

Treatment

The patient should be positioned so the head is tilted slightly backward. If the bleeding does not stop in a few minutes, cold compresses or an ice bag should be applied to the injury. A permanent deformity of the nose may occur as a result of the fracture, so medical attention should be obtained upon returning to port.

For pain, aspirin 600 mg with codeine sulfate 30 mg should be given by mouth. If aspirin is not well tolerated by the patient, acetaminophen may be tried at the same dosage and frequency. Before repeating the codeine sulfate, medical advice by radio should be obtained.

CLAVICLE (COLLARBONE)

Fractures of the clavicle are common and usually are the result of falling with the hand outstretched. The force from the fall is transmitted to the shoulder. Usually the fracture is easy to detect because the clavicle lies immediately under the skin and a deformity can be seen easily. Also, the fracture can be detected by feeling the bone with the fingers and noting a tender or swollen area. There is pain and tenderness, and a grating sensation can be felt. The shoulder on the injured side may droop downward and forward.

Treatment

Because splints for these fractures are difficult to apply, only a physician should put them on. If clavicle splints are applied tightly enough to immobilize the fracture, the compression of the blood vessels and nerves at the armpits might endanger the arm. The fracture should be treated by supporting the arm in a simple sling on the injured side. The sling will remove weight from the clavicle which helps to support the arm. The arm and sling should be secured to the body with a wide cravat bandage. (See Fig. 3–26.)

For pain, aspirin 600 mg with codeine sulfate 30 mg should be given by mouth. If aspirin is not well tolerated by the patient, acetaminophen may be tried at the same dosage and frequency. Before repeating the codeine sulfate, medical advice by radio should be obtained.

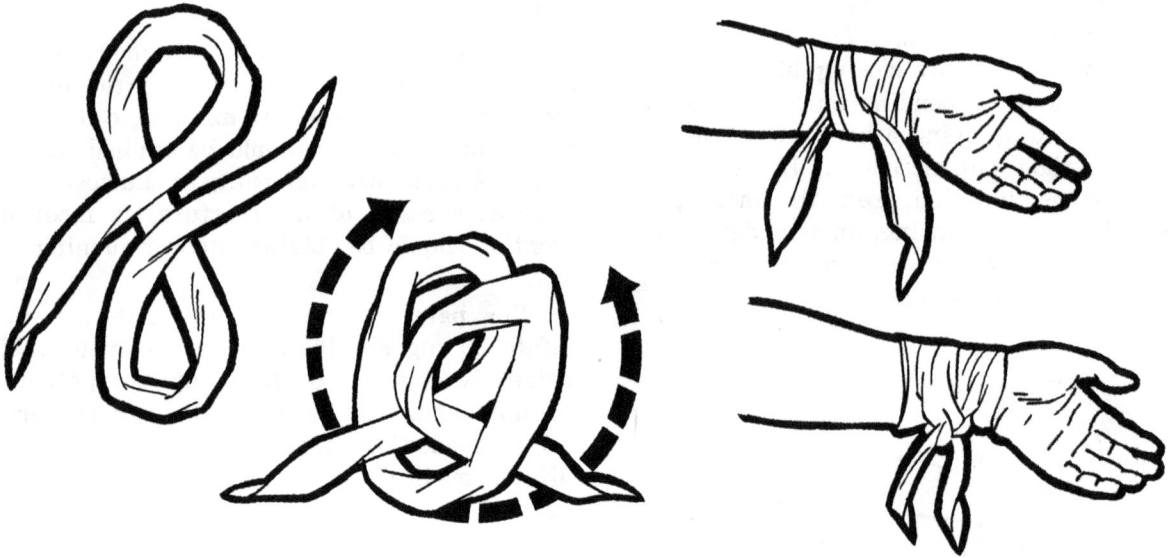

Fig. 3–30. Clove hitch bandage.

SCAPULA (SHOULDER BLADE)

Fractures of the scapula generally are due to direct trauma and are not common. Usually they are simple fractures with little displacement. There is pain and swelling, usually coupled with inability to swing the arm. The patient should be examined further, as there may be associated injuries from the blow.

Treatment

A sling should be applied to the arm on the injured side, and the sling and arm secured to the body by a wide cravat bandage. (See Fig. 3–26.)

For pain, aspirin 600 mg with codeine sulfate 30 mg should be given by mouth. If aspirin is not well tolerated by the patient, acetaminophen may be tried at the same dosage and frequency. Before repeating the codeine sulfate, medical advice by radio should be obtained for a patient with a fractured scapula.

DISLOCATION OF SHOULDER

An injury to the shoulder which results in complete loss of function is more apt to be a dislocation than a fracture. There is a sagging of the shoulder with the elbow held away from the body at an awkward angle. Extreme pain is present in the shoulder region. The head of the humerus often may be felt in an abnormal position. A history of previous dislocations may be described by the patient.

Treatment

No attempt should be made to reduce the dislocation, *if a physician can be reached within 24 hours.* The arm should be placed in a sling. (See Fig. 3–26.) If severe pain is present, morphine sulfate 10 mg may be given by intramuscular injection. To repeat the morphine sulfate, medical advice by radio should be obtained.

If the dislocation must be reduced, medical advice by radio should be obtained. Sometimes it can be reduced without active manipulation. The patient should be given 10 mg of morphine sulfate intramuscularly and allowed to rest quietly for 30 minutes to one hour before the reduction is attempted. A clove hitch bandage should be applied to the wrist on the side of the injury. (See Fig. 3–30.) Then the patient should be placed face down on a table with his shoulder and arm hanging over the side. A bucket with 10 to 15 pounds of weight in it should be attached to the clove hitch. (See Fig. 3–31.) The weight of his arm and the additional weight of the bucket will gradually stretch the tight muscles about the dislocated joint and pull it back into position. Often the dislocation will reduce in 10 to 15 minutes, but may require as long as 30 minutes to one hour.

To repeat the morphine sulfate, medical advice by radio should be obtained.

Following reduction of the dislocation, the arm should be placed in a sling, with the arm and sling secured to the body by a wide cravat bandage. (See Fig. 3–26.)

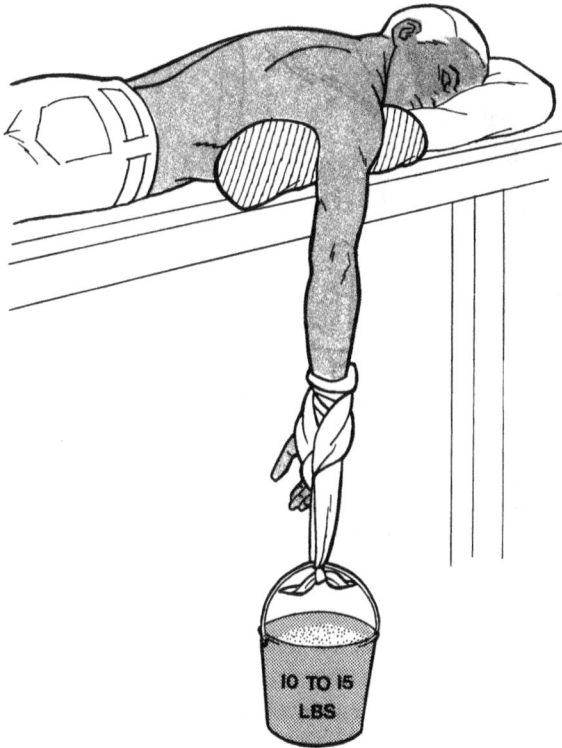

Fig. 3–31. Reduction of a dislocated shoulder.

HUMERUS (UPPER ARM AND ELBOW)

Complications may occur in fractures of the humerus because of the closeness of the nerves and blood vessels to the bone. There is pain and tenderness at the fracture site and an obvious deformity may be present. The patient may be unable to lift his arm or to bend his elbow.

Treatment

A full arm, inflatable air splint should be applied to the fracture. (See Fig. 3–32.) If inflatable splints are not available, the arm should be placed in a sling, with the sling and arm secured to the body by a wide cravat bandage. (See Fig. 3–26.) A short padded splint, applied to the outer surface of the arm, may be used in addition to the above procedure. (See Fig. 3–33.) The *elbow* should not be bent, if it does not bend easily. Long, padded splints should be applied, one to the outer surface and the other to the inner surface of the arm. If there is any possibility that the *elbow* is involved in the *fracture*, the joint should be immobilized with a splint. (See Fig. 3–34.)

For pain, aspirin 600 mg with codeine sulfate 30 mg should be given by mouth. If aspirin is not well tolerated by the patient,

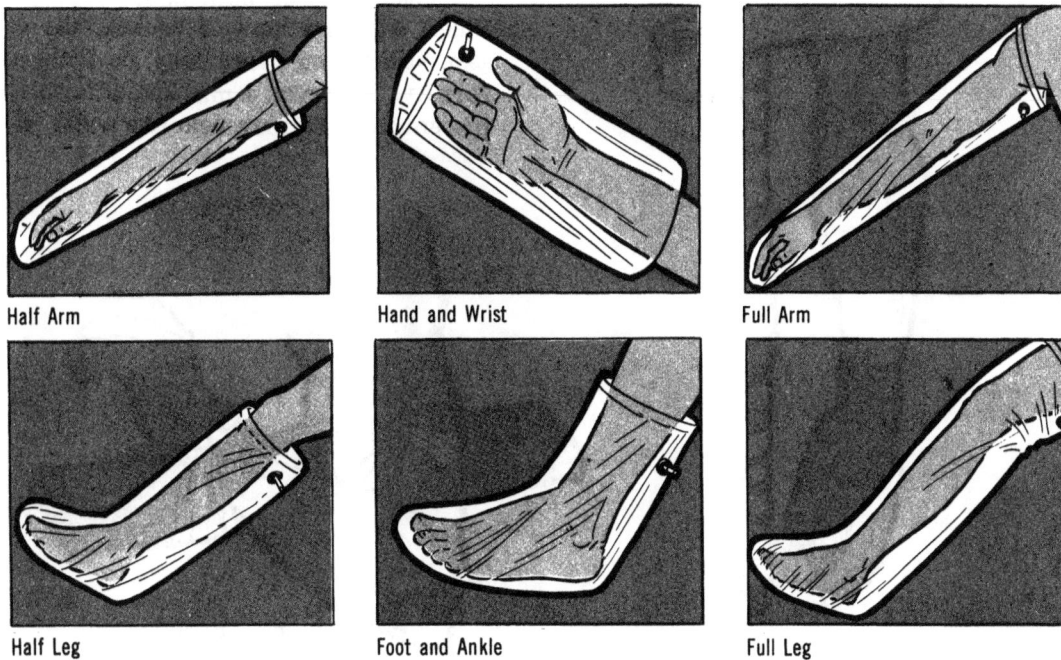

Half Arm

Hand and Wrist

Full Arm

Half Leg

Foot and Ankle

Full Leg

Fig. 3–32. Inflatable air splints.

a. Elbow Bending Easily

b. Elbow Not Bending Easily

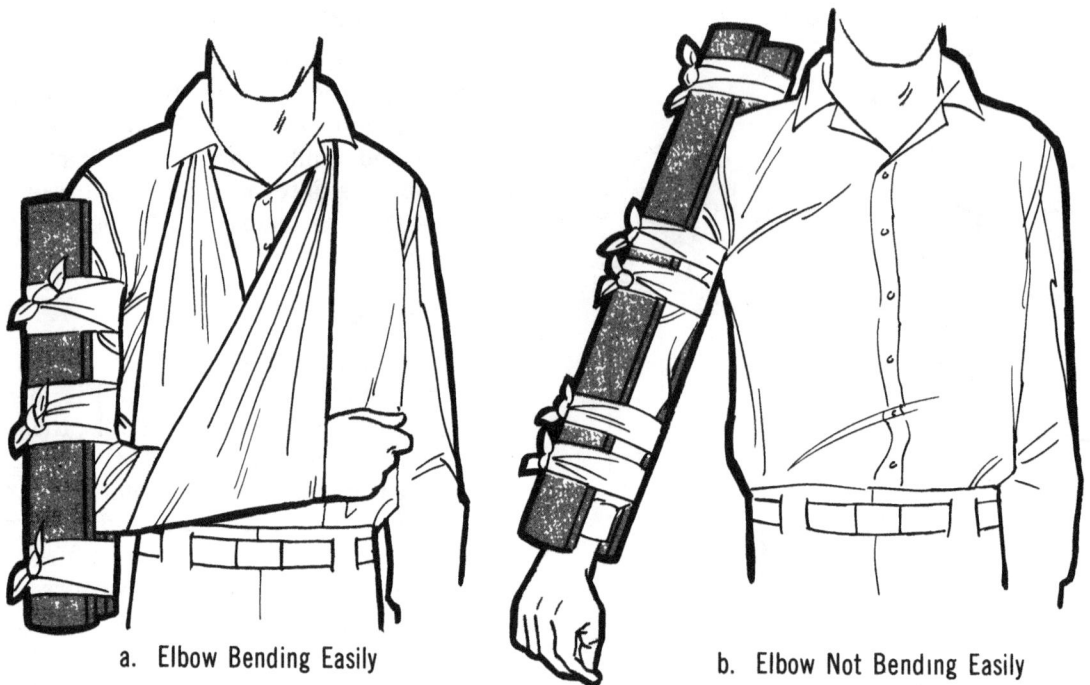

Fig. 3–33. Splinting a fractured humerus.

acetaminophen may be tried at the same dosage and frequency. To repeat the codeine sulfate, medical advice by radio should be obtained.

RADIUS AND ULNA (LOWER ARM)

There are two large bones in the forearm, and either one or both bones may be broken. When only one bone is broken, the other acts as a splint and there may be little or no deformity. However, a marked deformity may be present in a fracture near the wrist. When both

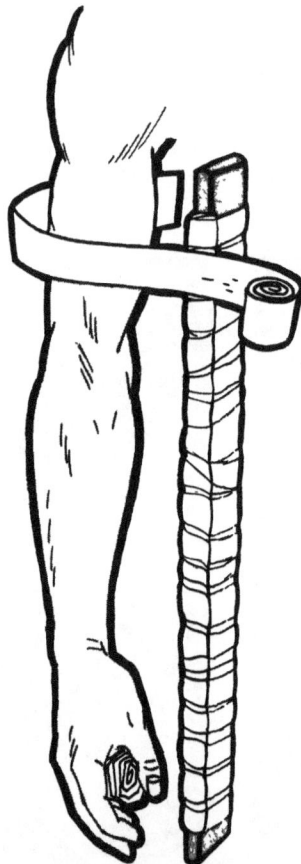

a. Straight Position

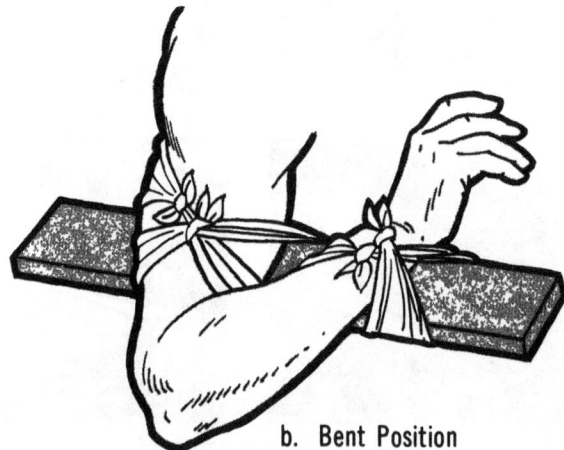

b. Bent Position

Fig. 3–34. Dislocated or fractured elbow.

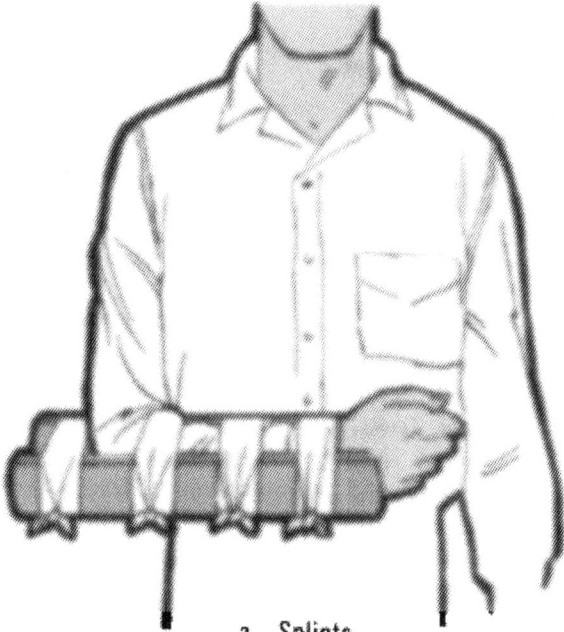

a. Splints

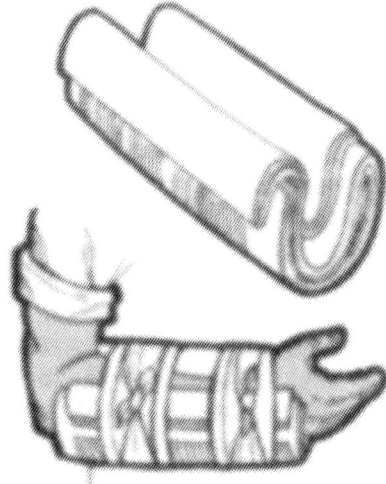

b. Magazine

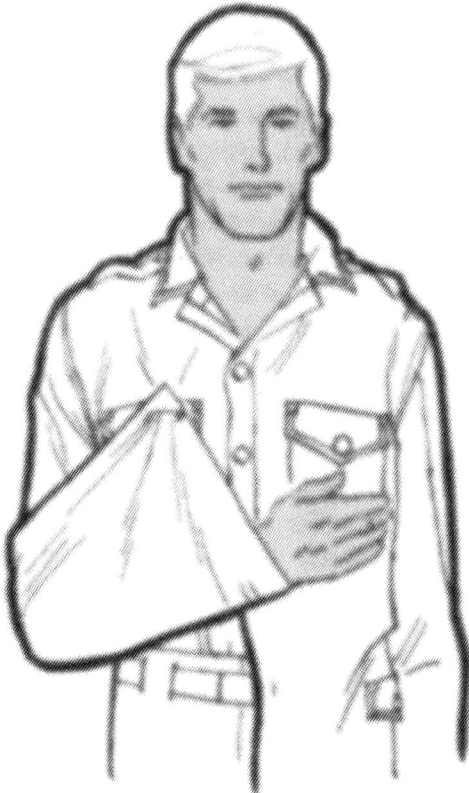

c. Jacket Flap

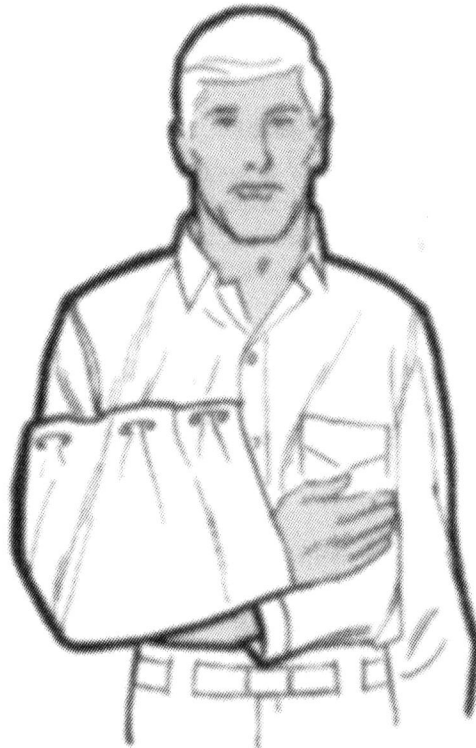

d. Shirttail

Fig. 3–35. Splinting a fractured forearm.

bones are broken, the arm usually appears deformed. In any fracture of the forearm, pain, tenderness, swelling, and inability to use the forearm may be present.

Treatment

The fracture should be straightened carefully by applying traction on the hand. (See Fig. 3–28.)

A half arm, inflatable air splint should be applied to the fracture. (See Fig. 3–32.) If inflatable splints are not available, two well-padded splints should be applied to the forearm: one on the top and one on the bottom. (See Fig. 3–35.) The splints should be long enough to extend from beyond the elbow to the middle of the fingers. The hand should be raised about four inches higher than the elbow, and the arm supported in a sling. (See Fig. 3–35.) An improvised splint could be applied, if other splints are not available.

For pain, aspirin 600 mg with codeine sulfate 30 mg should be given by mouth. If aspirin is not well tolerated by the patient, acetaminophen may be tried at the same dosage and frequency. To repeat the codeine sulfate, medical advice by radio should be obtained.

WRIST

The wrist usually is broken by falling with the hand outstretched. Usually a lump-like deformity occurs on the back of the wrist, along with pain, tenderness, and swelling.

Treatment

A fracture of the wrist should *not* be manipulated or straightened. In general, the fracture should be managed like a fracture of the forearm.

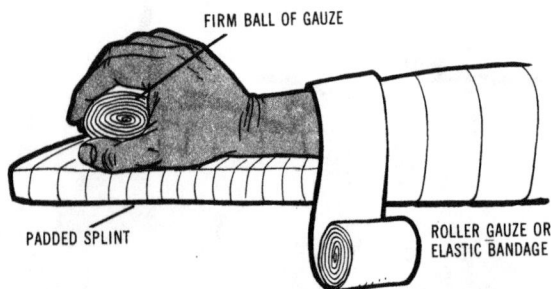

Fig. 3–36. Splint for crushed or fractured hand.

HAND

Crushed Hand

The hand may be fractured by a direct blow or may receive a crushing injury. There may be pain, swelling, loss of motion, open wounds, and broken bones.

Treatment

When there are open wounds, refer to Treatment of Wounds (p. 51+). The hand should be placed on a padded splint which extends from the middle to the lower arm to beyond the tips of the fingers. A firm ball of gauze should be placed under the fingers to hold the hand in a cupped position. Roller gauze or elastic bandage may be used to secure the hand to the splint. (See Fig. 3–36.) The arm and hand should be supported in a sling. (See Fig. 3–26.) Often, further treatment is urgent, regardless of the severity of the injury, to preserve as much of the function of the hand as possible. Medical advice by radio should be obtained.

Finger Dislocation

The fingers are injured easily and even a minor injury may cause a dislocation. The injury is recognized readily by the abnormal position of the two adjoining bones. There will be pain, swelling, and shortening of the finger; and the patient may be unable to bend the finger in the injured area.

Treatment

Before a reduction is attempted, morphine sulfate 10 mg may be given by intramuscular injection for pain, and the patient allowed to rest quietly for 30 minutes to one hour. To repeat the morphine sulfate, medical advice by radio should be obtained. The patient should be lying down before the procedure is started, and the hand should be placed in a position with the palm down. The finger should be grasped *above* and *below* the injured joint, with a small dressing to prevent slipping. Strong, steady traction should be applied, pulling straight out from the hand. The bone usually will slip into

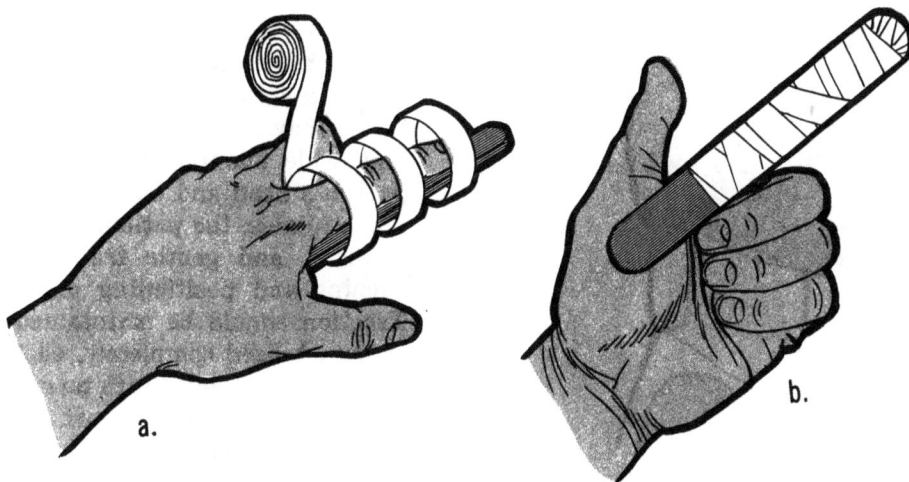

Fig. 3–37. Dislocated or fractured finger.

position with ease. If traction is applied to more than one joint, another dislocation could occur.

The injured finger should be immobilized with a splint. A padded tongue blade should be placed under the finger and secured in place with a roller gauze bandage. (See Fig. 3–37.) The arm should be placed in a sling. (See Fig. 3–26.) The patient should be examined by a physician on arrival in port.

Fractured Finger

The finger or thumb may be fractured by a direct blow, a crushing injury, a blow to the end of the finger, or when forced into sudden flexion or hyperextension.

Treatment

Only the fractured finger should be immobilized, and the mobility of the other fingers should be maintained. The finger should be straightened by grasping the wrist with one hand and applying traction to the fingertip with the other. The finger should be immobilized with a splint using the procedure described earlier for a dislocated finger. (See Fig. 3–37.) The patient should be examined by a physician as soon as possible.

For pain, aspirin 600 mg with codeine sulfate 30 mg should be given by mouth. If aspirin is not well tolerated by the patient, acetaminophen may be tried at the same dosage and frequency. Before repeating the codeine sulfate, medical advice by radio should be obtained.

SPINE (BACKBONE)

The treatment of a fractured spine should be aimed at minimizing shock and preventing further injury to the spinal cord. If a patient complains of acute pain in the back of the neck following an injury, it would be advisable to treat the injury as a fracture, even if no other symptoms appear.

Cervical (Neck)

Fractures of the neck are not common on shipboard. However, they may occur as a result of a fall from a high place, or from a blow to the neck or head by a heavy moving object.

The patient usually will complain of severe pain at the site of the fracture, with tingling or numbness. If the spinal cord has been damaged, there may be paralysis down from the site of the fracture. Usually there is severe shock which may be delayed for a period of time. Patients with neck paralysis may not be able to urinate; but they should not be catheterized, unless advised to do so by a physician. Medical advice by radio should be obtained.

Treatment

To treat a fractured neck one person should hold the patient's head straight and apply gentle traction, while another person applies a cervical collar. (See Fig. 3–38.) Using several people, the patient should be rolled onto his side while supporting the neck, and a long spine

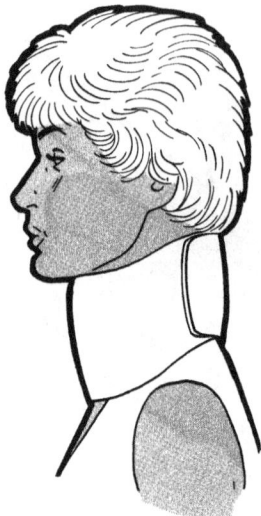

Fig. 3–38. Cervical collar.

board placed next to him. (See Fig. 3–39.) After he has been rolled onto the board, he should be strapped securely to it. (Fig. 3–40.)

If a spine board is not available, any long board may be used. This board should be long and wide enough to contain completely the patient's head and body. If a cervical collar is not available, the patient's head should be held straight, and gentle traction applied during turning and positioning on the spine board. Traction should be maintained until the head is immobilized completely. Clothing, about the thickness of a rolled bath towel should be placed under the neck to support it. A sandbag, or similar material, should be placed on each side of the head, and the head secured to the board with a cravat bandage. For cervical fractures,

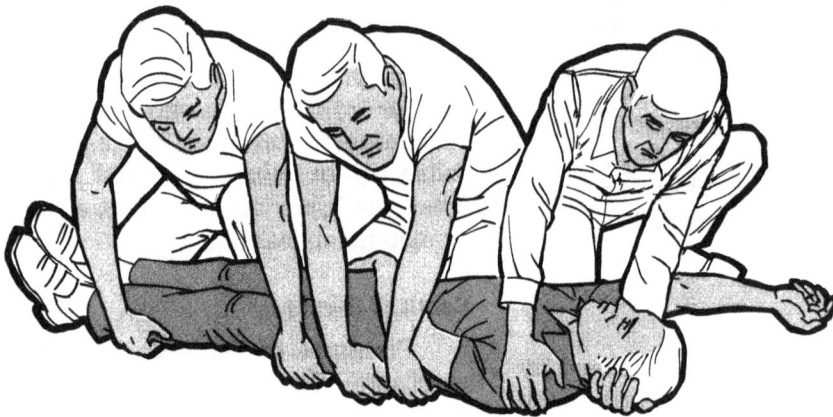

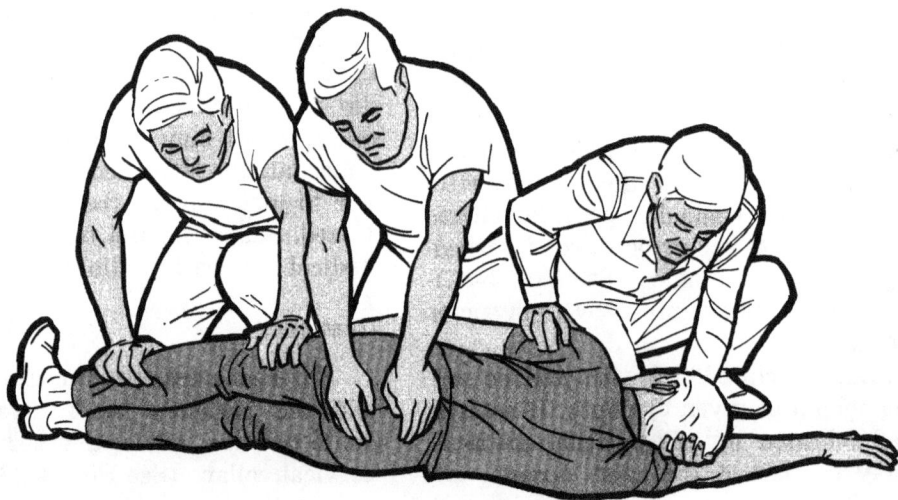

Fig. 3–39. Rolling a patient onto his side.

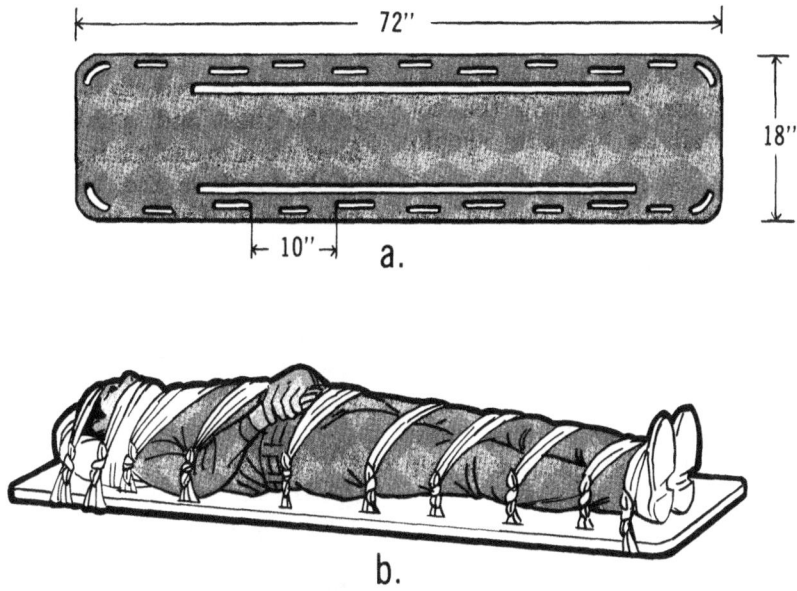

Fig. 3–40. Long spine board.

a short spine board also can be used, depending on the position and location of the patient. It should be placed behind the patient and all straps secured. (See Fig. 3–41.) Then the patient should be placed on a stretcher and transferred to a bed in his quarters or sickbay. The bed should have a board placed beneath the mat-tress. The cervical collar should be left in place, and the patient cautioned against undue move-ments. If the patient does not have a cervical collar, sandbags should be placed on each side of the head to assure immobilization.

For pain, aspirin 600 mg with codeine sulfate 30 mg should be given by mouth. If

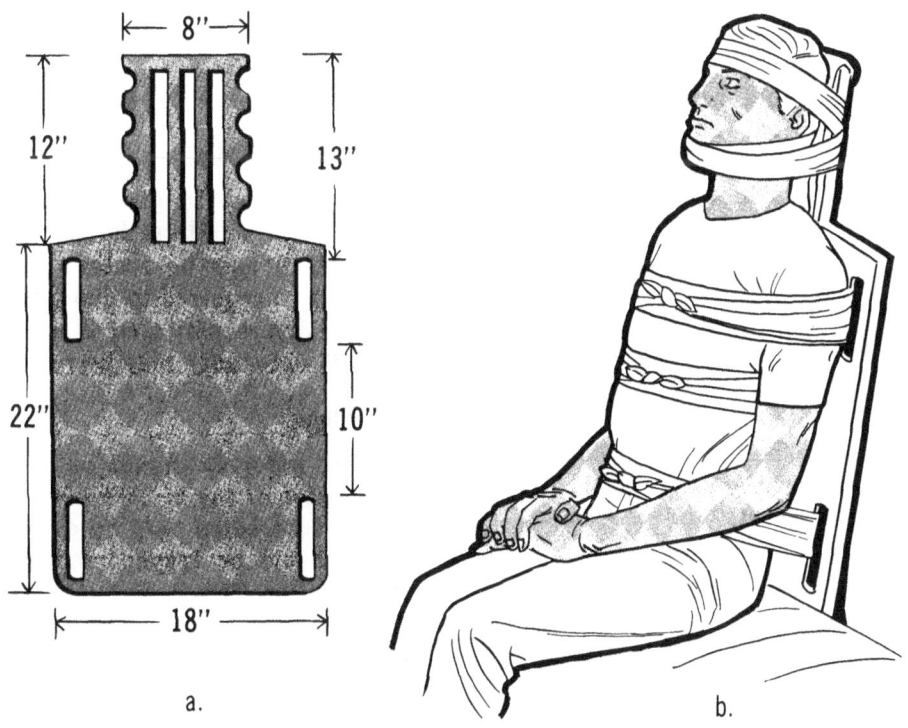

Fig. 3–41. Short spine board.

aspirin is not well tolerated by the patient, acetaminophen may be tried at the same dosage and frequency. Before repeating the codeine sulfate, medical advice by radio should be obtained.

Because medical attention is needed urgently, evacuation of these patients by helicopter should be discussed by radio.

Thoracic and Lumbar (Back)

Fractures of the back are not common but do occur occasionally aboard ship. They may occur as a result of a fall from a height, a fall across a rail, a crushing injury, or a sharp blow to the spine.

The symptoms of a fractured back are similar to the symptoms of a fractured neck. If the spinal cord is damaged, paralysis may occur below the site of the injury. Pain may be severe, or there may be a little discomfort with only a tender area around the spine. As with all spinal fractures, the danger lies in the possibility of damage to the spinal cord. *Correct handling of the patient is crucial.* The slightest displacement of a fractured vertebra may damage the spinal cord, producing paralysis below the point of injury.

Treatment

The patient should be transported lying in a face-down position. If this is not possible, padding should be placed under the small of the back to retain it in its natural position. Refer to Cervical (Neck) p. 85+ for rolling and positioning of the patient on a long spine board or any long board. *The patient's body must not be twisted or bent when moving him or further damage may occur to the spinal cord.* The patient may be placed on his back after he has been transferred to a bed with a large board under the mattress. The proper position must be maintained, and the patient should be cautioned against undue movement.

For pain, aspirin 600 mg with codeine sulfate 30 mg should be given by mouth. If aspirin is not well tolerated by the patient, acetaminophen may be tried at the same dosage and frequency. Before repeating the codeine sulfate, medical advice by radio should be obtained.

RIB

A fractured rib is the most common injury to the chest and usually is caused by a direct blow or a crushing injury. There will be pain at the fracture site, with little displacement or deformity. There may be severe pain when breathing, bending, or coughing. The patient may press his hands against the chest to prevent painful movement. If the lung has been punctured, bright red, frothy blood may be coughed up.

Treatment

If the patient is fairly comfortable, it will not be necessary to apply anything to the chest. If there is severe pain, the ribs can be immobilized somewhat by applying adhesive tape. If the patient should become short of breath, the tape should be removed. If necessary, an elastic bandage may be applied in place of the adhesive tape. (Refer to p. 95, for treatment of a Punctured Lung.)

For pain, aspirin 600 mg with codeine sulfate 30 mg should be given by mouth. If aspirin is not well tolerated by the patient, acetaminophen may be tried at the same dosage and frequency. Before repeating the codeine sulfate, medical advice by radio should be obtained.

HIP

Dislocation of Hip

A hip may be dislocated by a fall, a blow to the thigh, or direct force to the foot or knee. A fracture may be present as a result of the great force required to dislocate the hip. There will be severe pain and loss of motion, and a marked deformity may be present.

Treatment

No attempt should be made to reduce a dislocation of the hip. The injury is serious and should be treated only by a physician. The patient should be transported on a long spine board. (See Fig. 3–40.) A blanket, pillow, or other suitable padding should be used to support the legs in the position of the deformity. This position should be maintained after the patient has been transferred to a bed in his quarters or the sickbay.

For pain, aspirin 600 mg with codeine sulfate 30 mg should be given by mouth. If aspirin is not well tolerated by the patient, acetaminophen may be tried at the same dosage and frequency. Before repeating the codeine sulfate, medical advice by radio should be obtained.

Fracture of Hip

A fractured hip usually is caused by a fall. There is severe pain in the groin area, and the patient may not be able to lift the injured leg. The leg may appear shortened and be rotated, causing the toes to point abnormally outward. Shock generally will accompany this type of fracture.

Treatment

A fracture of the hip should be splinted with a half-ring traction splint—a Thomas or Hare Traction Splint. (See Fig. 3–42.) If one is not available, a well-padded board splint should be placed from the armpit to beyond

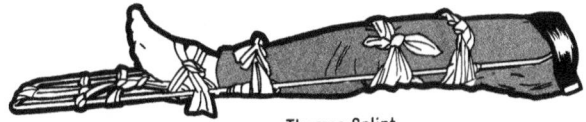

a. Thomas Splint

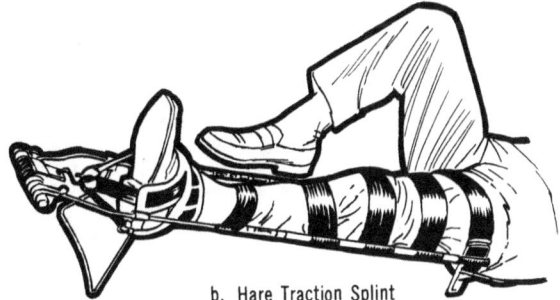

b. Hare Traction Splint

Fig. 3–42. Half ring traction splints.

the foot. Another well-padded splint should be placed on the inner side of the leg from the groin to beyond the foot. The splints should be secured in place with an adequate number of ties, and both legs tied together to provide additional support. (See Fig. 3–43.) The patient

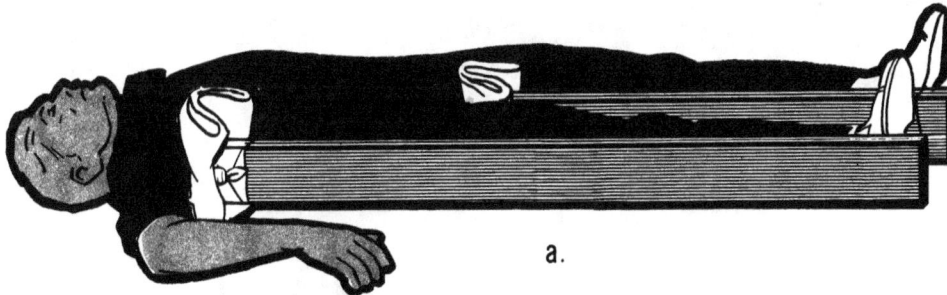

a.

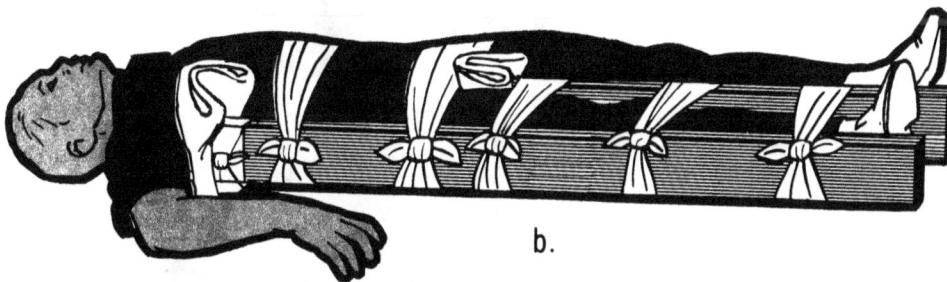

b.

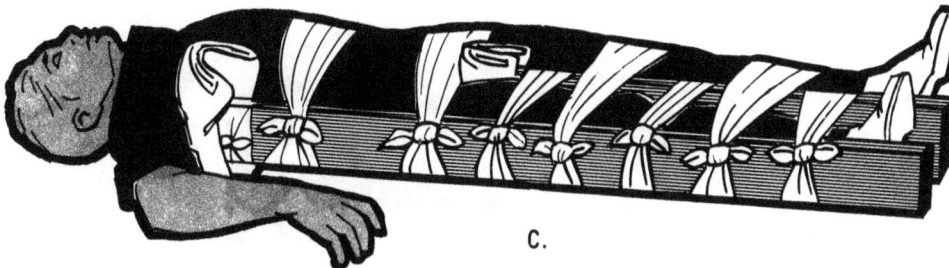

c.

Fig. 3–43. Fractured hip or femur.

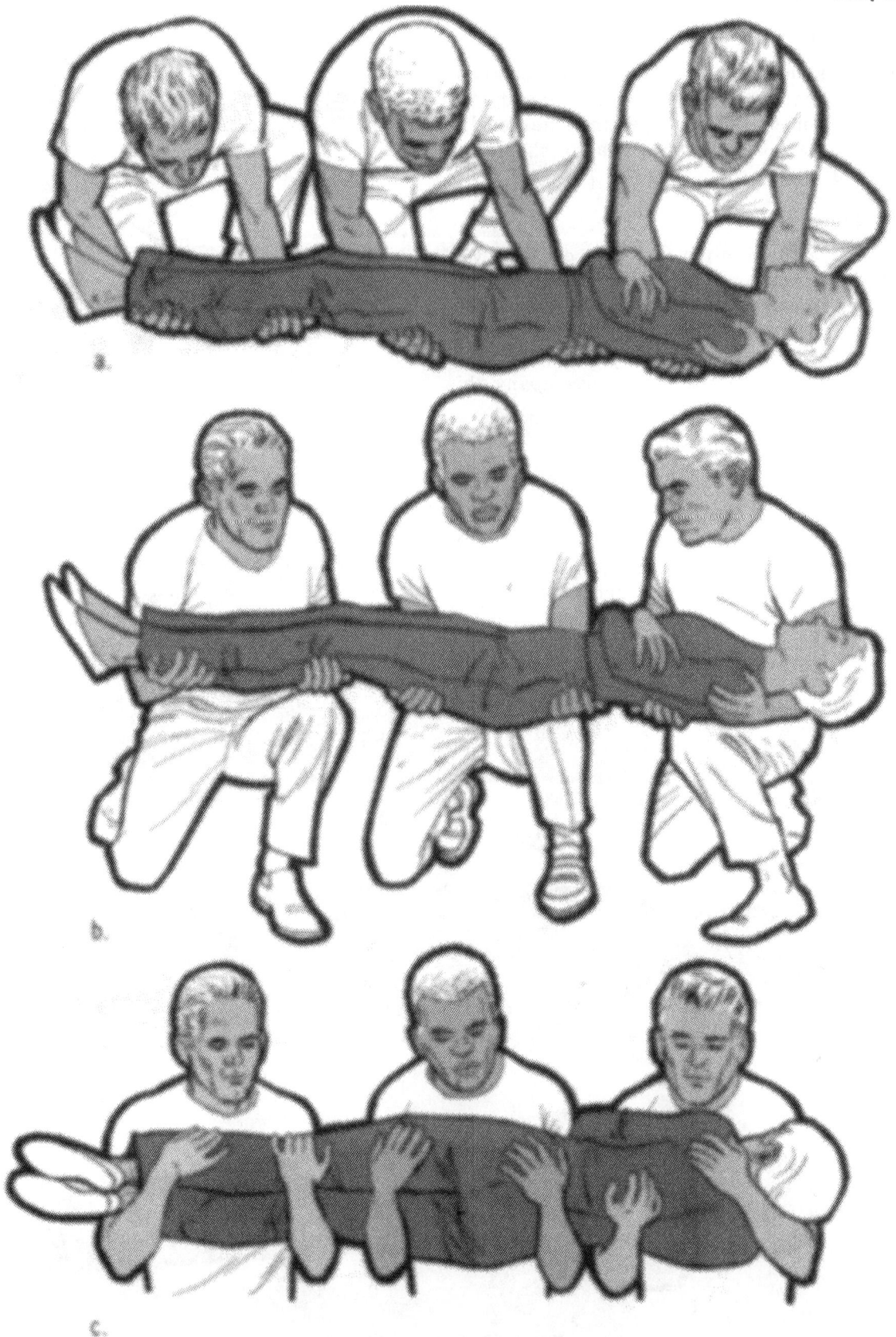

Fig. 3–44. Lifting a patient (three persons).

should be transported on a long spine board to a bed in his quarters or sickbay. (See Fig. 3–40.) If a backboard is not available, a stretcher may be used.

For pain, aspirin 600 mg with codeine sulfate 30 mg should be given by mouth. If aspirin is not well tolerated by the patient, acetaminophen may be tried at the same dosage and frequency. Before repeating the codeine sulfate, medical advice by radio should be obtained.

PELVIS

Pelvic fractures usually are caused by falls, crushing accidents, and sharp blows. Severe pain, shock, internal bleeding, and the loss of ability to use the lower extremities may be present. The bladder may be injured or ruptured, as well as other organs which are protected by the pelvis.

Treatment

The patient with a fractured pelvis should be treated for shock, but not placed in a shock position. A long spine board or rigid stretcher will provide the necessary support during transportation. If possible, four people should be used to lift the patient onto the spine board. (See Fig. 3–44.) Rolling the patient may cause additional internal damage. A pad should be placed between the patient's thighs, and the knees and ankles bandaged together. The patient may be placed on the spine board with the knees straight or bent, whichever position is more comfortable. If the knees are flexed, padding should be placed under them for support. The patient should be secured firmly to the spineboard both above and below the pelvis. (See Fig. 3–45.)

If medical care by a physician is to be delayed, the patient with a pelvic fracture is best treated by placing him on a bed that has a firm mattress or a board which is under the mattress.

For severe pain, morphine sulfate 10 mg may be given by intramuscular injection. Before repeating the morphine sulfate, advice by radio should be obtained.

FEMUR (THIGH)

A fracture of the femur usually is caused by a fall or direct blow. There will be severe pain, a shortening of the leg, deformity, and a grating sensation. The limb has a wobbly motion, and below the fracture, there is a complete loss of control. Severe damage to the nerves and blood vessels may occur.

Treatment

The injured leg should be straightened carefully by applying gentle traction on the foot. (See Fig. 3–28.) If available, the fracture should be splinted with a half-ring traction splint—a Thomas or Hare Traction Splint. (See Fig. 3–42.) The traction of the limb will reduce pain and tissue damage during transportation. If a traction splint is not available, a full leg, inflatable splint may be applied. (See Fig. 3–32.) If necessary, the fracture may be splinted with long, well-padded board splints. For the procedure, see fracture of the hip, p. 89+.

For pain, aspirin 600 mg with codeine sulfate 30 mg should be given by mouth. If aspirin is not well tolerated by the patient, acetaminophen may be tried at the same dosage and frequency. Before repeating the codeine sulfate, medical advice by radio should be obtained.

KNEE

A fracture of the knee generally occurs as a result of a fall or a direct blow. Besides the usual signs of a fracture, a groove in the kneecap may be felt. There will be an inability

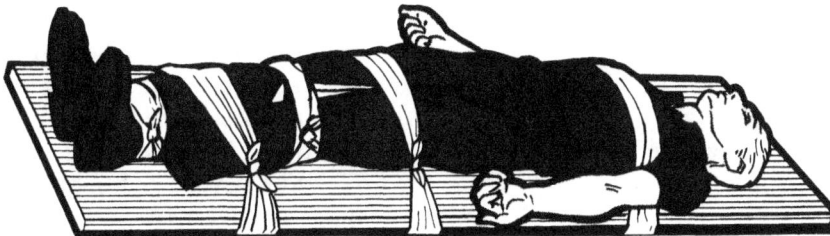

Fig. 3–45. Pelvic fracture.

to kick the leg forward, and the leg will drag if an attempt is made to walk.

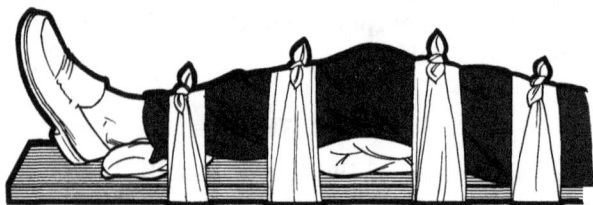

Fig. 3–46. Splinting fractured kneecap.

Treatment

The leg should be straightened carefully. (See Fig. 3–28.) A full leg, inflatable air splint should be applied. If other types of splints are used, a well-padded board splint should be placed with padding under the knee and below the ankle. The splint should be secured in place with ties. (See Fig. 3–46.) When splints are not available, a pillow or a blanket may be used to immobilize the knee.

For pain, aspirin 600 mg with codeine sulfate 30 mg should be given by mouth. If aspirin is not well tolerated by the patient, acetaminophen may be tried at the same dosage and frequency. Before repeating the codeine sulfate, medical advice by radio should be obtained.

TIBIA AND FIBULA (LOWER LEG)

Fractures of the lower leg are common and occur as a result of various accidents. There is a marked deformity of the leg when

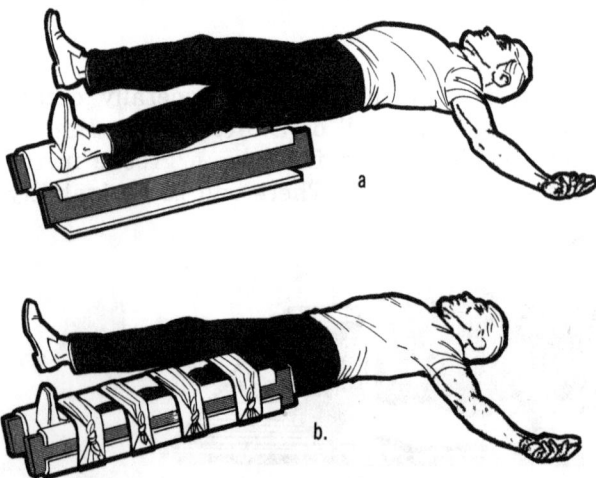

Fig. 3–47. Splinting fractures of tibia and fibula.

both bones are broken. When only one bone is broken, the other acts as a splint and little deformity may be present. When the tibia (the bone in the front of the leg) is broken, a compound fracture is likely to occur. Swelling may be present and the pain usually is severe enough to require morphine sulfate (see below).

Treatment

The leg should be straightened carefully, using slight traction. (See Fig. 3–28.) A full leg, inflatable air splint may be applied, if available. (See Fig. 3–32.) The air splint will assist in controlling the bleeding, if there is a com-

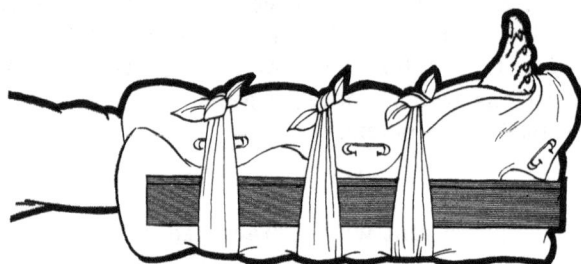

a. Splints

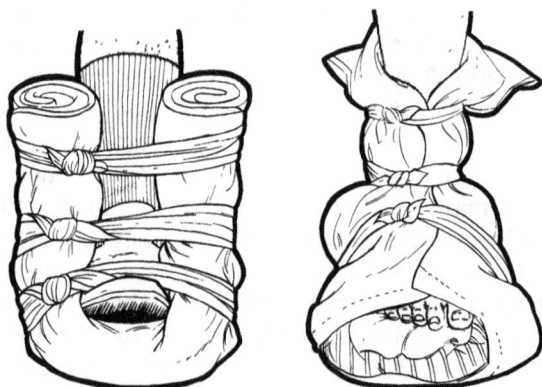

b Improvised With Blanket   c Improvised With Pillow

Fig. 3–48. Splinting fractures of ankle and foot.

pound fracture. If other types of splints are used, three should be applied. A well-padded splint should be applied to each side of the leg, and another should be placed under the leg. The splints should extend from the middle of the thigh to beyond the heel. (See Fig. 3–47.)

For severe pain, morphine sulfate 10 mg may be given by intramuscular injection. To repeat the morphine sulfate, medical advice by radio should be obtained.

ANKLE AND FOOT

A fracture of the ankle or foot usually is caused by a fall, twist, or a blow. Pain and swelling will be present, along with marked disability.

Treatment

If available, a half-leg, inflatable air splint should be applied. If conventional splints are applied, the ankle should be well-padded with dressings or a pillow. The splints, applied to each side of the leg, should extend from the midcalf to beyond the foot. (See Fig. 3–48.)

For pain, aspirin 600 mg with codeine sulfate 30 mg should be given by mouth. If aspirin is not well tolerated by the patient, acetaminophen may be tried at the same dosage and frequency. Before repeating the codeine sulfate, medical advice by radio should be obtained.

TOE

A fractured toe usually is caused by a crushing injury or by kicking the foot against a hard object. There is pain and swelling, and a deformity may be present.

Treatment

If necessary, the injured toe can be bandaged to the next toe to provide support, or splinted with a tongue depressor.

For pain, aspirin 600 mg with codeine sulfate 30 mg should be given by mouth. If aspirin is not well tolerated by the patient, acetaminophen may be tried at the same dosage and frequency. To continue the codeine sulfate, medical advice by radio should be obtained.

Chapter III

Emergency Treatment of Injuries

Section E

INJURIES TO SPECIFIC BODY AREAS

ABDOMINAL INJURIES

Open Wounds

A WOUND THAT PENETRATES the abdominal cavity is extremely dangerous because of possible damage to internal organs. The stomach or intestine may be perforated, internal bleeding may occur, and infection may develop. Bacteria may be introduced into the peritoneal cavity from the outside or from a perforated intestine.

Usually there is intense pain, severe shock, nausea, and vomiting; a spasm of the abdominal muscles may occur.

Treatment

As soon as possible, plans should be made to evacuate the patient from the ship to the nearest medical facility, because immediate surgical treatment generally is required.

The patient should be placed on his back. If the intestine is exposed or protruding, a pillow or bulky material should be put under his knees to relax the abdominal muscles. *No attempt ever should be made to push the protruding intestine back into the abdominal cavity, because of the danger of infection.*

The intestine should be covered with a sterile dressing that is dampened with sterile or cool, boiled water, or lactated Ringer's solution.

The dressing should be large enough to cover the wound and surrounding skin, and should be held in place with a bandage. Care should be taken *not* to fasten the bandage so tight that it interferes with circulation. When the intestines are not protruding, a dry, sterile dressing may be applied to the wound.

The patient should be treated for shock (see p. 57+). Morphine sulfate 10 mg intramuscularly may be given if the patient has no difficulty in breathing. To repeat the morphine sulfate, medical advice by radio should be obtained. *No fluids should be given by mouth* because surgery will be necessary as soon as the patient reaches a medical facility.

Closed Wounds

Closed wounds from severe blows or crushing injuries may be extremely dangerous. Serious injury to internal organs, internal hemorrhage, and shock may occur. Complications might develop within the first 48 hours that will be as serious as the immediate effects of the injury.

Treatment

Treatment for a closed wound should be the same as for an open wound, except for the application of a dressing.

BACK INJURIES

Treatment

Closed injuries to the spine are covered on p. 85. These injuries usually are the result of falls, crushing accidents, and sharp blows across the back. Severe pain in the side, blood in the urine, muscle spasm, and shock may indicate an injury to a kidney.

Open injuries to the back usually are the result of stabbings, bullets, and flying debris from explosions. The treatment for an open wound should be followed for this type of injury. (See p. 94.)

Medical advice by radio should be obtained, and plans should be made as soon as possible to evacuate the patient to a medical facility.

CHEST INJURIES

Sucking Wounds

Because of the lower internal pressure, an open wound into the chest cavity permits air to flow in and out as the patient breathes. (See Fig. 3–49.) This may cause the lung to collapse and fail to function. Also, there is a danger of internal hemorrhaging, if the lung, heart, or large blood vessels have been punctured. A sucking chest wound *always* should be suspected, when there is an open chest wound.

The patient may have increasing difficulty in breathing, blueness of the skin (cyanosis), faintness, dizziness, thirst, and a rapid pulse. If the lung, heart, or large blood vessels have been punctured, the patient may cough up frothy, bright red blood, have a weak pulse, faint heart sounds, and distention of the neck and arm veins. There may be a "sucking" or "hissing" sound as the air flows in and out of the chest cavity.

Treatment

The wound opening must be sealed off immediately. A large dressing of sterile gauze should be applied and the area sealed off with overlapping strips of 3-inch adhesive tape. (See Fig. 3–49.) If sterile gauze dressings are not available immediately, the palm of the hand could be used temporarily. The patient should be placed on the injured side so the uninjured lung can expand more freely. The patient can be treated for shock, if it occurs. (See p. 57+.) An airway should be maintained and artificial respiration administered, as necessary. (See p. 115+.)

Medical advice by radio should be obtained for additional treatment; and as soon as possible, plans should be made to evacuate the patient from the ship to the nearest medical facility.

Protruding Objects
Treatment

Never remove the wounding object, if it is still in place. Fatal bleeding may occur if it is removed. Dressings should be placed around the object to immobilize it, and a bandage applied to hold the dressings in place. Artificial respiration should be provided if the patient is having

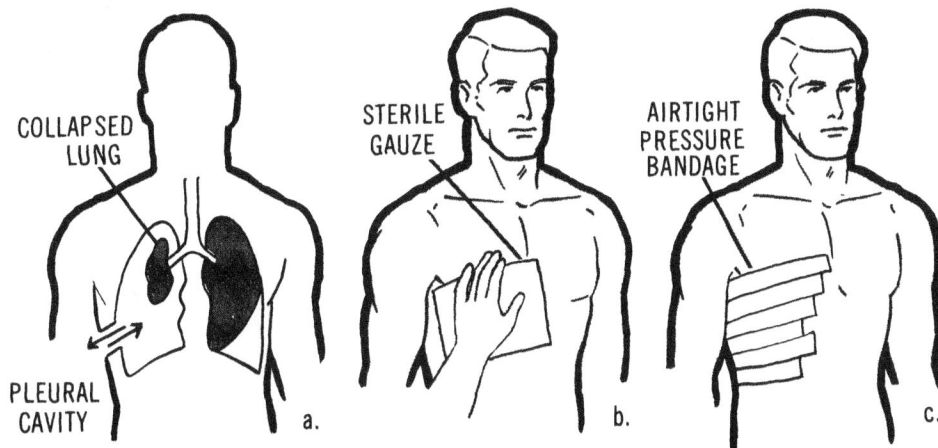

COLLAPSED LUNG

STERILE GAUZE

AIRTIGHT PRESSURE BANDAGE

PLEURAL CAVITY

a.

b.

c.

Fig. 3–49. Treatment of a sucking chest wound.

difficulty breathing, or is *not* breathing. (See p. 115+.) Treatment for shock should be given. (See p. 57+.)

Medical advice by radio should be obtained, and plans should be made as soon as possible to evacuate the patient from the ship to the nearest medical facility.

Compression of the Lung

Blood, air, and other fluids may enter the chest cavity and compress the lung. *Immediate medical attention is necessary* and plans should be made as soon as possible to evacuate the patient to the nearest medical facility.

Treatment

The patient may have difficulty breathing. An airway should be established (see p. 116); and artificial respiration applied, if necessary. (See p. 115+.)

Crushing Injuries

These injuries usually result from vehicle accidents and falls. The severe pain from the injuries, often intensified by broken ribs, tends to cause the patient to restrict breathing. Also, the chest wall may collapse between the multiple fractures on each side of the chest (flail chest), which prevents an adequate amount of air to be exchanged.

Treatment

To make breathing easier, the patient should be placed in a comfortable position with the head and shoulders elevated. If the patient has a flail chest, the rib cage should be splinted. (See p. 63.) Medical advice by radio should be obtained for additional treatment, and plans should be made to evacuate the patient to the nearest medical facility.

EAR INJURIES

Cuts and Lacerations

Cuts and lacerations of the ear occur frequently; and occasionally, a section of the ear may be severed. This section should be saved, placed in ice water, and sent to the medical facility with the patient. There, it may be sutured to the patient's ear.

Treatment

The treatment of these cuts and lacerations would be the same as for regular wounds. (See p. 51+.) If there is excessive bleeding, direct pressure should be applied (see p. 53+), and the bleeding controlled before the area is bandaged.

PERFORATION (RUPTURE) OF THE EARDRUM

An injury to the eardrum generally occurs as a result of a blow to the ear, explosion or blast, or a sudden change in the pressure on the ear, as from a dive into deep water. Also, an infection in the middle ear may cause the eardrum to rupture.

Treatment

The ear should not be tampered with and no instrument should be inserted into it. A small piece of cotton should be placed loosely into the ear canal to protect the injured area, until medical assistance can be obtained.

When the eardrum has been perforated as a result of a skull fracture, the flow of the cerebrospinal fluid should not be stopped. Also, nothing should be inserted into the ear canal because of the danger of causing a brain tissue infection. The patient should be placed on his injured side, with the shoulders and head propped up. This will allow the fluid to drain freely until medical assistance can be obtained.

EYE INJURIES

Emergencies

There are two ocular emergencies that require *immediate treatment* within seconds to minutes. They are chemical burns of the cornea (especially alkali burns) and closure of the central retinal artery.

Treatment

It is doubtful if anything can be done aboard ship to treat successfully the central retinal artery problem; but there is a possibility that the following measures may help. If a person complains of a sudden, complete or almost complete loss of vision in one eye, two things can be tried:

• Breathing and rebreathing into a paper bag may help to dilate retinal vessels due to the effect of carbon dioxide. Continue rebreathing the exhaled air from the bag for 15 minutes.

• Massage the eyeball through the closed eyelids with the fingers. Do this while the patient is breathing into the bag. There is a remote chance that by these measures, an embolus blocking the artery will move into the periphery of the retina.

Chemical Injuries
Treatment

Almost without exception, immediate first aid for a chemical injury to the eye is: *immediate gentle irrigation of the eye with large amounts of fresh clean water or a neutral fluid such as milk (at least two or three quarts).* Do *not* use boric acid solution. Sterile normal saline or 5% dextrose solution intended for intravenous administration can be used, when available. *Do not delay the irrigation to obtain these special solutions. Fresh clean water will do!*

Seconds count! The eyelids must be opened for irrigation. It may be necessary to use force to open the lids. However, care must be taken not to exert pressure on the eyeball if there is a penetrating injury. If a person is alone, the eye should be flushed over a fountain, in a shower, or under a faucet. The difference between retention of vision and possible future blindness can depend upon one's remembering to irrigate the eye gently with large amounts of fresh, cool water or milk.

After irrigation, homatropine hydrobromide 5% eye drops should be instilled into the injured eye. Then, antibiotic ophthalmic ointment should be applied and the eye covered with a dressing. For pain, acetaminophen 600 mg may be given by mouth alone or with codeine sulfate 30 mg, if necessary. To repeat the codeine sulfate, medical advice by radio should be obtained. The bandage should be changed daily. The patient should be evacuated immediately to the nearest medical facility. Corticosteroid drops should be used *only* on the advice of a physician.

Alkalies, such as sodium hydroxide (lye), ammonium hydroxide (ammonia), calcium hydroxide (slaked lime), toilet bowl cleaner, and other caustics cause many of the most serious chemical injuries to the eyes. *The eye should be irrigated immediately and medical advice*

by radio obtained. The patient should be evacuated to the nearest medical facility, as soon as possible.

Acids, such as sulfuric acid, hydrochloric acid, chromic acid, superphosphate fertilizers and sulfur dioxide gas (forms sulfurous acid when dissolved in water), also can cause severe injury. Early medical attention is indicated after irrigation of the eye.

Petroleum products, such as crude oil, gasoline, kerosene, and naphtha may cause local irritation of the eye. Usually they do not cause severe ocular damage. The immediate treatment is the same as with chemical injuries. In minor cases, it only may be necessary to irrigate the eye thoroughly.

Other chemicals generally require the same irrigation treatment. If the chemical is harmful, usually the eye will become painful, red, and teary. If these symptoms do not occur immediately or are only slight, the substance in question probably is not very injurious to the eye.

In all cases of injury to the eye, it is useful to evaluate the visual acuity in the injured eye after irrigation and before instilling any medication. If an eye chart is not available, the patient should be asked to read a newspaper at 14 inches. If this is not possible, "counting fingers" vision, hand motion or perception should be evaluated. This will give some idea of the visual capacity of the injured eye. The patient should be asked:

• If light can be perceived through the injured eye.

• If hand motion can be seen in front of his face.

• If the number of fingers held in front of his face can be identified.

Foreign Bodies

Common foreign bodies include eyelashes, sand, soot, cinders, chips of rust, paint, and metal shavings. Sometimes a chip of steel may come off a steel chisel or hammer, and strike the eye with such speed that it punctures the eye like a bullet. The only symptom, other than mild irritation, may be severe loss of vision. *In such a case immediate medical attention must be obtained.* Wearing safety glasses, whenever working with tools such as a chipping hammer or lathe, will help prevent such accidents.

Treatment

Most foreign bodies are flushed out of the eye by the large amount of tears produced by the irritation. However, sometimes the foreign body remains and must be removed. A small speck on the *conjunctiva* can be removed almost painlessly by irrigation, or by carefully lifting it up with the end of a moist, sterile, cotton-tipped applicator. *However, an attempt should not be made to remove a foreign body from the cornea with a dry unsterile cotton-tipped applicator.*

Foreign bodies on the cornea are often difficult to see and must be looked for carefully. A foreign body often lodges under the upper eyelid where it can be found by rolling back the lid and looking at its undersurface. Frequently, there is more than one foreign body in the eye at one time. When the foreign body is found, an attempt should be made to remove it by irrigating with a fine spray from a bottle of sterile eye irrigating solution. If the foreign body does not come off easily, it is best to patch the eye and try again in 12 to 24 hours. Medical advice by radio should be obtained for additional treatment.

The eye may remain somewhat irritated, even after the foreign body has been removed. The patient should be started on a course of polymyxin B - neomycin - gramicidin eye drops. (See p. 288.) Occasionally the patient will be more comfortable if the eye is patched with a sterile dressing for 24 hours.

Scratches, Cuts, and Abrasions

When a patient has rubbed something in his eye and injured it, the sensation of a foreign body (pain, redness, tearing) may be felt. Often in these cases a small scratch or abrasion has occurred on the cornea. Frequently this can be seen only when fluorescein is placed in the eye. The scratch or abrasion takes up the fluorescein and is outlined as brilliant green. (See p. 279.) It may be necessary to place a drop of anesthetic (proparacaine hydrochloride eye drops 0.5%) into the eye in order to examine for a scratch, cut, or abrasion. Do *not* use anesthetic ointments.

Treatment

The treatment for a scratch, cut, or abrasion of the eye consists of instilling polymyxin B-neomycin-bacitracin ophthalmic ointment and patching the eye. The bandage should be changed each day for two to three days. (Superficial abrasions and scratches of the cornea often heal overnight.) If the patient still is uncomfortable after this time period, medical care should be obtained.

A deep cut into the eye through the cornea and sclera is a severe injury. When this occurs, the inner portions of the eye may come out through the wound. These inner structures often look grey to black, and the anterior chamber may be filled with blood. These are very serious cases that require the immediate care of a skilled eye surgeon in order to save the eye. Two drops of the antibiotic polymyxin B-neomycin-gramicidin eye drops should be instilled immediately into the eye. The eye should be patched lightly, and emergency medical care obtained as soon as possible. *Do not exert pressure on the eyeball when opening the lids.* The contents of the eye might extrude if the wound extends through the cornea and/or sclera.

Contusions and Black Eyes

Severe contusions of the eyeball and extensive black eyes caused by blunt objects or fists should be seen by an eye physician on return to port, although the injured part may seem to be recovering satisfactorily. Damage to the lens or retina may be present and blowout orbital fractures can occur without obvious clinical evidence.

Treatment

If a blood clot (hyphema) can be seen behind the cornea and in front of the iris when the patient is upright, the patient should be placed into bed with both eyes patched for six days. Bleeding may recur if ambulation is allowed following contusion hyphema, with secondary glaucoma resulting as a hazard to vision. Subconjunctival hemorrhages without other findings need no treatment.

Thermal Injuries to Eyes

Flame Burns

Flame burns to the eyes may be of three types:

- First-degree (superficial)—reddening of the skin without blistering.
- Second-degree—blistering of involved areas.
- Third-degree—charring and more complete destruction of the tissues.

Treatment

Superficial burns of the eyelids may be left open to the air. If the patient experiences mild pain, cold compresses often provide sufficient relief.

Second- and third-degree burns of the lids should be covered with a sterile, dry dressing, *if the patient is to be evacuated immediately.* Blisters should not be opened. Early treatment and skin grafting often are necessary in these cases to prevent permanent scarring and deformity.

If the patient is not to be evacuated immediately, the following treatment should be administered. Considerable pain and sensitivity to light may be present, so a drop of anesthetic such as proparacaine hydrochloride 0.5% eye drops placed in the eye may be required to permit examination. Involvement of the eyeball is indicated by marked redness of the conjunctiva, or greyness and even charring of the conjunctiva and cornea.

To prevent infection, polymyxin B-neomycin-bacitracin ophthalmic ointment should be placed in the eye and a sterile patch taped in place over the closed lid. Additional ointment should be placed in the eye daily and the dressing changed. Medical advice by radio should be obtained and systemic pain medications administered as prescribed.

Contact Burns

Treatment

Matchheads, hot cinders, and fly ash often strike the cornea and produce a localized grey or yellow cloudy area. Even the smallest corneal break or injury can cause severe pain and requires treatment similar to that for flame burns to prevent infection and permanent scarring.

Molten metal of low melting points, such as lead or solder, often form a mold on the front of the eye. Removal of the metal, treatment with polymyxin B-neomycin-gramicidin ophthalmic drops, and patching the eye often result in complete healing in two to three days. The eye should be examined and the bandage changed every day.

Scalds by hot fluids and steam should be treated as flame burns after irrigation of the eye. Large amounts of sterile water or mild eye irrigating solution should remove traces of such fluids as gasoline and oil. The eyeball itself rarely is affected due to the protection of the blink reflex. However, it should be examined in every case.

Welder's (Ultraviolet) Keratitis

The most common ultraviolet injuries are the result of gazing without dark goggles into a welding arc or the arc from an electrical short circuit. The ultraviolet light often can affect the eye, even if the patient does not look directly at the arc.

Initial symptoms first appear after 30 minutes to 12 hours, depending upon the intensity of the rays and the length of exposure. Patients generally report pain about the eyes, sensitivity to light, and/or a gritty, burning sensation.

Treatment

These patients should rest in a darkened room. Cold compresses should be placed on the eyes and forehead, and medication by mouth for pain may be required. Anesthetic eye drops such as proparacaine hydrochloride 0.5% should *not* be used except when necessary to examine the cornea. *In no case* should eye drops or ointment be given to the patient for pain during the recovery phase. Eye patches may be necessary for comfort during the first 24 hours.

With the above treatment, patients usually recover completely within 24 to 48 hours.

HEAD INJURIES

Scalp Injuries

Open wounds of the scalp are prone to bleed profusely, and the wound edges usually tend to gape. Also, dirt, hair, glass, soil, or other foreign matter, and bone fragments may be found in deep wounds.

Treatment

Minor wounds of the scalp should be treated like regular wounds. (See p. 62.) If the skull is fractured, deep scalp wounds should not be cleansed because it may lead to serious bleeding or contamination of the brain tissues. Severe bleeding should be controlled by placing a sterile dressing on the wound. If a fracture is suspected, firm pressure should be applied, but *not* forcibly. Once the bleeding has been controlled, a bandage may be applied to hold the dressing in place.

For a severe wound or a suspected fracture, medical advice should be obtained by radio and plans made to evacuate the patient to the nearest medical facility as soon as possible.

Brain Injuries

An injury to the brain may be present in all head injuries. The extent of the injury may be estimated within limits by the severity of the symptoms.

An open skull fracture may be present with destruction of the covering membrane and brain tissues. For this type of injury, the risk of infection is very high, due to the probable contamination of the wound.

Immediately following a head injury, temporary loss of consciousness may occur, which may or may not indicate brain injury. However, when unconsciousness persists for a long period of time, some degree of brain injury probably has occurred. Also, a patient with this type of injury later may lose consciousness due to the progressive swelling of the brain within the skull.

Symptoms of brain damage, which may develop at any time before or after the initial unconsciousness, may include:

• Confusion which may persist for some time, then clear up, or develop into semiconsciousness, stupor, or deep coma.

• Paralysis or numbness of the limbs (opposite the side of the injury) ; and of the face (same side as the injury).

• Convulsions which may be general or local. (See p. 212.)

• Difficulty in speaking.

• Excitement, restlessness, and occasionally delirium.

• Pupils of the eyes may be unequal in size.

• Watery, blood-tinged discharge from the patient's nose, ear canal, or mouth.

• Vomiting.

• Headache.

• Slow and full pulse which becomes fast and weak.

• Flushed or pale face.

• Loss of bladder or bowel control.

Treatment

Any patient with a suspected concussion, or other brain injury from either a major or a minor accident, should be watched carefully for 24 to 48 hours. Medical advice by radio should be obtained for specific treatment, and plans made as soon as possible to evacuate the patient to a medical facility.

The patient should be placed in bed, kept warm, and handled as little as possible. If a neck injury is *not* suspected, a pillow or a pad may be placed under the head and shoulders. *Never* place a pillow under the head only, because it may obstruct the airway. An open airway should be maintained, and the patient's head turned to the side, so secretions can drain from the mouth. Artificial respiration should be administered, as necessary. (See p. 115+.)

Bleeding should be controlled (see p. 53+), and a sterile dressing applied. Although watery, blood-tinged cerebrospinal fluid may drain from the patient's ears or nose for several days following a skull fracture, *no* attempt should be made to insert gauze or cotton to stop the flow. However, the ear may be covered by a light, sterile dressing. The patient should be cautioned against nose blowing.

Ice bags may be applied to the head for pain. Morphine sulfate should *not* be given. Fluids should *not* be given by mouth except on the advice of a physician.

An accurate record should be kept of the extent and duration of unconsciousness, pulse rate, breathing rate, and the patient's progress.

Face and Jaw Injuries

Injuries to the face and jaw generally occur as a result of fights, falls, vehicle accidents, and other violent type accidents. Obstruction of the air passage with blood and other secretions is common and requires immediate treatment. Teeth may be loose, deformed, or missing. This type of patient may have difficulty opening and closing the mouth, speaking, and swallowing.

Treatment

An open airway should be established immediately (see p. 116+). Open wounds should be treated as regular wounds (see p. 51+). *Unless a neck injury is suspected, a conscious patient without a neck injury* should be positioned to lean forward, so secretions can drain out. Sterile dressings should be applied. An *unconscious patient without a neck injury* should be turned toward the side with the head and shoulders elevated, to let secretions drain out. Treatment for shock should be given (see p. 57+). Artificial respiration (see p. 115+) should be administered as required.

Nose Injuries

Nosebleeds may occur as a result of an injury, a disease such as hypertension (high blood pressure), exposure to high altitudes, and overactivity or strenuous exercise. Most nosebleeds are not serious and can be treated aboard ship.

If the nose is fractured, the patient should be evacuated to a medical facility. Unless the broken parts are positioned properly, distortion of the nasal bones may result in difficulty in breathing.

Treatment

When treating a nosebleed, the patient should be in a sitting position, leaning forward. If the patient cannot lean forward, and must lie in a reclining position, the head and shoulders should be raised. Pressure should be applied to the bleeding site, and cold compresses applied to the face and nose. If the bleeding continues, a small gauze dressing should be placed in the nostrils and pressure applied.

Always leave a corner of the dressing protruding from each nostril, so it can be removed easily. The patient should remain quiet, and avoid blowing the nose for an hour after the bleeding has ceased. If the bleeding cannot be controlled, medical advice by radio should be obtained for additional treatment.

Mouth Injuries

Treatment

Small wounds of the lips, tongue, and cheeks usually heal quickly without serious infection. Large lacerations and gaping wounds will require suturing. Plans should be made as soon as possible to evacuate the patient from the ship to the nearest medical facility.

If there is bleeding, it can be controlled by direct pressure (see p. 53+) with a sterile gauze dressing. When there is a small wound, the mouth should be rinsed well with sodium bicarbonate mouthwashes several times a day. Good oral hygiene must be maintained. (See p. 152 for the treatment on loss of a tooth.)

NECK INJURIES

Treatment

Because the jugular veins are on each side of the neck, plus other deeper major arteries and veins, lacerations and puncture wounds can be extremely serious. If one of these blood vessels is damaged, direct pressure must be applied immediately, and maintained until the patient is seen by a physician. *This patient must be evacuated immediately to save his life.* A small wound would be treated as a regular wound. (See p. 51+.)

If pressure is applied forcibly to the throat, or if the throat is struck by a blunt force—collapse, swelling, or a serious spasm of the larynx may occur. Artificial respiration should be administered immediately (see p. 115+). An oropharyngeal tube should be inserted, if necessary (see p. 71). The patient's head and shoulders should be elevated if there are no suspected fractures of the back or neck. If the condition appears serious, plans should be made as soon as possible to evacuate the patient to the nearest medical facility for treatment of a possible fractured neck.

HAND INJURIES

Treatment

Minor wounds to the hand are common and should be treated as regular wounds. (See p. 51+.) If there has been a crushing type of injury and a fracture is suspected, the hand should be treated for a fracture. (See p. 84.)

Extensive wounds should not be cleansed. A roll of gauze or fluffed-up gauze dressings should be applied over the injured area, and a pressure bandage applied (see p. 54) to control the bleeding. Then the arm should be placed in a sling and elevated above the level of the heart to reduce the swelling. If the patient is on his back, pillows should be placed under the hand to elevate it.

For additional treatment, medical advice by radio should be obtained. Plans should be made as soon as possible to evacuate any patient with an extensive wound or fracture of the hand to the nearest medical facility.

GENITAL INJURIES

Injuries to the genitalia usually are the result of kicks, blows, falling astride rails or similar objects, machinery accidents, and being struck by flying missiles. Severe pain, faintness or fainting, considerable swelling and bleeding usually occur. If the urethra or bladder are damaged, urine and blood will leak into the injured area. Severed tissue should be saved, placed in ice water and sent with the patient to a medical facility.

Treatment

Bleeding should be controlled by direct pressure. (See p. 53+.) To ease the pain and reduce the swelling, the patient should be placed in bed with cold compresses applied to the injured area. The patient should be treated for shock, as necessary. If there is an open wound, a dressing should be applied. (See p. 58+.) Medical advice by radio should be obtained, if the injury appears serious.

Chapter III

Emergency Treatment of Injuries

Section F
COLD AND HEAT EXPOSURE EMERGENCIES

COLD EXPOSURES INJURIES (LOCAL)

COLD INJURIES TO PARTS of the body (face, extremities) are caused by exposure of tissues and small surface blood vessels to abnormally low temperatures. The extent of the injury depends upon such factors as temperature, duration of exposure, wind velocity, humidity, lack of protective clothing, or the presence of wet clothing. Also, the harmful effects of exposure to cold are intensified by fatigue, individual susceptibility, existing injuries, emotional stress, smoking, and drinking of alcoholic beverages.

Cold injuries to parts of the body are broken down into *Chilblain*, *Immersion Foot*, *Trench Foot*, and *Frostbite*. These are descriptive terms which indicate the way the injury occurred.

Chilblain

This relatively mild form of cold injury occurs in moderately cold climates with high humidity and temperatures above freezing, 32°F to 60.8°F (0°C to 16°C). Chilblain usually affects the back of the hand; but it may affect the lower extremities, especially the anterior tibial surface of the legs.

It is characterized by a bluish red appearance of the skin and a mild swelling often associated with an itching, burning sensation which may be aggravated by warmth. If the exposure is brief these manifestations may disappear completely with no remaining signs. However, intermittent exposure results in the development of chronic manifestations, as increased swelling, deep reddish purple discoloration of the skin, blisters, and bleeding ulcers which heal slowly to leave numerous pigmented scars.

Treatment

For skin discomfort, apply a bland soothing ointment such as petrolatum. People susceptible to chilblain should avoid the cold or wear wool socks and gloves.

Immersion Foot and Trench Foot

These two forms of local cold injuries are related.

Immersion foot occurs by exposure of the lower extremities to water at above-freezing temperatures, usually below 50°F (10°C), in excess of 12 hours. This characteristically occurs among shipwrecked sailors existing on

103

lifeboats or rafts with a poor diet, inactivity, dependency of the legs, constricting clothing, wet clothing, and adverse weather circumstances. Clinical manifestations include swelling of the feet and lower portions of the legs, numbness, tingling, itching, pain, cramps, and skin discoloration.

Trench foot occurs at above-freezing temperatures, usually below 50°F (10°C). It generally happens in a damp environment in connection with immobilization and restriction of the extremities.

Treatment

In cases of Immersion Foot and Trench Foot uncomplicated by trauma there usually is no blistering or tissue destruction. One should prevent continued exposure and apply petrolatum for skin discomfort.

Freezing Injuries (Frostbite)

This is the term applied to cold injuries where there is destruction of tissue by freezing. It is the most serious form of local cold injury. Although the area of frozen tissue usually is small, a frostbite may cover a considerable area. Fingers, toes, cheeks, ears, and nose are the most commonly affected body parts. If the exposure is prolonged, the freezing may extend up the arms and legs. Ice crystals in the skin and other tissues cause the area to appear a white or greyish-yellow color. Pain may occur early and subside. Often, the part will feel only very cold and numb, and there may be a tingling, stinging, or aching sensation. The patient may not be aware of frostbite until someone mentions it. When the damage is superficial, the surface will feel hard and underlying tissue soft when depressed gently and firmly. In a *deep*, unthawed frostbite the area will feel *hard*, solid, and cannot be depressed. It will be cold and numb, and blisters will appear on the surface and in the underlying tissues in 12 to 36 hours. The area will become red and swollen when it thaws and later gangrene will occur and there will be a loss of tissue (necrosis). Time alone will reveal the kind of frostbite that has been present. It is fortunate therefore that the treatment for various degrees of frostbite is identical except for superficial frostbite. *A frostbite of the superficial dry freezing type should be thawed immediately to prevent a deepfreezing injury of the part involved. However, never thaw a frozen extremity until arrival at a facility with water, heat, and equipment where the extremity can be rewarmed rapidly.*

Treatment

All freezing injuries follow the same sequence in treatment: first aid, rapid rewarming, and care after first aid.

First Aid

The principles of first aid in local cold injury are relatively few. The two most important aspects are getting the patient to a place of permanent treatment as soon as possible, and then rewarming. It is important to note that a patient can walk for great distances on frostbitten feet with little danger. Once rewarming has started, it must be maintained. All patients with local cold injuries to the lower extremities become litter cases. Refreezing or walking on a partially thawed part can be very harmful. During transportation and initial treatment, the use of alcoholic beverages should not be permitted, because they affect capillary circulation and cause a loss of body heat. Ointments or creams should not be applied.

Rapid Rewarming

The technique of rewarming has two phases: (1) the treatment of exposure; and (2) the treatment of the local cold injury. *Treatment of exposure* consists of actively rewarming the general patient. This is done in principle by the removal of cold and the addition of warmth. *Removal of cold* is accomplished by removal of all cold and wet clothing and constricting items, as shoes and socks. *Addition of warmth* is provided from external and internal sources. External warmth is accomplished by providing the patient with prewarmed clothes and blankets. Giving a patient a cold change of clothes, a cold blanket, or a cold sleeping bag will cause a rapid dissipation of his residual heat. If necessary, it would be better to have someone donate the clothing that he is wearing to the patient. Someone should warm the sleeping bag prior to the patient's entrance into it. A good source of warmth is the body heat of other people. In general, internal warmth is provided by hot liquids and an adequate diet.

There are two techniques of *rapid rewarming:* wet and dry.

Wet rapid rewarming which is preferred is accomplished by completely immersing the local part in an adequate amount of water at a temperature between 104°F and 107.6°F (40°C and 42°C). The water bath should be tested frequently with a thermometer. If one is not available, some of the water should be poured over the inner portion of the wrist to make sure the water is not too hot. Warming should be discontinued when the part becomes flushed, usually within 20 minutes with the wet method. Further rapid wet rewarming is not necessary.

The dry rapid rewarming technique takes three to four times as long as the wet technique, and is best accomplished by the use of natural body warmth as exemplified by putting the patient's hands in another person's axilla or sharing warm clothing. Also, the patient can be exposed to warm room air.

Do not walk such a patient nor massage a body part. Do not use water hotter than 111°F (44°C), nor recool with ice or snow and do not expose the extremity near an open flame or fire.

Care After First Aid

After the rewarming of a cold injury of a lower extremity, the patient is treated as a litter case. All constricting clothing items should be removed, total body warmth should be maintained, and sleep should be encouraged.

After rewarming, the part should be cleansed carefully with povidone-iodine skin cleanser and water, or soap and water, taking care to leave the blisters intact. Sterile fluff dressing should be applied. Dry, sterile gauze should be placed between toes and fingers to keep them separated. The patient should be placed in bed with the affected part elevated and protected from contact with the bedding. If available, a bed cradle can be used, or one can be improvised from boxes to keep sheets and blankets from touching the affected area. Additional heat should *not* be applied.

Morphine sulfate 10 mg should be given intramuscularly for pain and repeated every four hours as needed, *only if medical advice by radio recommends it.*

Caution: Morphine sulfate is a dangerous depressant of respiration. After receiving a dose the patient must be watched for shallow or very slow breathing. If this occurs, mouth-to-mouth resuscitation should be given. (See p. 117+.)

Medical advice by radio must be obtained for additional treatment. As soon as possible, the patient should be evacuated from the ship to the nearest medical facility.

COLD EXPOSURE INJURIES (GENERAL)

For discussion of generalized hypothermia due to acute, wet cold from total immersion see Chapter VIII, p. 339+.

HEAT EXPOSURE INJURIES

Heat Exhaustion

(Heat Prostration, Heat Collapse)

Exhaustion or collapse in the heat is caused by excessive loss of water and salt from the body. It occurs commonly among persons working in hot environments such as furnace rooms, bakeries, and laundries, or from exposure to hot, humid heat while outdoors. The circulation to such vital organs as the heart and brain is disturbed by the pooling of blood in the capillaries of the skin in order to cool the body. The capillaries constrict to compensate for this deficient blood supply, so the patient's skin appears pale and clammy. (See Fig. 3–50.)

Weakness, dizziness, nausea, dim or blurred vision, and mild muscular cramps may signal the attack. There is profuse sweating. The pulse will be fast and weak, the pupils dilated, and the respirations rapid and shallow.

Treatment

To improve the blood supply to the brain when fainting has occurred or seems likely to occur, the patient should be placed in a sitting position with the head lowered to the knees. Then, the patient should be placed in a reclining position with all tight clothing loosened. Sips of cool water containing one teaspoonful of table salt per glass should be given orally;

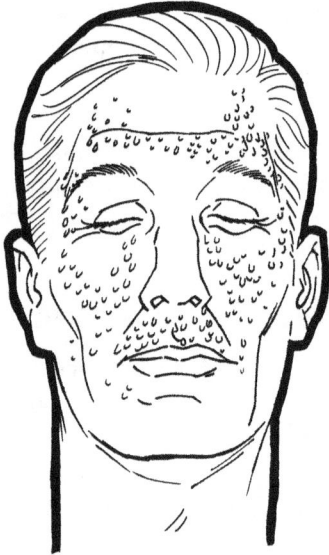

Fig. 3–50. Facial appearance in heat exhaustion.

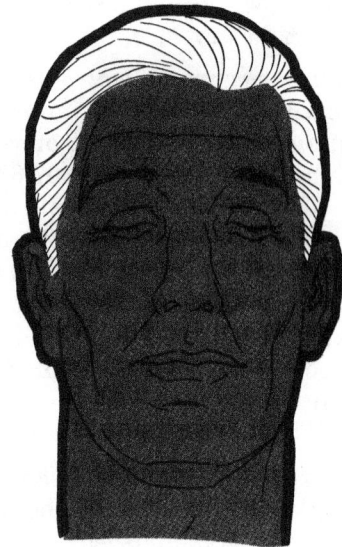

Fig. 3–51. Facial appearance in heat stroke.

approximately one-half glassful should be given every 15 minutes for an hour. If the patient vomits, fluids by mouth should be stopped. If oral fluids are discontinued and the patient is in a deep state of collapse, sodium chloride injection 0.9% should be given intravenously. Medical advice by radio should be obtained.

The patient should be instructed to remain off work for several days, and to avoid exposure to excessively high temperatures during that time.

Heat Cramps

(Stoker's, Miner's, or Fireman's Cramp)

Heat cramps is a condition that affects individuals working in high temperatures. The severe pain and spasms of the abdominal or skeletal muscles occur as a result of profuse sweating and a failure to replace the salt loss. The cramps usually are more severe when the individual has been drinking large amounts of fluids without replacing the salt.

The cramps begin suddenly and occur most frequently in the muscles that bend the arms and legs. The patient may be lying down with the legs drawn up, while crying out from the severe pain. The skin may be pale and wet, the blood pressure remains normal, and the rectal temperature runs about 98°F to 100°F (36.6°C

to 37.7°C). Usually there is no loss of consciousness. Although an untreated attack may last for hours, the condition is not considered dangerous.

Treatment

The patient should be moved to a cool place and given water with one teaspoonful of table salt added to each glass. A half glass of the salt water should be given initially; and repeated every 15 minutes for an hour, or until the symptoms are relieved. Manual pressure to the muscle or massage may help to relieve the cramp. If a more serious problem seems to be present, medical advice by radio should be obtained for patients with heat cramps.

Heatstroke (Sunstroke)

Heatstroke is a medical emergency that is associated with a potentially high mortality rate. *Heat exhaustion* may be regarded as the end result of overactive heat balance mechanisms which are still functioning. *Heatstroke* results when the body's heat regulatory activities are *not* functional, and the main avenue of heat loss (evaporation of sweat) is blocked. There may be early warning symptoms of headache, malaise, and excessive warmth, or a general picture of heat exhaustion. The onset usually is abrupt with sudden loss of consciousness, convulsions, or delirium. Sweating is absent in the typical case; and inquiry frequently reveals that this was noted by the patient prior to onset of the other symptoms.

On physical examination the skin is hot, flushed, and dry. (See Fig. 3–51.) In severe cases, tiny rounded hemorrhage spots (petechiae) may appear. Deep body temperature is high, frequently in excess of 106°F (41°C). A rectal temperature above 108°F (42.2°C) is not uncommon, and indicates a poor outlook (prognosis) for the patient's future. The pulse will be rapid and strong, and may go up to a count of 160 or more. Respiration may be rapid and deep, and the blood pressure elevated slightly. The pupils of the eyes first will contract, then dilate. Muscular twitching, cramps, convulsions, and projectile vomiting may occur, and may be followed by circulatory collapse and deep shock.

Due to the extreme seriousness of heatstroke, all members of the vessel's crew should be taught the importance of recognizing cessation of sweating, so that corrective measures can begin at an early reversible stage.

Treatment

Immediate treatment for heatstroke must be given to reduce the body temperature, or brain damage and death may occur. The patient should be undressed and placed in a tub of cold water; or covered with continuous cold packs such as wet blankets; or sponged with cold water until the temperature drops. The temperature should be taken every 10 minutes, and not allowed to fall below 101°F (38.3°C). The skin should be massaged during this procedure to prevent constriction of the blood vessels, to stimulate return of the cooled blood to the overheated brain and other areas, and to speed up the heat loss. After the body temperature has dropped, the patient should be placed in bed in a cool room with a fan or air conditioner blowing toward the bed. If the body temperature starts to rise, it will be necessary to begin the cooling procedure again. Do *not* give the patient morphine sulfate, epinephrine, or stimulants. *Sedatives are given only to control convulsions.* The patient should be kept on bed rest for several days, and cautioned against later exposure to heat.

Chapter III

Emergency Treatment of Injuries

Section G
POISONING

EMERGENCY AID FOR POISONINGS

It is a MEDICAL EMERGENCY when anyone swallows a poison! Every *non-food substance* should be considered a potential poison!

What To Do First

1. Try to determine the probable poison and the amount swallowed. Carefully assess the patient's condition.

2. If the poison container is available, read the label for *ingredients* of the poison.

3. Use the radio for medical advice on further treatment.

4. While waiting for medical advice by radio, provide the treatment stated below.

5. Keep the patient warm.

Swallowed Poisons

Make the patient vomit . . . but *remember* there are conditions in which the patient should NOT be made to vomit.

1. Do NOT make the patient vomit when:

• The patient is unconscious or convulsing.

• The poison swallowed is a strong corrosive, such as acid or lye.

• The swallowed poison contains kerosene, gasoline, lighter fluid, furniture polish, or other petroleum distillates, unless instructed to do so by radio.

(*Exception:* if these are mixed with dangerous insecticides, then the poison must be removed.)

2. Directions for making the patient vomit:

• Give two tablespoonfuls (30 ml) syrup of ipecac. Follow this with one to two cups of water. If no vomiting occurs after 20 minutes, this dose may be repeated one time only. To stimulate vomiting, gently tickle the back of the throat with a spoon or similar blunt object.

3. Administration of activated charcoal:

• Activated charcoal (two to four tablespoonfuls in a glass of water) may be given after vomiting has occurred or if ipecac has failed to cause vomiting within an hour. *Do not* give activated charcoal before ipecac has had an opportunity to cause vomiting.

Poison Contact of Eyes or Skin

• Wash or flush thoroughly with water.

When Poison is Inhaled

• Remove the patient from exposure to fumes.
• Support respiration.

Important

• *Under no circumstances should liquids be given to a patient who is unconscious or convulsing!*

INTRODUCTION

Poisoning usually occurs as a result of inhaled or swallowed poisons. Certain chemicals, particularly insecticides, can be absorbed by the skin and cause poisoning. The treatment of inhaled noxious gases (as carbon monoxide) is discussed in Chapter IV, p. 127+. Many organic solvents found in paint thinners and cleaning solvents may cause poisoning by inhalation. These should be used in well-ventilated areas. Persons overcome by fumes of solvents should be removed to fresh air. The treatment of poisoning by insecticides that can be absorbed by the skin is discussed on p. 114.

Often poisons are swallowed accidentally. *Never* store poisonous substances with foods or medicines. *Never* store poisons in discarded food or medicine containers. Poisons in mislabeled containers have been confused with food substances and used in cooking with lethal results.

Poisoning may be confused with other medical emergencies. Poisoning should be suspected in sudden, severe illness associated with violent vomiting, diarrhea, severe abdominal pain, and physical collapse with subsequent unconsciousness. Prolonged, deep sleep from which the individual cannot be aroused, or can only be partially aroused, may indicate poisoning. The patient should be examined for stained or burned areas on the lips and on the inside of the mouth. The breath may help to diagnose a poisoning, as well as identify the poison through its characteristic odor. A careful check of the individual's room, or place where he was found, may reveal a container from which a poison was taken.

GENERAL PRINCIPLES OF TREATMENT

Too much antidote,* sedative, or stimulant often does more damage than the poison itself. It is important that good judgment plus a calm attitude should prevail when drugs or therapeutic measures are administered.

See p. 108 for a ready reference chart entitled, *Emergency Aid for Poisonings.*

Give symptomatic treatment, first aid (as artificial respiration, CPR) and, as indicated, diazepam, 5 to 10 mg injection for excitement or convulsions.

Give supportive treatment, such as keeping the patient warm and comfortable, and administering oxygen if indicated.

In all cases, seek medical advice by radio.

Identify the poison as soon as possible. The label on the container may give the ingredients and may list specific antidotes.

If the poison was taken by mouth, *quickly remove the unabsorbed poison from the stomach.* Many poisons are emetics and cause vomiting. If this does not occur spontaneously, vomiting should be induced provided there are no special circumstances that make it unadvisable. *Do not induce vomiting* if the patient has taken a corrosive (acid or alkali), strychnine,

and petroleum distillates; or if the patient is unconscious or convulsing.

Vomiting may be induced by giving the patient syrup of ipecac in a dose of two tablespoonfuls (30 ml) followed by one or two glasses of water. If vomiting has not occurred in 20 to 30 minutes, this dose should be repeated.

Do not give syrup of ipecac at the same time that activated charcoal (a general antidote) is given because the activated charcoal will render the ipecac ineffective. The activated charcoal may be given after the patient has vomited, or 20-30 minutes after the last dose of syrup of ipecac. If vomiting does not occur after administering syrup of ipecac, gastric lavage should be started at once. (See p. 110 for instructions.)

GENERAL ANTIDOTE

If ipecac is not to be used, or if it has failed to work, give two to four tablespoonfuls of activated charcoal (a general antidote) mixed into a glass of water. Activated charcoal is safe to use, and will bind a large number of poisons, preventing them from being absorbed into the body. *Do not use the Universal Antidote**

---

* An *antidote* is a substance which neutralizes (counteracts) the effects of a poison or prevents its absorption.

* The *Universal Antidote,* a mixture of tannic acid, charcoal, and magnesium oxide, formerly considered a general antidote, should not be used because it is not effective.

GASTRIC LAVAGE (Stomach Washing)

Gastric lavage is a method used to withdraw some poisons from the stomach. Water or other lavage solutions are introduced into the stomach by means of a tube. Then the contents of the stomach are withdrawn through the tube and the washings are continued until the stomach is free from poison. The procedure is explained below.

Gastric lavage may be lifesaving, especially (1) if done within three hours after the ingestion of a poison; (2) if the patient did not vomit; or (3) if slowly absorbed drugs or poisons were ingested. *In most cases, vomiting induced by syrup of ipecac is preferable to gastric lavage. Gastric lavage or induced vomiting should not be used for the ingestion of strychnine and corrosive agents, as lye or mineral acids.*

Equipment

- Stomach tube
- Funnel
- Large pitcher (for irrigating solution)
- Large container for the return flow
- Cut strips of adhesive tape

Instruction

Explain the gastric lavage procedure to the patient. Wet the stomach tube before passing. The tube is best passed when the patient sits up with his head slightly forward. Pass the moist tube through the nose by gently pushing in a back and downward direction. Have the patient swallow continuously as the tube is passed, and instruct him to breathe deeply through his mouth. If the head is held slightly forward, swallowing is easier and the tube is passed more readily.

The following procedure should be used to make sure that the tube has not accidentally entered the trachea. Look into the back of the patient's mouth to determine that the tube passed down the throat. Before instilling any solution or antidote, the end of the tube should be placed in water. *Remove the tube at once if there is any bubbling, because the trachea (windpipe) has been entered, instead of the stomach. Usually coughing will signal any entrance into the trachea.* If neither bubbling nor coughing has occurred, continue passing the tube until it is inserted about 18 inches. The tube usually is marked about 46 cm (18 inches) from the gastric end.

The tube should be taped to the patient's nose to prevent it from slipping out of the stomach. The patient should be lying on his left side. Before pouring a large volume of any solution into the tube, always make a final check with a few drops of water to make sure that the tube is placed properly into the stomach. Attach the funnel to the end of the tube, hold the tube and funnel even with the patient's head, and pour a few drops of water down the tube. If this small amount of water does not cause the patient to cough, the tube most likely is in the stomach. However, if violent coughing occurs, the tube probably is in the trachea *and should be removed and reinserted as described in previous paragraphs.*

If the water does not cause the patient to cough, the tube should now be in the stomach properly placed to receive a larger volume of solution. Next pour the solution into the funnel. About a pint of water should be instilled into the tube. Do not allow the tube to empty of solution as this causes air to enter the stomach. The tube should be closed with the fingers or a clamp, when the last amount of solution from the funnel has been administered. Lower the tube and funnel below body level, invert, and allow the stomach contents to siphon out. This procedure should be carried out 10 or 12 times; or until the return fluid is clear. A record should be kept of the amount instilled into the stomach and the amount siphoned off.

TREATMENT OF SPECIFIC POISONINGS

Unfortunately, it may be very difficult to identify a specific poison without elaborate chemical tests. Not all poisons have a specific antidote. For treatment, poisoning may be divided into several types with similar prominent symptoms. General measures are applicable for the treatment of most types of poisonings. However, better results will be obtained if the cause of the poisoning can be classified into a specific group.

In general, poisons may be classified as follows:

Inhaled Carbon Monoxide and Other Noxious Gases

(See Chapter IV, p. 127+.)

Caustic or Corrosive Poisons

(Acids, Alkalis, and Iodine)

These poisons may produce burns and pain in the mouth, throat, or abdomen; vomiting; diarrhea which becomes bloody and contains mucus; and swelling in the throat may block breathing passages.

Treatment

Acids (as Mineral Acids, Phenol)
and Alkalis (as Lye, Ammonia)

The stomach should *not* be washed out and vomiting should *not* be induced. Large amounts of milk or water should be given by mouth as soon as possible. If a poison containing oxalic acid was taken, tetany (convulsions) from hypocalcemia might occur. Medical advice by radio may include intravenous calcium gluconate, 10% (10 ml ampul) to counteract the tetany (convulsions). It should be given very slowly until the convulsions are controlled. After the initial treatment, *medical advice by radio should be sought.* After poisoning by either alkalis or acids, the patient should be advised to have an esophageal examination by a physician at the earliest opportunity. (Also, see Chemical Burns, p. 73.)

Iodine (as Tincture of Iodine
or Lugol's Solution)

Starch water should be given immediately by mouth. Starch water is made by adding enough cornstarch or flour to water to make a thin mixture. If a large quantity of the poison were ingested, gastric lavage with starch water should be performed and arrangements made for immediate evacuation. Povidone-iodine, an organically bound, iodine complex, is relatively non-corrosive as compared to the elemental iodine preparations. Starch water or milk, taken orally, is used to treat ingestions of povidone-iodine.

Petroleum Distillates

(as Gasoline and Mineral Spirits)

A severe chemical pneumonia may occur if petroleum distillate is aspirated into the lungs. Although depression of the central nervous system is rare in adults, it may occur if four ounces or more of any petroleum distillates were taken.

Treatment

Large quantities of milk should be administered, and medical advice by radio sought immediately. If the patient experiences difficulty in breathing (possible chemical pneumonia), preparations should be made to give oxygen.

Central Nervous System Depressants

(as Barbiturates, Tranquilizers, Sedatives, and Alcohol)

Various preparations of these central nervous system depressants have been given descriptive synonyms by users which include the following, among others: knockout drops, downers, and sleeping pills. (See p. 210.)

These depressants affect the nervous and cardiovascular systems. Excitement and hallucinations may precede the depression, which varies from stupor to coma. Respiration decreases, blood pressure falls, urine output decreases, and shock may occur.

Treatment

If there is difficulty in breathing, oxygen should be administered. Artificial respiration should be administered if breathing has stopped. (See p. 115.) If the patient is conscious, induce vomiting unless the patient is very drowsy. Stimulants (such as caffeine or amphetamines) should not be used. If coma or stupor occur, medical advice by radio should be obtained.

Narcotics

(as Morphine, Meperidine, Codeine, Paregoric)

The drug propoxyphene is included in this group. Although it is not classified as a narcotic, the treatment is the same.

Respiratory arrest is the main cause of death with these compounds. Some of the symptoms of poisoning are drowsiness, respiratory depression, convulsions, and coma.

Treatment

Naloxone, a narcotic antagonist given by injection, is the specific antidote for treating respiratory depression in poisoning by narcotics. (See p. 284.) Oxygen and artificial respiration should be administered, if respiratory difficulties develop. Obtain medical advice by radio.

Stimulants

(as Amphetamine, Cocaine)

Various preparations in this group have been given descriptive synonyms which include the following: bennies, speed, meth, uppers, and snow.

These are central nervous system stimulants. Effects from an overdose include excessive activity, frenzied excitement, exaggerated reflexes, tremors, fever, dilated pupils, and sweating. Sometimes coma and convulsions, elevated blood pressure, very rapid heart action, and irregular heart beat will occur. These patients often display aggressive behavior and feelings of persecution, and are capable of violent action.

Treatment

Actions that might be interpreted as antagonistic should be avoided and one should remain calm while talking to the patient. Diazepam 5 to 10 mg may be given intramuscularly every 4 hours, for sedation. Medical advice by radio should be obtained on the dosage and frequency of medication.

Antihistamines

(as Cyclizine, Diphenhydramine)

Symptoms of poisoning with these drugs are lethargy or drowsiness, followed by coma. Some patients exhibit excitation, nervousness, and convulsions.

Treatment

If the patient is conscious, induce vomiting unless the patient is very drowsy. If respiratory difficulties develop, oxygen and artificial respiration should be given. If convulsions occur, the treatment given on p. 212 should be followed. Medical advice by radio should be obtained for additional treatment.

Hallucinogens

(as LSD, Peyote)

These chemicals cause intense visual and auditory hallucinations, alterations of body image, and an exaggerated sense of comprehension. The physical effects include dilated pupils, lack of coordination, numbness, tingling sensations, nausea, and sometimes vomiting.

Treatment

Rest, reassurance, sympathy, and support often are the best treatments. If there is a compelling need for sedation, diazepam 5 to 10 mg should be given intramuscularly every 4 hours. Depending upon the patient's response, a larger dose may be indicated on subsequent injection. A physician should be contacted by radio for advice.

Cyanides

Hydrogen cyanide or hydrocyanic acid (HCN) is a colorless liquid which boils at 77° to 78.8°F (25° to 26°C). It exists under ordinary conditions as a gas which is lighter than air. Hydrogen cyanide has a characteristic odor of "peach pits." The cyanides (the acid and its salts) are deadly to most living things. Hydrocyanic acid gas is one of the most effective fumigants available for vessels, but its use is extremely hazardous and it must be handled by specially trained individuals. Suicides and homicides account for most fatal cyanide poisonings but vessel fumigation has contributed a number of cases.

Hydrocyanic acid gas is absorbed readily through the lungs, the gastrointestinal tract, and the intact skin. Because of very rapid absorption, hydrocyanic acid gas exerts its toxic effects at once. Persons overcome by the gas may die very rapidly (within a few minutes) from respiratory failure. If removed within minutes from a sublethal exposure they will recover completely within a relatively short time.

Symptoms and signs develop very rapidly in cyanide poisoning. If the victim has been exposed to lethal amounts of hydrocyanic acid gas, the principal manifestation may be respiratory stimulation. The sequence of symptoms include immediate unconsciousness, convulsions, and death within a few minutes.

See Chapter XI, p. 378, on preventive measures which should be taken to avoid exposure to toxic gas hazards aboard ship.

Inhaling or absorbing hydrocyanic acid gas through the skin in an amount close to a lethal dose causes a marked respiratory distress, dizziness, headache, nausea, vomiting, drowsiness, irritated and scratchy throat, drop in blood pressure, rapid pulse, and unconsciousness. The odor of "peach pits" in the room or from the vomitus helps confirm a cyanide poisoning.

When taken orally, sodium cyanide, potassium cyanide, and other salts of hydrocyanic acid may give rise to acute or subacute poisonings with the above symptoms. With a lethal dose of a cyanide salt (for an adult about 250 mg), death occurs suddenly with or without convulsions.

It is important to know that workers handling cyanides may develop a rash which first occurs around the wrists, hands, and fingers associated with moderate scaling of the skin and itching which later may spread to all regions of the body.

Treatment

The emergency measures to follow for poisoning from hydrocyanic acid gas are:

• Quickly remove the victim into fresh air that is free of poison.

• Give amyl nitrite inhalation 0.2 ml every five minutes. This administration should be discontinued if the systolic blood pressure goes below 80 mm of mercury.

• Give oxygen and artificial respiration *other than* mouth-to-mouth resuscitation. *Mouth-to-mouth resuscitation can poison the rescuer.* (See p. 130+.)

Emergency measures for a person who has ingested a cyanide salt such as potassium cyanide, should include amyl nitrite inhalation, artificial respiration (*not mouth-to-mouth*), and oxygen. (Same as for the gas.) However, the ingestion of a cyanide salt is usually with suicidal or homicidal intent. Because of the rapid absorption of the cyanide, one can anticipate that a victim poisoned by cyanide probably will expire within the first 30 minutes. However, if the victim survives for four hours or more, there should be full recovery.

Medical advice by radio should be obtained promptly as to whether a physician should be put aboard ship, or the victim evacuated to a medical facility for follow-up care.

Methanol

(as Methyl Alcohol, Wood Alcohol, Columbian Spirit)

This poison is found in some paints, varnishes, paint removers, and "canned heat." A fatal dosage for methanol is between two and eight ounces.

The symptoms of poisoning by wood alcohol are the same as those for the depressants of the central nervous system (see p. 208). Also, there may be headache, nausea and vomiting, gastric pain; visual disturbances, eye pain, sudden blindness; acidosis; coma; and death from respiratory or circulatory failure.

Treatment

For methanol poisoning vomiting should be induced, followed by gastric lavage with two tablespoonfuls of sodium bicarbonate per liter (quart) of solution. Then, three to four ounces of whisky should be given every four hours for four days to inhibit the metabolism of methanol. If respiratory difficulties develop, oxygen and artificial respiration should be administered. Obtain medical advice by radio. Prompt evacuation of the patient from the vessel may be indicated.

Salicylates

(as Aspirin, Methyl Salicylate or Oil of Wintergreen)

Poisoning by a salicylate results in rapid, deep, and pauseless breathing because of the direct effect on the brain. Vomiting, extreme thirst, profuse sweating, fever, and convulsions or delirium may occur. Shock, coma, convulsions, a decreased urine output, and blood in vomitus may appear as the intoxication becomes severe.

Treatment

Unless the patient is convulsing or unconscious, vomiting should be induced immediately or a gastric lavage performed. For an adult, 50 or more tablets of aspirin, 300 mg (5 grains) would be a potentially poisonous quantity. Also, about 15 ml (½ ounce) of oil of wintergreen may be poisonous. If convulsions occur, the treatment given on page 212 should be followed. Seek medical advice by radio.

Pesticides

(as Arsenic, Sodium Fluoride, Organophosphates, Carbamates)

Pesticides are used to poison insects and other animals.

• Arsenic

After arsenic is ingested, symptoms develop in a few minutes or hours. Intense upper abdominal pain is followed by violent vomiting and profuse diarrhea. At first, the vomitus and stools usually contain blood and mucus; and later, the stools assume a "rice-water" appearance. There may be a garlic odor to the breath and stools. These symptoms are followed quickly by exhaustion and collapse.

Treatment

The poisonous arsenic should be removed by repeated vomiting or gastric lavage. A large amount of water should be given, followed by milk of magnesia. After initial treatment has been administered, arrangements should be made for prompt evacuation of the patient.

• Sodium Fluoride

Sodium fluoride poisoning causes nausea, vomiting, diarrhea, and abdominal pain. These symptoms generally are not as severe as those produced by caustic and corrosive poisons, or arsenic. These symptoms are followed by a twitching muscular movement related to hypocalcemia, and later by muscular weakness and collapse.

Treatment

Vomiting should be induced to remove sodium fluoride from the stomach. Repeatedly administer large quantities of milk. The patient should be placed in bed and kept as quiet as possible. On the advice of a physician, 2 to 10 ml of 10% calcium gluconate may be given very slowly intravenously, until muscular twitching stops. After the initial treatment, immediate evacuation of the patient from the vessel should be arranged.

• Organophosphate pesticides (as Parathion,® Diazinon®) and Carbamates (as Carbacryl®)

Organophosphates and carbamates are very toxic compounds that are absorbed by the skin, lungs, and gastrointestinal tract. The symptoms include all or some of the following: weakness, blurred vision, contraction of the pupil of the eye, and tightness in the chest. These are followed by vomiting, cramping, diarrhea, salivation, weeping eye, sweating, tremors, difficult breathing, bluish color to skin and mucous membranes, coma, and convulsions.

Treatment

For organophosphate and carbamate poisoning treatment includes maintaining respiration, administering oxygen, and injecting 2 to 4 mg of atropine intramuscularly at 5- to 10-minute intervals, until the patient's skin is flushed and dry, and mild tachycardia (rapid pulse) occurs. Contaminated clothing should be removed and the contaminated skin washed thoroughly with soap and water. In cyanotic patients, oxygen should be given to overcome cyanosis (bluish tint to skin) before administering atropine. Obtain medical advice by radio. After the initial treatment, arrangements should be made for prompt evacuation of the patient from the vessel to a medical facility.

Heavy Metals

(as Lead, Mercury and their Salts)

Heavy metal poisoning and its treatment are usually chronic; however, single ingestions or exposures, or symptoms may be acute. Generally, the salts of heavy metals, rather than actual metallic lead or mercury are most poisonous if ingested. *Mercury chloride (corrosive sublimate) is extremely poisonous if ingested.* Inhalation of vapors of these substances or skin or eye contact may also be harmful.

Treatment

Following ingestion of heavy metals or their salts, vomiting should be induced with syrup of ipecac. Follow with activated charcoal and/or milk. Appropriate symptomatic and supportive care should be given. If vapors have been inhaled, remove the patient from the contaminated area and administer oxygen. For skin or eye contact, flush with large amounts of water. *In all cases, seek medical advice by radio.*

Chapter IV

Cardiopulmonary Resuscitation (CPR)*

INTRODUCTION

RESUSCITATION IS THE TERM which covers measures taken to reverse the dying process in acute, life-threatening conditions. These measures include artificial respiration (manual and mechanical) that are performed to restore breathing, plus external cardiac compression to restore circulation.

Beginning CPR

Speed is essential once the need for resuscitation has been recognized. After four to six minutes without respiration or circulation, irreversible brain damage probably will have occurred. Because the duration of absence of heartbeat and breathing usually is not known by the rescuer, resuscitation efforts should be started at once. The two exceptions would be the patient with a terminal illness (as determined by a doctor), and the patient known to have been dead for ten minutes.

* Derived from *Standards for Cardiopulmonary Resuscitation (CPR) and Emergency Cardiac Care (ECC)*, JAMA, Vol. 27, No. 7, Feb. 18, 1974. © 1974 by the American Medical Association. Reprinted with permission from the American Heart Association.

Contraindications to CPR

External cardiopulmonary resuscitation may be ineffective when certain conditions exist. These include crushing injuries to the chest, internal chest injuries, cardiac tamponade (symptoms due to a large accumulation of pericardial fluid), tension pneumothorax, or emphysema with enlargement and fixation of the rib cage. If external cardiac compression is required, it may be the only alternative to death. It should be performed with the knowledge that internal injuries may be compounded.

Patients exposed to toxic or caustic materials can be a hazard to a rescuer performing mouth-to-mouth resuscitation, so another method of artificial ventilation should be used. (See p. 130+.)

Examination of Patient

A collapsed or unconscious patient must be examined immediately to determine the adequacy or absence of breathing and circulation. Follow the ABC's; Airway, Breathing, and Cir-

---

CARDIOPULMONARY RESUSCITATION (CPR)
Some Points To Remember

***Don't Delay!* Place victim flat on his back on a hard surface.**

$$\text{Cardiopulmonary Resuscitation (CPR)} = \text{Artificial Ventilation} + \text{External Cardiac Compression}$$

A. Airway—If unconscious, open the airway; thereafter make sure it stays open.

> Lift up neck.
> Push forehead back.
> Clear out mouth with fingers.

B. BREATHING—If *not* breathing, begin artificial breathing:

> Mouth-to-mouth or Mouth-to-nose resuscitation.

>> Before beginning CPR, check *carotid pulse* in neck. Then it should be felt after the first minute of CPR, and checked every 5 minutes, thereafter.

>> Give 4 quick breaths and continue at a rate of 12 inflations per minute.

>> Chest should rise and fall. If it does not, check to make sure the victim's head is tilted as far back as possible. If necessary, use fingers to clear the airway.

C. Circulation—If pulse is absent, begin artificial circulation:

> If possible, use two rescuers. *Don't delay!* One rescuer can do the job.

>> Locate pressure point (lower half of sternum).
>> Depress sternum 1½ inches to 2 inches (60 to 80 times per minute).
>> If *one rescuer*—15 compressions and 2 quick inflations.
>> If *two rescuers*—5 compressions and 1 inflation.

> *Pupils of Eyes* should be checked during CPR. A pupil that constricts on exposure to light shows that the brain is getting adequate blood and oxygen.

---

culation in examining and in setting the priorities for action. *Listen* and *feel* for any movement of air, because the chest and abdomen may move in the presence of an *obstructed airway*, without moving air. The rescuer's face should be placed close to the patient's nose and mouth so that any exhaled air may be felt against his cheek. Also, the rise and fall of the chest can be observed and the exhaled breath heard.

A partially obstructed airway is characterized by noisy breathing. There is usually a "snoring" sound when the airway is obstructed by the tongue, and a "crowing" sound when it is obstructed by foreign matter, as phlegm, blood, or vomit. *Repiratory failure* is characterized by little or no respiratory effort and movement, and the absence of air movement through the mouth or nose.

Quickly check the carotid (neck) pulse by placing the tips of the four fingers of one hand into the groove between the windpipe and the large muscle at the side of the neck. (See p. 120.) The carotid pulse normally is a strong one; if it cannot be felt or is feeble, there is insufficient circulation.

Check the pupils of the eyes to see if they are dilated or constricted. When the heart stops beating, the pupils will begin to dilate within 45 seconds to one minute. They will stay dilated and will not react to light.

AIRWAY

Establishing an open airway is the most important step in resuscitation. Spontaneous breathing may occur as a result of this simple measure. Place the patient in a face-up position on a hard surface. Put one hand beneath the patient's neck and the other hand on the forehead. Lift the neck with the one hand, and apply pressure to the forehead with the other to tilt the head backward. (See Fig. 4–1.) This extends the neck and moves the base of the tongue away from the back of the throat. *The head should be maintained in this position during the entire resuscitation procedure.* If the airway still is obstructed, any foreign material in the mouth or throat should be removed immediately with the fingers.

Occasionally, there may be an incomplete opening of the air passages even with a properly performed "head-tilt." In such cases, further opening of the air passages can be achieved by displacing the patient's jaw forward so that his lower teeth are in front of his upper teeth. This may be accomplished by grasping the lower jaw between the thumb and index finger and lifting, or by placing the fingers behind the angles of the lower jaw and pushing forward. Any further obstruction will be evident upon the first effort to inflate the lungs.

BREATHING

If the patient does not resume adequate, spontaneous breathing promptly after his head has been tilted backward, artificial ventilation should be given by mouth-to-mouth or mouth-to-nose ventilation or other techniques. Regardless of the method used, preservation of an open airway is essential.

Equipment Isn't Necessary. No special equipment is required for effective artificial ventilation. There should be no delays caused by seeking such equipment, or by putting it into use. When available and properly employed, various devices (masks, airways) may be useful.

Mouth-to-Mouth Ventilation

• Keep the patient's head at a maximum backward tilt with *one hand* under the neck. (See Fig. 4–1b.)

• Place the heel of *the other hand* on the forehead, with the thumb and index finger toward the nose. Pinch together the patient's nostrils

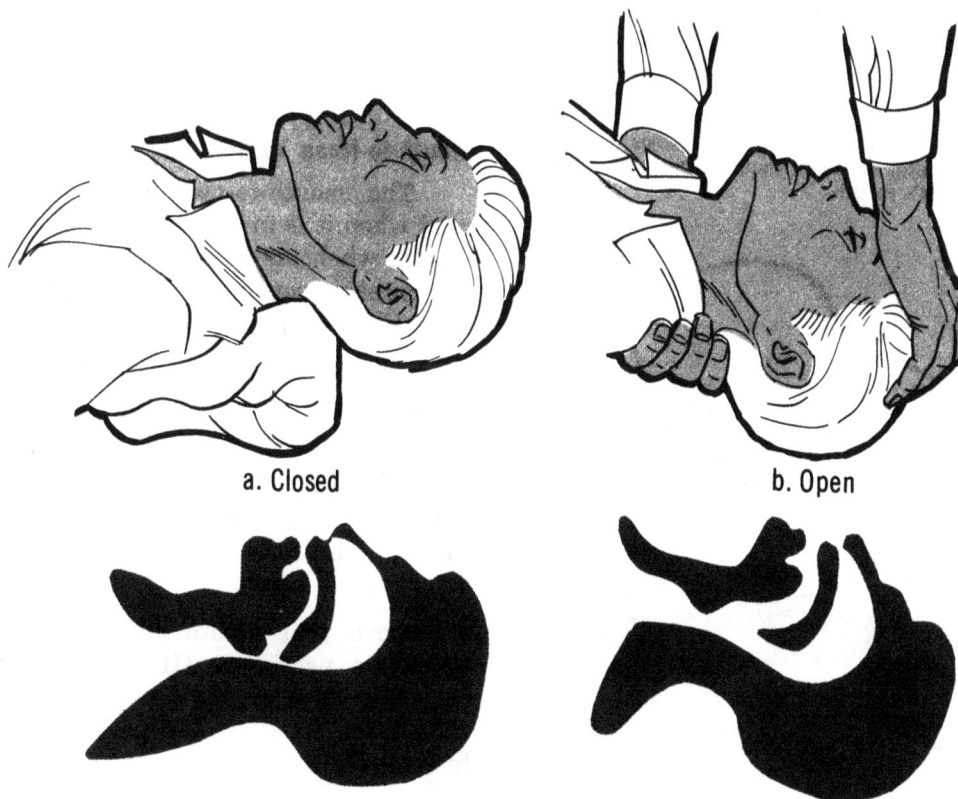

a. Closed   b. Open

Fig. 4–1. Establishing an open airway.

with the thumb and index finger to prevent air from escaping. Continue to exert pressure on the forehead with the palm of the hand to maintain the backward tilt of the head.

• Take a deep breath, then form a tight seal with your mouth over and around the patient's mouth. (See Fig. 4–2a.)

• Blow 4 quick, full breaths in first without allowing the lungs to deflate fully. Then, continue the procedure.

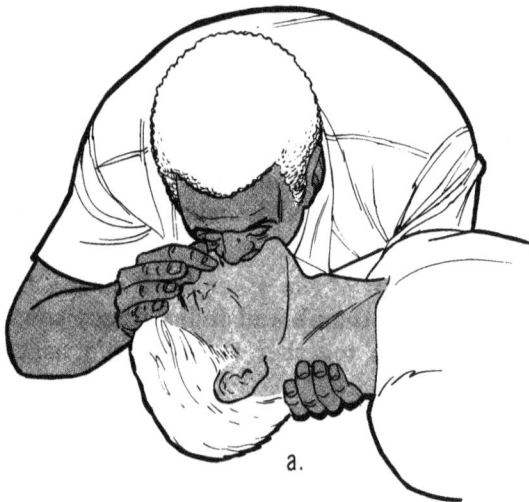

Fig. 4–2a.
Mouth-to-mouth ventilation. Attendant blows forcefully into patient's mouth, after his mouth forms a tight seal around the patient's mouth.

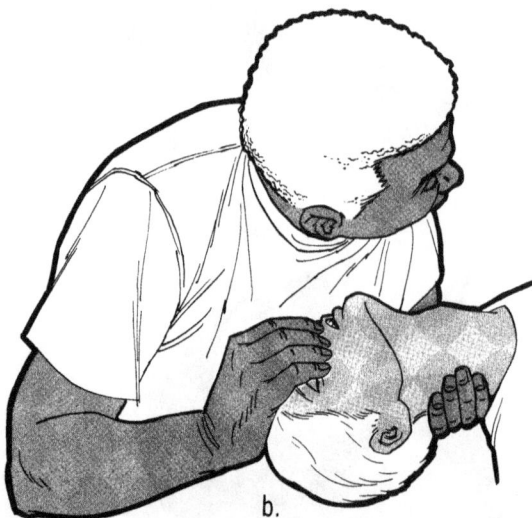

Fig. 4–2b.
Mouth-to-mouth ventilation. Attendant removes his mouth and allows the patient to exhale.

• Blow forcefully and smoothly into the victim's mouth. Do not use sudden, excessive force. Too much sudden pressure might damage the person's lungs.

• Watch the patient's chest while inflating the lungs. If adequate ventilation is taking place, the chest should rise and fall.

• Remove your mouth and allow the patient to exhale passively. If in the right position, the patient's exhalation will be felt on your cheek. (See Fig. 4–2b.)

• Take another deep breath, reform a tight seal around the patient's mouth and blow into the mouth again. Repeat this procedure 10 to 12 times a minute, once every 5 seconds, for adults and children over 4 years.

• If there is no air exchange and an airway obstruction exists, make sure the head is tilted well back and the jaw is jutting up and out. If there is still no exchange of air, roll the victim to one side and pound firmly between the shoulder blades to try to dislodge any blocking material. If necessary, reach into the patient's throat to remove foreign matter that will not fall free. Clean any vomit from the patient's mouth and resume artificial ventilation.

Mouth-to-Nose Ventilation

The mouth-to-nose technique should be used when it is impossible to open the patient's mouth, when the mouth is severely injured, or a tight seal around the lips cannot be obtained. (See Fig. 4–3.)

• Keep the patient's head tilted back with one hand. Use the other hand to lift up the patient's lower jaw to seal the lips.

• Take a deep breath, seal your lips around the patient's nose, and blow in forcefully and smoothly until the patient's chest rises. Repeat quickly four times.

• Remove your mouth and allow the patient to exhale passively. (If possible, it may be necessary to open the patient's mouth during exhalation, to allow the patient's exhaled air to escape.)

• Repeat the cycle 10 to 12 times per minute, or approximately every 5 seconds.

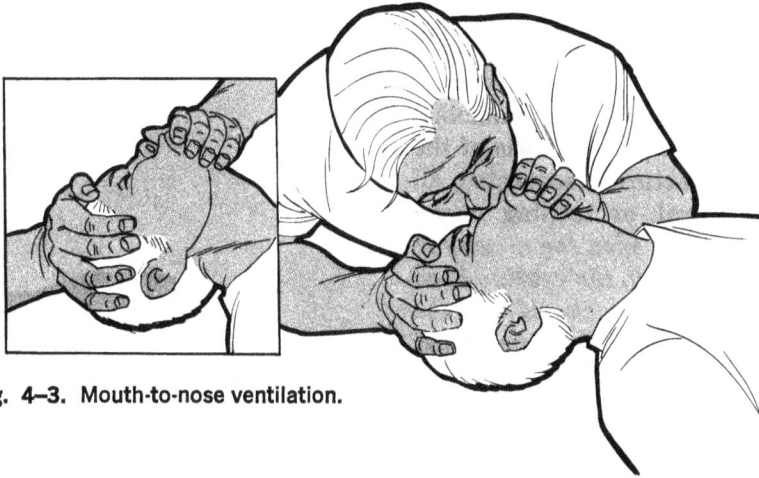

Fig. 4–3. Mouth-to-nose ventilation.

Special Situations

Children—Resuscitation is performed in essentially the same way for children. For infants and small children, the patient's nose and mouth should be covered with the rescuer's mouth. (See Fig. 4–4.) The rescuer should blow gently, using less volume to inflate the lungs. Babies require only small puffs of air from the rescuer's cheeks. The rate of inflation should be 20 to 30 times per minute, or once every 3 seconds. The neck of an infant is so pliable that forceful backward tilting of the head may obstruct breathing passages. Therefore, the tilted position should not be exaggerated.

Foreign Bodies —A foreign body should be suspected if you are unable to inflate the lungs, despite proper positioning and a tight air seal around the mouth or nose. The first blowing effort should tell you whether or not any obstruction exists. The patient should be rolled quickly onto his side. Firm blows should be delivered over the spine between the shoulder blades to try to dislodge the obstruction. Then the material causing the obstruction should be removed from the mouth with the rescuer's fingers. The patient should be rolled back quickly and artificial ventilation resumed. This procedure may need to be repeated in order to dislodge the foreign bodies. (See Heimlich maneuver, p. 132.)

A small child with an obstructive foreign body in the airway should be picked up quickly and held over the rescuer's forearm. Firm blows should be delivered between the shoulder blades and ventilation resumed quickly.

Stomach Distention—Artificial ventilation (exhaled air ventilation) frequently causes distention of the stomach, especially in children. It is most likely to occur when excessive pressures are used for inflation, or if the airway is not clear. Slight stomach distention may be harmful because it promotes vomiting, reduces lung volume by elevating the diaphragm, and may start harmful nerve reflexes.

Obvious gross distention should be relieved whenever possible. In the unconscious patient, this is accomplished by using one hand to exert moderate pressure over the patient's abdomen between the navel and the rib cage. A second rescuer, if available, can prevent recurrence of stomach distention by maintaining moderate pressure in this area. During this maneuver, the victim's head and shoulders should be lowered or turned to one side to prevent aspiration of the stomach's contents.

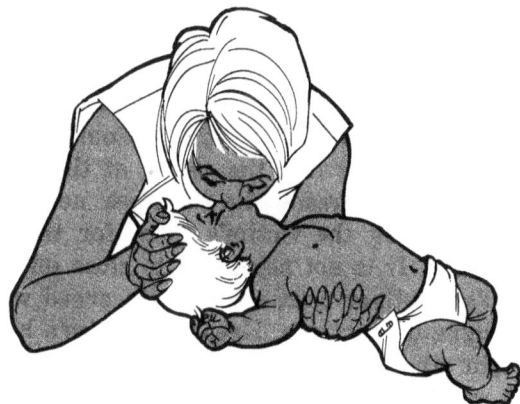

Fig. 4–4. Artificial ventilation (small children).

Suspected Neck Injuries—In accident cases, it is imperative that caution be used to avoid extending the victim's neck, when there is a possibility of a neck fracture. A fractured neck should be suspected in diving or automobile accidents when the victim has lacerations of the face and forehead. If a fracture is suspected, all forward, backward, lateral, or turning movements should be avoided. *To open the airway in cases of suspected neck injury, the routine head tilt and jaw thrust technique should not be used. Instead, the following* **modified jaw thrust** *technique should be used:*

• Place a hand on either side of the victim's head to maintain it in a fixed neutral position without the head extended.

• Use the index fingers to displace the jaw forward. Do not tilt the head in any direction.

• Artificial ventilation usually can be successful in this position. If not successful, tilt the head back very slightly and make another attempt to ventilate, using the modified jaw thrust.

Laryngectomees (Mouth-to-Stoma Method Used)—In the United States several thousand individuals have had the larynx completely or partially removed by surgery. The surgical operation is called a *laryngectomy.* Persons who have had the operation are called *laryngectomees.* Laryngectomees breathe through an opening (stoma) that is made into the front of the neck to connect with the windpipe (trachea). They do not use the nose or mouth for breathing.

Direct mouth-to-stoma artificial ventilation should be used to resuscitate people who have had a laryngectomy. Neither head tilt nor jaw thrust maneuvers are required. The same general procedure for mouth-to-mouth resuscitation is used except that the rescuer's mouth is placed firmly over the victim's stoma. Then the rescuer blows into the stoma at the same rate as for a person who breathes normally while watching the victim's chest for the inflow of air. It is not necessary to close off the victim's mouth or nose, or to be concerned with his tongue or dentures. Keep the victim's head straight and avoid twisting it. Twisting the head might change the shape of the stoma or close it.

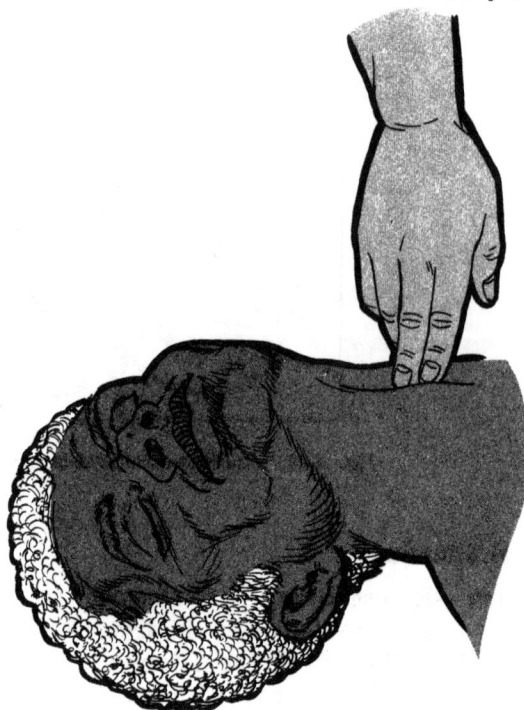

Fig. 4–5. Carotid pulse.

CIRCULATION
(External Cardiac Compression)

After three to five effective lung inflations, the pulse of the carotid (neck artery) should be checked. A head-tilt should be maintained with one hand. With the index and middle fingers of the other hand, gently locate the voice box, and slide the fingers flat to the side of the neck where the carotid pulse can be felt. The carotid pulse area should be "felt," not squeezed. (See Fig. 4–5.)

External cardiac compression should be started when the presence of the carotid pulse is absent or questionable. Rhythmic pressure should be applied over the lower half of the sternum (breastbone). This compresses the heart between the sternum and spine and produces some blood circulation. When properly performed, it can produce enough blood pressure to support life.

CARDIOPULMONARY RESUSCITATION (CPR)

Dangers in CPR Performance

CPR may be ineffective in providing basic life support when performed improperly. The following points should be remembered when performing cardiopulmonary resuscitation:

• Never interrupt cardiopulmonary resuscitation (CPR) more than five seconds for any reason except when moving a patient up or down a stairway. In this situation effective CPR can be performed best at the head or foot of the stairs. On a given signal, interrupt CPR and move quickly to the next landing where it can be resumed. Such interruptions should only occur under emergency conditions when the patient must be relocated and then never to exceed 15 seconds.

• Never move a patient for convenience until he has been stablized or until arrangements have been made for uninterrupted CPR during movement.

• *Never* compress the xiphoid process at the tip of the sternum. Pressure on it may tear the liver and lead to severe internal bleeding.

• Although pressure *must* be completely released between compressions, the heel of the hand should remain in constant contact with the chest wall over the lower half of the sternum.

• The attendant's fingers must *never* rest on the patient's ribs during compression. This increases the possibility of rib fractures. Interlocking the fingers of the two hands may help avoid this.

• *Never* use sudden or jerking movements to compress the chest. The action should be smooth, regular, and uninterrupted, with 50% of the cycle compression and 50% relaxation.

• *Never* maintain continuous pressure on the abdomen to decompress the stomach. This traps the liver and may cause it to rupture.

• The attendant's shoulders should be directly over the patient's sternum, elbows straight, and pressure applied vertically downward on the lower sternum. This provides maximum thrust, minimal fatigue for the attendant, and reduces the chance of complications to the patient.

• The lower sternum of an adult *must* be depressed 1½ to 2 inches to be effective.

• Chest compression usually is ineffective if the patient is on a bed or spring mattress.

• Improperly applied CPR may cause trauma, such as rib fractures. Careful adherence to details of performance will minimize complications. It must be remembered that effective CPR is required during cardiac arrest even if traumatic conditions do result, because the alternative is death.

Technique for External Cardiac Compression

Compression of the sternum produces some artificial ventilation, but not enough for adequate oxygenation of the blood. For this reason, artificial ventilation always is required whenever external cardiac compression is used.

Effective external cardiac compression requires sufficient pressure to depress the patient's lower sternum 1½ to 2 inches in an adult. *For chest compression to be effective, the patient must be on a firm surface. If he is in bed, a board or improvised support should be placed under his back. However, chest compression must not be delayed to look for a firmer support.*

Kneel close to the side of the patient and place only the heel of one hand over the lower half of the sternum. Avoid placing the hand over the tip (xiphoid process) of the breastbone which extends down over the upper abdomen.

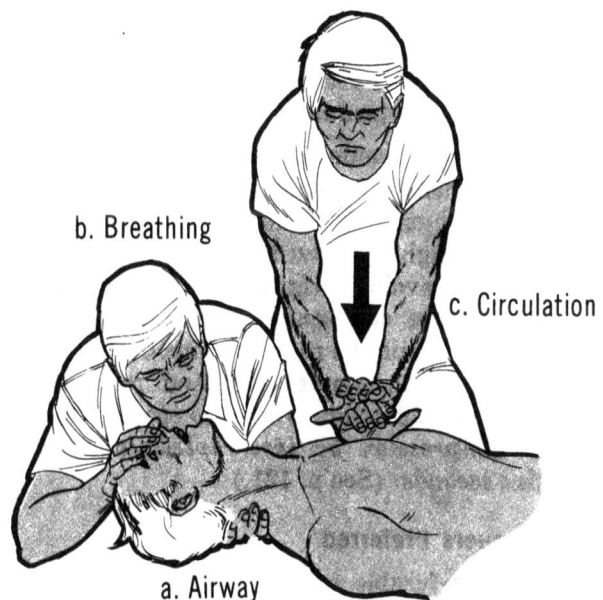

Fig. 4–6.
Two-rescuer cardiopulmonary resuscitation (CPR)
• 5 chest compressions
  —At rate of 60 per minute
  —No pause for ventilation
• 1 lung inflation
  —After each 5 compressions
  —Interposed between compressions

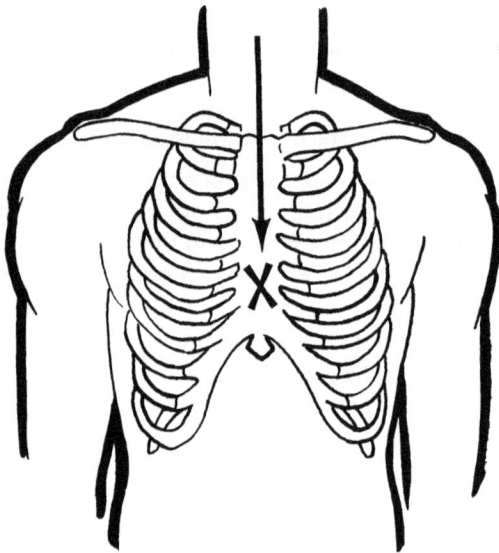

Fig. 4–7. Artificial circulation (pressure point).

Feel the tip of the sternum and place the heel of the hand about 1½ inches toward the head of the patient. (See Fig. 4–7.)

• Place the heel of the other hand on top of the first one.

• Rock forward so that your shoulders are almost directly above the patient's chest.

• Keep your arms straight and exert adequate pressure almost directly downward to depress an adult's lower sternum 1½ to 2 inches.

• Depress the sternum 60 times per minute for an adult (when two rescuers are used). This is usually rapid enough to maintain blood flow, and slow enough to allow the heart to fill with blood. Also it avoids fatigue and aids timing at the rate of one compression per second. The compression should be regular, smooth, and uninterrupted, with compression and relaxation being of equal duration. *Under no circumstance should compression be interrupted for more than five seconds.* (See p. 121.)

Two Rescuers Preferred

It is preferable to have *two rescuers* because artificial circulation must be combined with artificial ventilation. (See Fig. 4–6.) When possible, the rescuers should not be on the same side of the patient. The most effective ventilation and circulation are achieved by giving quickly one lung inflation after each five chest compressions (5:1 ratio). *The compression rate should be 60 per minute for two rescuers.* One rescuer performs external cardiac compression while the other remains at the patient's head, keeps it tilted back, and continues rescue breathing (exhaled air ventilation). *Supplying the breaths without any pauses in heart compression is important, because every interruption in cardiac compression results in a drop of blood flow and blood pressure to zero.*

Single Rescuer

A *single rescuer* must perform both artificial ventilation and artificial circulation using a 15:2 ratio. (See Fig. 4–8.) *Two very quick lung inflations should be delivered after each 15 chest compressions, without waiting for full exhalation of the patient's breath. A rate equivalent to 80 chest compressions per minute must be maintained by a single rescuer* in order to achieve 50 to 60 actual compressions per minute because of the interruptions for the lung inflations.

Children and Infants

The *technique is similar for children,* except that the heel of only one hand is used for small children and only the tips of the index and middle fingers for babies. The heart of

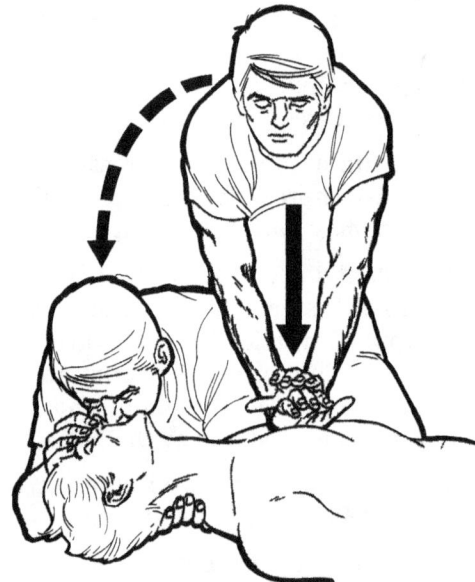

Fig. 4–8.
One-rescuer cardiopulmonary resuscitation (CPR)
• 15 chest compressions
    —At rate of 80 per minute
• 2 quick lung inflations

infants and small children lies higher in the chest so external pressure should be applied over the midsternum. The danger of injuring the liver is greater in children because of the smallness and pliability of the chest and the high position of the liver under the lower sternum.

In an *infant*, the midsternum should be compressed one-half to three-fourths of an inch; and in a *child*, three-fourths to one and one-half inches. The compression rate should be 80 to 100 times per minute with breaths placed between each five compressions. A backward tilt of the head arches (lifts) the back in infants and small children. A firm support for external cardiac compression can be provided if the rescuer slips one hand beneath the child's back, while using the other hand to compress the chest. An alternative method for small infants is to encircle the chest with the hands and compress the midsternum with both thumbs.

Checking Effectiveness of CPR

The reaction of the pupils should be checked during cardiopulmonary resuscitation. A pupil that narrows when exposed to light indicates that the brain is receiving adequate oxygen and blood. If the pupils remain widely dilated and do not react to light, serious brain damage is likely to occur soon or has occurred already. Dilated but reactive pupils are less threatening. Normal reactions of the pupils may be altered by the administration of drugs.

The carotid (neck) pulse should be felt after the first minute of cardiopulmonary resuscitation, and every five minutes thereafter. The pulse will indicate the effectiveness of the external cardiac compression or the return of a spontaneous effective heartbeat.

Other indicators that show CPR effectiveness are the following:

• Expansion of the chest each time the operator blows air into the lungs.

• A pulse which can be felt each time the sternum is compressed.

• Return of color to the skin.

• A spontaneous gasp for breath.

• A return of a spontaneous heartbeat.

Terminating CPR

The decision to stop cardiopulmonary resuscitation is a medical one that depends upon an assessment of the cerebral (brain) circulation. Deep unconsciousness, the absence of spontaneous respiration, and fixed, dilated pupils for 15 to 30 minutes indicate cerebral death and further resuscitative efforts are usually futile.

In the absence of a physician, CPR should be continued until:

• Spontaneous circulation and ventilation have been restored.

• Resuscitation has been transferred to another responsible person to continue basic life support.

• Responsibility has been assumed by a physician.

• The patient is transferred to the care of properly trained and designated medical or allied health personnel responsible for emergency medical care.

• The rescuer is unable to continue because of fatigue.

OXYGEN ADMINISTRATION

Oxygen should be given as soon as it is available. If the patient is breathing without assistance but is unconscious or cyanotic (bluish skin), oxygen inhalation should be started. Also, oxygen should be given to all carbon monoxide and toxic gas patients even when conscious.

Because a mask provides the highest concentration (approaching 100%) of oxygen, it is the preferred method. A well-fitting mask made of clear plastic should be selected so the patient can be observed for vomiting. Some patients are afraid of the mask and it is important to overcome this fear. If able, the patient should be allowed to breathe a few times with it, and a few times without it. The instructions given with the mask and oxygen tank should be followed carefully. *No open flames or smoking should be allowed in the area where oxygen is administered.*

Relatively low concentrations of oxygen should be sufficient for many patients, but high concentrations may be required. Medical advice by radio should be obtained.

SUCTION (ORAL AND NASAL)

The air passages may be blocked by mucus, vomitus, or foreign material in the mouth or nose, or both. The head of the patient should be turned to one side to allow the fluids to drain away and the fingers of the rescuer should be swept through the mouth to remove the blockage. The rescuer's fingers may be wrapped in a piece of cloth or gauze to help remove the mucus and slippery objects. If these methods are not successful, suction will have to be used.

Suction is negative pressure (drawing pressure, vacuum) created by a mechanical or hand-operated apparatus (aspirator). When the suction tip (suction catheter or rigid pharyngeal suction tip) is placed in the mouth, the fluids are drawn through the tube into a catch jar. This jar is located between the patient and the source of the vacuum. While suction will remove fluids from the mouth and throat, fingers may have to be used to wipe out solid matter.

Either a suction catheter or a rigid pharyngeal tip can be used to suction the mouth. The following recommended suction catheter sizes* should be used:

Newborn _____ 6 French
6 months to 3 years _____ 8 French
5 years to 16 years _____ 10 French
Adult (Female) _____ 12 French
Adult (Male) _____ 14 French

Oral Suction

When suctioning the mouth, this procedure should be followed:

• Use one hand to open the mouth for the insertion of the catheter or pharyngeal tip.

• Do *not* insert the catheter or pharyngeal tip too far into the mouth and throat as it may make the patient vomit or may produce a laryngospasm.

• Perform the suctioning quickly in a few seconds and repeat as needed.

Nasal Suction

• Do *not* attempt to suction the nose by inserting the catheter or pharyngeal tube into the

---

* One size smaller or larger should be allowed for individual variations.

nose. Serious bleeding may develop from nasal injury.

• If nasal suction is essential, place the suction tip at the opening of the nostrils.

When suctioning, the tubing must be rinsed frequently to avoid clogging. The tube should be immersed in a jar of water and a short spurt of water allowed to clear the tube. The suction equipment should be kept clean by washing it with hot water and soap; and if possible, sterilize it after use.

RESUSCITATION IN ELECTRIC SHOCK

The type and the extent of an injury from electric shock will depend upon the amount and frequency of the current, the duration of contact with the current, and the pathway through the tissue. The resistance of the body primarily is centered on the skin. A dry, well-keratinized, intact skin provides a higher resistance to electricity than moist thin skin and electrical contact is more easily established.

The resulting injuries from electric shock may range from benign to fatal ones. Other than burns and injuries from falls, the possible emergency conditions include:

Tetany (painful spasms) of the musculature of breathing. This usually is limited to the duration of the shock. However, it may cause secondary cardiac arrest to occur when the shock is a prolonged one.

Prolonged paralysis of respiration. This may last for minutes after the shock as a result of massive convulsions.

Heart flutter (ventricular fibrillation) or other serious disturbances of heart rhythm (arrhythmias).

The *cardiopulmonary status* of the patient should be determined as soon as the electrical object has been cleared. Cardiopulmonary resuscitation should be started immediately if spontaneous respirations or circulation are absent. The procedure for CPR is given on p. 120+.

Effective CPR only can be performed with the patient in a horizontal position on a hard surface. In cases where the patient cannot be placed immediately into a horizontal position, but where the rescuer can reach the victim within one minute after the accident, a precordial thump should be delivered and mouth-to-mouth ventilation started immediately. The *precordial thump* is a sharp, quick single blow delivered over the midportion of the sternum, hitting with the bottom, fleshy portion of the fist, 8 to 12 inches from the victim's chest. *Then* the patient should be moved quickly to a flat surface and CPR started. If more than 60 seconds elapse between electric shock and rescue, the precordial thump should not be given. Instead, the victim should receive artificial ventilation and be moved as quickly as possible to a horizontal position, prior to initiating CPR.

RESUSCITATION IN DROWNING

Drowning is a type of suffocation caused by a breathing in of fluids or a spasm of the voice box (larynx). Basic life support resuscitation principles are the same as presented previously on p. 116+, and should be performed immediately.

A drowning victim must be rescued as quickly as possible. Most incidents occur within reach of the rescuer, thus, even a non-swimmer can be of assistance. If the drowning occurs near a dock, pool side, shore, or a boat, the rescuer should lie down and extend a hand, foot, piece of clothing, towel, fishing pole, rope, stick, or other objects to the victim. (See Fig. 4–9.) A ring buoy also may be used to pull the victim to safety, if available. If the drowning occurs too far from shore to extend an object, a boat or surfboard should be used to rescue the victim. The life of the rescuer should *not* be endangered while attempting to rescue a drowning person.

Artificial ventilation should be started *immediately*. Although mouth-to-mouth ventila-tion may be performed while in the water, it may be difficult or impossible because of the depth of the water. In such situations, a flota-tion device may be used to support the head of the victim, while performing mouth-to-mouth ventilation. The rescuer may have to postpone artificial ventilation until he can stand in shal-low water. *Effective cardiac compression can-not be performed in the water.*

Whenever a neck or back injury is sus-pected, the victim *must* be removed from the water on a back support. If available, a back-board should be slipped under water and al-lowed to float up to the victim. (See Fig. 4–10.) If a backboard is not available, such items as a wide board or door may be used. The victim should be secured to the support with any avail-able material to prevent sliding or rolling. (See Fig. 4–11.) The victim should be kept as level as possible while being removed from the water. When materials or assistance are not available, the victim should remain in the water until they do arrive. If removal is urgent because of ex-cessive bleeding, cardiac arrest, or very cold water, the victim's back should be kept as level as possible. See p. 120, for *modified jaw thrust* that should be used in cases of suspected neck injuries.

Stomachs of drowning victims usually be-come distended due to the large amount of water swallowed. The water may be forced out and distention relieved by turning the victim on the side and compressing the upper abdomen. Also, the victim may be turned into a prone (face downward) position and lifted under the stomach with the rescuer's hands to force the water out.

All patients saved from drowning should be evacuated to a medical facility for additional care.

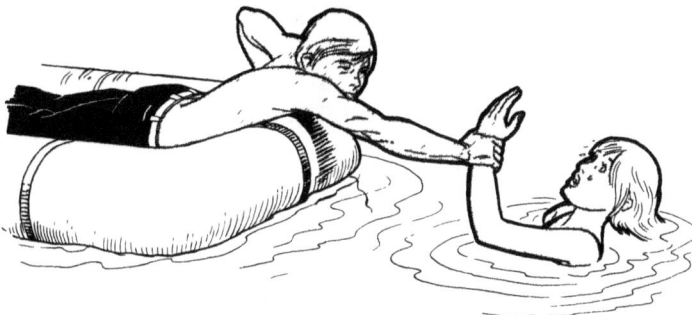

Fig. 4–9.
Rescuing a drowning victim.

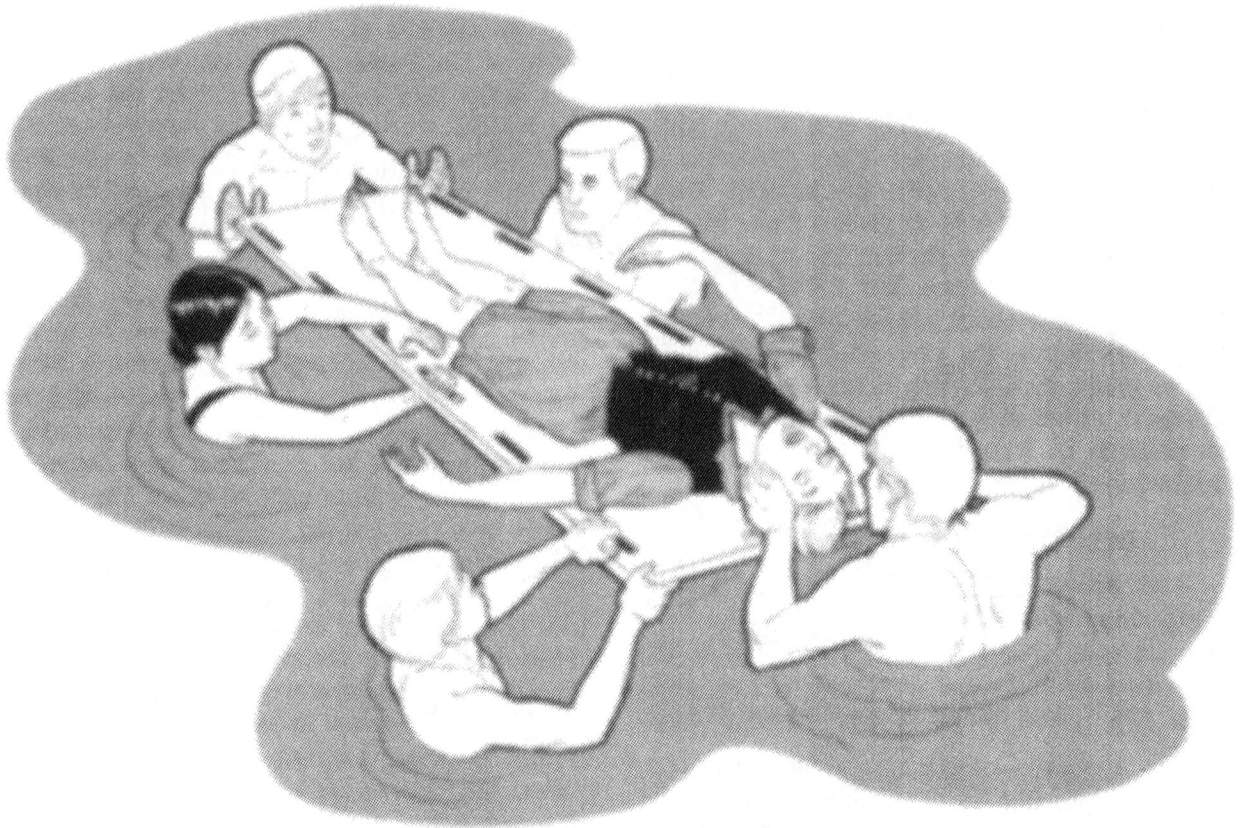

Fig. 4–10. Placing a backboard under a drowning victim.

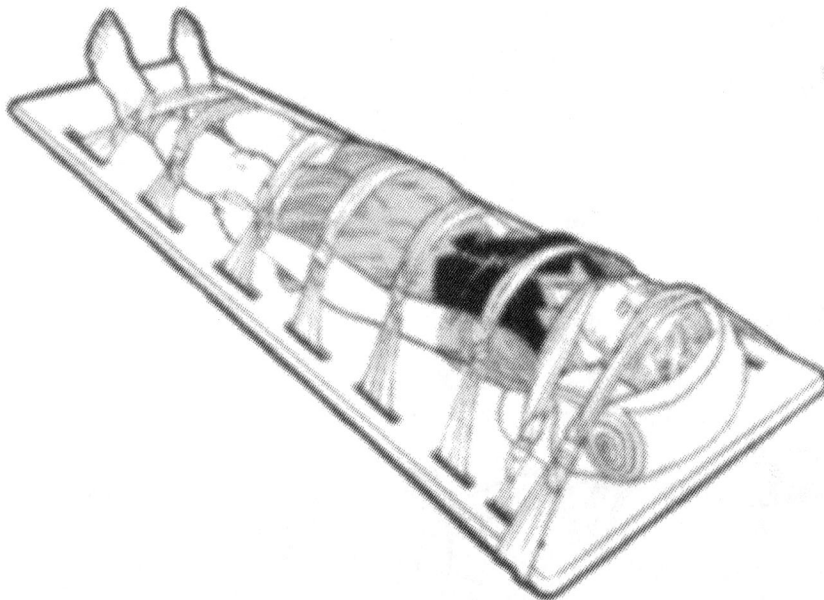

Fig. 4–11. Drowning victim secured to a backboard.

NOXIOUS GASES

Suffocation (asphyxia) may occur when the air we breathe contains noxious (harmful or poisonous) gases as carbon monoxide; carbon dioxide; carbon tetrachloride; petroleum products (as gasoline, kerosene, benzene, ether); and refrigerants (as Freon®, ammonia, carbon dioxide, methyl chloride). These and other noxious gases cause asphyxiation because they block the air passageway to the lungs, or unite with the hemoglobin in red blood cells so that insufficient oxygen is carried to the brain.

General Treatment

When smoke or noxious gases are inhaled, some general rules for first aid are: (1) remove the victim as quickly as possible from the contaminated area of the vessel to a section that has plenty of fresh air; (2) administer oxygen if the person is breathing; (3) if breathing has stopped, give mouth-to-mouth resuscitation (see p. 117+); (4) if both spontaneous circulation and respiration are absent, apply cardiopulmonary resuscitation (see p. 120+); (5) treat for shock (see p. 57+); (6) remove clothing that absorbed the gas; and (7) keep the patient lying down, covered, and quiet.

Caution: For a victim of toxic gas inhalation, as hydrogen cyanide, mouth-to-mouth resuscitation is not recommended because of the potential danger to the rescuer. Instead, a manual resuscitation procedure should be used. (See p. 130+ for a description of the Back Pressure-Arm Lift Technique.)

Medical advice by radio should be obtained. As a general rule, medications other than oxygen should be administered only upon competent medical advice.

Rescue Precautions

Many noxious gases (as carbon monoxide, carbon dioxide, hydrogen, Freon®) have no odor to warn anyone of their presence. Also, safety measures against fire and explosion must be made for combustible gases as hydrogen, carbon monoxide, and methyl chloride, among others.

If the victim of gassing is in a closed compartment or at the bottom of a hold, *a rescuer should go down only if he has a lifeline attached around his chest and under the armpits.* Another lifeline should be taken to be attached in a similar manner to the casualty. Also where victims are exposed to gas or lack of oxygen, rescuers should use a breathing apparatus, smoke helmet, or smoke mask with a tube attached to open air. Nothing should be done that will jeopardize the safety of the rescuer or victim. If the victim will not be rescued quickly, a breathing appartus should be taken down to him.

When no breathing apparatus is carried aboard ship, extreme care must be taken if a rescuer goes below to bring up a victim. The rescuer should be pulled up immediately if contact is lost by voice or by line and the lifeline goes taut. *A gas mask gives little or no protection and is of no value as a breathing apparatus.*

Ammonia Gas in Air

Ammonia is an alkali. It is used as a refrigerant.

Breathing ammonia vapor in low concentrations will cause watering and irritation of the eyes and catching of the breath or coughing. Highly concentrated ammonia vapor causes choking, and intense irritation and corrosion of the air passageway. Collapse, respiratory arrest and death can result. Other symptoms may be excessive salivations, nausea, vomiting, diarrhea, abdominal pain, shock, and convulsions.

Treatment

Remove the victim to a well-ventilated space. Flush the eyes with water for at least five minutes. Give a dilute solution of citrus fruit juice or vinegar diluted with equal parts of water to act on gastrointestinal irritation. Apply artificial respiration. If the patient is breathing, have oxygen inhaled under positive pressure to prevent excessive accumulation of fluid in the lungs. Respiratory depressant narcotics as morphine sulfate and codeine sulfate should *not* be given. *Medical advice by radio should be obtained* on ammonia inhalation.

Carbon Dioxide

This colorless, odorless gas is heavier than air and may collect in holds and compartments of vessels. Suffocation from carbon dioxide may occur while fighting a fire in a hold. The gas may be used as a refrigerant. Grain in the hold that ferments and refrigerated cargoes of certain foods may produce the gas. Exposure to carbon dioxide causes giddiness, headache, breathing difficulties, and loss of consciousness.

Treatment

The victim should be removed to fresh air and oxygen inhalation administered. If respiration has ceased, mouth-to-mouth resuscitation should be given. (See p. 117+.) *Medical advice by radio should be obtained* on handling exposure to carbon dioxide gas.

Carbon Monoxide

This gas is colorless, odorless, lighter than air, and combustible. Carbon monoxide is produced from incomplete combustion of organic matter in fires that may occur in the hold of a vessel, from some explosions, and the exhaust gases of gasoline and oil-driven engines. It can form in ill-ventilated stokeholds when refrigerated meat cargoes decompose. Carbon monoxide reacts with the hemoglobin of the red blood cells to cut off the body's oxygen supply. Exposure to this gas produces dizziness, intense headache, muscular weakness, throbbing in temples, dilated pupils, and breathing difficulty that results in unconsciousness. In severe cases the lips may be bright red, and the skin of the face and body has a pink color. In high concentrations of carbon monoxide, a person will die in a few minutes.

Treatment

The patient should be removed from the contaminated air as quickly as possible with little or no exertion on his part. Artificial respiration by mouth-to-mouth should be applied. If the patient is breathing, inhalations of 100% oxygen should be given. He should be kept in bed and chilling avoided. *Medical advice by radio should be obtained on caring for those exposed to carbon monoxide.*

Cyanides

Hydrogen cyanide or hydrocyanic acid is used to fumigate ships. Both the solid cyanides and the gaseous form are extremely poisonous.

Refer to p. 112+ for detailed information. *Medical advice by radio should be obtained.*

Carbon Tetrachloride
Other Chlorinated Hydrocarbons

Carbon tetrachloride is a poison that affects the nervous system. Prolonged exposure causes loss of consciousness. Low level exposure causes headache, dizziness, and a feeling of depression and confusion with loss of coordination. Extensive liver and kidney damage can follow one high-level exposure or repeated exposures to low level concentrations. The symptoms of poisoning often are delayed. A victim exposed to a toxic concentration of the vapor often does not realize his condition, until he becomes dangerously ill several hours later. Signs of poisoning include nausea, headache, mental confusion, and occasionally drunken behavior like that caused by alcohol. Eyes, nose, throat, and lungs will show considerable irritation.

The chlorinated hydrocarbons have had wide usage as solvents for dissolving oils, fats, and waxes. They have been used for dry cleaning, degreasing metal articles, and cleaning electric and electronic equipment. However, this type of usage is being restricted because of the poisoning potential of these chemicals.

Carbon tetrachloride in the past has been used in some fire extinguishers, but this use is not widespread now. Not only is inhalation of its vapor poisonous, but fire and heat will decompose it to form phosgene gas—a deadly irritant that has been used as a chemical warfare agent.

Treatment

For inhalation of carbon tetrachloride (and other chlorinated hydrocarbons) move the victim from the toxic area. Remove contaminated clothing. If he is breathing, give oxygen. If necessary, apply artificial respiration. Keep the patient lying down, quiet, and warm. (*Caution:* DO NOT USE ALCOHOL OR STIMULANTS!) Wash the body with soap and water to remove the contaminant.

Freon ®

Freon is a colorless, odorless gas that has extensive use as a refrigerant. It is a registered trademark for selected halogenated compounds containing fluoride. The trademark is used only with compounds that are nonflammable and low in toxicity. Although generally classed as non-poisonous, it is toxic in high concentrations. Dangerous conditions may be created in closed space areas aboard ship when large quantities of Freon gases leak from refrigeration units.

In confined or unventilated sections, Freon may displace the air and produce asphyxiation in anyone caught in the areas. After prolonged inhalation of Freon gases, a patient may have serious disruption of normal heartbeat if subjected to fear or excitement, which causes the body to release adrenalin. The liquid form of some types of Freon in contact with eyes and skin may cause frostbite or freezing of tissues.

In a fire aboard ship, Freon gases in contact with an open flame or hot metal surfaces may undergo chemical change to produce poisonous gases that tend to collect in low places. These toxic gases are easily detected by their intensely irritating effect on the nose and eyes.

Rescue: There should be forced air ventilation of the areas where Freon gas is present. Those who must enter the danger area should use mechanical breathing apparatus with an independent air supply and a lifeline. Gloves, protective clothing, and special eyeglasses also should be worn to prevent frostbite.

Treatment

Remove a patient from the toxic atmosphere. Take off the contaminated clothing. Give artificial respiration, if necessary. Pay special attention to the victim's eyes because Freon is a powerful freezing agent that can freeze delicate eye tissues. Flush the eyes for several minutes with running water. Keep the patient at rest for several hours to avoid excitement or emotional stress. *Do not give any medication that contains epinephrine or similar heart-stimulating drugs. Medical advice by radio should be obtained.*

Methyl Chloride

Methyl chloride is a colorless, combustible gas with an ether-like odor. It has been used as a refrigerant. It is a dangerous substance which may cause drowsiness, nausea, vomiting, mental confusion, convulsions, coma, and death. The gas is absorbed rapidly through the skin, adding to its toxicity. Accumulation of fluid in the lungs and bronchial pneumonia are most often the cause of death from methyl chloride.

Because of its explosive nature, the gas is dangerous in low concentrations. Therefore, no naked flame or light should be exposed to its vapor. If an accident occurs that involves methyl chloride, electric motors should be stopped to avoid risk of sparking.

Treatment

The victim exposed to methyl chloride should be removed from the contaminated area. Take off the patient's clothing, and administer oxygen and/or artificial respiration. Restrain an overactive patient. Medical advice by radio should be obtained at once on further treatment or evacuation.

Petroleum Gases

Extremely dangerous concentrations of fumes or gases from various petroleum products may be encountered aboard vessels carrying these cargoes. In addition to being on the alert for possible suffocation or poisoning, strict precautionary measures against fire and explosion are necessary.

Gasoline, benzene, naphtha, and other petroleum products are poisonous if swallowed or inhaled, or if there is prolonged contact with the skin. If gasoline is swallowed, see p. 111 for treatment.

Inhalation of gasoline fumes produces a kind of intoxication like that caused by alcohol. At first, the victim has a false sense of well-being and security. Then his ability to think is lessened, giddiness sets in with uncoordinated and unsteady movements. Because he is likely to fall, he should be kept away from moving machinery. The face becomes flushed or mucous membranes develop a bluish tint because of reduced hemoglobin in the capillaries. Exposure to concentrated fumes causes dilated pupils, labored breathing, followed by coma and death from asphyxiation.

Treatment

Assist the victim to a well-ventilated area and remove contaminated clothing. If he is breathing, give oxygen or an oxygen-carbon dioxide mixture. If breathing is not evident, give artificial respiration.

Medical advice by radio should be obtained before administering any medications. The patient should be kept in bed, warm, and quiet. When he begins to recover, he may become violent and almost uncontrollable. He should be carefully guarded to prevent self-injury or harm to others.

ALTERNATE METHOD OF ARTIFICIAL VENTILATION

In some instances mouth-to-mouth resuscitation cannot be used. For instance, certain toxic and caustic materials create a hazard to the rescuer. Also, facial injuries may prohibit the use of mouth-to-mouth or mouth-to-nose resuscitation. This section describes an effective alternate method of artificial respiration, the *Back Pressure—Arm Lift Technique.* However, a rescuer must remember that this method should be used only when circumstances prohibit the use of the more desirable exhaled air technique.

Back Pressure—Arm Lift Method

The rescuer should place the victim who has stopped breathing in the position shown in Fig. 4–12, clear the patient's mouth and throat, and begin artificial respiration at once.

Step 1. *Position of the Victim*

Place the victim in a face-down position. Bend his elbows, placing one hand on the other. Turn his face to one side and place his cheek on his hands, with his chin jutting out. If there is a second rescuer available to assist, have him hold the victim's chin in the jutting-out position. Remove foreign matter from the mouth and pull his tongue forward. Always make sure that the tongue does not block the air passage.

Step 2. *Position of the Rescuer*

The rescuer should kneel on either the right or left knee at the head of the victim, facing him. Place the knee at the side of the victim's head, close to his forearm. Place the opposite foot near the victim's elbow. If it is more comfortable, the rescuer can kneel on both knees, one on each side of the victim's head.

Next, the rescuer should place his hands on the flat of the victim's back in such a way that the heels of the hands lie just below a line running between the armpits. With the tips of the thumbs just touching, the rescuer's fingers should be spread downward and outward.

Step 3. *Compression Phase*

The rescuer rocks forward until his arms are about vertical, and allows the upper part of his body to exert slow, steady, even pressure downward upon the hands in contact with the victim's back. This forces air out of the lungs. The rescuer's elbows should be kept straight and the pressure exerted almost directly downward on the victim's back. Do not exert sudden or too heavy pressure. The rescuer's hands should not be placed high on the victim's back or shoulder blades.

Step. 4. *Position for Expansion Phase*

The rescuer should release the pressure by "peeling" his hands from the victim's back without giving any extra push with the release. The rescuer should rock slowly backward while gliding his hands along the victim's arms, until he is able to grasp the arms with each hand, just above the elbows.

Step 5. *Expansion Phase*

The victim's arms should be drawn upward toward the rescuer. While doing this, the rescuer should keep his arms straight. Just enough lift should be applied on the victim's arms by the rescuer so that resistance and tension can be felt at the victim's shoulders. The arm lift pulls on the victim's chest muscles, arches his back, and relieves the weight on his chest. The victim's arms are placed gently on the floor to complete the cycle.

Step 6. *Repeat Previous Five Steps*

The above cycle should be repeated about 12 times per minute at a steady rate to the rhythm of (a) *press,* (b) *release,* (c) *lift,* (d) *release.* The counts for *press* (compression) and *lift* (expansion) should occupy about equal time, with the *release* periods being of minimum duration. The emphasis is placed on *press* and *lift* because these are the action steps. *Artificial respiration should be continued for two hours; longer if there are signs of life.*

The rescuer may use either or both knees, and the knees may be shifted during the procedure with no break in the steady rhythm. Remember to rock *forward* with the back pressure and *backward* with the arm lift. The rocking motion helps to sustain the rhythm and adds to the ease of operation. If the rescuer gets tired and another person is available, take turns with him. In making the change, be sure that the rhythm is not broken.

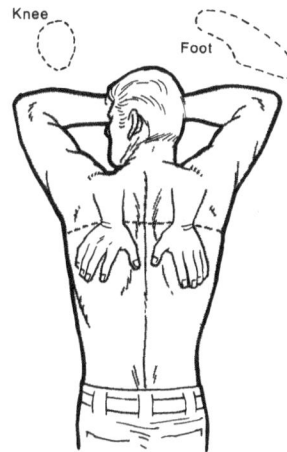

a. Position of the Subject

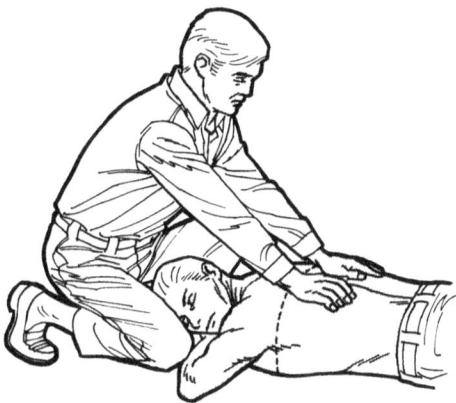

b. Position of the Operator

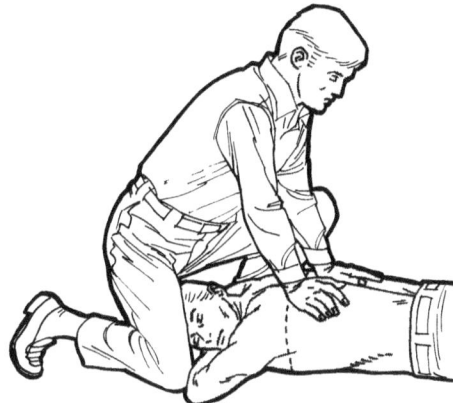

c. Compression Phase

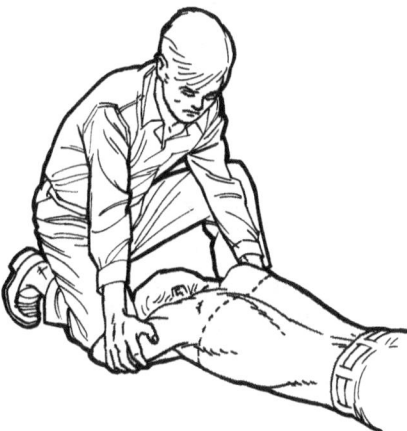

d. Position for Expansion Phase

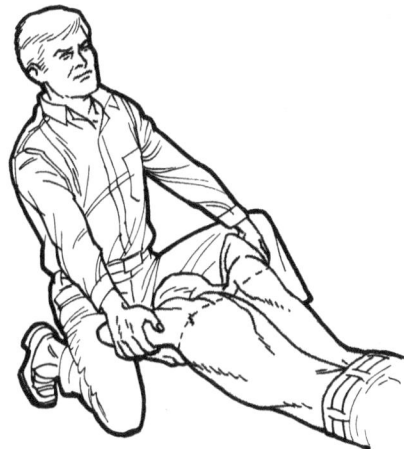

e. Expansion Phase

Fig. 4–12. Back pressure—arm lift method of resuscitation.

CHOKING EMERGENCIES

An estimated 4,000 people in the United States today choke to death from food and other materials that lodge in the windpipe (trachea).

The middle-aged and the elderly have been found to be prone to choking on food, especially if they have had several alcoholic drinks, or have ill-fitting artificial teeth. However, choking incidents can strike people at all ages, it commonly occurs among children who swallow small toys and other objects.

Usually the incident occurs at the dinner table from meat or other food that the victim cannot swallow. *The person chokes suddenly and cannot breathe, turns blue or black, cannot speak, and dies in 4 or 5 minutes.* Usually those who witness the incident stand by helplessly and often think that the victim is having a heart attack. Thus the choking incident has become known as a *cafe coronary*. Artificial respiration and slapping the victim's back have been found to be futile motions for this type of emergency.

A physician at the scene could cut an opening into the throat to reach the trachea, or he could insert a large-caliber hypodermic needle to provide a temporary airway. Such expertise seldom is available to provide the immediate action required. Dr. Henry J. Heimlich at the University of Cincinnati College of Medicine developed a procedure that anyone can perform to save a choking victim's life.

Heimlich Maneuver*

The Heimlich procedure is performed as follows: The rescuer stands behind the choking victim and puts both arms around him just above the belt line. The victim's head, arms, and upper torso are allowed to hang forward. Then the rescuer grasps his fist with his other hand, and presses upward quickly into the victim's abdomen. This action below the rib cage forces the diaphragm upward to compress the lungs and expel air that removes the obstructing food mass. (See Fig. 4–13.) When the choking victim is sitting, the rescuer kneels behind the chair and wraps his arms around the back of the chair and the victim, then

*Adapted from "Pop Goes The Cafe Coronary," by Henry J. Heimlich, M.D. *Emergency Medicine*, Vol. 6. No. 6, pp. 154–5, June 1974.

performs the Heimlich maneuver in the same manner.

The same effect can be obtained with the victim lying face up on the floor and the rescuer kneeling astride the victim's hips or thighs. The rescuer presses quickly with both hands—one on top of the other—into the navel and below the rib cage). (See Fig. 4–14.)

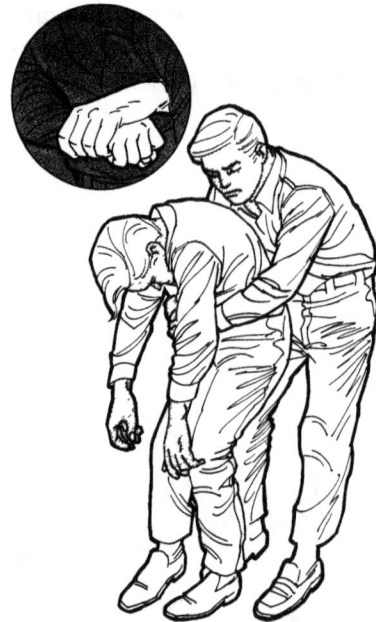

Fig. 4–13. Heimlich maneuver (rescuer standing and victim standing or sitting). Standing behind the victim, wrap your arms around his waist. Grasp your fist with your other hand and place the fist against the victim's abdomen. Press the abdomen with a quick upward thrust.

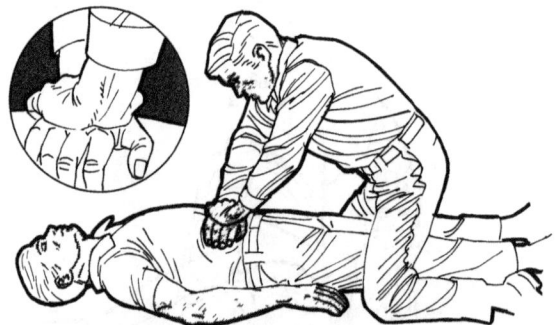

Fig. 4–14. Heimlich maneuver (rescuer kneeling and victim lying on his back). Kneel astride the victim's hips. Put one hand on top of the other and place the heel of the bottom hand on the abdomen. Press in with a quick upward thrust. Repeat, if necessary.

In both situations described above, the rescuer must remove the food from the victim's mouth with his fingers—especially if the victim is on his back.

It has been reported there have been incidents when it was necessary to perform the procedure eight or nine times to dislodge the foreign body. Once or twice was not enough. In a few instances, a poorly informed rescuer did not succeed, only to be followed by a second rescuer whose efforts expelled the offending food mass. Also, there have been many occasions when choking victims have self-administered the Heimlich maneuver—punching the upper abdomen with the fists, or pressing the abdomen against the edge of a sink or table, or the back of a chair.

Misapplication of the maneuver has resulted in several cases of cracked ribs caused by crushing embraces applied by overzealous rescuers. Such injuries may be avoided if the rescuer remembers to press INWARD and UPWARD with his HANDS—he should not squeeze with his arms.

Near-Drowning Victims

Dr. Heimlich states that the Heimlich maneuver has been successful in saving the lives of near-drowning victims, after usual resuscitative efforts failed. The maneuver forced water out of the lungs to gush forth from the mouth. As one rescuer stated: "You can't get air into the lungs, until you get the water out."

WHEN PATIENTS NEED OXYGEN

Delay Can Be Fatal!

When breathing is impaired during medical emergencies, the patient usually requires some method of artificial ventilation. (See p. 116.) However, some patients may have illnesses or accidents that require highly concentrated oxygen—as in heart attacks, shock, severe burns, heavy loss of blood, or extreme breathing difficulties. To save a person's life, it may be necessary to use a resuscitator or mask to supply oxygen.

To administer oxygen effectively, medical attendants aboard ship should have received prior training in resuscitation and the care and use of oxygen apparatus or equipment. Ship owners and Masters of vessels should consult with State and local health departments and emergency medical care units on (1) the training of all concerned; and (2) the purchase and maintenance of reliable oxygen therapy equipment.

CARDIOPULMONARY RESUSCITATION (CPR)

Lifesaving Procedure!

Cardiopulmonary resuscitation (CPR) is a lifesaving technical procedure, which requires exactness and good physical coordination. *Book knowledge only* on how to administer CPR is not enough. Correct practice at frequent intervals is required. A mannikin—not a healthy person—should be used during practice sessions on CPR. Personnel should receive supervised training in a formal course of instruction, certified by either the American Heart Association or the American National Red Cross.

Thus aboard ship, it is desirable that several people will have received training in first aid and be certified to apply CPR. Also, it is essential that retraining and recertification be carried out periodically.

All text on cardiopulmonary resuscitation (CPR), stated previously in Chapter IV, should be used primarily to refresh the memories of personnel who are certified to apply CPR.

Chapter V

Treatment
of
Diseases

Section A
INTRODUCTION

IF THIS TEXTBOOK IS STUDIED CAREFULLY, a medical attendant will be able to provide essential treatment promptly. Those who become familiar with the entire text will find it useful as a ready reference for specific problems. Also, it carries reminders on when to consult with a physician by radio.

It is important for the ship's Master and other concerned personnel to remember that many symptoms are common to several diseases. For example, a large number of communicable diseases start with the same group of symptoms: general malaise, headache, constipation, sore throat, running nose, inflamed eyes, and slight fever. The specific symptoms of the disease, on which a definitive diagnosis can be made, may not develop for hours or days. The treatment is much the same during the early stages of these diseases. This is referred to as "symptomatic treatment" and consists of relieving the unpleasant symptoms or complaints of the patient. Common examples of symptomatic treatment are aspirin for headache and rest for malaise.

The material on the following pages should help the ship's Master and other responsible personnel to treat most medical emergencies at sea. The medicines considered to have a priority in the treatment of these emergencies are described in Chapter VI. If possible, medical advice by radio should be obtained before administering any medication that requires a doctor's order or prescription. Such a medication will include a statement on the label affixed to the container that a prescription (physician's order) is required.

When a seaman is in good physical condition, an illness that he is likely to get at sea should improve under simple treatment. Therefore, to assure maximum body resistance to disease, a seaman should have an annual physical examination and have all immunizations current.

The index at the end of this book should be referred to freely. Symptoms and diseases are cross-indexed to provide a broader and safer check beyond the alphabetical list of references in this chapter.

This book is only an elementary guide. However, it should enable the reader to acquire a certain skill in the following essentials of diagnosis and treatment:

• Ability to make a primary diagnosis and to know the application of symptomatic treatment.

• Ability to further refine a diagnosis by observation of the patient and from medical advice by radio.

• Ability to recognize a communicable disease and to take steps to prevent its spread.

• Ability to recognize serious conditions that require additional medical advice by radio.

135

Chapter V

Treatment
of
Diseases

Section B

CARDIOVASCULAR
DISEASES

ACUTE MYOCARDIAL INFARCTION
(Heart Attack, Coronary Occlusion)

THE PATIENT FREQUENTLY is a heavy cigarette smoker over 40 years of age. A history of hypertension, diabetes, angina pectoris, or a previous myocardial infarction will help confirm the diagnosis of a heart attack. The pain usually is centered behind the breastbone and is not intermittent or pulsating. Generally it is described as a pressure or squeezing sensation. The pain builds in intensity over the first minutes and lasts from a half hour to several hours. Pain may travel to the left shoulder or left arm, the lower jaw, or upper abdomen. Less often, it radiates to the right shoulder or right arm. Sweating, nausea, and a feeling of impending death often are associated features. The pain is not relieved by changes in body position nor affected appreciably by breathing. If the patient goes into shock or acute heart failure, he may not survive.

Some patients with acute myocardial infarction do *not* have chest pain. They may have fainting, shortness of breath, or palpitations. Because belching and vomiting are common with heart attacks, one should not be mislead and attribute the chest pain to "indigestion."

Treatment

The conscious patient suspected of having a myocardial infarction should be put to bed in a half-sitting position.

For severe pain, morphine sulfate 10 mg by intramuscular injection should be given. If additional doses of morphine sulfate are required, medical advice by radio should be obtained before continuing the medication. If the patient's skin or mucous membranes show a bluish tinge in color (cyanosis), reduced oxygen in the blood or lungs is indicated. If oxygen is available, it should be administered. (See p. 123.)

Medical advice by radio always should be obtained. Evacuation should be arranged as soon as possible.

ANGINA PECTORIS

Angina pectoris occurs when the blood flow to the heart is temporarily inadequate to meet its oxygen needs. The major importance of angina pectoris is that it indicates a patient is prone to myocardial infarction.

The pain of angina pectoris resembles that of myocardial infarction. Usually it is a squeezing, steady pain, centered behind the breastbone. Pain may radiate to the same body areas as in myocardial infarction. However, the pain is different in that it is brought on by physical exertion, exposure to cold, emotional stress, or by the ingestion of food. It seldom lasts longer than ten minutes and almost always responds to nitroglycerin. Acute myocardial infarction is as likely to occur at rest as during activity. This pain lasts much longer than ten minutes and does not respond to nitroglycerin.

Treatment

Nitroglycerin dissolved under the tongue is the most commonly used medication for angina pectoris. After a definitive diagnosis of angina has been made, nitroglycerin can be used freely, especially before activities known to have provoked past attacks. Nitroglycerin tablets should not be swallowed because the acid juices of the stomach destroy the therapeutic effect. Patients should make note of situations that have brought on attacks in the past and try to avoid these.

The patient who is suffering his first attack of angina pectoris should be treated the same as the patient with a myocardial infarction. The same treatment should be given to patients with a long history of angina pectoris whose attacks are more frequent or more easily triggered. Frequent easily provoked attacks often precede an acute myocardial infarction. Medical advice by radio always should be obtained. Evacuation should be arranged as soon as possible.

CONGESTIVE HEART FAILURE

Congestive heart failure occurs when the heart is unable to perform adequately its usual functions. This results in a lessened supply of blood to the tissues and congestion of the lungs. In acute failure, the heart muscle fails quickly and the lungs become congested rapidly. In chronic failure, the heart muscle fails gradually and the body has time to compensate. However, when compensation is no longer adequate, fluid will begin to accumulate in the lower parts of the body. Swelling most often appears in the legs and feet but it may occur in other parts of the body. Although, there are many underlying causes of congestive heart failure, the most common are chronic coronary, hypertensive, and arteriosclerotic heart disease.

The signs and symptoms of the disease depend on whether the onset of failure was sudden or gradual. Generally, a gradual loss of energy and a shortness of breath (dyspnea) occur upon exertion. In more acute cases, the patient may cough up frothy, bloodstained, or pink sputum. Later, shortness of breath may appear during periods of lesser activity, and the patient may need to sit up in bed, or sleep on several pillows at night to breathe more easily. Ankle swelling may occur due to the accumulation of fluid in the tissues and as failure progresses, the swelling may involve the hands, legs, and abdomen. The liver may become enlarged due to congestion which results in discomfort and tenderness. In more advanced cases, there may be a blueness of the skin (cyanosis), especially at the lips, ears, and fingernails.

Treatment

For *acute* failure, see acute myocardial infarction on p. 136. In severe cases of chronic failure, the patient should be placed on absolute bed rest in a sitting or semisitting position. Heavy meals should be avoided, and the food kept as salt-free as possible. Smoking should be prohibited. Medical advice by radio must be obtained. *A patient with chronic heart failure should receive medications only upon medical advice.*

CYANOSIS (Blueness of the Skin)

This bluish discoloration is a result of the body's lack of oxygen and shows up best in the lips, ears, inside of the mouth, and under the nails. Common causes are injury to the chest that impairs breathing, inhaling air with decreased oxygen (as in smoke inhalation), obstruction of breathing channels by foreign objects or by infection (pneumonia), drowning or other causes of suffocation, heart disease, stroke, heavy sedation by alcohol or drugs, and severe infection.

Sometimes cyanosis occurs when the blood supply is decreased to a part of the body. For instance, cold weather may cause cyanosis of the hands and/or feet in susceptible people. When this is the case, the parts involved (usually the fingers and toes) will be blue, while the lips and inside of the mouth will be pink.

Treatment

The underlying disease should be treated. If the cyanosis is due to a lack of breathing, mouth-to-mouth breathing should be started immediately. Oxygen should be administered, if it does not interfere with other forms of treatment. (See Cardiopulmonary Resuscitation, p. 115+.)

EDEMA

Edema means the accumulation of excess body fluid. This fluid usually accumulates in the legs, abdominal cavity, or chest. Edema may be secondary to a variety of causes, the most common being congestive heart failure. Swelling of the patient's ankles and occasionally an increase in the size of his abdomen may be noted. There may be shortness of breath either after exertion or when lying down. A history of high blood pressure, angina pectoris, heart murmur, or a variety of other symptoms related to heart disease may be present. Other common causes of edema include chronic liver disease, kidney disease, varicose veins, or previous vein inflammations (phlebitis). Also, frostbite may cause localized leg swelling.

Treatment

The amount of salt in the patient's diet should be limited. When the edema is caused by a leg problem, swelling will diminish if the legs are elevated. However, if heart failure is suspected, the legs should not be raised as this may aggravate shortness of breath. *Medical advice by radio should be obtained before administering any medications.* (See Angina Pectoris, p. 136.)

HEART RATE IRREGULARITIES
(Skipped Beats and Palpitation)

At times some individuals are conscious of a racing or fluttering (palpitating) heartbeat, or a skipped beat. These irregularities are likely to occur when a person has consumed too much food, alcohol, or coffee; smoked to excess; or is emotionally excited or depressed. These spells of rapid pulse and skipped beats may cause considerable apprehension. Unless they are associated with symptoms of heart disease, there usually is no cause for alarm. However, the patient should be advised to consult a physician.

Treatment

If there are frequent attacks of palpitation or skipped beats, the amount of food eaten at each meal should be reduced to remove the possibility that the stomach has been overloaded. Small quantities of food may be taken between meals if the patient feels hungry. Coffee, tea, alcoholic beverages, and tobacco should be reduced or discontinued to see if they have any relationship to the condition. The patient should have adequate sleep and additional rest. Phenobarbital 30 mg by mouth should be given at bedtime if the patient is unable to sleep.

The patient may have a serious heart disease if the pulse is very irregular, or the heart rate is very slow (less than 50 beats per minute), or very rapid (150 or more beats per minute). This is especially true if these occur with fainting attacks or other symptoms indicating heart disease or heart failure. One should look carefully for other signs of a failing heart. If found, the patient should be treated as indicated under Congestive Heart Failure (p. 137). If the irregularities persist, medical advice by radio should be obtained.

HIGH BLOOD PRESSURE
(Hypertension)

When the heart beats, blood is forced into the arteries and pressure is exerted against their walls. The amount of pressure is determined by the strength of the heartbeat and by the resistance offered by the arteries.

The pressure exerted by the blood on the artery wall can be estimated by a measuring apparatus, the sphygmomanometer. (See procedure for taking blood pressure, p. 306.)

Anything that increases arterial resistance increases blood pressure. A gradual rise in pressure is associated with advancing age. The rise usually is due to increasing rigidity of the arteries and a thickening of the arterial wall. The heart has to pump harder to force the same amount of blood through the hardened arteries.

In general, high blood pressure may be suspected when the diastolic pressure is 90 mm of mercury or above. High blood pressure usually takes years to develop and often is associated with or is a complication of many other diseases.

Hypertension symptoms may include: pain in the back of the head and neck, usually starting early in the morning; flushing of the face; and dimness of vision. It may be associated with heart disease or kidney disease. If high blood pressure is not treated adequately, a stroke may occur due to rupture of blood vessels in the brain.

Treatment

The symptoms should be treated and unnecessary physical and mental strain should be avoided. The patient should eat lightly, restrict salt intake, and maintain bowel regularity. If the patient is restless, phenobarbital 30 mg by mouth should be given two or three times a day as needed.

Medical advice by radio should be obtained when the patient exhibits symptoms of high blood pressure, or has a diastolic pressure of 110 or higher.

LYMPH GLAND ENLARGEMENT

The lymph glands are small, kernel-like nodes found in such places as the neck, armpits, or groins (See Chapter I, p. 19.) The most important ones and the areas they drain are listed below. When a lymph gland becomes swollen and painful, infection must be looked for in the area it drains.

Glands in the groins drain the lymph from the penis, foot, and leg. An infected wound of one leg causes enlargement of the glands on the same side. However, venereal disease, a common cause of enlargement, may cause enlargement of the glands in both groins.

The lymph glands in an armpit drain the lymph from the arm and side of the chest. Those in the front and sides of the neck drain the lymph from the tonsils, adenoids, teeth and gum areas; and those in the back of the neck drain the scalp and neck. Enlargement of all lymph glands in the neck may indicate secondary syphilis or a serious blood disease.

Treatment

The illness causing the infection should be treated. For pain, aspirin 600 mg should be given by mouth every three to four hours. If the patient does not tolerate aspirin, acetaminophen 600 mg should be tried. If the swelling persists, the patient should be referred to a physician.

PHLEBITIS
(Thrombophelebitis)

Phlebitis, sometimes referred to as thrombophlebitis, is an inflammation of the wall of a vein due to the presence of blood coagulation or a clot. It usually occurs as a result of the slowing down of the blood flow in varicose veins. However, phlebitis may occur as a complication of surgery, pregnancy, trauma, and incorrect posture, such as prolonged sitting or crossed legs.

There may be pain and tenderness along the vein, usually in the lower limb, and a hard core may be felt. Frequently, the skin may be red over the hard core area. If a large vein is involved, swelling (edema) may develop in the limb below the level of the clot. Also, a rise in body temperature of two to three degrees may develop. In some acute conditions the patient may complain of a feeling of heaviness or an aching pain in the limb. Patients who have infectious diseases such as typhoid fever or typhus, or have recovered from such diseases, are much more susceptible to phlebitis.

Treatment

The patient should be placed on bed rest (usually for five to ten days). The foot of the bed should be elevated from 6 to 8 inches so that the extremity is on a higher level than the heart. To ease the discomfort, warm moist compresses or a heating pad should be applied to the involved area. The calf of the extremity *never* should be massaged.

If pain or fever is present, aspirin 600 mg may be administered by mouth every four hours. If the patient does not tolerate aspirin, acetaminophen 600 mg should be tried.

Medical advice by radio should be obtained.

PULMONARY EMBOLISM

Pulmonary embolism is caused by a blockage in the arteries of the lung by a fragment of blood clot usually originating in the leg veins. The pain may resemble that of pleurisy (made worse by breathing) or that of myocardial infarction (a constant squeezing pain). The patient may be breathless, quite anxious, and cough up blood. The calves of the legs may be swollen, warm, and tender.

Treatment

If this potentially fatal disease is suspected, the patient should be placed in bed and medical advice by radio should be obtained. Oxygen may be administered for a pulmonary embolism while awaiting advice by radio.

VARICOSE ULCERS

The formation of ulcers or sores is a common complication of varicose veins. They are formed as a result of some trauma which would heal without a problem in a limb with normal circulation. The ulcer may become infected and itching is a common complaint which compounds the problem. The area around the sore is discolored and the ulcer surrounded with a raised dull red border. The center and bottom of the sore is covered with a yellow discharge and the limb is usually swollen.

Treatment

The circulation of the blood in the area should be improved and the ulcer kept clean. In severe cases, bed rest is important and the limb should be elevated on a pillow. The ulcer should be cleansed twice daily with soap and water, and a sterile dressing applied. When the floor of the sore becomes a healthy red color and the pus has disappeared, the healing process has begun. At this point, the sore should be kept clean with sterile dressings. The patient

should be made ambulatory at this time but should avoid standing in one position for any extended period of time. The dressings should be kept fresh and clean.

VARICOSE VEINS

Varicose veins are abnormally dilated veins occurring most often in the lower extremities and the lower trunk. Often they are found in people whose work requires prolonged standing. This places a strain on the valves in veins because muscle action is not helping to return the blood. Chronic systemic disease, as heart disease and cirrhosis of the liver, may interfere with effective return of blood to the heart and contribute to varicosities.

Varicosities of superficial veins appear as darkened, tortuous, raised blood vessels that become more prominent when the patient stands. The patient may have pain, fatigue, a feeling of heaviness in the legs, and muscular cramps. The discomfort is increased greatly by prolonged standing and is worse during hot weather or when the patient is in high altitudes.

Treatment

The patient with varicose veins should be advised to elevate his feet for a few minutes at regular two-hour to three-hour intervals throughout the day to improve circulation in the legs. An elastic stocking or elastic bandage should be worn. If an elastic bandage is used, it should be applied before the patient gets out of bed while the leg is elevated. Rest in bed is essential if there is increased swelling of the leg or foot. The patient should be instructed to seek medical advice when convenient.

Chapter V

Treatment of Diseases

Section C

EAR AND EYE DISEASES

EAR

Earache

AN EARACHE MAY BE CAUSED by infection of the middle ear; an inflammation, abscess, or a boil of the external auditory canal; inflammation of the eustachian tube; dental conditions; mumps; and inflammation of the mastoid bone or other nearby structures.

The ears frequently ache, feel sore, or have a feeling of fullness during a head cold or some other disease in which the respiratory passages are affected. Acute infection of the middle ear causes severe earache and usually results in the formation of an abscess.

Neuralgia is one of the causes of earache and is characterized by a sudden stabbing pain. The patient feels as though someone had stabbed a knife into the eardrum or the canal. Usually, the pain stops suddenly. This fairly rare disease is mentioned to indicate that not all sudden, sharp, stabbing ear pains are due to the common causes listed previously.

Treatment

The upper part of the ear should be pulled upward and backward to inspect the ear canal.

Any swelling, redness, or localized boil should be treated by rest in bed and hot wet compresses applied over the ear. For pain, aspirin 600 mg should be given by mouth every three to four hours as needed. If aspirin is not tolerated by the patient, acetaminophen may be tried at the same dosage and frequency.

Symptoms similar to earache may result from dental conditions. The mouth and teeth should be inspected for dental defects, and if necessary treated as described under Dental Emergencies (see p. 152).

If the throat is inflamed, it should be treated as described under Sore Throat (see p. 230). The sides of the face should be felt beneath the ears for tenderness or swelling that would be suggestive of mumps (see p. 182).

Middle Ear Infection

Bacteria from the nose and throat reach the middle ear through the eustachian tube. Middle ear infections usually develop as a complication of a common cold, tonsillitis, or an acute infection as measles and scarlet fever.

Forcible blowing of the nose may drive infected mucus through the eustachian tube into the middle ear. A patient with nasal con-

141

gestion (stuffy nose) should be instructed to blow his nose gently, preferably with both nostrils open. In acute inflammation of the nose and throat, the measures for relieving nasal stuffiness and sore throat are outlined under the symptomatic treatment of Common Cold (see p. 225). These measures will help prevent infection of the middle ear.

Acute infection of the middle ear causes severe earache. Usually it is accompanied by fever and pus often forms behind the eardrum. If the eardrum is under great pressure, there is a throbbing pain. Spontaneous rupture of the eardrum, with the release of pus, usually gives dramatic relief from pain. If all goes well, the infection clears up in about a week and the hole in the eardrum heals.

The chief danger from a middle ear abscess is the spread of infection to the mastoid bone behind the ear. The signs of mastoid involvement are pain, tenderness on pressure behind the ear, possible swelling behind the ear, continued earache even after rupture of the drum, and usually an increase in fever.

Treatment

For an infection of the middle ear, an initial dose of penicillin V potassium 500 mg should be given by mouth followed by 250 mg every six hours. If the patient is suspected of being allergic to penicillin, oral erythromycin should be used in the same dosage and frequency. The patient should be kept on the antibiotic for at least four days after the temperature becomes normal.

For pain, aspirin 600 mg should be given by mouth every three to four hours as needed. If aspirin is not tolerated by the patient, acetaminophen may be tried at the same dosage and frequency.

Phenylephrine hydrochloride 0.25% nasal drops or nasal spray should be used in the nostrils every eight hours to assist in opening the eustachian tube.

Chronic low grade inflammation of the middle ear, without the formation of pus, may be a complication of repeated or persistent colds. The usual symptoms are a nagging pain, a feeling of dullness or fullness, ringing in the ear, and impaired hearing. Because chronic inflammation of the middle ear is an important cause of loss of hearing, the patient should be

urged to consult a physician when the ship reaches port. Three drops of hydrocortisone-neomycin-polymyxin B eardrops should be used twice a day in the affected ear, until the patient sees a physician.

Earwax, Impacted *(Impacted Cerumen)*

There is a normal secretion of brownish wax (cerumen) in the canal of the external ear. Excessive amounts of this wax is an important cause of deafness. Some persons produce large quantities of earwax. Pain in the ear may occur suddenly because of accumulated hard wax.

Treatment

Hard earwax may be softened by placing a few drops of olive oil or cooking oil into the ear and leaving it in for 24 hours. Then it should be removed by gently syringing the ear with a hypertonic sodium chloride (table salt) solution (one tablespoonful to a glass of lukewarm water). Earwax never should be removed by forcible instrumentation. After irrigation, the external ear canal should be dried thoroughly with cotton-tipped applicators.

The patient should be advised to see a doctor at the next port of call if the problem persists.

EYE

This section on eye problems is not intended to cover all possible problems which might occur at sea. Generally anyone who develops sudden loss of vision, pain in the eye, red eye, or a discharge from the eye deserves medical attention as soon as possible.

Chronic Eye Diseases

Cataracts

A cataract is a clouding of the lens of the eye. This usually occurs as an aging process in people over age 60, but cataracts may occur at a much younger age or even at birth. Cataracts may develop without an obvious cause but some result from severe injuries. In advanced cases, cataracts may be cloudy enough to make the pupil appear white instead of black. Persons with possible cataracts should have a complete eye examination. In almost all cases the cure for cataracts is surgical removal.

Glaucoma

Glaucoma is a category of eye diseases in which the fluid substance in the eyeball is under higher pressure than usual. The glaucomas are probably the most common cause of blindness in the United States. *Primary glaucomas* develop without known cause and include two main types; *chronic simple glaucoma* and *acute congestive glaucoma*. *Secondary glaucomas* may develop as a result of damage due to previous injuries or inflammations of the eye.

Chronic Simple Glaucoma

Chronic simple glaucoma is the most common form of primary glaucoma. It is painless and may go undetected by the patient until severe loss of vision has occurred. It is sometimes called the "sneak thief of vision." This form of glaucoma is detected only by careful professional eye examination. If detected early, vision can be saved. Thus adults should be encouraged to have eye examinations which include glaucoma screening every two years, even in the absence of symptoms.

Treatment

Because signs and symptoms of chronic simple glaucoma generally are not present, it will not be detected aboard ship. However, some crew members already may be under a physician's treatment for the condition. Pilocarpine hydrochloride eye drops in various concentrations are commonly used to treat this form of glaucoma, often in combination with other medications. Because medical treatment of chronic simple glaucoma is of lifelong duration, the patient will be familiar with the specific diagnosis and medication program. Two percent pilocarpine hydrochloride eye drops should be carried aboard ship for temporary use by any of the crew who may run out of the medication. If a crew member is not certain of his diagnosis, or if he is under glaucoma treatment with a different medication, obtain medical advice by radio before substituting pilocarpine.

Acute Congestive Glaucoma

Acute congestive glaucoma is the less common form of primary glaucoma, but it is an extremely serious condition requiring immediate treatment by an eye specialist. The eye pressure increases suddenly accompanied by extreme pain, redness of the eye, and slight cloudiness of the cornea. The pupil does not react to light. In addition to severe pain, which may be accompanied by nausea and vomiting, the patient experiences somewhat decreased vision and perceives colored halos around bright lights.

Treatment

Emergency surgery often is required to lower the pressure in the eye to prevent irreversible loss of vision. Management of acute congestive glaucoma always should be referred to a physician, so medical advice by radio should be obtained in suspected cases. If professional treatment cannot be provided immediately to the patient, the physician giving advice by radio may direct the temporary use of pilocarpine hydrochloride eye drops, and oral administration of acetazolamide tablets (commonly in dosage of 250 mg every 4 to 6 hours).

For pain, aspirin 600 mg should be given by mouth every three to four hours as needed. If aspirin is not well tolerated by the patient, acetaminophen may be tried at the same dosage and frequency. If pain is very severe, a 10 mg dose of morphine sulfate may be given intramuscularly upon medical advice by radio.

Secondary Glaucoma

Secondary glaucoma may develop as a complication of other eye conditions, such as keratitis, corneal ulcer, iritis, and previous surgery or injury.

Treatment

The most important treatment for secondary glaucoma which can be provided aboard ship is prevention. Serious eye disorders should have adequate professional treatment. Crew members should be directed to have professional follow-up of persistant eye problems even if reported as mild. Specific management of secondary glaucoma varies with the cause, often requires surgery, and cannot be generalized. Medical advice by radio should be obtained in suspected cases.

Contact Lens Problems

All contact lens wearers should bring a pair of spectacles aboard ship. If there is any unusual irritation of the eyes, contact lenses should be removed and spectacles worn until the patient is examined by an eye physician. Antibiotic eye drops may be given for irritation that lasts more than a few hours after removing the lenses. Before any medication is used, the patient should be questioned about possible allergies to its ingredients. Any injury or infection to the eye is another indication to discontinue wearing a contact lens until seen by an eye physician. With chemical injuries, the immediate removal of the lenses is indicated. Although the contact lens may tend to protect the cornea from some foreign materials, liquids will flow rapidly under the lens to create a more hazardous situation.

Removal of Contact Lens—The wearer may need assistance if he has difficulty removing his contact lenses, or if a lens becomes dislodged from the cornea under the lid and cannot be repositioned. If the lens is under an eyelid, the wearer should look in the opposite direction, lift the lid and try to slide the lens onto the cornea.

A lens cannot slip behind the eyeball. If it cannot be located, no harm will occur if it remains under the eyelid until the patient can be examined by an eye doctor. However, to prevent possible infection, antibiotic eye drops as polymyxin B-neomycin-gramicidin should be instilled four times daily.

Infectious Eye Diseases

The most common infectious eye diseases that might be encountered aboard ship include blepharitis (infection of the eyelid margins), conjunctivitis (infection of the conjunctiva), sties (infection of the glands in the lid margins), and more rarely, keratitis (infection of the cornea). Also discussed are orbital cellulitis and trachoma.

Before any medication is used in the eye or elsewhere, the patient should be questioned about possible allergies to ingredients in the medication.

Blepharitis

Blepharitis is an inflammation of the margins of the eyelids with redness and thickening, plus crusting that resembles dandruff. There is itching, burning, loss of eyelashes, tearing, and

sensitivity to light. There may be shallow marginal ulcers.

Nonulcerative blepharitis—This scaly type may be caused by allergies or associated with seborrhea (dandruff) of the scalp or face, which should be treated. The scales on the margins of the lids may be greasy and easily removable.

Ulcerative blepharitis—This is a bacterial infection (usually staphylococcal) of glands on the lids and follicles of the eyelashes. Removal of the crusts causes bleeding. Pus forms in the follicles of the lashes and ulcers appear. While the patient sleeps, the lids become glued together. Often there is a history of repeated sties and chalazions. (A chalazion is a small cyst or tumor on the margin of an eyelid that is caused by an infection of an oil gland.) Both types are slow to heal, resist treatment, and may recur.

Treatment

For the *nonulcerative type*, dandruff of the scalp or facial dermatitis should be eliminated. Then polymyxin B-neomycin-bacitracin ophthalmic ointment should be applied with a sterile applicator or clean fingertip directly to the lashes at the lid margins.

For *ulcerative blepharitis*, hot compresses may be applied during the acute phase and in the morning if the lids are stuck together. Crusts may be removed with a moistened sterile applicator. Then polymyxin B-neomycin-bacitracin ophthalmic ointment may be massaged with the fingers on the lashes along the lid margins as described above. Polymyxin B-neomycin-gramicidin eye drops may be used during the day and the ointment applied at night and upon arising.

Medical advice by radio should be obtained. If the condition persists, the patient should consult an ophthalmologist upon reaching shore.

Conjunctivitis, General

Conjunctivitis is an infection of the conjunctiva of the eyes. Somewhat different signs and symptoms may be present depending on the specific bacterium or virus that causes the infection. As a rule, the patient will have a red eye, a variable amount of pus, discharge, and tearing, and at times slight pain or sensitivity to light. The eyelids often stick together in the morning and it may be necessary to soak the eyes before they can be opened.

Treatment

The treatment of conjunctivitis consists of applying antibiotic eye drops or ointment, as polymyxin B-neomycin-gramicidin. Before any medication is used in the eye, the patient should be questioned about possible allergies to ingredients in the medication. Care should be taken to keep washcloths, towels, and linen from being used by other members of the crew. Food handlers should be relieved of duty until well. Most cases respond to treatment in three or four days. Even without treatment most of the cases clear by themselves within ten to 12 days with the exception of gonococcal conjunctivitis.

Conjunctivitis, Gonococcal

Gonococcal conjunctivitis is differentiated from other kinds of conjunctivitis by the presence of an acute purulent (with pus) inflammation of the eye and marked swelling, redness, and firmness of the lids. Untreated gonococcal conjunctivitis may cause corneal ulceration and scarring with loss of vision. It is usually unilateral but may spread to the other eye. The mode of transmission almost always is by fingers from the genitalia to the eye. Concurrent infection of the genitalia if present will aid in the diagnosis. Medical advice by radio should be obtained to help confirm the diagnosis before local or systemic anti-infective therapy is initiated.

Treatment

Warm saline soaks to the infected eye and antibiotic eye drops as polymyxin B-neomycin-gramicidin instilled every two hours are good supportive therapy for possible gonococcal conjunctivitis, while awaiting medical advice by radio. If gonococcal infection is confirmed, the patient should be treated with antibiotics as directed by radio medical advice. Before antibiotic eye drops are used, the patient should be questioned about possible allergies to ingredients in the medication.

Sty

A sty is an abscess of the small oil glands along the margin of an eyelid. There is usually a painful red lump in the eyelid which may increase in size, finally open, and drain pus.

Treatment

Treatment for a sty consists of (1) frequent hot moist soaks (at least four times daily, for 15 minutes each time); (2) antibiotic eye drops as polymyxin B-neomycin-gramicidin four times a day, following a hot soak; and (3) antibiotic eye ointment as polymyxin B-neomycin-bacitracin at bedtime for one week after the sty drains. A sty should not be squeezed or lanced. After the infection subsides, a small lump occasionally remains which usually disappears slowly in a period of several weeks. The lump may persist and if it is large enough will require drainage by a physician.

Keratitis (Inflammation of the Cornea)

There are several kinds of keratitis, an inflammatory condition that affects the cornea, the transparent part of the eyeball. It is more serious than conjunctivitis because scarring of the cornea may result in a serious loss of vision. Keratitis may be due to primary or secondary infections from bacteria (staphylococcal, streptococcal, or pneumococcal). A viral form is caused by the *herpes simplex type 1* (cold sore or fever blister) *virus.* Another type of keratitis is one that may accompany *shingles* (*herpes zoster*) when facial nerve cells are involved.

Corneal inflammation may be associated with ulcers that arise from abrasions or other injury. A foreign body in the eye, a scratch from a finger, or a contact lens may erode the corneal surface to set the stage for an infection that leads to keratitis. One must be careful when foreign bodies are being removed from the eye, because infectious microorganisms could be introduced into the cornea at the same time. A foreign body imbedded in the cornea should be removed with a spud* or a sterile needle—not with a cotton swab—because the cotton will destroy the surface epithelium.

Eyespud is an ophthalmic instrument used to remove foreign bodies from the eye. Prior training is recommended for those who intend to use it.

A small flashlight may be used to detect ulcers or other imperfections in the cornea. These imperfections produce irregular reflections, much as an irregularity would on a convex mirror. The patient should be examined in a semidarkened room. If the light from the flashlight is shined from the side onto a normal corneal surface, a clean, smooth reflection will be noted. However, if the medical attendant changes the position of the flashlight so as to vary the angle of incidence while observing the reflection of the light from the cornea, a damaged epithelium often can be identified as an irregular reflection. An antibiotic as polymyxin B-neomycin-gramacidin eye drops and protection of the eye will be necessary until the epithelium heals.

Systemic infections as tuberculosis or syphilis may be carried by the blood to the eye to infect the cornea and cause keratitis. Burns from chemicals or ultraviolet rays may produce a form of keratitis. Allergies also are a cause.

Although symptoms may vary between the several types of keratitis, usually there is a scratchy pain that is moderate to severe, redness, excessive watering of the eye, a conjunctival discharge, and blurred vision.

Treatment

For suspected keratitis, medical advice by radio should be sought. For all types of confirmed keratitis, only an ophthalmologist should provide the treatment.

For superficial abrasions of the epithelium of the cornea, local application of antibiotic eye drops as polymyxin B-neomycin-gramicidin are recommended. Drops are preferred to the ointment because the latter delays healing. An eye patch will help the patient to feel more comfortable.

For a minor corneal abrasion it is not necessary to use a cycloplegic to dilate the pupil. If medical advice by radio recommends cycloplegia, a drop of 5% homatropine hydrobromide may be instilled into the eye along with the polymyxin B-neomycin-gramicidin antibiotic eye drops. (*Do not use homatropine hydrobromide on a patient who has glaucoma; it could aggravate the glaucoma and cause serious damage.*)

The form of keratitis caused by the *herpes simplex virus* produces a superficial corneal ulceration that may be identified by using fluorescein strips. (See p. 279.) The fluorescein often will show a stain pattern on the cornea as a branching arrangement like veins on a leaf, with knoblike terminals. *For keratitis patients with herpes simplex virus as the suspected cause, NEVER use medication that contains cortisone or cortisone-like drugs, such as the anti-inflammatory prednisolone sodium phosphate eye drops stocked in the ship's medicine chest. It may increase the infection and cause blindness.*

Today there is specific antiviral drug therapy—idoxuridine (IDU) — for corneal ulcers caused by the *herpes simplex virus;* but this is not stocked in the ship's medicine chest.

Cortisone or cortisone-like drugs, such as the anti-inflammatory prednisolone sodium phosphate *may* be used for *herpes zoster keratitis*, if medical advice has been obtained.

Orbital Cellulitis

Abnormal protrusion of the eyeball (exophthalmos) with fever, pain, tenderness, redness, and swelling of lids and conjunctivitis may indicate probable orbital cellulitis. The protrusion may be caused by penetrating injuries, extension of infection from the paranasal sinuses and rarely by organisms carried by the bloodstream from a remote site of infection. Meningitis may become a serious complication. Inflammation of the internal tissue of the eyes (endophthalmitis) may result in permanent loss of vision.

Treatment

Antibiotic treatment should be initiated for orbital cellulitis. Penicillin G procaine 1.2 million units should be given intramuscularly twice daily. Medical advice by radio should be obtained on continuing the medication and possible evacuation of the patient. When a history of an allergy to penicillin exists, tetracycline hydrochloride 500 mg should be given by mouth, four times daily for six days.

For pain, aspirin 600 mg should be given by mouth every three to four hours as needed. If aspirin is not tolerated by the patient, acetaminophen may be tried at the same dosage and frequency. If pain is not controlled by aspirin or acetaminophen alone, oral codeine sulfate 30 mg may be given concurrently with either of these medications. To repeat the dosage of oral codeine sulfate, medical advice by radio should be obtained. The patient should be placed on bed rest.

Trachoma

Trachoma remains the leading cause of blindness in the world. In the United States trachoma is relatively rare, except among the Indians of the southwest. Poor diet, unsanitary conditions, and lack of medical care are factors that contribute to the prevalence of this viral disease. It usually begins insidiously with slight redness and irritation and smolders for years, gradually causing severe scarring of the cornea and eyelids. Precautionary measures should be taken to prevent infecting others.

The diagnosis should be made by an eye doctor.

Treatment

A patient suspected of having trachoma should be referred to a doctor at the next port of call. In the meantime, tetracycline 250 mg should be given by mouth four times a day for three weeks, or until the ship reaches port.

Chapter V

Treatment of Diseases

Section D

GASTROINTESTINAL DISEASES

ABDOMINAL PAIN (Stomachache)

THE LOCATION, direction, and characteristics (as cramps that are steady, dull or sharp) of abdominal pain are important in determining its cause. For simplicity, pain above the umbilicus should be considered in the *upper abdominal region* and below the umbilicus in the *lower abdominal region*.

Upper abdominal pain usually is due to conditions of the stomach, upper small intestine (duodenum), pancreas, or bile ducts. Specific causes include food poisoning, gastritis, gastroenteritis (dysentery), gastric and duodenal ulcer, stone in the bile duct (usually with jaundice), and pancreatitis or pancreatic cancer. Medical advice by radio should be obtained when sudden severe pain occurs.

Upper abdominal pain on the right side generally signifies a spasm in the colon, a gall-bladder attack, or a problem of the muscular wall of the abdomen. Other causes would include hepatitis and disease of the right kidney.

A common cause of *lower abdominal pain* on the right side is appendicitis. Other causes would include muscular strain or a stone in the right kidney. Such pain in females may be caused by a twisted ovary, inflamed fallopian tubes, ovarian cyst, or an ectopic pregnancy.

Pain in the left lower abdomen can occur from the causes stated in the previous paragraph with the addition of acute diverticulitis (a type of colitis). Although appendicitis rarely causes pain on the left side, it cannot be ruled out.

Pain across the entire lower abdomen or especially at the midline may be caused by enterocolitis or bowel obstruction. When the pain is mild and not associated with diarrhea, it usually is due to intestinal spasms or excessive intestinal gas. Other causes would include a urinary bladder inflammation (cystitis), inflammatory disease of the pelvic organs, and menstrual cramps in females.

Medical advice by radio should be obtained when the pain is sudden, severe or progressive, and not relieved by an antacid. Laxatives *never* should be given to a patient with abdominal pain without the advice of a physician.

APPENDICITIS

Appendicitis is an inflammation of the appendix. The appendix is a small pouch which is attached to the large intestine in the lower right portion of the abdominal cavity. The usual signs and symptoms of appendicitis include cramps or pain in the abdomen accompanied or followed by loss of appetite, nausea, and occasionally vomiting. The cramps gradually cease and the pain becomes steady and localizes in the lower right quadrant of the abdomen. Nausea and vomiting usually decrease when the pain localizes. There may be fever, a rapid pulse, constipation, or occasionally diarrhea.

If the inflamed appendix lies in the usual position, finger pressure by the medical attendant on the lower right quadrant of the abdomen may produce pain. Sometimes this pain is extremely severe. Often, one will feel tenseness or resistance in the abdominal muscles in this region while the rest of the abdomen is normally soft. Occasionally, when pressure is applied with the palm of the hand on the left side of the lower abdomen and released suddenly, a twinge of pain is felt by the patient on the right side in the region of the appendix. The patient may be extremely uncomfortable and apprehensive.

An attack may either subside or the appendix may rupture and peritonitis may develop. When peritonitis occurs, the patient may show the symptoms and signs of shock. (See Shock, p. 57.) Generally, the temperature is elevated but very little fever may be present if the patient is in shock. In peritonitis, the area of tenderness and muscle tenseness spreads to almost the entire abdomen. The muscles may become rigid as a board.

Treatment

More lives are lost when unqualified persons perform abdominal surgery than when applying proper treatment while waiting for a physician. When evacuated by a helicopter within 300 miles of the U.S. coastline, a seaman is less than eight hours from a well-equipped modern U.S. hospital.

A laxative *never* should be given to a patient suspected of having appendicitis.

The following instructions should be carried out while waiting for medical advice by radio or for evacuation:

• Keep the patient on absolute bed rest.

• *Do not give the patient morphine sulfate if a surgeon will be available within a few hours.* Morphine sulfate may cover up symptoms and make a diagnosis more difficult. If a physician will not be available, a single dose of morphine sulfate 10 mg may be given intramuscularly, if the patient has severe pain, great discomfort, or shows extreme apprehension. Morphine sulfate will reduce or stop the muscular movement of the intestinal walls (peristalsis). To repeat the morphine sulfate, medical advice by radio should be obtained.

• Keep an ice bag over the appendix area.

• *Do not give anything by mouth* for at least 24 hours or until severe acute symptoms have subsided. Then give small amounts of liquid food as water, jello, broth, or fruit juice. As the patient convalesces, this liquid diet can be changed to a soft diet, which may be continued until all symptoms subside.

COLITIS, DIARRHEA, DYSENTERY

Colitis is an inflammation of the large intestine (colon). Usually there is diarrhea, with or without lower abdominal cramps. *Enterocolitis* is inflammation of both the small and large intestines.

Diarrhea is defined as an abnormal increase in the amount, frequency, and fluidity of the evacuations from the intestine. Diarrhea is not a disease itself but a symptom of trouble in the intestinal tract. In this respect, it is like cough, chills, and fever, which are general symptoms of many diseases.

Dysentery is an inflammation of the intestines, particularly of the large bowel. There may be griping abdominal pains and frequent stools often containing blood and mucus.

Colitis, diarrhea, and dysentery often are used interchangeably to describe a variety of conditions with diarrhea. Normally, during the process of digestion, food is moved slowly through the intestines to allow for the absorption of the food. In diarrhea, the motion of the intestines (peristalsis) is speeded up and the stools are soft or semisolid, but may become watery, possibly frothy, and may have a very foul odor.

There are many different causes of diarrhea, colitis, and dysentery. Generally, the symptoms are caused by an infectious organism or its toxic products. Infection may be caused by viruses, a wide variety of bacteria, one-celled animals as amoebic and malarial parasites, and many-celled organisms as intestinal worms.

The non-infectious causes include poisoning from heavy metals as mercury, allergies to certain foods, inability to digest foods or absorb the digested foods, and emotional upsets.

In most cases of diarrhea there is inflammation of the intestines. The loss of fluid through large watery stools may cause serious complications. Dehydration leading to coma or death may occur when extreme diarrhea is combined with vomiting. This will cause a loss of the water taken in and of water stored in the body. Severe dehydration may occur rapidly. In addition to loss of water, the loss of various chemicals normally dissolved in body fluids may cause complications and death.

Signs which may be useful in determining the cause of intestinal illness and its severity include:

• *Character of stools*—Are they watery? What is the color? Is there blood, odor, mucus, or pus? Are worms visible? Is it all liquid, or are there some formed pieces?

• *Frequency of stools*—How often does the patient pass stools?

• *Signs of dehydration*—Is the mouth very dry? Do the eyeballs seem unusually sunken? If you pinch the skin, does the fold return slowly to its former position?

• *Other signs*—Is there a rash on the skin, or vomiting?

• *History*—Has the patient ever had intestinal symptoms before, if so when? Does the patient have any idea what might be causing the symptoms?

• *Epidemiology*—Is anyone else sick? What symptoms do the patients have in common?

There are methods of controlling the incidence of diarrheal illness. In foreign ports, it is important to drink pure or boiled water, and to avoid uncooked foods and unclean eating places. Good hygiene should be maintained aboard ship. Appropriate immunizations should be kept current.

Treatment of Diarrhea

Because the mechanism governing diarrhea is basically the same, regardless of the cause, the means of controlling this symptom need not be extensive. The patient should be placed on bed rest and made as comfortable as possible. A liquid or low-residue diet should be given that includes soft drinks and broths containing salt. Milk will be helpful if it can be tolerated by the patient. Spicy, fatty, or greasy foods should be avoided. If there is blood in the vomitus or in the stools, signs of dehydration (especially a daily weight loss of 3 or more pounds), or decreasing urinary output (less than 500 ml in 24 hours), *prompt medical advice by radio should be obtained.* Intravenous fluids, isotonic sodium chloride solution or 5% dextrose and 0.45% sodium chloride solution may be ordered by the physician.

The patient's feces should be flushed into the ship's sewage treatment system or retention tank. Eating utensils and plates should be boiled for 10 to 15 minutes to disinfect them if an automatic dishwater is not available.

Although adsorbents as kaolin-pectin mixture are of limited effectiveness, they should be given for mild to moderate diarrhea. In the acute disease, diphenoxylate hydrochloride with atropine should be administered promptly. Initially, two tablets of diphenoxylate with atropine should be given four times a day. Most patients will require this dosage level until control is achieved. Then a downward adjustment of the dosage should be made. Control may be obtained from two tablets of diphenoxylate with atropine per day.

Caution

The drug diphenoxylate may make more effective the action of barbiturates, tranquilizers, and alcohol. Therefore, the patient should be observed closely when these medications are administered together. Do not give this drug to young children.

Specific causes of diarrhea and some special treatments are outlined below:

Viruses. Several viruses produce enterocolitis with or without gastritis (vomiting and upper abdominal discomfort). Usually, there is little or no fever, the onset lasts several hours and the illness is over within two or three days. The vomitus and stools are watery without blood and mucus. The patient often feels well between bouts of diarrhea or vomiting. Epidemics or single cases may develop.

Salmonella. The salmonella organism, which may be carried in powdered eggs, powdered milk, or other food, as well as by livestock and some pets, produces one kind of food poisoning. (See p. 157.) A shipboard epidemic of salmonelosis could occur if the organism is food-borne.

The clinical picture of salmonellosis resembles that of viral enterocolitis. Without a stool examination the diagnosis is uncertain. Mucus may be present in the stool, vomiting is absent or insignificant, and a faint rash (rose spots) may appear on the abdomen and trunk. The illness may last several days.

Shigella. These bacteria produce shigellosis, clinically similar to salmonellosis. Bloody diarrhea is more apt to occur with shigella than with salmonella. If the illness is severe, medical advice by radio should be obtained.

Staphylococcus. Staphylococcal food poisoning (see p. 157) is caused by the toxins of staphylococci bacteria which are produced in poorly refrigerated foods as pastries, custards, and mayonnaise. The symptoms begin rapidly and violently within 1 to 6 hours after eating the contaminated food. There is considerable vomiting and diarrhea, and abdominal cramps and prostration occur.

Amoeba. Amoebic dysentery is caused by *Entamoeba histolytica,* a parasite that infects the bowel. Amoebiasis tends to be a chronic diarrheal illness that on occasion produces an acute colitis which is indistinguishable from salmonellosis or shigellosis. The diagnosis requires laboratory identification of the amoeba in the feces. Usually a fever is present and abcesses may form in the liver or elsewhere, which may prove fatal in exceptional cases.

Cholera. This is a severe acute enterocolitis caused by *Vibrio cholerae* bacteria. Epidemics still occur in the Orient, Africa, and recently in the Mediterranean. The diarrhea has the appearance of rice water and several quarts of stool may be produced per day. This may cause rapid dehydration, shock, and kidney failure if not treated with adequate intravenous fluid replacement. (See p. 174.) *Prompt medical consultation by radio is essential and the patient should be evacuated to a hospital as soon as possible.*

Chronic ulcerative colitis. This is usually a long-standing disorder with a slow onset but it may start with acute diarrhea. The stools often are bloody and vomiting is rare. It is hard to distinguish from other forms of colitis without special diagnostic tests.

Regional enteritis. This is a chronic inflammatory condition of the small intestine and occasionally of the colon. The cause, as in ulcerative colitis, is unknown. It may begin with acute diarrhea or abdominal pain similar to acute appendicitis.

Functional or spastic colitis. This may be caused by emotional or nervous factors. Usually the disease is a long-standing disorder with alternating constipation and diarrhea. It is not an acute, prostrating condition as with the infectious types of colitis. Stools are not bloody and may or may not contain mucus.

Malabsorption and maldigestion. These conditions occur when food is not broken down (digested) so that it can be absorbed into the blood; or when digested food cannot be absorbed properly by the bowel. This is usually a chronic condition with a slow onset. The stools are bulky, foul-smelling, and sometimes frothy, often leaving an oil slick on the water of a toilet bowl. Generally, the condition does not respond to ordinary measures used for diarrhea. Malabsorption is rarely if ever a problem requiring emergency measures.

CONSTIPATION

Constipation is a symptom and not a disease. Rarely is constipation an acute or serious medical problem.

Treatment

Frequently changes in diet, environment, type of work, degree of physical activity, and emotional or nervous upsets may result in constipation. The patient should be advised to eat regularly, drink ample amounts of water, and exercise regularly. A gentle laxative such as milk of magnesia may be given. Prunes or prune juice could be added to the patient's diet.

Persistent constipation of recent onset or a change in bowel habits may indicate a serious underlying bowel condition such as cancer. The seaman should be advised to seek medical attention when port is reached.

DENTAL EMERGENCIES

The following dental first aid procedures are to relieve pain and discomfort until professional care is available.

Bleeding

Bleeding normally occurs following a tooth removal. However, prolonged or profuse bleeding must be treated.

Treatment

To treat bleeding, excessive blood and saliva should be cleared from the mouth. Then, 2″ × 2″ gauze should be placed over the extraction site and biting pressure applied. It is important to fold the gauze to a proper size well adapted to the extraction site. The pack should be left undisturbed for 3 to 5 minutes, then replaced as necessary. Once bleeding has stopped, the area should be left undisturbed. If bleeding is difficult to control, a 2″ × 2″ gauze twisted into a thin cone shape should be packed into the site, with a second 2″ × 2″ gauze pressure pack placed over it. The patient should apply biting pressure for 30 minutes to

1 hour and continue biting if necessary. The mouth should not be rinsed for 24 hours. A soft diet should be maintained for two days.

Lost Fillings

Fillings may come out of teeth because of recurrent decay around them or a fracture of the filling or tooth structure.

Treatment

If pain is absent, no treatment will be required for a lost filling and the patient should be advised to see a dentist when in port. If the tooth is sensitive to cold, a temporary dressing should be placed into the cavity. First, the tooth is isolated by placing a 2″ × 2″ gauze on each side. A cotton pellet can be used to dry the cavity. A drop of oil of cloves or eugenol should be placed on cotton and gently pressed into the cavity. Pain is usually controlled. This may be repeated 2 or 3 times daily as necessary.

Toothache Without Swelling

This condition usually is caused by irritation or infection of the dental pulp from a cavity, lost filling, or a recurrent problem in a tooth that has a filling in place.

Treatment

The patient who has a toothache without swelling of the gums or face should be advised to chew on the opposite side of his mouth. Foods should not be too hot or too cold. Pain may be relieved with aspirin 600 mg by mouth or with codeine sulfate 30 mg if the pain is severe. If the patient does not tolerate aspirin, acetaminophen at the same dosage and frequency should be given. The patient with a toothache should be told to swallow the aspirin and never to hold the tablets in the mouth as this will burn the soft tissues. If the aching tooth has a large cavity, the instructions for placing a sedative cotton dressing, described under *Lost Filling,* should be followed.

Toothache With Swelling

Toothache with swollen gums or facial tissues often results from infection by tooth decay that involves the dental pulp and spreads into the tissues of the jaws through the root canals. The condition also is common as a result of infections associated with diseases of the gums, periodontal membrane, and the bone that supports the teeth. In all cases, frequently there is pain, swelling, and the development of an abscess with pus formation.

Treatment

The patient with mouth-facial swelling should be observed closely and the following findings noted: (1) the exact area of the swelling, initially and during the illness; (2) the type of swelling, whether soft, firm, or fluctuant (movable tissue containing a pus-filled cavity); (3) difficulty in opening and closing the mouth; and (4) the oral temperature, morning and night. These findings are important for following the patient's progress and evaluating the effectiveness of the medication used.

The pain should be controlled with analgesics as described under *Toothache Without Swelling*.

For infection, an initial dose of penicillin V potassium 500 mg should be given by mouth followed by 250 mg every six hours. If the patient is allergic to or suspected of being allergic to penicillin, oral erythromycin should be used in the same dosage and frequency. The patient should be kept on the antibiotic for at least four days after he becomes afebrile (without fever). Instructions should be given to see a dentist at the earliest opportunity.

The patient should be advised to rinse the mouth with warm saline solution (a quarter teaspoonful of table salt in 8 ounces of warm water) for five minutes of each waking hour. This will cleanse the mouth and help to localize the infection in the mouth. Also, saline solution may produce earlier drainage and relief from pain. After the pain and swelling subside, the oral rinsing should be continued until the patient is seen by a dentist.

Dental Infection

Dental infection usually occurs when decay extends into the pulp of teeth. Bacteria from the mouth will enter the tissues of the jaws via the canal in the tooth's root. The infection may remain mild or may progress to a swelling in the mouth or face, after producing fever, weakness, and loss of appetite.

Treatment

Discomfort from a dental infection may be controlled with aspirin 600 mg by mouth or with codeine sulfate 30 mg, if the pain is severe. If the patient does not tolerate aspirin, acetaminophen at the same dosage and frequency should be given. Antibiotics are used as described in the section, *Toothache With Swelling*. *Medical advice by radio should be obtained* to repeat the codeine sulfate or to use antibiotics.

Painful Wisdom Tooth (*Pericoronitis*)

Pericoronitis is an infection and swelling of the tissues surrounding a partially erupted tooth, usually a wisdom tooth (third molar). Often a small portion of the crown or a cusp of the offending tooth can be seen through the soft tissues. The soft tissues appear swollen and the degree of inflammation or redness may vary considerably. When the infection is severe, the patient may complain of difficulty in opening the mouth. When the area is examined carefully, pus may be found coming from underneath the soft tissues in the area of the partially erupted tooth.

Treatment

For a painful wisdom tooth, the area between the crown of the tooth and the soft tissues should be flushed with warm saline solution (a quarter teaspoonful of table salt in 8 ounces of warm water). Also, the patient should be treated as directed under *Toothache With Swelling*.

Trench Mouth (*Vincent's Infection*)

Vincent's infection, a generalized infection of the gums, is more common in young and physically run-down individuals. During the acute stage it is characterized by redness and bleeding of the gums. Usually there is a film of grayish tissue around the teeth. There is usually a very disagreeable odor and a foul metallic taste in the mouth. The acute stage may be accompanied by a moderately high fever. Lymph glands in the neck may be swollen.

Treatment

For Vincent's infection a mouthwash of equal parts of 3% hydrogen peroxide and water should be prepared. The patient should be instructed to swish the solution vigorously within the mouth several times a day, especially after meals. A fresh solution must be prepared each time it is used.

The teeth and gums should be cleaned gently several times daily with cotton swabs moistened with the mouthwash solution. When tolerated, a soft toothbrush may be used carefully. *Although often uncomfortable, cleaning the gums and teeth is an essential phase of treatment.*

The patient should be advised to eat an adequate diet but avoid hot or spicy foods. The fluid intake should be increased.

For pain, aspirin 600 mg should be given by mouth every three to four hours as needed. If aspirin is not well tolerated by the patient, acetaminophen may be tried at the same dosage and frequency. If the pain is not controlled by aspirin or acetaminophen alone, codeine sulfate 30 mg should be given by mouth with aspirin or acetaminophen. To repeat the codeine sulfate, medical advice by radio should be obtained.

For infection, an initial dose of penicillin V potassium 500 mg should be given by mouth followed by 250 mg every six hours. If the patient is allergic to or suspected of being allergic to penicillin, oral erythromycin should be given at the same dosage. The patient should be kept on the antibiotic until at least four days after the fever has left. He should be instructed to see a dentist at the earliest opportunity.

Denture Irritation
(Partially or Fully Removable Dentures)

Generalized inflammation in the denture area usually is due to poor oral hygiene. Inflammation in localized areas usually requires some alteration or adjustment of the denture by a dentist. These localized areas usually are located where the border of the denture rests against the tissues.

Treatment

The patient should avoid using the denture until the soft tissues have healed. The denture should be cleaned carefully with mild soap and water, and stored in a water-filled container to avoid dehydration of the base material of the denture. The patient should be referred to a dentist for appropriate denture adjustment.

DIABETES MELLITUS (Sugar Diabetes)

In diabetes mellitus, the body is unable to use or to store all of the sugar derived from the carbohydrates normally eaten. The excess sugar remains in the blood and spills over into the urine, carrying water with it. This loss of sugar and water from the body causes increased appetite and thirst, frequent urination, and loss of weight.

Diabetics do not produce enough insulin which is a hormone secreted into the blood by the pancreas. Adjustments in the metabolism of sugar have to be made by changing the diet and/or the amount of insulin. Urine sugar (glucose) determinations help to determine the proper adjustment of diet and insulin needs. There are two basic methods for testing the urine, with each having its place in the control of the diabetic. One is the *glucose oxidase method* with such brands available as Testape,* Clinistix,* and Ketodiastix.* The other is a *copper reduction test method* with a brand such as Clinitest* tablets. When tests show large amounts of sugar in urine taken from diabetics before they have eaten breakfast, the diabetes is not well controlled. Testing should be done on arising before breakfast, and more frequently if indicated. If acetone is present in the urine, the patient may go into a diabetic coma. (See p. 155.)

Most diabetics prefer to use the *glucose oxidase test method* which is quick, convenient, easy to use, and requires no special equipment. However, should accurate determination of the amount of glucose in the urine become necessary to adjust the insulin intake, the *copper reduction test method* should be used.

Treatment

Diabetics generally are divided into three categories for treatment: (1) the diabetic treated with diet alone; (2) the diabetic treated with diet plus insulin; and (3) the diabetic who is treated with diet and oral blood sugar lowering agents (hypoglycemic agents).

• Diet

The initial treatment consists of adjusting the diet to eliminate the need for insulin. Many

---

* Trade names.

diabetics are treated successfully by diet alone. In the diabetic diet, special emphasis is placed on weight control, regular habits of eating, and avoidance of excess starches and sugars. The final diet consists of a varied and satisfying menu that is equally acceptable to a non-diabetic.

• Diet Plus Insulin

If diet alone does not control the disease, injections of insulin generally are prescribed. Insulin is used as replacement therapy. It supplements deficient levels of insulin in the body and temporarily restores the ability of the body to utilize properly carbohydrates (sugars and starches), fats, and proteins. The patients on insulin will have been instructed about the technique of administration and the kind and amount of insulin to be used. To meet an individual patient's needs, a variety of insulin preparations are available. However, for use in an emergency such as diabetic coma, regular insulin is used.

• Diet and Oral Blood Sugar Lowering Agents (Hypoglycemic Agents)

In selected cases, oral medications may be prescribed to lower the blood sugar. Most of these preparations help the pancreas to release more insulin. Five common medications of this type are: acetohexamide, chlorpropamide, phenformin hydrochloride, tolazamide, and tolbutamide.

Insulin Reactions

Insulin Shock (Hypoglycemia)

Insulin shock will occur if too much insulin is given, too little food eaten, a meal delayed too long, or an unusual amount of exercise or work is done. Prior to becoming unconscious, the patient may have emotional changes, a headache, numbness and tingling, poor coordination, a staggering gait, and slurred speech. Also, convulsions may occur. When the blood sugar falls below the normal level, the patient may appear pale, break out in a cold sweat, and have a rapid heart beat. Many of these symptoms suggest alcoholic intoxication. The treatment for insulin shock occasionally has been delayed with fatal results, because the odor of alcohol was on the diabetic's breath.

Treatment

When an insulin reaction occurs or when there is doubt as to the cause of unusual behavior or unconsciousness, the *conscious patient* should be given a rapidly absorbable carbohydrate by mouth as orange juice or a candy bar. *Fluids should not be given to an unconscious person.* Glucagon 1 mg should be given intramuscularly immediately. Glucagon will return the glucose blood levels to normal or near normal within 30 minutes in most adults. Fifty ml of dextrose 50% in water should be injected intravenously if the coma deepens or continues after 30 minutes, if the patient convulses, or a physician recommends it. A large bore needle (20 gauge) should be used for the injection. If a lump begins to rise under the skin, the injection must be stopped and the old needle discarded. Then a new sterile needle should be used to enter a vein at a different site. The lump in the skin showed that the needle did not enter a vein.

Emergency treatment *must be administered first,* and medical advice obtained by radio. Other causes of coma should be considered.

Diabetic Coma (Ketoacidosis, Hyperglycemia)

Overindulgence in food, too little insulin, injury or burns, infection, pain, anxiety, or decreased activity can lead to increased blood sugar (*hyperglycemia*) and an increased loss of sugar and water in the urine. With insufficient insulin the body is not able to convert all of this sugar into energy. Then fat normally stored in the body is broken down for energy, and poisonous acidlike substances accumulate.

Some of these substances excreted in the urine as acetone or ketones can be detected with commercial products as Acetest * tablets or Bili-Labstix.* The acetone test should be performed whenever a diabetic has a high level of glucose in the urine. Some of these acid products are exhaled from the lungs and give the breath a peculiar sweetish odor. These substances also cause dryness of the mouth and rapid, deep respirations (air hunger). The patient may be thirsty, the skin dry, and the eyeballs soft and sunken due to the loss of

---

* Trade names.

fluid. Abdominal pain, slight fever, nausea, and vomiting may occur. Urine tests for sugar and acetone are very important and should be performed before medical advice is sought by radio.

Treatment

If not treated, diabetic acidosis may cause unconsciousness (diabetic coma) and eventually death. *The most important step in treatment is to give fluids and insulin.* Crystalline (regular) insulin should be given according to medical advice received by radio. If there is any delay in obtaining medical advice, an initial dose of regular insulin should be administered subcutaneously. The results of the *urine test for sugar and acetone* should be used as a guide for the following initial dose:

If urine sugar is	and acetone is	then give this insulin
3+	negative	10 units
3+	positive	15 units
4+	negative	15 units
4+	positive	20 units
4+	strong positive	30 units

Fluids should be given to replace the excessive loss of salt and water from the body. The patient should be encouraged to drink large quantities of water, broth, soup, and fruit juice. Sodium chloride injection 0.9% should be started intravenously while awaiting medical advice by radio for further treatment.

The Diabetic and the Job

During the physical examination at the time of signing-on, a diabetic should be evaluated and accepted for sea duty in accordance with the facilities available.

Diabetes, a common disease, may first appear or become exaggerated under such trauma as burns, infections, diarrhea, vomiting, and emotional disturbances. Medically-trained crew members should watch for excessive thirst and urination following any of these events.

To maintain good control of their disease, diabetics require a great deal of self-discipline. They learn the type of food that they should eat and the quantity. They must maintain a balance between their food intake and insulin dosage. Adult diabetics may control their disease with diet alone or with diet plus oral medication. (See p. 332.)

The diabetic treated with diet alone or with diet and oral medications will not need any employment restrictions and may be assigned to both hazardous and non-hazardous jobs. On the other hand, diabetics who require insulin should not be assigned a job where an unexpected insulin reaction will physically endanger either themselves or their co-workers. They should not be assigned to potentially hazardous jobs, such as working on scaffolding or near unshielded machinery.

DIGESTIVE DISORDERS

The signs and symptoms of illness of the digestive tract include stomach pain, nausea and vomiting, diarrhea, bloating, belching and gas, vomiting of blood, bleeding from the bowel, constipation, and jaundice (yellow skin and eyes). The stomach and intestines may be upset by many kinds of sickness or injury.

Treatment

Until appendicitis is ruled out, a cathartic or laxative should not be given if the patient complains of pain in the abdomen. (See Appendicitis, p. 149, and Abdominal Pain, p. 148.) Appendicitis probably can be excluded if several members of the crew have pain in the stomach at the same time. Under such circumstances, the cause may be due to food poisoning (see p. 157), or an epidemic intestinal infection as dysentery. (See Diarrhea, p. 150.)

If the diagnosis for a digestive condition is uncertain, frequent small feedings should be given instead of occasional large meals. Until a definitive diagnosis is made, the diet should be limited to foods that are digested easily. Pepper, spices, coffee, fried or greasy foods, leafy vegetables and roughage (except in simple constipation) should be avoided. Usually, soft-boiled eggs, creamed soups, milk, chipped beef, baked potato, toast, crackers, custard, gelatin, and small amounts of fruit juice are well tolerated.

The diet should be limited to liquids until the fever goes down or nausea passes. Often a jaundiced person cannot tolerate fat (butter, cream, or grease) and should be given plenty of sugar and lean boiled or broiled meat.

Medical advice by radio should be obtained before treating a patient with severe abdominal complaints.

Food Poisoning

Bacteria account for most cases of food poisoning in the United States. Food poisoning as discussed in this section relates to intestinal symptoms usually caused by certain bacteria that seem to thrive in the gastrointestinal tract, especially the intestines. Usually these bacteria are transmitted by fecal contamination of food or water in areas with poor sanitation or situations where people neglect to practice good hygienic procedures.

Food poisoning is a general term applied to various illnesses that begin in the intestine(s) after contaminated food or water have been consumed. Not included here are intoxications caused by chemical contaminants (as fluorides, lead and other heavy metals); or intoxications caused by organic substances present in natural foods as mushrooms, eels, mussels, or other seafood. (See pp. 108, 160.)

Bacterial Food Poisoning

Food poisonings caused by bacteria are classified either as *food intoxications* or *food infections*. A *food intoxication* results from harmful toxins (poisons) formed by bacteria in contaminated food before it is eaten. In a *food infection* bacteria produce their harmful effects directly in the intestines after being ingested with the food. No matter whether it is a food infection or a food intoxication, the effects on the body are much the same. After eating the contaminated food, there is a sudden onset of symptoms, as diarrhea, cramps, nausea, and sometimes vomiting, headache, fever, or chills.

A common cause of food poisoning is the handling of food by people with cuts or wounds, sore throats, and intestinal diseases. Or food may become infective from bacteria carried by flies, cockroaches, rats, and mice. Bacteria will multiply at a rapid rate in food mixtures that are prepared several hours before a meal and allowed to stand unrefrigerated at room temperature. This high rate of bacterial growth is likely to occur in unrefrigerated protein foods, as meats, processed meats or meat mixtures, seafoods, milk and milk products, eggs (especially dried eggs), custard cream fillings in pies and other pastries, chicken and potato salads, and salad dressings.

Prevention

In most outbreaks of food poisoning, the infected food will not have changed in appearance, taste, or smell. So prevention of food poisoning should begin when meats or other foods are first inspected. Foods should be condemned and discarded if found to be below standard. Canned foods showing gas formation (the bulging or swelled can), or food that is unnaturally soft and mushy, should not be eaten. Equally important is proper, sanitary handling of food in the galley, storerooms, and mess hall. All those who handle food or utensils for food preparation aboard ship are directly responsible for the health of their shipmates. All food handlers should take extra care to keep themselves, the gear they work with, and the food they handle, as clean as possible. After soiling the hands, whether in the ship's head or elsewhere, thorough washing with soap and water must be done. If in doubt about whether a food is *safe*, do not rely on tasting the contents. If in doubt throw it out.

Staphylococcal Food Poisoning

This type of food poisoning is called staphylococcus toxin gastroenteritis. It is caused by a preformed enterotoxin that grows on a variety of foods (custards, cream-filled pastry, milk, processed meat, and fish) prior to ingestion. It is probably the principal cause of food poisoning in the United States. Food handlers with staphylococcal skin infections usually are responsible for its spread.

About two to four hours after the contaminated food is eaten, the onset of symptoms will be abrupt: diarrhea, cramps, nausea, vomiting, occasional headache and fever. In severe cases acid-base imbalance, prostration, and shock may occur. At times the temperature will be subnormal with a noticeable drop in blood pressure. Occasionally, blood and mucus may be found in the stools. The attack may last only a few hours, and at the most a day or two.

Usually diagnosis is based on recognition of several cases with the usual acute GI (gastrointestinal) symptoms occurring shortly after eating a common item of food, with an attack that lasts only a short time, followed by rapid recovery.

The human being usually is the source of infection. The toxin-producing staphylococci can originate from the infected hands, abscesses, or nasal discharges of food handlers, or from apparently normal skin on arms and forearms. Contaminated milk or milk products also are sources of the bacteria. The following foods when unrefrigerated may harbor staphylococcal bacteria: custards, pastries, salads and salad dressings, sandwiches, sliced meats, and meat products. Ham and bacon, milk from cows with infected udders, and at times dried milk have been implicated in outbreaks of staphylococcal food poisoning.

Prevention

The following measures will help to prevent staphylococcal food poisoning:

(1) Promptly refrigerate potentially hazardous foods to avoid multiplication of staphylococci accidentally introduced into the food; (2) Leftover foods should be refrigerated promptly or disposed of at once; (3) Persons with skin infections should not be allowed to handle food; (4) Food handlers with respiratory infections, who cannot be replaced, should be issued face masks. Disposable gloves should be given to salad mixers and other workers who use the hands to prepare foods; (5) Food handlers should give strict attention to sanitation and cleanliness of kitchens, including proper refrigeration, handwashing, attention to fingernails, plus being on the alert to the dangers of working with foods while having a skin infection; and (6) Custards prepared commercially should be pasteurized.

Treatment

For acute staphylococcus food poisoning, usually no specific treatment is required. In mild cases, cure follows such measures as rest in bed with general nursing care. Cleansing enemas should be given to remove any toxin that remains in the colon. Light liquids as water, tea, barley or rice water, or bouillon with added salt may be given. For mild to moderate diarrhea, although of limited effectiveness, kaolin mixture with pectin may be given according to directions on the container. Initially in the acute stages of diarrhea, two

tablets of diphenoxylate hydrochloride with atropine sulfate should be given four times daily. After control is achieved, a lower dosage of one tablet three or four times daily may be indicated for several days.

In severe cases or when marked dehydration of the patient results from prolonged vomiting or diarrhea, medical advice by radio should be obtained. Intravenous administration of fluids such as dextrose 5% and sodium chloride 0.45% injection may be recommended. (See p. 314 for information on intravenous administration procedure.)

Food Poisoning by Clostridium perfringens (C. welchii)

This is an intestinal infection (not an intoxication) caused by strains of *Clostridium perfringens* (*C. welchii*) bacteria. There is an abrupt onset of abdominal pains or spasms followed by diarrhea. Nausea is common but vomiting is absent. Usually this is a mild disorder of one day or less.

The infection is transmitted by eating food contaminated with feces. Outbreaks of the disorder usually are associated with meats: at times with fresh meats not thoroughly cooked, but generally from stews, meat pies, reheated meats, or gravies made from beef, turkey, or chicken. Outbreaks have been traced to catering firms, restaurants, and cafeterias.

Prevention

Preventive measures against *Clostridium perfringens* food poisoning are as follows: (1) After meat dishes have been cooked, they should be served immediately while hot—or cooled rapidly until eating time, then rapidly reheated, if necessary; (2) Large cuts of meat should be cooked adequately; (3) Stews and similar dishes prepared in bulk should be divided into small lots for cooking and refrigeration; and (4) Food handlers should be taught about the risks connected with large-scale cooking—especially of meats.

Treatment

For *C. perfringens* food poisoning the treatment is the same as that stated above for staphylococcal food poisoning.

Salmonellosis Food Poisoning

Salmonella bacterial strains cause this food infection (not an intoxication). The incubation period in the body takes 6 to 48 hours before symptoms appear. The infection is characterized by acute gastroenteritis of sudden onset that includes abdominal pain, diarrhea, nausea, and vomiting. Dehydration may be severe and fever nearly always is present. There is a loss of appetite and loose bowels may persist for several days. Some patients have difficulty in urinating and shock may develop. For most people the attacks are mild, but in some cases the infectious bacteria may produce localized abscesses in any part of the body, affect the gallbladder, heart, kidneys, or cause pneumonia, arthritis, or meningitis. Some patients remain carriers for several months after recovery.

The infection is transmitted by eating food contaminated by feces of humans or other animals. Suspect foods may be whole eggs or egg products, meat and meat products, and poultry. Pharmaceuticals of animal origin, animal feeds, and fertilizers can become contaminated. Epidemics have been traced to working surfaces or tables previously contaminated by foods, as poultry products.

Prevention

To prevent food poisoning by salmonella, the following should be done: (1) Cook thoroughly all foodstuffs from animal sources, especially poultry, egg products, and meat; (2) Avoid eating raw eggs and avoid using dirty or cracked eggs; (3) Refrigerate prepared foods whenever stored before use; and (4) Instruct food handlers on the necessity for refrigerating foods, washing hands before and after food preparation, maintaining a sanitary kitchen, and protecting all stored foods against insect and rodent contamination. Domestic animals and pets may become infected with salmonella.

Treatment

For food poisoning or infection from *Salmonella* organisms, the treatment is the same as that for staphylococcal food poisoning. (See p. 158.)

Botulism Food Poisoning

Botulism is a highly fatal food poisoning (an intoxication, not an infection) that is caused by the bacterium, *Clostridium botulinum*. In improperly preserved foods these germs grow in the absence of air to produce one of the most potent poisons known. In the United States the toxin usually is found in poorly preserved non-acid vegetables as string beans, corn, spinach, olives, beets, asparagus, and seafood, beef, and pork products.

Signs or symptoms can begin in a few hours or as late as eight days after ingestion of the contaminated food. The usual time lapse is 18 to 36 hours. Generally, persons with an early onset of illness (within 24 hours) will be affected severely, be more likely to die, and if they survive, will have a slower recovery period.

Symptoms of botulism are body weakness, headache, and nerve paralysis that causes difficulties in breathing, seeing, and swallowing. Visual disturbances include double vision, loss of acuity, drooping of upper eyelids, and a diminished or total loss of the pupillary light reflex. Usually intestinal symptoms are absent, although some outbreaks have resulted in early nausea and vomiting. Difficulty in swallowing may lead to aspiration pneumonia. Muscular movements may be uncoordinated, and dizziness and restlessness may be present. Usually the body temperature remains normal, unless the patient also has another disease.

Mortality may be as high as 65%. Most fatalities occur from the second to the ninth day following ingestion of the toxin. Death usually results from respiratory paralysis or secondary pneumonia. In survivors the disease reaches its peak in 10 days, after which recovery is slow and the eye muscles may be weak for months. There should be no permanent aftereffects.

The diagnosis of an isolated case of botulism is suggested by the pattern of the neuromuscular disturbances. However, a likely food source provides an important clue. The diagnosis is simplified when two or more cases occur after eating the same meal. Further confirmation can be gotten if the same symptoms occur in pets that have eaten the contaminated food.

Prevention

The spores of *C. botulinum* are highly resistant to heat. However, heat rapidly destroys the toxins, so cooking food at 176° F

(80° C) for 30 minutes before eating it, will safeguard against botulism.

All foods that show evidence of spoilage should be discarded—as commercially prepared canned foods that show bulging at the ends of the can. When such cans are found, they should be reported to health authorities and grocers.

Treatment

When botulism is suspected aboard ship, medical advice by radio should be obtained at once. It is important that the polyvalent antitoxin (as a minimum types A, B, and E) be given intravenously to those ill or exposed within 12 to 18 hours. Appropriate tests for sensitivity should be made. If evacuation is not possible within this time period, consideration should be given to using an airdrop to get the antitoxin.

The patient should be kept in a darkened room and watched constantly. Only those concerned with his care should be admitted to the room. If breathing stops, artificial respiration should be given and attendants should be prepared to administer it for hours. If severe vomiting persists or the patient cannot swallow, dextrose 5% and sodium chloride 0.45% injection may be recommended to be infused intravenously to manage dehydration and acid-base imbalance.

Morphine sulfate should be avoided because it will make difficult respiration even worse. To relieve anxiety, phenobarbital may be administered orally or pentobarbital administered intramuscularly in a dose of 30 to 60 mg., three to four times daily.

Oral medication and feeding should be carried out with caution because of the danger of aspiration; and rectal and parenteral routes of administration will have to be used if the patient cannot swallow. It may be necessary to feed the patient intravenously for several days. The patient should be encouraged to force fluids to maintain a daily urinary output of at least 800 ml.

When the patient has difficulty swallowing, mouth secretions must be removed by suction because their accumulation may result in aspiration, followed by pneumonia. If the patient cannot swallow at all, a tracheostomy may be lifesaving. If necessary, oxygen can be given

through the tracheostomy tube. To prevent lung collapse, the patient should be turned frequently from side to side.

As signs of recovery are noted and the patient is able to swallow, medical advice on diet should be gotten by radio.

Nonbacterial Food Poisoning*

Some plants and animals have naturally occurring poisons. It is possible to contact these on and off the ship. Examples discussed here are certain fish, mushroom-like toadstools, and mussels.

Fish Poisoning

Some fish are naturally poisonous. Other varieties that are safe to eat in some localities may be found highly toxic in other regions of the world, because they feed on poisonous plankton. Highly suspect should be fishes living in reef areas.

These classes of poisonous fish include:

• *Pacific type*—Barracuda, black ulna, red snapper, sea bass, and trigger fish.

• *Caribbean type*—Cavallas, amberjack, great barracuda, groupers, and sierra, among others.

• *Tetraodon type*—balloon fish, globe fish, puffers.

Symptoms that may develop immediately or within 30 hours after eating the food are numbness of limbs, tingling sensation around the mouth, diarrhea, nausea, vomiting, abdominal pain, aching joints, fever, sweating, chills, itching, painful urination, and extreme exhaustion. Muscle weakness, incoordination, and paralysis are common. The severity of the attacks varies greatly. The Caribbean type is usually nonfatal. The overall mortality for the Pacific type is not greater than 3%, while that for the Tetraodon type is over 70% in Japan.

Treatment

Bed rest is required for patients with fish poisoning. If vomiting or diarrhea have been violent, stomach lavage or use of an emetic will

---

* Adapted from the *Merck Manual of Diagnosis and Therapy.* Published by Merck & Co., Inc., Rahway, New Jersey. 12th edition, copyright 1972. pp. 714-6.

not be necessary. However, if diarrhea or vomiting were little or none, gastric lavage should be used to remove the bulk of the poison. An emetic such as ipecac syrup 15 ml with one to two glasses of water should be given by mouth *for mild cases only of fish poisoning, but never in mussel and mushroom poisoning.* If nausea and vomiting continue, fluids such as dextrose 5% and sodium chloride 0.45% may be injected intravenously to combat dehydration and acid-base imbalance. For pain 50 to 100 mg of meperidine hydrochloride may be given intramuscularly every four to six hours.

Mussel Poisoning

From June to October, especially on the Pacific coast, clams and mussels may ingest a poisonous protozoan (dinoflagellate) that produces mytilotoxin which is not destroyed by cooking. In 5 to 30 minutes after ingestion, the first symptoms appear—a burning, tingling sensation around the mouth. Nausea, vomiting, and abdominal cramps occur, followed by muscle weakness and paralysis along the outer surface of the body. Death may occur from respiratory failure.

A shellfish poison called "venerupin" has been isolated following outbreaks of food poisoning in Japan after the ingestion of asari (*Venerupis semidecussata*) and the oyster (*Otrea gigas*). In 24 to 48 hours gastrointestinal symptoms develop with increased numbers of leukocytes in the blood, retardation of blood coagulation, and disturbances in liver function. About one-third of the patients die. This shellfish toxin does not affect nervous tissue like mussel poison does (described above).

Treatment

For mussel poisoning the treatment is the same as that described above for fish poisoning. Get medical advice by radio.

Mushroom (Toadstool) Poisoning

For suspected mushroom poisoning medical advice by radio should be gotten at once. There are several poisonous varieties of mushroom-like fungi, but two species cause most of the illlness: *Amanita muscaria* and *Amanita phalloides.*

Amanita Muscaria

A. muscaria produces the toxic drug muscarine that has a harsh action on parts of the nervous system. It causes death less frequently than *A. phalloides* (see below). Muscarine symptoms appear within a few minutes to two hours after ingestion: excessive saliva is secreted, tears flow, pupils of the eyes constrict, there is profuse sweating, vomiting, abdominal cramps, diarrhea, thirst, dizziness, confusion, collapse, coma, and occasionally convulsions.

Treatment

For muscarine poisoning by *Amanita muscaria*, atropine sulfate 1 mg should be given subcutaneously or intravenously every 1 or 2 hours until the symptoms are controlled. Otherwise, treat as described above for fish poisoning.

Amanita Phalloides

A. phalloides poisoning is due to a toxin that liquifies various body cells, especially red corpuscles in the blood. Symptoms begin six to 15 hours after ingestion with sudden onset of nausea, vomiting, diarrhea, and abdominal pain. Stools and vomitus often are streaked with blood. Dehydration is extreme and kidney function may be affected with reduction in the quantity of urine produced. Jaundice due to liver damage follows in one or two days. Symptoms of damage to the central nervous system (CNS) usually are present, as jaundice, an enlarged tender liver, and diminished tendon reflexes.

Treatment

For poisoning from *A. phalloides*, to prevent severe liver damage, a high carbohydrate diet should be given supplemented by an intravenous injection of dextrose as recommended by radio medical advice. Otherwise, treat the same as for fish poisoning (described above).

Gallbladder Disease, Acute

Acute inflammation is the most frequent complication of a chronically inflamed gallbladder with stones. Acute cholecystitis (inflammation of the gallbladder) may be the first manifestation of gallbladder disease, but ordinarily it occurs after repeated attacks of biliary colic. Although acute inflammation of the gallbladder may occur at any age, it is most common after 40. Pains in the right upper quadrant of the abdomen develop, persist, and become steady; these usually are associated with nausea and vomiting and intensified by deep breathing. Tenderness is present in the right upper abdomen. Involuntarily, the patient may tighten the abdominal muscles when gentle firm pressure is applied.

Treatment

Many cases of acute inflammation of the gallbladder subside with treatment. However, some cases develop complications. If the symptoms are severe, the patient should be placed on bed rest and oral fluids. Foods should be withheld until the acute symptoms subside. If there is considerable vomiting, dextrose 5% and sodium chloride 0.45% should be administered intravenously to replace body fluids. To relieve pain, meperidine hydrochloride 75 mg to 100 mg may be given intramuscularly every four to six hours as required.

Belladonna tincture 0.2 ml (approximately 10 drops) by mouth may be given in a half glass of water, two or three times a day to help control the gallbladder spasm. This medication should be discontinued if the patient complains of blurred vision. (See p. 273.)

Gallstone Colic

Gallstone colic is caused by the passage of a stone through the bile duct leading from the gallbladder to the small intestine. The pain which is sharp, knifelike, severe, and associated with vomiting, starts in the right upper quadrant of the abdomen. Usually, a sore spot will be found that is tender to pressure. The pain may be intense, and the patient may groan, toss about the bed, and gasp for breath. The attack, which may last several hours, stops after the stone works its way through the bile duct and is discharged into the intestine. Attacks may recur as new stones enter the duct. The pain may spread to the back, beneath the right shoulder blade, and sometimes to the right shoulder.

When the stone or stones block the duct, bile is prevented from following its normal path from the liver to the small intestine. If blocked long enough, a sufficient amount of bile is absorbed and the whites of the eyes become yellowish, the urine dark colored, and the stools light- or clay-colored. (See Jaundice, p. 164.)

While the acute attack of pain usually ceases as soon as the stone passes out of the bile duct, other symptoms of gallbladder disease may remain. Jaundice gradually disappears after the stone is passed.

If the stone becomes lodged permanently in the bile duct, the pain will persist but may become less severe. When the stone blocks the bile duct, jaundice will continue. Infection of the gallbladder, which causes chills and fever, is an additional complication.

Treatment

Medical advice by radio should be obtained for patients exhibiting symptoms of gallbladder disease. The patient should be advised to see a doctor at the first convenient port.

The patient should be placed in bed and vital signs checked every hour or two. Food and liquids should be withheld during the acute attack. If the abdominal pain is severe or persists, the patient should be given meperidine hydrochloride and/or belladonna tincture as described previously for acute gallbladder disease. After the severe attack has diminished, aspirin 600 mg should be given by mouth for pain every three to four hours as needed. If aspirin is not well tolerated by the patient, acetaminophen may be given in the same dosage and frequency. The patient should be started on belladonna tincture 0.2 ml (approximately 10 drops) by mouth in a half glass of water two or three times a day, to help relieve any discomfort. During the acute stage, dextrose 5% and sodium chloride 0.45% solution should be administered intravenously to replace body fluids. Medical advice by radio should be obtained.

After the patient becomes more comfortable and vomiting stops, cracked ice should be given by mouth every 15 minutes. Then quantities of clear fluids should be given gradually. A soft diet, which is as fat free as possible, should be started as the patient recovers.

Gastritis, Acute

Acute gastritis or inflammation of the lining of the stomach accompanies dietary or alcoholic indiscretion, food or chemical poisoning, acute infectious diseases, ulcer, or cancer.

There is nausea and vomiting and possibly pain, thirst, fever, and coated tongue. Distention and tenderness may be present in the middle of the upper abdomen. Vomiting may be excessive and tinged with blood.

Treatment

In the first 24 hours only sips of water or hot tea should be given. Aluminum hydroxide gel, with magnesium hydroxide or magnesium trisilicate oral suspension, 15 ml may be given for any discomfort. Liquids, followed by a soft diet, are advisable. The patient should be kept at bed rest, quiet, and warm. (See Indigestion, below.)

Indigestion

Indigestion occurs when food fails to undergo the normal changes of digestion in the alimentary canal. It is a symptom rather than a disease. Occasional indigestion may be of no consequence, but when chronic it may indicate such serious maladies as cancer or an ulcer.

The symptoms may include discomfort after eating, fullness in the upper stomach, bloating, belching, gas, heartburn, pain beneath the breastbone, nausea, headache, foul breath, coated tongue, constipation, or inability to sleep.

The causes of occasional attacks of acute indigestion are:

• *Overeating,* excessive drinking or smoking, and eating irritating foods.

• *Emotional upset.* The digestive secretions, intestinal peristalsis and other functions of the digestive tract are disrupted if a person eats when angry, depressed, or emotionally upset.

Food allergies (See p. 220.)

Treatment

For mild attacks of indigestion, aluminum hydroxide gel with magnesium hydroxide or magnesium trisilicate oral suspension, 15 ml should be given every hour until the symptoms subside. If the patient is distressed sufficiently but has not vomited, vomiting should be in-

duced. This may be accomplished by having the patient drink one or two pints of warm salt water (1 to 2 teaspoonfuls of table salt to a pint) and having him touch the back of his throat with his finger. It severe pain is present, a hot water bag should be applied to the upper abdomen.

For chronic indigestion, the diet should be limited as far as possible to foods that will cause the least distress to the patient. The patient should be advised to eat slowly and chew his food thoroughly. Bowel regularity should be maintained. It is important to find the underlying cause of the indigestion because it may point to a very serious disease. The patient should be advised to consult a physician at the next port of call.

Intestinal Obstruction

Complete blockage of some portion of the intestines may be caused by the accumulation of hard fecal matter, a strangulated hernia, adhesions (sticking together) of the coils of the intestines, tumors, or kinks in the bowel. There is usually a sudden onset of severe abdominal pain, without fever, accompanied by constipation. There may be nausea, vomiting, and after a matter of hours or days, the abdomen may become distended with gas.

Treatment

Medical advice by radio should be obtained. In the meantime, the patient should be kept at absolute bed rest. Food and water should be withheld except for ice chips which may be taken by mouth.

The obstruction may be a fecal mass in the rectum which can be removed by an enema (sodium biphosphate and sodium phosphate solution). Sometimes it is necessary to remove pieces of the hard fecal matter from the rectum by hand. A rubber glove or a rubber finger-cot should be worn. However, the bare finger can be used. The gloved finger should be lubricated with petrolatum and inserted gently into the patient's rectum. If a mass of hard fecal matter is felt low in the rectum, it should be broken up by gentle movement of the finger so that it can be passed by the patient, or helped out by the finger or the enema.

163

Applying a hot water bottle to the abdomen may relieve pain. Fifteen drops (0.3 ml) of tincture of belladonna may be given in a quarter glass of water every six hours. If the pain is severe and the patient's condition seems to be getting worse, morphine sulfate 10 mg should be given intramuscularly. To repeat the morphine sulfate, medical advice by radio should be obtained.

If the patient goes into shock, he should be treated as described on p. 57. If vomiting continues, it may be necessary to replace the fluid by giving 1,000 ml dextrose 5% and sodium chloride 0.45% solution intravenously. *Medical advice by radio should be obtained.*

Jaundice

Jaundice refers to the yellowish discoloration of the whites of the eyes and skin that occurs when bile is absorbed into the blood, instead of passing from the liver through the bile duct into the intestine.

Jaundice is a symptom of an illness and not a disease. It may indicate acute infectious hepatitis. Jaundice may accompany yellow fever, liver diseases, cancer, gallbladder disease, gallstones, malaria, and certain blood diseases.

In a typical case, the skin and the whites of the eyes are yellowish, greenish-yellow, or brownish-yellow. However, medications like quinacrine and atabrine also may cause a yellowish color. The urine may be dark mahogany in color and when shaken the froth is yellowish or brownish instead of white. The stools may be light in color and have the appearance of clay or putty. Also, the skin may itch.

Treatment

When medical advice by radio is requested on jaundice, specific information should be given as the presence or absence of pain in the stomach, chills and fever, and blood in the stools. Until advice is received, a soft and fat-free diet should be given and the patient placed on bed rest. (See p. 331.)

If there is any reason to suspect yellow fever, the patient should be isolated and the case reported to the authorities. (See p. 193.) When the ship reaches port, the patient should be advised to see a physician.

Ulcers, Peptic (Gastric or Duodenal)

A peptic ulcer is an open sore, usually benign, that occurs in the mucous membrane of the inner wall of the digestive tract in or near the stomach. Peptic ulcers are of two types: (1) *gastric ulcers* that occur in the stomach and (2) *duodenal ulcers* that form in the duodenum, the first section of the small intestine that is separated from the stomach by the pylorus. Although the cause of these ulcers is obscure, excessive secretion of hydrochloric acid and gastric juice in the stomach is an important factor in their production.

In normal digestion, both the stomach and duodenum are exposed to the action of the gastric juice. Oversecretion of the acid-gastric juice is a prime factor in the production of duodenal ulcers and the reactivation of healed ulcers. Emotional strain, as suppressed anger or other psychological problems, is a contributing factor to ulcer formation. Certain medications (as aspirin and the salicylates, phenylbutazone, prednisone) or excessive use of alcoholic beverages may cause ulcers.

The symptoms of peptic ulcer often follow a predictable pattern. However, these symptoms can be deceptive because they mimic other disorders of the digestive tract such as hiatal hernia, simple gastritis, and diseases of the liver, gallbladder, large intestine, pancreas, and right kidney. The various organs involved with these diseases are located near the stomach and duodenum.

Pain, the most common symptom of a peptic ulcer, is felt in the middle of the upper abdomen, at times under the tip of the breastbone. Usually the pain is steady, but it can be intermittent. At times it merely may be an annoying, burning pain. The pain is relieved when food is eaten, but tends to recur two or three hours after a meal or during the night when the stomach-duodenum region is empty and the gastric juice irritates the sore. Other symptoms are heartburn, gastric distention, nausea, vomiting, belching, loss of appetite, diarrhea, and weight loss.

Serious complications other than the recurrence of the peptic ulcer are: excessive bleeding, perforation of the walls of the organs involved, or obstruction, especially in the duodenum. If ulcers are neglected, increased bleeding can lead to anemia. An ulcerating lesion of the stomach raises the possibility of cancer, whereas malignant ulcers of the first part of the duodenum are almost unknown.

Dark brown particles like coffee grounds in vomitus indicate a bleeding ulcer. Black tarry stools also point to upper gastrointestinal bleeding. Each stool passed by a patient should be observed and its color noted. If there is a hint of bleeding, a rectal examination should be done and the glove inspected for a black stool. Blood pressure and pulse rate should be measured *while the patient is lying down, and repeated after the patient stands or sits for three minutes. A 15 mm drop in either systolic or diastolic blood pressure (lying down vs standing or sitting), or a 15-beat rise in the pulse rate (lying down vs standing or sitting), suggests a significant loss of blood.* With a 15% or greater loss of blood volume, there often is a drop in blood pressure and a rise in the pulse rate when the patient assumes the sitting position from recumbency.

The usual diagnostic aid for peptic ulcers is X-ray examination and fluoroscopic examination after the patient swallows barium sulfate. A careful history and use of a trial treatment with an antacid (see below) will establish the diagnosis well enough for shipboard treatment.

Treatment

Before initiating any medication, medical advice by radio should be obtained.

When perforation (see below) and hemorrhage (see p. 166) have been ruled out, initial treatment aboard ship should be aimed at getting the ulcer to heal and preventing its recurrence. This should include use of an antacid to neutralize excessive digestive acid; medication to slow down secretion of gastric juice; other medication to reduce motility and muscular spasm in the stomach-duodenum areas; frequent small feedings to take gastric juice away from the ulcer; and provision of a restful atmosphere that will reduce emotional tension for the patient.

The patient should be put to bed in the acute phase when pain and apprehension are prominent. In uncomplicated cases several days of rest usually will control acute symptoms, and ambulation may begin as pain is controlled.

Although special diets were used in the past, there is no evidence they are beneficial in the treatment of peptic ulcer. The patient should be the best judge on what agrees with him. However, in the acute phase hourly feedings of skim milk (100 ml) are recommended. After pain subsides, bland foods, excluding whole milk and cream, can be added. Highly seasoned, greasy, and fried foods, and roughage should be avoided. Also, alcohol and coffee should be avoided.

When the patient is able to tolerate solid foods, to control hyperacidity frequent light meals are preferable to a few heavy daily meals; also occasional use of antacids after meals and between feedings are required. A combination of aluminum hydroxide gel and magnesium hydroxide or magnesium trisilicate suspension (antacid), administered in 10 to 15 ml doses every 30 to 60 minutes in the acute phase while awake and every two hours at night, will help to neutralize the gastric juice. Some antacids cause constipation; this may be relieved by giving occasional doses of magnesium hydroxide suspension. Aluminum hydroxide (combined with magnesium hydroxide or magnesium trisilicate) is also available in chewable tablet form. Although somewhat less effective than the suspension, this may be more convenient for the patient to use, particularly while working. One or two tablets should be chewed thoroughly, then swallowed, every two to four hours. To reduce the intestinal spasms and delay emptying of the stomach, belladonna tincture, 15 drops in a half glass of water may be given three or four times daily, preferably before each meal and at bedtime. This will help to relieve pain. (Before administering belladonna tincture, review the dosage and warning information on p. 273.)

Perforated Peptic Ulcers (Peritonitis)

Perforation is a very serious complication, so medical advice by radio should be requested immediately. When an ulcer eats its way through the walls of the stomach or duodenum, the partly digested contents pass into the abdominal cavity to cause peritonitis, which is an inflammation of the smooth membrane that lines the abdominal cavity. The patient suffers sudden onset of intense pain in the abdomen. Usually bowel sounds will not be heard through a stethoscope placed on the abdominal wall. The abdomen will have a hard boardlike feeling to the touch. If pressure is applied gently to the abdomen, increased gradually, then abruptly released, there will be severe pain.

Treatment

Perforation of a peptic ulcer requires early surgery. Medical advice by radio should be obtained to arrange for evacuation of the patient to a medical facility and on use of the medication indicated below.

The patient should be placed in bed and kept warm. *Nothing* should be given by mouth. Morphine sulfate 10 mg intramuscularly may be given once for pain, and medical advice by radio will be needed for any additional doses. When possible, sodium chloride injection 0.9% or lactated Ringer's injection should be given intravenously at a rate of 1000 ml every eight hours; if shock is present, the rate should be increased.

Hemorrhage from Peptic Ulcer

A hemorrhaging peptic ulcer is a very serious complication. Medical advice by radio should be sought. The patient will feel faint, dizzy, weak, and will perspire profusely. There may be vomiting of blood or partly digested material (like coffee grounds) or black tarry stools may be passed. The pulse becomes weak and rapid. Thirst will develop. The patient may faint if he sits up or stands.

Treatment

The patient should be placed in bed and kept warm. Medical advice by radio should include arrangements for a prompt evacuation to a medical facility. Diazepam 5 mg may be given intramuscularly every 4 to 6 hours to control restlessness or anxiety. *Morphine sulfate generally should not be used because it may cause nausea or vomiting.* For severe pain, meperidine hydrochloride 50 mg should be given intramuscularly every four hours.

An infusion of sodium chloride injection 0.9% or lactated Ringer's injection, 1000 ml every 12 hours, may be given intravenously.

This is mainly a safety precaution. If shock is present or impending, medical advice should be sought by radio for a possible increase in the rate of the infusion.

At least every hour the patient's pulse and blood pressure should be checked; then both should be rechecked with the patient sitting, if he is able. (See p. 275 for possible use of Dextran infusion.)

Skim milk, 100–200 ml may be given every hour. Liquid antacids may be used, as discussed previously, if the patient does not tolerate milk.

Obstruction from Peptic Ulcer

Obstruction of the outlet of the stomach may be partial or complete. It may be due to a spasm, a narrowing of the channel or aperture, or an inflammatory swelling about a pyloric or duodenal ulcer. Symptoms of obstruction include vomiting of foods eaten at previous meals and foul belching. Also in patients with thin abdominal walls, very active visible peristalsis may be seen travelling from the left upper quadrant of the abdomen to the navel area. If there is pronounced vomiting, there may be evidence of dehydration and increased alkalinity of the blood (alkalosis). If obstruction is suspected, medical advice by radio should be sought at once. Discussion should deal with possible evacuation to a hospital and management of the patient prior to and during evacuation.

Treatment

Before any medication is given *for suspected obstruction, medical advice by radio should be obtained.*

Give nothing by mouth. To control thirst, 1000 ml sodium chloride injection 0.9% should be given intravenously over a four to eight hour period. If necessary, follow this over eight hours with 1000 ml dextrose 5% and sodium chloride 0.45% injection intravenously. Medical advice by radio should be obtained on the administration of fluids pending evacuation. If there is complete obstruction, without intravenous fluids the patient can live for only a few days; with intravenous fluids, severe imbalances in body chemistry are likely within three days.

For severe pain, meperidine hydrochloride 75 mg should be given intramuscularly every four hours.

Vomiting

Vomiting is a symptom of most diseases of the digestive tract and may occur with other diseases.

The amount, forcefulness, frequency, and regularity of vomiting are clues to diagnosing its cause. Projectile (extremely forceful) vomiting without nausea suggests increased pressure within the skull due to brain injury. Also, the contents, color, and odor of the vomitus (material vomited) are clues in diagnosing why a person vomits. The vomitus may be clear and watery (gastric juice) or contain varying amounts of undigested or fully digested food. Blood may be present in the vomitus as streaks, bright red hemorrhage, or material resembling coffee grounds which suggests a slowly bleeding ulcer.

The blood from a hemorrhage in the respiratory tract may be swallowed and vomited. The odor of vomitus resembles feces when a bowel obstruction is present; or urine, in a serious kidney condition. Vomiting accompanied by fever and headache suggests the onset of a communicable disease. The patient should be isolated and observed carefully.

Treatment

The stomach should be rested when there is nausea and vomiting due to overeating or a "morning after" sick stomach.

For the vomiting from seasickness, stomach ulcer, systemic disease, or mechanical irritants (poisons), the treatment described in the text under those headings should be given. In general, rest, liquid diet, and warmth are indicated.

HEMORRHOIDS (Piles)

Hemorrhoids are enlarged veins surrounding the last inch or so of the rectum and its outlet, the anus. Not all hemorrhoids bleed, but bleeding occurs sooner or later in most untreated cases.

The enlarged veins may occur internally above the anal sphincter muscle or externally below the muscle. Although external hemor-

rhoids can be seen, internal hemorrhoids cannot be seen unless they are forced through the anus by straining.

Hemorrhoids may be painful or painless, and may be as large as an almond or even larger. Bleeding hemorrhoids may produce a few drops or a tablespoonful of blood. Internal protruding hemorrhoids may pose a very serious medical problem when they become engorged and inflamed. They may not be able to be pushed back easily into the rectum.

Common causes of hemorrhoids include constipation, straining at the stool, excessive use of cathartics, and heredity.

Treatment

A patient with hemorrhoids should be advised to consult a physician to make sure that other conditions are not present as an abscess, fissure, or possibly cancer.

To relieve pain in acute cases, warm compresses made by wringing out cloths with warm saline solution (one teaspoonful of sodium chloride in 1,000 ml of water) may be applied. The patient should sit in a tub of warm water for 20 to 30 minutes, every two to three hours for relief of pain and itching. After the baths he should return to bed rest. Hemorrhoidal suppositories may be inserted rectally, as directed on the package, to supply relief. Medical advice by radio should be obtained on whether local application of hydrocortisone ointment 1% may be prescribed.

To keep the stools soft, milk of magnesia should be administered once or twice daily.

HERNIA (Rupture)

A hernia is a protrusion of an organ or a part of the intestine through a wall of the cavity in which it is normally enclosed. Ordinarily, a hernia means the protrusion of the intestine through a weak place in the abdominal wall.

Treatment

The patient should be placed on his back with hips higher than the shoulders. The knees should be drawn up to relax the abdominal muscles. Then, by gentle manipulation with the fingers, a gradual effort should be made to work the sac back into the abdomen. If a rupture has been protruding for a long time, adhesions may have formed and may prevent its reduction.

To reduce the more difficult hernias, morphine sulfate 10 mg should be given intramuscularly to relax the abdominal musculature and to relieve pain. About 45 minutes after giving this medication, an attempt should be made to reduce the hernia. Once the hernia has been reduced, the patient should be kept at bed rest on a liquid diet and given milk of magnesia to prevent constipation. Before repeating the morphine sulfate, medical advice by radio should be obtained.

When the rupture cannot be reduced, the protruding intestine may become compressed by adhesions or swelling to such a degree that its blood supply is shut off. This strangulated hernia is very serious. Symptoms are similar to those of obstruction of the bowel (see p. 163). Gangrene of the bowel may cause general peritonitis and death within a few days unless properly treated. *Medical advice by radio should be obtained promptly.*

SEASICKNESS (Motion Sickness)

Motion sickness aboard ship is called seasickness. Fatigue, food, gastrointestinal disturbances, and other factors may increase the tendency to be seasick. There may be nausea, weakness, inability to concentrate, and giddiness. The patient may break out in a cold sweat and experience dizziness for a short period of time.

Treatment

The patient should be kept quiet and warm. Small amounts of dry food as crackers, dry bread, toast, or a piece of lean meat may settle his stomach. The attack often disappears after a few hours. The symptoms may be diminished by placing the patient in a reclining position with his head on a pillow and eyes focused on a fixed distant point.

Cracked ice may be given to help check the vomiting and to relieve thirst. An excess amount of liquids should be avoided. Phenobarbital 30 mg may be given by mouth to help the patient sleep and recover.

Seasickness may be avoided if cyclizine hydrochloride 50 mg is taken by mouth several hours before going aboard ship. It may be given every 4 to 5 hours as needed.

WORMS

Intestinal worms usually occur as a result of eating uncooked or undercooked infected meat or fish. Most intestinal worms are relatively harmless and rarely require emergency treatment. There is a specific treatment for most worms which may be postponed until port has been reached.

Tapeworm. This infection may be contracted by eating raw or inadequately cooked pork, beef, or fish. Although these three food sources will show several varieties of tapeworms that may differ from each other in some ways, each can cause digestive disturbances, abdominal pain, nervousness, sleeplessness, and loss of appetite. However, the symptoms often are absent or vague. The diagnosis can be confirmed when flat tapelike segments of the worm are found in the stool.

Roundworm. This infection may be contracted by drinking contaminated water or eating contaminated food. Acute intestinal symptoms with sharp pains and diarrhea may occur. However, no disturbing symptoms may occur and the patient may not be aware of the existence of the worms. Roundworms resemble earthworms and are about the size of an average lead pencil.

Pinworm. This infection may be contracted through contaminated food, bedding, and clothing. Usually, the symptoms are mild and consist of restlessness, irritability, sleeplessness, and loss of appetite. However, if the infection is severe, there may be itching around the anus, often during sleep.

A diagnosis may be obtained by applying a tongue blade (with cellophane tape wound around it so that the sticky side is on the outer surface) to the anal area before bathing or passing a stool. If pinworms are present, they will appear as short pieces of white thread.

Due to anal scratching, reinfection often occurs. The fingers may pick up worms or their eggs and carry them to the mouth. Therefore, hands should be washed frequently, particularly after going to the bathroom and after sleep.

Hookworm. In an infected area, the eggs are found in soil contaminated by human feces. The young worms that hatch from these eggs penetrate the skin of the feet, and rarely are swallowed. They cause a serious and disabling anemia, diarrhea, and retarded mental and physical development in children. The infection is confirmed when eggs of the worm are found in the stool.

Trichina. This infection called trichinosis is contracted by eating undercooked pork contaminated with the trichina worm. The worms burrow through the bowel wall and, eventually, reach the muscles where they form small cysts. Usually, the first symptom is swelling (edema) of the upper eyelids, followed by muscular soreness and pain, profuse sweating, thirst, chills, weakness, fever, and collapse. A mild infection, however, may go unrecognized.

Chapter V

Treatment of Diseases

Section E
GENITOURINARY DISEASES

KIDNEY STONE COLIC

STONES COMPOSED OF CRYSTALS of various salts and other solid particles may form in the kidneys. Some people seem to be susceptible to the formation of these stones. Once they are formed, the stones usually must be "passed out" from the kidney through the ureter and into the bladder, which is an extremely painful experience. The pain caused by the passage of kidney stones is called kidney stone colic.

The pain of kidney stone colic usually begins suddenly and is agonizing. It radiates from the back in the region of the lower ribs on one side, down through the abdomen, and frequently into the area of the genitalia and inner sides of the thigh. The extreme pain usually is accompanied by nausea and vomiting. The patient doubles up and writhes with each spasm. The pulse becomes weak and rapid. The patient may have a pale face and be covered with a cold and clammy sweat. The pain may subside in an hour or it may last several hours. Pain may come intermittently with temporary relief between seizures.

Usually there is no fever. If infection is present, fever and chills are prominent symptoms. Blood may be passed in the urine. There is almost a constant desire to urinate. However, the frequent attempts to urinate cause pain but produce little urine.

Usually there is little or no tenderness over the painful area, when pressure is exerted on the abdomen. Lack of tenderness and rigidity differentiates kidney stone colic from appendicitis and other infections in the abdomen. When the stone is discharged from the ureter into the bladder, the pain suddenly stops.

Treatment

The first objective for kidney stone colic is relief of pain. Changes in position may help pass the stone. A hot water bottle should be applied to the painful area.

Usually the pain is so acute that morphine sulfate is essential. If the pain persists, morphine sulfate 10 mg should be given intramuscularly and repeated in one and a half to two hours. If more than the two doses are needed, medical advice by radio should be obtained. The patient should be encouraged to drink a glassful of water every half hour or hour to increase the flow of urine. The urine should be filtered through gauze to see if the stone or stones have been passed.

When the stone is passed, the patient should continue to drink fluids freely. The diet should be liquid or soft for a day or two, or longer if the patient continues to feel ill. If chills and fever occur, indicating infection of the genitourinary tract, sulfisoxazole may be indicated (see Urinary Tract Infection, p. 172). Medical advice by radio should be obtained. The patient should be advised to see a doctor at the next port. The stone, if passed, should be given to the doctor.

NEPHRITIS
(Bright's Disease, Glomerulonephritis)

This inflammation or degeneration of the kidneys may occur in acute or chronic forms.

Acute Nephritis

The acute inflammation interferes with the removal of waste products from the bloodstream. A marked decrease in the amount of urine passed, swelling (edema) of the ankles, and a pale pasty skin may occur suddenly. Also the usual symptoms of acute diseases may occur as malaise, pain in the small of the back, headache, fever (usually slight), shortness of breath, nausea, and vomiting.

With reasonable care, acute nephritis may clear up in a few weeks to a few months. However, the disease always is serious. Aggravated cases may terminate fatally in a relatively short time, or they may go on to chronic nephritis despite the best treatment.

Prolonged exposure to cold temperatures (without proper clothing or other protection) or overindulgence in alcohol also may be associated with kidney damage. Other common causes of kidney damage and acute nephritis are: toxins from such focal infections as abscessed teeth, pyorrhea, and infection of the prostate gland; toxins and other products from acute infectious diseases as syphilis, measles, typhus, tonsillitis, mumps, meningitis, typhoid fever, and gastro-intestinal diseases; chemical poisoning as mercury, or poisonous plants as mushrooms; physical injury to the kidney, as from a direct blow or fall; or extensive burns that destroy large areas of the skin, throwing an extra heavy excretory burden on the kidneys.

Treatment

There is no specific treatment for Bright's disease. The patient should be kept at rest in bed. The sickroom should be comfortably warm, well-ventilated, and without drafts.

The diet should be soft and easily digested and the patient should be careful not to overeat. Both salt intake and water intake should be kept low, especially if there is swelling of the ankles. *In most diseases with fever the patient is urged to drink a lot of water, but in acute nephritis it should be discouraged.*

If the patient is restless, cannot sleep, or is bothered by headache or other symptoms, phenobarbital 30 mg may be given by mouth once or twice a day. For pain in the back, a hot water bag often gives much relief.

In acute nephritis that follows an infection, especially by a streptococcus organism, penicillin G, procaine, sterile suspension, 600,000 units should be given intramuscularly each day for 10 days. Oral erythromycin 250 mg four times daily for ten days may be substituted in penicillin-sensitive individuals.

The patient should be watched for symptoms of systemic poisoning (uremia) which include increased headaches, drowsiness, twitching of the muscles, and convulsions associated with marked decrease in the amount of urine passed. A patient with uremia usually is critically ill. Medical advice by radio should be obtained.

Chronic Nephritis

The onset of chronic nephritis usually is slow and without obvious symptoms except when it follows acute nephritis. When symptoms occur, they include swelling of the ankles and perhaps other parts of the body, puffiness around the eyes, pale pasty skin indicating anemia, chronic indigestion, malaise, headache, irritability, sleeplessness, nausea, vomiting, and either a marked increase or a marked decrease in the amount of urine. Also, there may be signs of a failing heart, high blood pressure, cramps in the muscles (especially of the legs), attacks of shortness of breath, and diarrhea.

Chronic nephritis may be a rapidly crippling disease; or the patient may be able to live a useful life for many years without much disability. A seaman with chronic nephritis should be sure to obtain competent medical advice before returning to sea.

Treatment

The emergency treatment for chronic nephritis is symptomatic and follows the same general plan outlined above for acute nephritis. An accurate measure of the urine over 24-hour periods will assist the doctor in giving medical advice by radio. Medical assistance should be sought early.

Patients with chronic nephritis must lead a moderate, carefully regulated life. All excesses should be avoided especially in the use of alcohol and in food, work, and exposure to rough weather. Warm clothing should be worn to maintain comfort at all times.

URINE RETENTION (Anuria)

The patient with acute retention of urine complains of severe pain in the lower part of the abdomen. Although he has an urgent desire to urinate, he cannot. In cases of prostatic enlargement, the retention may be chronic and patients may suffer from constant dribbling away of the urine, a condition known as retention with overflow. The distended bladder may be visible as a rounded swelling rising out of the pelvis in the middle line.

Inability to pass urine may be due to congestion at the base of the bladder; stricture of the urethra, usually associated with a history of previous gonorrhea; paralysis of the muscles of the bladder in an unconscious patient with a brain or spinal injury; a stone lodged in the urethra; conditions of the prostate gland that constrict the neck of the bladder and the urethra; and alcoholic excesses.

Treatment

Preferably the bladder should be emptied by natural means without the aid of a catheter. Passing a catheter involves introducing an instrument into a urinary tract that is already inflamed and prone to infection. Even if the retention is relieved, the bladder may become infected and cystitis result. For this reason, effort should be made to help the patient to urinate normally. Reassurance is an important part of treatment. Pentobarbital sodium 100 mg may be given orally once, if the patient is highly apprehensive. It may be helpful to have the patient sit in a warm bath for a half hour or take a warm shower. Such relaxation may relieve the spasm, allowing the patient to urinate. If this procedure fails, a phosphate solution enema should be given. When the patient's bowels move, urine also may pass. If this fails, a catheter will need to be passed. Medical advice by radio should confirm the need for catheterization. (See p. 325.)

URINARY TRACT INFECTION

Chills and fever, pain and soreness over one or both kidneys, and frequent, painful or burning urination may indicate an infection of the urinary system. (See Kidney Stone Colic, p. 170, Venereal Disease, p. 246.)

Treatment

The treatment for infection of the urinary tract consists of bed rest, liberal fluids by mouth (water, fruit juices), no alcohol or coffee, a liquid or nonirritating soft diet, and a course of sulfisoxazole. Sulfisoxazole 3 g (six 500 mg tablets) should be given as the first dose with a full glass of water. Follow this with 1 g (two 500 mg tablets) with a full glass of water every six hours, for a period not to exceed five days without medical advice by radio.

Chapter V

Treatment of Diseases

Section F

INFECTIOUS DISEASES

ANTHRAX

Incubation Period: Within 7 days (usually 2 to 5 days).

Isolation Period: Until lesions are free of anthrax bacilli.

ANTHRAX IS AN ACUTE, infectious bacterial disease that is caused by *Bacillus anthracis*. It is rare in the United States and most western countries. Primarily a disease of sheep, cattle, and horses, it occurs most commonly among wool sorters, felt makers, tanners, and others who work with animals or their products. If cattle or hides are shipped by sea, exposure to anthrax is a possibility.

When anthrax appears as a skin disease, it may look like an ordinary boil or carbuncle. However, the surrounding skin may become swollen and break down. There may be severe systemic symptoms such as fever or prostration.

It is difficult to distinguish anthrax from an ordinary boil. Someone with a severe skin reaction surrounding a boil plus other bodily symptoms should be treated with antibiotics.

Treatment

If the patient is not allergic to the penicillins, penicillin G, procaine, sterile suspension, 600,000 units should be given intramuscularly every twelve hours until oral medication can be retained. Then penicillin V potassium 250 mg should be given by mouth every six hours, either one hour before or two hours after meals. The treatment should continue until all signs and symptoms disappear or until the patient has seen a physician. If the patient is allergic to the penicillins, erythromycin in the same dosage and frequency may be used instead of penicillin V potassium. (See Boils, p. 235, and Carbuncles, p. 236.) *Medical advice by radio should be obtained.*

173

CHICKENPOX (Varicella)

Incubation Period: 14 to 21 days (usually 13 to 17 days).

Isolation Period: Until scabs are no longer present.

Chickenpox is a highly contagious viral disease that produces a typical rash. The disease begins with a running nose, tearing eyes, slight fever about 101°F (38.3°C), occasional sore throat, loss of appetite, decreased energy, and restlessness. Within 24 hours of these symptoms, an eruption appears mostly on the trunk and face, and occasionally on the arms and legs. The skin lesions are vesicles (clear fluid-filled blisters on a slightly raised red base). These blisters frequently become pus-filled and crust in a few days. Finally as healing occurs, the crusts or scabs fall off.

Lesions of chickenpox typically appear in crops. Lesions of different ages are seen at the same time in a given area of the body surface. *This helps to distinguish chickenpox from smallpox.* In smallpox, the lesions in a given area of the body surface are of the same age and stage of development. They usually begin and are most extensive on the face and/or extremities.

The disease is communicable from a few days before the rash appears until all vesicles have crusted (five to 10 days). In adults, there may be serious complications of chickenpox, including viral pneumonia and meningoencephalitis.

Treatment

There is no specific therapy. Patients should be kept in bed and isolated from the rest of the crew. For fever, aspirin 600 mg should be given by mouth every three to four hours as needed. If aspirin is not well tolerated by the patient, acetaminophen may be tried at the same dosage and frequency. Diet and liquids should be given as tolerated. For persistent itching, diphenhydramine hydrochloride 50 mg should be given by mouth four times daily. The patient's fingernails should be scrubbed daily to prevent bacterial contamination of the lesions by scratching. *In all cases of suspected chickenpox, medical advice by radio should be obtained.*

CHOLERA (Asiatic or Epidemic)

Incubation Period: A few hours to 5 days (usually 2 to 3 days).

Isolation Period: Until declared free from infection by a physician.

The term cholera sometimes is used to cover any acute disease that has copious discharges of watery material from the bowels, vomiting, and prostration. Usually, the term refers to Asiatic (or epidemic) cholera, which is a bacterial disease caused by the organism *Vibrio cholerae.*

The disease is transmitted from one person to another by discharges from the intestinal tract. It is extremely serious and highly infectious. Cholera exists throughout the year in many areas of Asia. In North America, it exists only when introduced from abroad.

With proper precautions, merchant vessels should be able to proceed in and out of cholera ports without picking up the infection either in the intestinal tracts of crew members, or in fresh water, fresh vegetables, and other articles taken on board.

Cholera is spread (1) by food or water that is polluted with cholera germs; (2) by contact with articles soiled with the discharges of patients or carriers (persons who harbor the germs but have no apparent disease); and (3) by flies or vermin that have contacted infectious material.

The crews of ships sailing for a port where cholera is known to be present should be protected against it by immunization. If crew members go ashore in a cholera port, it is preferable that they should not eat or drink anything while ashore.

Cholera is an official quarantinable disease. Regulations require the Master, as soon as practicable, to notify local health authorities at the next port of call, station, or stop. The Master shall take such measures as the local health authorities direct to prevent the spread of disease. (See Appendix C, p. 436.)

The local health authorities (port, medical and American Consular) should be consulted when food, especially fresh vegetables, and fresh water are taken aboard anywhere in a cholera area. At ports where cholera is known to exist, food must be cooked and protected from flies. If there is the slightest question about the safety of water for drinking, washing, and cooking, it should be chlorinated aboard ship. (See p. 376.)

The symptoms of cholera usually begin about five days after the germs have entered the body (incubation period). Diarrhea may be the only symptom in mild cases. Most cases, however, are marked by violent diarrhea, vomiting, abdominal cramps, and prostration or collapse. Typical stools are almost clear water with shreds of mucus, which give them the appearance of rice water. Usually, there is intense thirst. Drinking water or other liquids often increases the tendency to vomit. There may or may not be fever and the pulse is weak.

Treatment

The patient with cholera should be kept in bed under strict isolation technique. If possible, the medical attendant charged with the care of the sick patient should have been inoculated against cholera within the past six months. *Medical advice on treatment should be obtained promptly by radio.*

The patient should be kept comfortably warm (not overheated) with blankets and hot water bottles. To control diarrhea, tablets of diphenoxylate hydrochloride 2.5 mg with atropine sulfate should be administered by mouth, two tablets, three or four times daily until the symptoms are controlled. Then the dosage should be reduced as required. Small amounts of cracked ice taken by mouth may help to check vomiting. Hot applications may relieve abdominal pain. If severe abdominal pain continues, morphine sulfate 10 mg may be given once only by intramuscular injection, *if recommended by radio medical advice.*

If the patient is severely dehydrated, intravenous sodium chloride 0.9% solution may prove lifesaving. *As a general rule, the amount of fluids given intravenously should equal that lost each day through diarrhea.*

When port is reached, stools should be examined for cholera germs. Usually, the entire crew should have stool examinations.

Food should not be given during the first few days of a severe case of cholera. Small sips of fluids should be forced, as long as they are tolerated; larger amounts may induce vomiting. If cold liquids are more nauseating than hot liquids, then hot tea, hot black coffee, or hot water should be tried. As the patient shows signs of recovery after the initial severe stages, he may be given soup, boiled milk, cooked cereal, and other bland easily digested liquid or soft foods, if he is able to tolerate them.

Stools and vomited matter should be flushed into the ship's sewage treatment system or retention tank. All articles used by the patient, as dishes, other eating utensils, bedpans, urinals, bed linens, and towels must be soaked in a disinfecting solution or boiled. (See p. 318.) All attendants must wear gowns while in the sickroom and the hands must be washed and rinsed in a disinfectant solution (see p. 321) each time after contact with the patient. The medical attendant must not eat or drink anything while in the patient's room.

The patient's room and his personal effects should be disinfected following the illness. Also any part of the ship that may have been contaminated through contact with the patient, his body excretions, clothing, or other personal effects should be disinfected very carefully. (See p. 321.)

DENGUE FEVER (Breakbone Fever)

Incubation Period: 3 to 15 days (usually 5 to 6 days).

Isolation Period: In a screened room at least 5 days after onset.

Dengue fever is an acute viral disease of tropical and subtropical climates. The disease is transmitted by the bite of infective *Aedes aegypti* mosquitoes, the same type that spreads yellow fever; *Aedes albopictus;* and one of the *Aedes scutellaris* complex. It is characterized by the sudden onset of high fever 102°F to 105°F (38.8°C to 40.5°C), severe muscle aches and pains, and a blotchy red rash. Many patients develop a second rise in temperature 12 to 72 hours after the initial rise. The disease lasts from three to 12 days.

Treatment

There is no specific treatment for dengue fever. Complete bed rest and good nursing care are important. Fluids should be forced. The temperature elevation and pain usually can be controlled effectively with aspirin and/or codeine sulfate.

For severe pain, aspirin 600 mg with codeine sulfate 30 mg should be given by mouth every four hours as needed. Aspirin alone may control the pain after four or five doses. If additional codeine sulfate appears to be needed after four or five doses, medical advice by radio should be obtained. If aspirin is not well tolerated by the patient, acetaminophen 600 mg, with or without codeine sulfate, may be effective at the same frequency.

Differentiating this disease from other viral illnesses is difficult without specific blood tests.

Control

Dengue fever usually occurs in epidemics. Control of the disease is based on preventing carrier mosquitoes from biting both infected and noninfected persons. Patients should be kept under mosquito netting until the second fever has abated (at least five or six days after onset).

DIPHTHERIA

Incubation Period: 2 to 5 days.

Isolation Period: 14 days after onset.

Diphtheria is a serious acute infectious disease that is caused by the *Corynebacterium diphtheriae* bacillus. The bacteria grow in the throat, nose or windpipe, and give off a toxin (poison) that causes an illness of the entire body.

Diphtheria once was a very common cause of sickness and death among infants and children, but it is now a rare disease in the United States. It may be prevented by diphtheria toxoid injection with booster doses every ten years. Most crew members have been inoculated as children. Before signing on, a check should be made to assure that booster doses have been maintained.

The early symptoms of diphtheria are like those in most communicable diseases: overall body discomfort, restlessness, weakness, loss of appetite, headache, chilliness, and constipation. Soon there is a sore throat or sore mouth with increasing fever to 103°F (39.4°C), prostration, vomiting, and convulsions in some cases. In the laryngeal (windpipe) type of the disease, dirty gray patches of an adherent membrane form in the back of the nose and throat, over the tonsils and in the windpipe itself. These patches resemble dead skin. If attempts are made to brush off patches with a cotton swab, they come away with difficulty and leave tiny bleeding points in the uncovered mucous membrane. There may be a bloody nasal discharge and a "croupy" cough.

The most serious complications include (1) suffocation, due to the mechanical blocking of the windpipe by the diphtheritic membrane; and (2) an overwhelming systemic poisoning due to the toxin. Because of a special affinity for certain nerves, the toxin may produce paralysis of the throat, eyes, or extremities; or death from heart failure.

Making the diagnosis of diphtheria at sea is difficult. Anyone with a severe sore throat, together with the severe systemic symptoms mentioned earlier, should be considered to have diphtheria until examined by a physician. *Medical advice by radio should be obtained.*

Treatment

If diphtheria is suspected, the patient should be placed on absolute bed rest and in strict isolation. Gargles of warm salt water (one teaspoonful of table salt to one pint of water) may help to ease pain in the throat.

Antibiotics are considered to have little effect on the clinical course of diphtheria. However, a ten day course of penicillin is indicated *if the patient is not allergic to it.* It is believed that penicillin cuts down on the toxin produced, is a useful treatment for associated infections as beta-hemolytic streptococcal pharyngitis, and hastens the clearing of the carrier state in the patient. Penicillin V potassium 500 mg should be given by mouth as an initial dose followed by 500 mg every six hours. If the patient is unable to retain medication taken orally, penicillin G, procaine, sterile suspension 600,000 units should be given by intramuscular injection every 12 hours, until the patient is able to take penicillin V potassium by mouth.

The patient should be evacuated by air to the nearest port as soon as possible. The entire crew should report to health authorities at the next port.

HEPATITIS, VIRAL

Viral hepatitis is an acute infection that destroys liver cells. There are two forms of the disease presumed to be caused by different viral agents that produce more or less identical symptoms. *Infectious hepatitis* whose virus has a short incubation period often can be prevented by injections of immune serum globulin. *Serum hepatitis* has a longer incubation period and immune serum globulin injections will *not* protect against the disease. Cases of either disease cannot be distinguished on clinical grounds only because jaundice is the dominant physical finding; and laboratory tests of liver function show similar abnormalities. However, a study of the patient and his environment will help to differentiate one disease from the other.

A diagnosis of *infectious hepatitis* can be made if (1) the patient's history shows contact with another case of jaundice within a 15 to 50-day incubation period; (2) the patient belonged to a defined neighborhood as a housing project or a ship where a localized epidemic occurred that was related to a person-to-person spread; or (3) there was a common exposure to contaminated water, food, or raw shellfish. In contrast, a diagnosis of *serum hepatitis* can be made if the history shows inoculation with blood or blood products, or exposure to contaminated hypodermic syringes and needles within a period of 50 to 180 days.

Infectious Hepatitis (*Virus A Hepatitis, Epidemic Hepatitis, Epidemic Jaundice*)

Incubation Period: 10 to 50 days; commonly about 30 to 35 days.

Isolation Period: First 14 days of illness and at least 7 days after jaundice shows up.

Infectious hepatitis in some patients may be so mild that a correct diagnosis never is made. Most recognized cases last about two or three weeks, followed by a prolonged convalescence. About 10 percent suffer permanent damage to the liver. About one percent may die

during the acute stage or after a year or two of chronic illness due to liver damage. Severity varies from a mild illness of one or two weeks, to a very disabling attack that demands several months of convalescence. Generally severity increases with age, but usually there is complete recovery with no lasting ill effects or recurrences.

Early detection and diagnosis of infectious hepatitis is important. There are no specific diagnostic measures. Differential diagnosis depends on clinical and epidemiological evidence that will exclude other causes of jaundice coupled with fever.

The disease has an abrupt onset with a fever of 100°F (37.7°C), severe headache, loss of appetite, vomiting, and lethargy. The virus is carried to the liver where it multiplies rapidly with widespread destruction of cells. The liver becomes swollen and tender with aching in the center and upper right abdominal areas, plus acute pain from pressure just below the ribs. At this stage the patient may think he has a touch of intestinal flu that can be ignored. On the contrary, the patient has a very infectious acute illness, and in three to seven days after onset he shows a yellowish (jaundiced) color in the eyes and skin due to excess liver bile in the blood. The color of the urine becomes dark brown because of excess bile in the kidneys, the stools show a pale grayish-white color, and the breath has a foul sweetish odor.

In some cases the onset resembles an acute attack of influenza, when the patient feels ill all over the body with severe abdominal pain, prostration, and a temperature that reaches 105°F (40.5°C). The illness will last about three or four weeks, after which there will be a slow convalescence during which the patient is listless, depressed, and shows little interest in food.

Treatment

Medical advice by radio should be obtained. Because infectious hepatitis may be transmitted through the stool and urine, all excretions must be disinfected. The patient must be isolated and instructed to apply good hygiene procedures after using the bathroom. The virus is excreted in feces and urine 14 to 21 days before the appearance of jaundice and 7 days thereafter. The patient's blood also is infectious. There is no specific treatment.

Enforced bed rest and strict adherence to a low-fat, high-carbohydrate diet no longer are considered essential. Diet and activity should be adjusted to the clinical condition of the patient. He should be given plenty of fluids. The very ill patient will not want to be out of bed and may have severe nausea and vomiting that will require fluid supplements of dextrose 5% and sodium chloride 0.45% injection administered intravenously. Headache and sleeplessness may be relieved by 30 mg of codeine sulfate by mouth. For additional doses and their frequency, *medical advice by radio should be obtained*. A mild laxative such as milk of magnesia may be given. A hot water bottle applied to the sensitive liver area may provide relief. Alcoholic drinks should not be used by the patient during the course of the disease and for many months after recovery.

When a member of the crew is known to have infectious hepatitis, others who have not had the disease should receive *immune human serum globulin* injections as soon as possible. Medical advice by radio should be sought on whether this medication can be made available at the next port of call or by airdrop. Those who have contacted the infection will receive short-term protection from the globulin for a period of six to eight weeks. However, its effectiveness depends on how soon after exposure the injection was administered. Disposable inoculation equipment should be used whenever possible.

Serum Hepatitis *(Virus B Hepatitis, Homologous Serum Jaundice)*

Incubation Period: 50 to 180 days, usually 80 to 100 days. In post transfusion hepatitis it may range from 10 to more than 180 days.

Isolation Period: Same as that for infectious hepatitis. (See above.)

Unlike the virus of infectious hepatitis, the serum hepatitis virus is not transmitted through contaminated water, food, or close personal contact. Instead it usually is spread from person to person only by the use of contaminated hypodermic needles, medical or surgical instruments, or by the transfusion of blood or blood products taken from a donor who is a carrier of the virus. Cases have been traced to tattoo parlors.

Serum hepatitis is practically identical with infectious hepatitis except its incubation period is longer. Symptoms may not occur for six months after inoculation. Its onset develops quickly with vague abdominal discomfort, loss of appetite, nausea and vomiting often leading to jaundice. Severity varies widely from inapparent cases detected only by liver function tests to those with extremely rapid development with liver cell destruction that causes death.

Many cases of serum hepatitis have been found among drug addicts, teenagers, and young adults who share contaminated hypodermic equipment when they experiment with drugs. Use of illicit drugs and narcotics is extremely perilous and few users are aware of the additional threat of death from serum hepatitis because inadequately sterilized needles and syringes were used. *Those who recover from the disease can become apparently healthy carriers who carry the live virus in their blood for years.*

Treatment

Medical advice should be obtained by radio. Because the disease is infectious, the patient must be isolated.

Disposable inoculation equipment should be used whenever possible. If not available, springes and needles that were used should be destroyed and discarded after being autoclaved for 30 minutes.

MALARIA
(Bilious Fever, Swamp Fever, Marsh Fever, Ague)

Incubation Period: 10 to 30 days.

Isolation Period: None.

One of the most common and important of all the infectious diseases, malarial fever is both an acute and a chronic disease. There is destruction of red blood cells and interference with the normal functioning of vital body processes. Chronic malaria may last for years.

The symptoms may interfere greatly with the patient's well-being and with his ability to function normally, or they may not be severe enough to keep the patient in bed all or even a part of the time.

The geographic distribution of malaria depends on the species of mosquito that transmits it. Females of the *Anopheles* group of mosquitoes act as intermediary hosts for the *Plasmodium* protozoal parasites that cause malaria. These live part of their life in the mosquito and part in the blood of the infected person. When a female *Anopheles* mosquito bites a person who has malaria, she sucks in some of these parasites with the blood on which she is feeding. The parasites go through a stage of development in the body of the mosquito. It takes at least two weeks before the mosquito can pass the parasites to another person. When the young parasites are ready to start the part of their life cycle that takes place in a human host, they enter the mosquito's saliva and are injected into the blood of any person bitten by the mosquito. In the blood of the new victim, the parasites go through another stage of development which takes about 10 to 14 days. Then the parasites are ready to cause the *chills and fever typical of malaria*. These attacks occur every day, every other day, or every third day, depending upon the type of infecting parasite.

Malaria may occur as a relatively mild or as a severe and fatal disease. In the *mild type*, the temperature rises above normal and falls below normal with each attack. In the *severe type*, it rises higher above the normal but does not drop back to normal before the next attack. To distinguish between these two types, the temperature should be taken at least every four hours for several days.

The typical attack of malaria has *three stages*. The *first or cold stage*, usually is ushered in by a preliminary period of malaise (feeling ill and tired), chilliness, headache, aching in the bones, loss of appetite, nausea, and possibly vomiting. Sometimes the chills begin without any of these warning symptoms. In the cold stage, the patient feels cold, shakes all over, his teeth chatter, and he has accompanying pains in the head and body. He yawns, usually is nauseated, may vomit, and the pulse is rapid and feeble. Despite his chilliness, the temperature will be above normal, sometimes as high as 104°F or 105°F (40°C to 45.5°C). The patient will get into bed and pile covers over himself, but he will not get warm. This stage lasts for a half hour or longer.

In the *second or hot stage*, the patient loses the chilliness, becomes uncomfortably warm, and throws off the bedclothing. The skin is hot and dry, the temperature remains elevated, the face is flushed, the pulse is rapid and full, and respirations are quickened. The patient becomes very thirsty, headache increases (often becoming agonizing), and frequently there is vomiting. This stage lasts from one to four hours or longer.

Then the fever begins to fall. The patient enters the *third or sweating stage*. He begins to perspire freely, first on the face and then over the entire body. Perspiration may be so profuse that the sheets are literally soaked. A feeling of comfort takes the place of the acute misery of the first and second stages. Headaches and other symptoms disappear and he may fall into a deep sleep. Afterwards, he feels fairly well until the next attack.

The patient should be watched for the following complications: (a) excessively high temperature 108°F to 110°F (42.2°C to 43.3°C); (b) coma, or delirium followed by coma; (c) heart failure following sudden exertion; and (d) severe distress in the stomach region, a tender abdomen, incessant vomiting, and collapse.

Some forms of malaria follow an unusual pattern. One form simulates heatstroke, acute mania, or an acute alcoholic mental disturbance. Headache, mental excitement, and/or prostration are prominent. All symptoms are relieved by antimalarial treatment. In another form, there is dimness and clouding of vision with headaches of long duration, usually over the temporal or frontal areas.

Treatment

Chloroquine phosphate remains the drug of choice for terminating acute attacks caused by the parasites *Plasmodium vivax*, *P. malariae*, or *P. ovale*. 1000 mg (four 250 mg tablets) of chloroquine phosphate should be given at once, followed by 500 mg six hours later; then 500 mg once daily for the next two days. Chloroquine phosphate ends acute attacks of malaria fairly quickly and may be given for *P. falciparum* strains that are not resistant. If some parasites develop resistance to a drug, then another drug must be tried.

For patients with a chloroquine-resistant *P. falciparum* infection, or any patient developing clinical malaria while on chloroquine prophylaxis, 600 mg (two 300 mg tablets or capsules) of quinine sulfate should be administered orally every eight hours for 14 days. On each of the first three days of treatment, 50 mg of pyrimethamine should be administered concurrently with the quinine sulfate.

Before treating any malaria patient, medical advice by radio should be obtained.

Prevention

To prevent malaria, travelers should take 500 mg of chloroquine phosphate by mouth, weekly on the same day each week, beginning two weeks before possible exposure, and continuing for eight weeks after the last possible exposure to malaria.

MEASLES (Rubeola)

Incubation Period: 8 to 13 days.

Isolation Period: From diagnosis until 7 days after the rash appears.

Measles, an acute viral disease, is the most contagious of all communicable diseases. The virus is found in secretions of the nose, mouth, throat, and lungs of infected persons. Most adults in childhood have had the disease, and one attack provides lifelong immunity. However, measles must be feared because of complications, mainly to the eyes, kidneys, and brain; and secondary infections as bronchitis, bronchial pneumonia, and inflammation of the middle ear.

Symptoms begin about ten days after exposure. The onset is sudden with a general overall feeling of not being well, sneezing, runny nose, headache, sore throat, cough, soreness of the eyes, dislike of bright light, and a rise in temperature to about 102°F (38.8°C). Symptoms are apt to be severe with copious tears, swollen lids, and bloodshot eyes. During this stage the disease is most contagious. On the sec-

ond and third day of the disease the symptoms become more marked and the face gets a puffy look. On the inner side of the cheeks, near the junction of the upper and lower jaws, where the back teeth meet, tiny whitish spots (Koplik's spots) may be seen. These spots confirm the diagnosis of measles. The patient now should be isolated, if not already done. After three to five days of the disease the temperature rises to about 104°F (40°C) and the typical measles rash appears. The rash of a reddish hue with slightly raised irregular blotch patches starts on the forehead and behind the ears, and gradually spreads to the face, body, and limbs. The rash remains about four or five days, then fades from the body regions in the same sequence that it appeared. This is followed by a fine peeling of the skin. As the rash disappears, the temperature drops to normal.

Because of its extremely infectious nature, measles usually cannot be kept from spreading to crewmen who have not had it. However, a measles patient should be isolated to protect him from exposure to germs of other communicable diseases, as the common cold or pneumonia, that are carried by many apparently healthy individuals. Secondary respiratory infections are so dangerous to a measles patient that masks should be worn by the patient and everyone attending to his needs.

Treatment

Treatment is symptomatic as there is no specific medicine that will cure measles. *Medical advice by radio should be obtained.*

The patient should be cared for in strict isolation (see p. 321) and in a well-ventilated cabin screened from bright light, comfortably warm, and without drafts. Close attention should be paid to cleanliness of the mouth and teeth. To protect the eyes, the patient should wear dark colored glasses. The room should be darkened but not completely blacked out. The eyelids and margins should be cleansed several times a day with cotton balls moistened with sterile isotonic eye irrigating solution.

If the rash causes irritation or itching, calamine lotion should be applied freely three times a day. If the patient develops a troublesome cough, 5 ml or one teaspoonful of dextromethorphan hydrobromide syrup 15 mg/5 ml, with glyceryl guaiacolate should be given every four to six hours, as needed. For headache, aspirin 600 mg should be given by mouth every three to four hours. If aspirin is not well tolerated by the patient, acetaminophen may be tried at the same dosage and frequency.

The patient should be kept in bed at all times. Exercise, even such slight exertion as going to the head while fever or malaise is present, may encourage kidney and other complications. The patient should drink plenty of fluids and the diet should be liquid or soft foods.

During convalescence one should watch for complications and secondary infections and try to avoid them. The patient should not engage in anything but the lightest tasks for two or three weeks after the attack. *At the first convenient port, he should be referred to a physician for a medical checkup.* (See German Measles, below.)

MEASLES, GERMAN (Rubella)

Incubation Period: 14 to 21 days (usually 18 days).

Isolation Period: 7 days after temperature returns to normal.

German Measles usually is a mild, acute, highly infectious viral disease, sometimes called three-day measles. If a woman develops German measles during the early months of pregnancy, there is a great risk of a spontaneous abortion, stillbirth, or the child may be born with birth defects. The disease is common among children and young adults.

The first sign usually is a rose-pink rash that does not appear until the fourth day, which may resemble measles or scarlet fever (see p. 187). However, there is no sore throat or pallor around the mouth as found in scarlet fever.

The rash of German Measles may be accompanied or followed by a general feeling of bodily discomfort, headache, symptoms of a common cold, eye soreness, stiffness of joints, tender swollen glands at the sides and back of the neck, and a slight fever about 102°F (38.8°C). The rash usually lasts about three days and the temperature may go to 104°F (40°C). The temperature will drop to normal as the rash fades.

Treatment

There is no specific therapy for German Measles. Treatment should be symptomatic, the same as for measles (Rubeola). Medical advice by radio should be obtained.

MONONUCLEOSIS, INFECTIOUS

Incubation Period: 14 to 42 days.
Isolation Period: Until a physician states the patient is free of infection.

The cause of infectious mononucleosis has not been definitely proven, although a herpes-like virus is suspected. It occurs among children and young adults and is a diagnostic challenge because of the wide variety of symptoms shown by its victims. It may occur as sporadic cases or localized epidemics and is common among college students and hospital personnel. Because it is spread by close upper respiratory contact, it has been called the "kissing disease."

Almost every organ of the body is involved. The first symptoms can mimic those of an upper respiratory infection: with fever, chills, headache, cough, and general malaise. The patient may have vague complaints of fatigue, loss of appetite, sleeplessness, and a sore throat. After about three days, swollen lymph glands may appear on the sides and back of the neck, in the armpits and groin. A reddish skin rash like that of typhoid fever or eruptions like German Measles occur. The spleen may enlarge considerably. Liver function is impaired and the skin and whites of the eyes become jaundiced (yellow-colored).

It may be necessary to obtain laboratory tests of the blood to confirm the diagnosis of mononucleosis. *The patient should be referred to a physician as soon as possible.*

Treatment

Medical advice by radio should be obtained. There is no specific treatment for infectious mononucleosis except bed rest during the acute phase. Bed rest should be extended in cases that resemble hepatitis. Fever, headache, itching of the skin, abdominal pain and other symptoms should be treated as they arise. The disease may run its course in a few days, a few weeks, or occasionally several months. The acute stage averages three to four weeks, but the side effects may prolong recovery. There is a risk that the disease will recur.

In a small percentage of patients there may be complications such as enlargement of the spleen; and unnecessary palpation of this organ and exercise by the patient increases the potential for rupture.

Because of the prolonged bed rest, taking fluids by mouth should be encouraged. For fever and pain, aspirin 600 mg may be given orally every four to six hours if needed. If aspirin is not tolerated by the patient, acetaminophen may be given at the same dosage. Complications should be treated as recommended by radio medical advice.

MUMPS (Epidemic Parotitis)

Incubation Period: 12 to 26 days.

Isolation Period: 21 days.

Mumps is an acute, contagious, viral disease identified by tenderness and swelling of one or more of the salivary glands. Usually the parotid pair of salivary glands is affected. The virus may be spread by direct or indirect contact with nose and throat discharges from an infected person.

Mumps is most prevalent in the winter and spring, and occasionally cases are seen in cities the year around. It is apt to occur in camps, training stations, and among new members of a ship's company recruited from rural districts and never previously exposed to mumps. One attack usually gives immunity for life.

At first there is a general feeling of malaise, headache, stiff neck, a slight rise in temperature, and at times nausea. In severe cases the temperature may reach 104°F (40°C) and last as long as a week. On the second day the swelling usually begins on one side and increases greatly in size. In a couple of days, there is considerable enlargement at the side of the neck, the posterior part of the cheek, and underneath the side of the jawbone. The patient complains of pain and stiffness on moving the lower jaw. The opposite side of the face usually becomes affected in a few days. The swelling lasts about ten days.

In the average case in childhood, the patient has little trouble beyond stiffness of the jaw, discomfort from swelling, and pain on opening the mouth. However, in young adult males, the infection may spread to one or both testicles to produce a painful inflammation and swelling called orchitis. This is a serious condition because in some adult males there may be long term damage to the testes that could cause one or both to cease to be functional.

Treatment

The patient should have bed rest with strict isolation nursing technique followed, because the infecting virus may be spread by coughing and sneezing. There is no specific medicine for the cure of mumps and symptoms should be treated as they arise.

Petrolatum rubbed gently over the swelling may relieve the stiffness and tightness of the stretched skin. A hot water bottle or heating pad may help to relieve pain. Cold applications should not be used. Mouthwash may be used several times a day. For pain or extreme discomfort, aspirin 600 mg should be given by mouth every three to four hours as needed. If aspirin is not well tolerated by the patient, acetaminophen may be tried at the same dosage and frequency.

Nourishing liquids and soft diet with an abundance of water should be given. Milk of magnesia should be administered as needed to avoid constipation.

If the testicles become involved, they should be supported on a towel or pillow. Keep the patient at absolute rest in bed until the swelling and tenderness have disappeared. When the patient is allowed up, he should wear a suspensory. *If there is unusual pain or indication of further complication, medical advice by radio should be obtained.*

PLAGUE

Incubation Period: 2 to 12 days (usually 3 to 4 days).

Isolation Period: Until declared free from infection by a physician.

Plague is an extremely serious bacterial disease caused by the bacillus *Pasteurella pestis*, which is transmitted to man by the bite of a flea that normally lives on a rat. Primarily a disease of rodents, plague only secondarily is a disease of human beings. Plague in the past has been a maritime disease because of the rat population aboard ships.

Federal regulations require that vessels be maintained free of rodent infestation through the use of traps, poisons, and other generally accepted methods of rodent control. Ships must be inspected periodically by the U.S. Public Health Service and a certificate of non-rat infestation given. (See Appendix, p. 436.)

This disease is still endemic (always present) in most countries and occasionally assumes epidemic proportions in other areas. The epidemic disease is associated with a rise in infestation by the domestic rat population.

Three types of human plague exist:

(1) The *bubonic type* that affects the lymph glands; (2) the *pneumonic type* that affects the lungs; and (3) the *septicemic type* that affects the blood. All three forms are marked by sudden violent onset, high fever, staggering gait, incoherent speech as in drunkenness, and severe prostration.

Bubonic Plague

The bubonic type, the more common form, is transmitted by the bite of an infected flea from rat to rat, from rat to man, or from man to man. The flea bites a person, rat, or squirrel whose blood contains the bacterium that causes plague. The plague germs pass through the flea's gastrointestinal tract without being killed and are excreted in its feces. The flea travels from the infected person or rat to a healthy person or rat. The flea bites the healthy person or rat, and while feeding, defecates on the skin. The fecal germs when rubbed into the flea bite or into a scratch or other break in the skin, will get into the bloodstream. The germs multiply in the blood and the individual has plague.

The patient suffers intense headache and drowsiness. His face becomes drawn and haggard with an expression of fear or anxiety.

The fever may rise as high as 105°F (40.6°C) on the first day, then fluctuates. The pulse is rapid and weak and the thirst is intense. Delirium and convulsions may follow. About the second or third day, the characteristic buboes develop. The bubo is a swelling of a lymph gland, and is most commonly found in the groins. Buboes may form in other areas, especially in the armpits and neck. A bubo may be as large as a hen's egg.

If untreated, about 70% of patients with bubonic plague will die. In cases that are going to recover, the patient begins to improve after the bubo appears. The temperature falls rapidly with profuse sweating. The bubo or buboes will continue to enlarge, soften, and usually discharge pus. The temperature becomes normal after the sixth to tenth day. Convalescence is rapid.

Pneumonic Plague

Spread by coughing, talking or sneezing, pneumonic plague is the most serious form and resembles pneumonia. Recovery is rare if the patient does not receive care soon after onset. Chills and vomiting often mark the onset. Cough, difficult breathing, and blueness of the skin and lips occur, accompanied by profuse watery, bloodstained sputum (not like the rusty, sticky sputum of ordinary pneumonia). The sputum, alive with plague bacilli, is extremely dangerous. Poisoning of the whole system develops rapidly, breathing becomes rapid, and death occurs in one to four hours.

Septicemic Plague

Septicemic plague, a rare form, resembles an overwhelming general blood poisoning. The patient is prostrated rapidly and hemorrhages often occur into the skin. Death occurs in two to four days; it is preceded by stupor, coma, or delirium. The infection at onset may be so overwhelming that the temperature may rise little, if at all; yet the patient may be dead in 48 hours.

Prevention of Spread

Plague is an official quarantinable disease (see Appendix, p. 436). Federal regulations require that the Master, as soon as practicable, shall notify the local health authority at the next port of call, station, or stop, and take such measures to prevent the spread of the disease as the local health authority directs.

Plague vaccine will give some protection. If the ship is proceeding to a port where plague is present, it is advisable to vaccinate the crew. Specific advice should be obtained from the port authorities as to regulations about entering and leaving the port.

Bubonic Plague—If *bubonic plague* occurs on shipboard, the patient should be isolated in a screened room that is free of vermin. The sickroom and the crew quarters should be treated with an insecticide to kill the fleas. (See p. 378.) A systematic rat hunt should be organized. Dead rats found aboard ship should not be handled with bare hands. The rats should be sprayed with a strong disinfectant solution to kill any fleas; then they should be picked up with a shovel or tongs and incinerated.

Discharges from buboes are infectious. Disposable surgical supplies such as gauze used on the buboes should be burned or sterilized prior to disposal. Attendants should wash and disinfect their hands with liquid povidone-iodine skin cleanser each time after giving care.

Pneumonic Plague—In *pneumonic plague*, which is spread by the patient's sputum, isolation nursing technique must be observed strictly. Attendants should wear a mask, cap, and gown; these articles must be kept in the sickroom after use and disinfected at the termination of the illness. The medical attendant's hands must be washed with liquid povidone-iodine skin cleanser before leaving the sickroom. Discharges from the patient's mouth must be caught in tissue and disposed of in an appropriate manner for infectious waste material by autoclaving or incineration. All nondisposable articles soiled with mouth discharges, which cannot be sterilized by autoclaving must be boiled or chemically disinfected. At the end of the illness, disinfection of the room must be carried out. (See p. 318.)

Treatment

Radio confirmation of the diagnosis should be made at the first suggestion of symptoms of plague. Also, plans should be made to evacuate the patient and arrangements made to obtain any necessary antibiotics not carried aboard ship.

Cold compresses should be applied to the buboes. When the buboes are open, dressings should be used as for boils. For the average adult, give tetracycline hydrochloride by mouth in an initial dose of 2,000 mg (eight 250 mg capsules), followed by 500 mg every six hours for 10 days. If the patient cannot retain the medication by mouth, the tetracycline hydrochloride will have to be given intravenously. *Before giving intravenous tetracycline hydrochloride, medical advice should be obtained by radio on the need to administer, plus action to get it aboard ship, if not already available.*

For severe pain or delirium, morphine sulfate 10 mg should be given by intramuscular injection. *To repeat the morphine sulfate, medical advice by radio will be needed.* For cough, dextromethorphan hydrobromide syrup with glyceryl guaiacolate, 5 ml (one teaspoonful) should be given by mouth every six to eight hours.

Diet in the acute stages should consist of forced fluids only. As symptoms lessen, the diet may be increased gradually by adding easily digested food.

The patient should be sent to a medical facility ashore at the first opportunity after consultation with the port's health authorities.

POLIOMYELITIS (Infantile Paralysis)

Incubation Period: Commonly 7 to 12 days, with a range from 3 to 21 days.

Isolation Period: Isolation precautions not more than 7 days in hospital management. Of little value in home or ship conditions because the spread of infection is greatest when symptoms first appear.

Poliomyelitis is an acute viral disease that occurs chiefly in children with most of the cases occurring in the first three years of life. Adults usually are immune. Today polio is wholly preventable with two types of vaccine available: the injectable Salk vaccine and the newer Sabin oral vaccine.

Polio may start with no recognizable symptoms or it may resemble a head cold with fever, vomiting, and irritability. The symptoms last about three days and the temperature may rise to 104°F (40°C). From the fourth to the tenth day the condition will seem to be clearing. However, the symptoms return with a feeling of apprehension, headache, stiff neck and back, and deep muscle pains. Varying degrees of paralysis follow. Thereafter improvement is gradual either with complete recovery or paralysis to some degree.

Treatment

No specific treatment is effective. *When poliomyelitis is suspected, medical advice by radio should be obtained.* The patient should be put to bed and isolation nursing technique observed. For paralysis of body parts, hot moist heat may be applied coupled with gentle, active or passive, motion as soon as the patient can tolerate it.

If urine is retained, a catheter should be inserted (see p. 325). All stools and urine are infectious, so bedpans and urinals should be disinfected (see p. 318).

RABIES (Hydrophobia)

Incubation Period: 10 days to 12 months (usually under 4 months). Patients bitten about the head and those with extensive bites will have shorter periods.

Isolation Period: Duration of the illness.

Rabies is an acute infectious viral disease that almost always is fatal. When a rabid mammal bites humans or other animals, its saliva transmits the infection into the wound where it spreads to the central nervous system. Rabies is primarily an infection of wild animals as skunks, coyotes, foxes, wolves, raccoons, bats, squirrels, rabbits, and chipmunks. The most common domestic animals reported to have rabies are cattle, dogs, cats, horses, mules, sheep, goats, and swine. It is possible for rabies to be transmitted if infective saliva enters a scratch or fresh break in the skin.

Human rabies begins with fever, nausea, headache, loss of appetite, and sore throat. The temperature may rise to 103°F (39.4°C). Because these symptoms are common to other viral infections, the condition may be misdiag-

nosed if the patient's history does not indicate a recent bite by an animal. At the bite wound, there is a tingling or burning feeling. As the infection progresses, the brain and the rest of the central nervous system become involved. Paralysis and muscle spasms occur, with especially painful spasms of muscles in the mouth and throat that control swallowing. The term hydrophobia (fear of water) derives from the refusal to drink by infected animals and humans. They may be thirsty and want the water badly, but efforts to swallow are too painful. The patient becomes very weak and his mental outlook changes. He becomes apprehensive, irrational, even maniacal. He suffers from widespread muscular twitching, severe pain, and convulsive seizures provoked by any stimulus, especially by attempts to drink. The voice becomes hoarse and thick ropy saliva drips from his lips because he cannot swallow. Eventually there are breathing difficulties, coma, and general paralysis. Once symptoms of rabies develop death is virtually certain to result. Thus prevention of the disease is of the utmost importance.

When a human is bitten by a dog or other animal, circumstances surrounding the attack frequently furnish vital information on whether or not use of rabies treatment is indicated. Most bites by domestic animals are provoked attacks; if the history obtained indicates this, usually rabies treatment can be withheld, if the animal appears to be healthy. The dog that bites without apparent cause or provocation should be considered rabid. Each case must be analyzed carefully before a conclusion can be reached on whether or not to proceed with treatment to prevent the disease.

Domestic animals that bite a person should be captured and observed for symptoms of rabies for ten days. If symptoms are not present, the animal may be assumed to be nonrabid. If the animal dies or is killed, the animal's head, undamaged, should be sent promptly under refrigeration but not frozen to a public health laboratory. Any wild animal that bites or scratches a person should be killed at once and the head kept under refrigeration during transportation to a public health laboratory.

Rubber gloves should be worn by the attendant for protection against infective saliva when the head is being prepared for laboratory examination. Then the gloves should be washed thoroughly with disinfectant solution and boiled in the sterilizer for five minutes before discarding. Finally the attendant's hands should be washed with disinfectant solution.

Treatment

As soon as an individual aboard ship is known to have been bitten by a dog or other possibly rabid animal, medical advice by radio should be obtained at once. Usually suspected cases are sent ashore to obtain the expert treatment and nursing care needed to prevent the disease. If it is determined that rabies preventive measures will be started aboard ship, it must be decided how the necessary medications will be put aboard.

Immediate local care should be given. Vigorous treatment to remove rabies virus from the bites or other exposures to the animal's saliva may be as important as specific antirabies treatment. Free bleeding from the wound should be encouraged. Other local care should consist of (1) thorough irrigation of the wounds with large amounts of sodium chloride injection 0.9%; (2) cleansing with liquid povidone-iodine solution; (3) removal of bruised or devitalized tissue from the wound; (4) if recommended by radio, giving an antibiotic to prevent infection; and (5) administering adsorbed tetanus toxoid, if indicated.

Generally, immediate suturing of the wound is not advised because it may contribute to the development of rabies. However, if exposure to rabies is unlikely, a severe laceration secondary to a bite may be sutured.

RELAPSING FEVER
(Tick-, Spirillum-, Famine-, or Recurrent Fever)

Incubation Period: 5 to 15 days (usually 8 days).

Isolation Period: None, if the patient's clothing, immediate environment, and all household contacts have been deloused or freed from ticks.

Relapsing fever is an acute infectious disease, caused by several species of spirochetes of the genus *Borrelia*, that is transmitted by lice and ticks. The first attack shows rapid heart-beat, fever, chills, dizziness, headache, muscle and joint pains, vomiting, and at times delirium. The fever remains high for two to nine days, then ends suddenly by crisis. This is followed by a week of fair health without symptoms, after which a relapse occurs with the same symptoms, plus jaundice in many cases. There may be three, four, or more recurrent attacks, each decreasing in severity, as immunity develops. The actual duration of immunity is unknown, probably less than two years.

A sick member of the crew should be suspected of having the disease if the ship recently had been in a port where relapsing fever was prevalent, or the disease had been diagnosed in any of the crew by a shore physician. With known relapsing fever suspects aboard, a thorough search should be made for ticks, lice, and bedbugs. If these are found, the crew's quarters should be treated with an insecticide (see p. 378).

Lice are infected when they feed on patients during the fever stage. After the lice are crushed on a person's body, the spirochetes can enter any scraped skin or be carried by contaminated hands that rub the eyes. Ticks become infected when they feed on wild animals that carry the disease.

Treatment

Medical advice by radio should be obtained. Tetracycline hydrochloride 500 mg should be given by mouth every six hours for one day; then 250 mg every six hours for seven days.

RHEUMATIC FEVER

Rheumatic fever is characterized by fever up to 103°F (39.4°C) and painful swelling of the large joints. The swelling migrates from one joint to another. A knee may be hot, painful, and swollen one day and the next day appear normal, when a wrist, ankle, or shoulder may be involved. Several joints may be affected at the same time. These symptoms may follow a sore throat, a general feeling of not being well, vague pains in joints, a rapid irregular heartbeat, and pain in the abdomen or chest.

This disease is a complication of Group A streptococcal infections. The greatest danger of the disease is the frequency with which it affects the heart. Both the prevention of rheumatic heart disease and its treatment require weeks or months of bed rest. The only way to tell when it is safe for the patient to get out of bed is by certain laboratory tests.

Treatment

Medical confirmation of a rheumatic fever diagnosis should be obtained by radio. The patient should be kept totally at rest in bed to protect the heart. Antibiotics should be given only on the advice of a physician. Aspirin should be given in large doses, 1200 mg every four hours, to help control joint symptoms and fever. Local gastric reaction usually can be avoided or controlled by giving milk or an antacid with the aspirin, or between doses of the aspirin. The aspirin dosage should be reduced if the patient develops nausea or ringing in the ears.

Woolen strips wrapped around the affected joints will help. A swollen knee can be made more comfortable if a pillow is placed underneath the joint. Menthol compound ointment can be applied gently to the skin around sore joints to afford some relief. If the patient cannot sleep, pentobarbital sodium 100 mg should be given by mouth at bedtime.

Until four weeks after all joint pains and temperature have subsided, there should be strict bed rest, careful nursing, and special attention to symptoms including heart complications. At the earliest opportunity arrangements should be made to transfer the patient to a hospital ashore.

SCARLET FEVER (Scarlatina)

Incubation Period: 1 to 7 days.

Isolation Period: Until declared free from infection by a physician.

Scarlet fever is an acute infectious disease caused by streptococci bacteria invading the nose and throat. The symptoms appear suddenly and consist of general discomfort, runny nose, fever, headache, nausea, vomiting, and sore throat.

The typical rash does not appear until later —12 to 36 hours or more after symptoms occur. The rash is most intense at the creases of the body, such as the groins and armpits. The face

is relatively free of it. The rash consists of pinpoint red spots scattered on a flushed skin. Occasionally, the spots may be so elevated that they can be felt with the hand. A sign of less importance, the so-called "strawberry tongue," is a furring of the tongue with prominent red, pinpoint spots at the edges.

The complications from scarlet fever may be severe. These include discharging ears, swollen glands of the neck, rheumatic fever, and kidney disease. *Medical advice by radio should be obtained.*

Treatment

The patient should be strictly isolated. Absolute rest in bed is necessary to protect the heart and kidneys. All dishes, silverware, and other utensils used by the patient should be disinfected. (See p. 321.)

For the infection, an initial dose of penicillin V potassium 500 mg should be given by mouth followed by 500 mg every six hours. If the patient is suspected of being allergic to penicillin, oral erythromycin should be used in the same dosage and frequency. The penicillin or erythromycin treatment must be continued for ten days.

For pain and fever, aspirin 600 mg should be given by mouth every three to four hours as needed. If aspirin is not well tolerated by the patient, acetaminophen may be tried at the same dosage and frequency.

The patient should have a liquid diet and other supportive treatment as necessary. As the patient improves, he may have a soft or regular diet. However, meats should be restricted until all risk of kidney damage is past. He should be kept in bed longer than the usual patient with fever (several days to a week or two after the fever has disappeared), depending upon the severity of his illness.

SMALLPOX (Variola)

Incubation Period: 9 to 16 days (usually about 12 to 14 days).

Isolation Period: Until declared free from infection by a physician.

Smallpox is a highly contagious viral disease with general bodily symptoms and a typical skin eruption that results in permanent scarring.

Smallpox still is prevalent in parts of the world. In many ports, quarantine and health authorities will request evidence of a recent successful vaccination. Therefore, every seaman should carry with his papers a written certificate showing dates of vaccination and types of reaction. (See Appendix, p. 450.) The type of reaction is important, because it indicates whether a vaccination is successful or not. Some countries will not admit aliens who have not been vaccinated successfully within periods of two, six, or 12 months or longer (depending upon the laws of the country in question). Seamen who lack satisfactory evidence of compliance (vaccination certificate as described) may be denied shore liberty at ports in such countries.

A *successful* vaccination is defined as one that is followed by an immune reaction, a modified immune reaction, or a successful "take." An *unsuccessful vaccination* is one without any reaction. The reaction must be read by a physician, three to nine days following vaccination.

Smallpox usually develops in 9 to 16 days (usually 12 days) following exposure to the disease. The onset is sudden with violent chills, intense headache, severe pains in the back, vomiting, strong rapid pulse, and a quick rise of temperature to 103°F (39.4°C) or 104°F (40°C). On the third or fourth day, coarse red spots appear, usually first on the forehead and wrists, then spreading over the body. After four days the spots become blisters. Four days later, the blisters become filled with pus that has a foul odor. At this stage, the fever rises again, later dropping as crusts form over the pustules, which begin to dry up and scale off. If the pustules have been deep enough, permanent scars (pockmarks) are left on healing.

In smallpox, all skin lesions in an area of the body are similar in appearance, whereas in chickenpox they vary. (To differentiate smallpox from chickenpox, see p. 174.)

Medical advice by radio should be obtained at once if the patient appears to have smallpox, because of the severity of the disease and the possible spread to susceptible crewmen. Smallpox is an official quarantine disease. (See Appendix, p. 436.) Federal regulations require that the Master, as soon as practicable, notify the local health authority at the next port of call, station, or stop, and take such measures to prevent the spread of the disease as the local health authority directs.

Treatment

There is no specific treatment for smallpox. The patient should be isolated and careful isolation nursing techniques followed. (See p. 321.) A sponge bath should be given twice a day with warm water in which sodium bicarbonate has been dissolved (one teaspoonful to a pint of water). Zinc oxide paste should be applied to the eruptions. A warm alkaline aromatic solution should be used as a mouthwash and gargle. The eyelids should be cleansed with sterile isotonic eyewash solution, as often as they become encrusted.

An ice bag on the head may help relieve headache or an excessive rise in temperature. For severe pain, aspirin 600 mg with codeine sulfate 30 mg should be given by mouth every four hours as needed. Aspirin alone may control the pain and discomfort after four or five doses; *if additional doses of codeine sulfate appear needed, medical advice by radio should be obtained.* If aspirin is not well tolerated by the patient, acetaminophen 600 mg, with or without codeine sulfate, may be tried at the same dosage and frequency. To control constipation, milk of magnesia should be administered by mouth as necessary. Plenty of fluids should be given. The liquid diet should be changed to a soft diet as convalescence begins.

TETANUS (Lockjaw)

Incubation Period: 3 days to 21 days or longer (dependent on the character, location, and extent of the wound).

Isolation Period: Until there are no more symptoms.

Tetanus is an acute infectious disease caused by toxin produced by the bacillus *Clostridium tetani,* a bacterium that grows in the absence of air at the site of an injury. Tetanus bacteria are found in the intestines of horses, cows, and other animals; also in animal manure and soil into which it has been dropped. Spores formed by tetanus bacilli are hard to kill; they can stay alive for years in the soil of gardens and farms, on country roads and city streets, ready to be transplanted into humans or other favorable environment for growth.

Tetanus bacteria almost always enter the body through wounds. They are likely to thrive in deep puncture wounds, from a nail, splinter, bayonet, or pitchfork; or those in which the flesh is bruised, crushed, or torn; abrasions into which dirt or soil is forced; or wounds from foreign objects driven deeply into the flesh, as gunpowder, bullets, or pieces of clothing.

The wound may not show any change when the beginning symptoms of tetanus develop; in fact it may seem to be healed. The toxin produced by the bacilli is carried to the central nervous system to produce the symptoms of tetanus. Early symptoms are aches and pains in the muscles, a general feeling of fatigue, and some headache. Soon the characteristic signs appear: stiffness of the neck and jaw which gradually extends to the muscles of the back and the extremities. The forehead is wrinkled, the corners of the mouth are drawn upward, and the jaws are tightly closed (lockjaw). The body is held rigidly straight or arched so that the patient when placed on his back may touch the bed only with his head and heels.

There is such extreme nerve sensitivity that the slightest jar, touch, or noise may cause spasms of the back and other muscles with agonizing pain. The temperature varies; usually it is high during the state of convulsions, rising to 103°F (39.4°C).

Prevention

A person can be protected (immunized) against tetanus by injections of adsorbed tetanus toxoid. Every seaman should obtain his primary immunizations and booster shots as required. (See Tetanus Toxoid, Adsorbed, p. 292.)

Treatment

If the medical attendant suspects that a patient has tetanus, immediate medical advice by radio should be obtained on diagnosis and treatment. First the wound should be cleaned, all foreign matter removed with a sterilized forceps, and a sterile dressing applied. Expert medical care and the administration of tetanus immune human globulin should be provided in the quickest possible manner. Medical advice by radio should be gotten on the dosage of tetanus immune human globulin.

Treatment with an antibiotic is felt to have no definite beneficial effect on the course of tetanus. However, penicillin G procaine sterile suspension 600,000 units should be given intramuscularly every twelve hours, *if the patient is not allergic to it.* The penicillin will help to minimize or control the development of pneumonia or secondary invasive wound infections.

If a case of tetanus should develop aboard ship, prompt evacuation to an appropriate medical facility is indicated. The patient must have constant nursing care and utmost quiet is essential to prevent the exhausting painful spasms.

There will be need for treatment with sedative and muscle relaxant drugs such as diazepam by injection. *Medical advice should be obtained for specific drugs and dosage.* During a convulsion, the jaws should be separated with a pencil wrapped in gauze to keep the patient from biting his tongue. A liberal fluid diet should be given, if tolerated; otherwise, no attempt should be made to give fluids or food by mouth. (See Delirium and Convulsions, p. 204+.) *However, medical advice by radio should dictate the treatment aboard ship and during an evacuation to a medical facility.*

Federal regulations require that the Master, as soon as practicable, shall notify the local health authority at the next port of call, station, or stop that a tetanus case is aboard ship. The Master should take such measures as directed by the local health authority to prevent spread of the disease.

TYPHOID FEVER (Enteric Fever)

Incubation Period: Variable, 3 to 25 days (usually 7 to 14).

Isolation Period: Until declared free from infection by a physician.

Typhoid fever is an acute infectious bacterial disease caused by *Salmonella typhosa.* It can be acquired by eating or drinking food or water contaminated by infective human feces or urine. The disease occurs worldwide, especially among individuals and groups who do not practice good sanitation in restaurants, shops where food is displayed, town sewage systems, or local water supplies. Flies and other insects can spread the disease if they crawl on milk or other foods after contacting infective stools. Uncooked shellfish, especially raw oysters, often are a source of infection. There are people with active typhoid germs in their bodies, whose urine or stools can infect others, yet they show no signs of the disease. Individuals with careless habits of hygiene, who do not wash the hands thoroughly after using the toilet, may spread the infection, especially if they are food handlers.

The disease begins slowly with a chilly feeling, and diarrhea or constipation. The patient complains of a constant severe headache and possibly some nosebleeding. The pulse rate is slow. He feels tired, listless, exhausted from minor exertion, and loses his appetite. During the first few days, he has some fever, higher at night than in the morning. After a few more days, the temperature rises to 103° to 104°F (39.4° to 40°C), and remains high. His face indicates mental dullness. The tongue is heavily coated. The abdomen becomes painful, tender, distended, and full of gas.

Usually there is a reddish rash (rose spots) that appears on the abdomen first, from the seventh to the tenth day. Slightly raised and flattened, the spots can be felt with the finger; their rose color disappears on pressure. From one-twelfth to one-sixth of an inch in diameter the spots come in successive crops, disappearing in two or three days, perhaps leaving a brownish stain. The rash may extend over the entire body.

During the third week, there may be bleeding from the bowels, due to ulcers of the intestines. When an ulcer eats through a large artery or through the intestinal wall, hemorrhage or peritonitis occurs.

In mild cases, the patient begins to improve at the end of the second or the beginning of the third week. At times, the disease persists for six, eight, or more weeks before convalescence begins.

Treatment

For typhoid fever, ampicillin by mouth in a high dosage is indicated. *Medical advice by radio should be obtained to determine the dosage regimen.*

The patient should be kept quiet in bed and given a liquid or semisolid diet. He should drink plenty of water. The mouth and teeth should be cleaned daily. A bedpan and urinal should be used. A large catheter inserted in the rectum may enable gas to escape to provide abdominal relief. An ice bag applied to the head will relieve the headache. Cool sponge baths should be given once or twice a day when the temperature is above 103°F (39.4°C).

Isolation procedures should be followed. (See p. 321.) Excretions from the bowels and bladder can be flushed down the toilet, if the ship has a sewage treatment system or retention tank. Linens can be disinfected through routine commercial laundering procedures. Other equipment should be cleaned with hot soapy water, rinsed, and wiped with a good disinfectant.

TYPHUS FEVER (Epidemic Typhus Fever)

Incubation Period: 10 to 20 days.

Isolation Period: Until declared free from infection by a physician.

The term typhus fever is applied to several worldwide forms of the disease that are caused by various strains of rickettsiae (organisms smaller than bacteria but larger than filterable viruses). These diseases are transmitted to humans by body lice, ticks, fleas, mites, and possibly bedbugs.

A comparatively mild form of typhus is transmitted from the rat to man by the rat flea. This form does not occur in epidemics but breaks out where rats, fleas, and humans live together. In the past it was the only form of typhus prevalent in the United States when several thousand cases occurred annually. The current level is less than 100 scattered cases reported yearly. Symptoms are the same as those for louse-borne typhus.

In *epidemic typhus fever* which is the most severe form, the disease is transmitted directly from person to person by body lice. Uncleanliness and crowded living conditions favor the spread of body lice from one person to another. Epidemic typhus always had been the scourge of armies and populations in war-devastated areas. However, since World War II the combination of dusting with insecticides to kill the lice, successful vaccination, and the highly effective treatment with broad-spectrum antibiotics has brought control of the disease.

Louse-borne epidemic typhus is an acute infectious disease. In suspected cases it is important to look for lice on the patient's body or clothing and to find out if recently he had been in an area where typhus was prevalent. For a day or two before the actual onset, the patient may feel ill and have a slight headache, dizziness, and loss of appetite. The onset may be sudden and violent with chills, severe headache and backache, loss of appetite, a bruised feeling in the limbs, with sweating and great thirst. The fever starts high, 103°F to 105°F (39.4°C to 40.5°C) and returns to normal in two weeks.

A rash breaks out on the fourth to the seventh day. It appears first near the front of the armpits and the sides of the abdomen; then spreads gradually over the entire trunk and extremities. Usually it does not affect the face and neck. At first the rash resembles that of measles, of a color that varies from dirty pink to bright red. Usually it disappears when the skin is pressed down with the fingers. In most cases the rash darkens as the disease progresses and begins to fade as the fever drops.

Signs of general toxemia—intense headache, mental confusion or stupor, muscular twitching, a dry brown trembling tongue, and exhaustion—are common by the end of the first week. At the beginning of the second week, the headache may be replaced by violent delirium, at times accompanied by suicidal tendencies. Toward the end of the second week, the patient may fall into a stupor from exhaustion, and continue in this condition until either he dies, or the temperature drops suddenly and he begins to get well. The crisis as a rule occurs on the fourteenth to the eighteenth day. From then on, the mental condition clears, the appetite returns, and the patient convalesces.

Typhus sometimes is confused with typhoid fever; and before the rash appears, with meningitis, influenza, smallpox, and other severe infectious fevers. However, a history of louse infestation, the sudden and violent onset of the disease, the character and distribution of the skin eruption, and the characteristic duration of fever with termination by crisis, make up a distinctive set of signs and symptoms.

Typhus is an official quarantinable disease. Federal and international regulations require that the Master, as soon as practicable, notify the local health authority at the next port of call, station, or stop. To prevent the spread of the disease the Master should take such measures as the local health authority directs. (See Appendix, p. 436.)

Treatment

The patient with typhus fever must be isolated in a vermin-free room. There is no danger of infection from him if there are no lice or other insect vermin to transmit the disease to others. Measures should be begun to kill any lice present. (See p. 378.)

Epidemic typhus fever is a serious disease that requires careful nursing. Patients may be irrational, agitated, and injure themselves or attempt self-destruction. Close observation and restraints may be required. (For treatment of Delirium, see p. 205.)

For the infection, tetracycline hydrochloride 500 mg should be given by mouth every six hours. *As soon as typhus is suspected, medical advice by radio should be obtained, particularly as it relates to the duration of treatment with tetracycline hydrochloride.* Intravenous administration of tetracycline may be necessary, if the patient is uncooperative or vomiting. Before giving intravenous tetracycline hydrochloride, medical advice by radio should be gotten on the need to administer, plus planning to get it aboard ship, if not already available.

Sedatives may be required. Pentobarbital sodium 50 mg should be given by mouth every four hours during the day and phenobarbital 90 mg given by mouth at bedtime.

For pain, codeine sulfate 30 mg and/or aspirin 600 mg may be given by mouth every three to four hours, if recommended by radio. If aspirin is not well tolerated by the patient, acetaminophen may be tried at the same dosage and frequency.

To prevent constipation, milk of magnesia should be given daily as needed.

Because typhus fever exerts a severe strain on the patient's heart, he should be kept in bed until a doctor sees him. His strength should be conserved in every way possible, so a urine bottle and a bedpan must be used.

Typhus fever and typhoid fever should not be confused. These are two different diseases that have no connection with each other.

UNDULANT FEVER (Malta Fever, Brucellosis)

Incubation Period: Variable; usually 5 to 21 days, at times several months.

Isolation Period: Until convalescence begins.

Undulant fever is an infectious disease that strikes both humans and animals, but symptoms differ for both groups. It is caused by several bacterial strains of the genus *Brucella*. The disease is contracted mainly from milk and milk products obtained from dairy cattle with Bang's disease (infectious abortion).

At first fever may be the only symptom, but the patient will not appear acutely ill. Then there is a gradual onset with irritability, a general feeling of discomfort, weakness, headache, pains in joints, with sweating and chills. In early stages, it may be confused with rheumatic fever, tuberculosis, typhoid fever, or malaria. The temperature may rise to 104°F (40°C) and remain elevated for one to four weeks followed by a fall to normal for a few days, and then a relapse. The intermittent periods of fever, separated by days when symptoms are absent or reduced, may last for months, even years. It is these repeated waves (undulations) of fever with intervening remissions that give the disease its name.

As the disease becomes chronic, enlargement of the spleen and lymph nodes occurs. Other symptoms in the later stages include weight loss; constipation; loss of appetite; aches in head, back, joints, abdomen; insomnia; and mental depression.

Exact diagnosis will be dependent upon laboratory procedures, so a suspected case should be transferred to a doctor's care as soon as possible. The patient should be asked if he drank goat's milk, and any found aboard should be discarded. Cow's milk obtained in foreign ports should be boiled before use.

Treatment

Medical advice by radio should be obtained, especially on the medication. The patient should be isolated and the symptoms treated as they arise. All utensils used by the patient should be disinfected. Headache and pains in the joints and limbs may be relieved by aspirin 600 mg or codeine sulfate 30 mg, administered orally every four to six hours. Tetracycline hydrochloride 500 mg may be given orally every six hours for 21 days to treat the infection. For relapses this treatment may be repeated. Fluids should be forced.

WHOOPING COUGH (Pertussis)

Incubation Period: 7 to 14 days.

Isolation Period: 4 weeks after the "whoop" begins.

Whooping cough is a highly communicable bacterial disease of early childhood that is caused by the bacillus *Bordetella pertussis*. Although it is unlikely to occur among the crew, it should be suspected if the patient had been exposed to a case of whooping cough one to three weeks previously, develops a cold with a cough, the coughing causes vomiting, and the typical "whoop" develops. The disease is spread by the patient's coughing, sneezing, and through contact with anything he has touched.

The disease often starts like an ordinary cold with runny nose, sneezing, and coughing. Usually there is no fever. Then listlessness shows with a loss of appetite and a persistent hacking cough that occurs at night but gradually includes the daytime as well. This catarrhal stage lasts about two weeks. In the next stage the patient will exhibit chilling and a thick mucus forms in the respiratory tract with increased coughing in spasms. There will be coughing spells 6 to 12 or more times in rapid succession all in one breath. This forces air from the patient's lungs and his face turns bluish from the extreme effort and the lack of air. The patient catches his breath in a long noisy deep inhalation (the whoop). During these coughing spasms much mucus is brought up but the irritation continues. The combined coughing and gagging often leads to vomiting.

The characteristic whooping type of cough reaches its worst stage about two or three weeks after symptoms begin. Then the convalescent stage occurs when coughing reduces in frequency and severity and vomiting decreases.

Treatment

No specific treatment for whooping cough is known. *Medical advice by radio should be obtained, especially on the repeated dosage of codeine sulfate described below.*

The patient should be isolated. This will protect others from the disease and there will be less likelihood for the patient to develop serious complications as pneumonia, middle ear infection, chronic bronchitis, or encephalitis, among others. There always is the threat of suffocation, plus inhalation of vomitus while coughing. Use of suction may be lifesaving.

Antibiotic therapy has not been proven to be beneficial in uncomplicated whooping cough. Treatment should be symptomatic, with aspirin 600 mg and/or codeine sulfate 30 mg given by mouth every six hours, if needed. If aspirin is not well tolerated by the patient, acetaminophen may be tried at the same dosage. Phenobarbital 30 mg may be given every eight hours by mouth, if mild sedation is warranted. Between periods of nausea, it is important to maintain the patient's intake of fluids and soft foods.

YAWS

Incubation Period: 14 to 90 days; generally 21 to 42 days.

Isolation Period: Until a physician declares the patient free from infection.

Yaws is a highly infectious, nonvenereal, bacterial tropical disease caused by *Treponema pertenue,* a species of spirochete similar to that of syphilis. Although the disease strikes all age groups, it is mainly a disease of children. The organism that causes yaws can enter the body through a slight scratch or other break in the skin. The disease may be spread through physical contact with sores of infected patients or their clothes; or by insects contaminated by discharges from the patient's skin.

About a month after a person becomes infected, the first symptom appears as a pain-less inflamed raspberry-red elevation of the skin. This is called the "mother yaw" which enlarges and forms an ulcer in its center. The primary lesion may heal in a few weeks or persist for months if left untreated.

Two to eight weeks after the appearance of the "mother yaw," open oozing sores occur on the face, scalp, trunk, hands, or feet. The patient may show a slight rise in temperature, an overall unwell feeling, headache, and pains in bones and joints. There may be a fine peeling on the skin. Wartlike lesions that arise may run together in masses that project about a half inch above the surface of the skin. In two or three weeks as the discharges lessen, the lesions get smaller and finally heal. Ulcers on the soles of the feet may be very painful and resist healing. Skin lesions may disappear in untreated cases and recur after several years with disfiguring aftereffects to the nose and facial tissues—and deformities to the hands and feet.

Treatment

Medical advice on treating yaws should be obtained by radio. The patient should be isolated and the lesions covered with a simple dry dressing. Soiled dressings should be discarded carefully. (See p. 324.) The infection rarely is fatal and antibiotic treatment should be withheld if the patient will reach port soon. This will not jeopardize the general health of the patient. If treatment aboard ship is necessary, an intramuscular injection of 1.2 million units of penicillin G procaine should be administered at one time for an adult. Medical advice by radio should be sought for the dosage appropriate for an infected child.

YELLOW FEVER

Incubation Period: 2 to 6 days.

Isolation Period: About 6 days. Screen the patient's room, use a bednet, and spray quarters with insecticide that has a residual effect.

Yellow fever is a generalized often fatal viral disease that is transmitted by the bite of an infective female *Aedes aegypti* mosquito. In tropical forests several other species of mosquitoes are able to transmit it.

To spread the disease a female mosquito must feed on the blood of an infected person about two days prior to onset through the third or fourth day of the attack. The virus develops in the mosquito's blood for 9 to 12 days during which time she cannot transmit the disease. Thereafter for the rest of the female mosquito's life, she can give yellow fever to any nonimmunized person that she bites.

The disease has a swift severe onset with chills and high fever, intense headache, plus pains in the limbs and back. There is constipation, nausea, vomiting, and the patient is prostrated. The eyes are watery with the lining of the eyelids an inflamed red. The fever usually reaches a maximum 104°F (40°C) within 24 hours. Muscle pains get worse and the patient is restless, anxious, and sleepless. The tongue is bright red along the edges with a furred coating in the middle. As the disease progresses and the temperature increases, the pulse rate may show a drop from a rate of 120 per minute to 50–60 per minute.

In three to five days the fever may go down and there will be a lull of a few hours to a day or two. The patient feels better and may begin to recover. In severe cases, however, the lull is followed by a return of the vomiting and fever. Three characteristic clinical symptoms appear: (1) marked jaundice (yellow color) of the eyes and skin about the third day because the virus destroys liver cells; (2) albumin in the urine because the kidneys are affected; and (3) "coffee grounds vomitus" from blood that has seeped through mucous membranes into the stomach. Other signs of hemorrhage are tarry stools; nosebleed; blood from tongue, lips, and gums; and purple spots in the skin. The urine flow lessens and may contain blood. Interference with kidney and liver function can lead to delirium, convulsions, coma, and death in some cases. However, these symptoms may subside and the patient recover.

An attack of yellow fever may be very mild, with only slight backache, headache, and a fever that lasts about two days. It may be severe as just described, or there may be a sudden violent attack with rapid development of the worst symptoms. The death rate ranges from 10% to 85%. One attack provides immunity thereafter.

In combating yellow fever the emphasis must be on prevention rather than cure. Crews of ships bound for yellow fever areas should be immunized. One inoculation will produce immunity that will last for ten years. All countries in yellow fever areas require that persons entering ports of that country be immunized before entry. All measures described under malaria (see p. 178) for the control of mosquito-borne diseases should be carried out when the ship is in a port where yellow fever prevails.

Federal regulations require that the Master, as soon as practicable, shall notify local health authorities at the next port of call, station, or stop that he has a suspected case of yellow fever aboard. The Master shall take such measures to prevent the spread of the disease as the local health authorities direct.

If a case occurs aboard ship, the patient must be isolated in a screened room. Mosquito netting must be placed over his bunk for at least six days after onset. Nonimmune members of the crew who report mosquito bites should be isolated to the extent possible and inspected daily for symptoms.

The ship must be freed from mosquitoes by the use of residual insecticide sprays or other means of control (see p. 378).

Medical advice by radio should be obtained.

Treatment

There is no specific treatment for yellow fever. Complete bed rest in isolation in a mosquito-proof area with the best of nursing care are necessary. Forced fluids are needed to prevent dehydration; if continued vomiting prevents this, dextrose 5% and sodium chloride 0.45% injection should be administered intravenously. For fever, an ice cap or cold compresses should be applied to the head, and the body sponged with cool water. For restlessness, phenobarbital 30 mg should be given by mouth three times a day, and to induce sleep pentobarbital sodium 100 mg by mouth at bedtime.

For severe pain, aspirin 600 mg with codeine sulfate 30 mg should be given by mouth every four hours as needed. Aspirin alone may control the pain after four or five doses. If more than five doses of codeine sulfate appear to be needed, medical advice by radio should be obtained. If aspirin is not well tolerated by the patient, acetaminophen 600 mg, with or without codeine sulfate, may be tried at the same dosage and frequency. To relieve mouth dryness, cracked ice may be given.

When the patient is able to eat, he should have a diet high in carbohydrates (bread, toast, crackers, potatoes, cereals, and sweets) and low in protein and fats. However, cheese, milk, and eggs are permissible.

Chapter V

Treatment
of
Diseases

Section G

MUSCULOSKELETAL
DISEASES

ARTHRITIS

ARTHRITIS, WHICH IS AN INFLAMMATION of a joint, often causes pain, deformity, and disability. It occurs as a result of aging, infection, irritation around a joint, scurvy, allergy, gout, and rheumatic fever.

Treatment

Rest and aspirin are the basic treatments for the acute pain of arthritis. Aspirin 600 mg should be given by mouth every three to four hours as needed. If aspirin is not well tolerated by the patient, acetaminophen may be tried at the same dosage and frequency. In mild cases, an elastic bandage may ease the pain.

Mild heat applied to a painful arthritic joint may give relief. A heating pad carefully wrapped with towels may be applied to the joint. Also, a bath at usual bathing temperature is beneficial. If this is not possible, the limb can be immersed in warm water, or warm soaks can be applied. These treatments may be repeated two or three times a day if they are well tolerated by the patient.

In some types of acute inflammatory arthritis, it is common to have pain, redness of the skin over a joint, and the joint may be swollen and hot to the touch. When such a condition occurs, ice packs applied for 15 minutes at 2-hour intervals may give more relief than the heat applications.

Complete immobilization also is a standard form of treatment for an acutely painful joint. The joint should be wrapped in cotton and supported on each side. Also the joint can be immobilized by loosely binding it to a well-padded, wooden splint. As a joint improves, the patient may move it by himself and work as long as the movement does not cause pain.

An acutely painful joint, especially if accompanied by fever, calls for absolute rest in bed. The patient while awake should be encouraged frequently to drink water, tea, fruit juice, or similar fluids. This fluid intake should be two quarts or more in 24 hours. A nourishing diet should be provided.

In cases of acute arthritis, medical advice by radio should be obtained. The patient should be referred to a physician at the next port, especially if the joint is infected. An infected joint is a serious condition which may develop complications and result in disability.

GOUT

Gout is a disease caused by a breakdown in the body's ability to act on some protein food substances, especially compounds called *purines* that are found in meats and seafoods. This defect in body chemistry causes a buildup of excess uric acid in the blood because the kidneys cannot excrete it fast enough. Some of the excess uric acid salts may be deposited in joints and other body tissues. At times, the kidneys may be affected. About 95% of the patients are men, usually over 30 years of age. The disease also seems to be hereditary in certain families.

The major symptoms of gout are the same as those of severe arthritis. Usually an *acute attack* occurs without warning, often at night, with excruciating pain in the affected joint. Most often the big toe is affected, but the ankle, knee, or any other joint may be the site of the attack. The joint will become swollen, tender, warm, and the skin reddish in color. The patient may have a headache or fever, and may not be able to walk because of the pain. In fact the person might not be able to bear the weight of bedclothes on the affected area.

An acute attack of gouty arthritis may last three or more days after which it gradually subsides and the patient becomes symptom-free. At first, attacks may occur every four months or more and only one joint is affected. As the attacks occur more often, several joints may become involved. If treatment is neglected, the attacks occur more often and deposits of urates are made at the joints to form chalky nodules (*tophi*). These deposits can lead to permanent deformities at the joint.

Treatment

In cases of a suspected acute gout attack, acetaminophen may be administered by mouth at a dosage of 600 mg every four hours. If the patient has been treated previously for gout and has a supply of medication prescribed by his physician for either maintenance or acute treatment, he should continue to follow the prescribed regimen until further medical advice by radio can be obtained.

The patient should be kept in bed with the affected joint protected. Walking too soon after an attack may cause another attack to occur. Foods high in purines (as liver, kidney, sweetbreads, sardines, anchovies) should be eliminated from the patient's diet. While bedfast and thereafter, the patient should force fluids— drink about 8 or 10 glasses of water daily to help flush the uric acid from the kidneys. On reaching shore, the patient should seek medical advice. Under the care of a physician, a cooperative gout patient may use several drugs available today to help him lead a very comfortable life.

BACKACHE

Lower back pain is common and can result from many causes. An underlying anatomic problem often exists. Lower back pain may be from muscle strain or inflammation. It may result from stresses which tend to lower the resistance of the back and make it easier for the joints to become inflamed and painful, as in chronic lumbosacral strain. Pain can be referred to the back from a diseased internal organ. This may result from gallbladder and kidney disease, and ulcer of the stomach or intestine.

Other causes of a lower backache include simple fatigue, nervous exhaustion, bone disease, lead poisoning, hemorrhoids, varicocele, enlarged prostate, and acute infectious diseases. An ache in the lower back (lumbosacral) may be caused by a fall or jump from a height, a blow, twisting, lifting, prolonged standing, sustained stooping, sleeping on a sagging mattress, a heavy or pendulous abdomen, unnatural curvature of the spine, hip disease, or by certain foot conditions.

Pain in the upper back (thorax) may be associated with heart disease, inflammation of the lungs (pneumonia) or pleura (pleurisy), gallbladder disease or gallstones, or stomach trouble (indigestion or stomach ulcer). Careful questioning and examination of the patient will help to establish a diagnosis.

Treatment

For back pain, the symptoms should be treated. The back should be massaged with menthol ointment compound or a smiliar product, and a hot water bottle or electric heating pad applied. The patient should be instructed to rest in bed on a firm hard mattress if the pain is severe and there is a spasm of the back muscles. For pain, aspirin 600 mg should be given by mouth every three to four hours as needed. If aspirin is not well tolerated by the patient, acetaminophen may be tried at the same dosage and frequency. The patient should be referred to a physician.

BURSITIS

Bursitis is the inflammation of a bursa. A bursa is a small fluid-filled sac, which is located between moving parts of a joint and certain other areas of the body to reduce friction upon movement. When a bursa becomes inflamed from injury or infection, movement of the parts around the bursa is impeded by the pain and swelling. The walls of the sac may stick together (adhesions). Bursitis often resembles arthritis so closely that it may require an X-ray study and other examinations for differentiation.

Of the many bursae in the body, only the few most likely to become inflamed are discussed here. When the bursae around the shoulder joint are inflamed, they may cause pain and limit motion. Inflammation of the bursae in front of the kneecap may cause a red, painful swelling (housemaid's knee). Pain in the heel or elbow may be caused by inflammation of the bursae in these regions.

Treatment

Resting the bursitis area is important during the first few days of acute inflammation. Local heat should be applied, such as an electric heating pad. For pain, aspirin 600 mg should be given by mouth every three to four hours as needed. If aspirin is not well tolerated by the patient, acetaminophen may be tried at the same dosage and frequency. If pain is not controlled by aspirin or acetaminophen alone, codeine sulfate 30 mg by mouth may be given concurrently with either of these medications. To repeat the codeine sulfate, medical advice

by radio should be obtained.

After the first few days as pain begins to decrease, the patient should be instructed to try active movements, especially if the shoulder joint is involved. Exercising the disabled joint should be done even with a mild degree of discomfort. But exercise sufficient to produce a great deal of pain is not indicated and may be harmful.

MUSCULAR PAINS
(Soreness, Stiffness, Myositis, Muscular Rheumatism, Charleyhorse, Stone Bruise, Muscle Bruise, Myalgia, Lumbago)

Muscle ills are due to physical strain, overwork, direct violence, exposure, toxins of diseases, other poisons, and direct infection as with pus-forming organisms. Stiffness and painful swelling of the muscles are among the symptoms that characterize the disease *trichinosis* that is caused by eating undercooked or raw pork containing the parasitic roundworm trichina. (See p. 169.) Aching pains in the muscles, small of the back, and joints usually occur in the early stages of most acute communicable diseases.

Treatment

If symptoms are severe enough, the affected muscles should be rested. Heat should be applied and gentle massage given. Bowel regularity should be maintained. (See Constipation, p. 152.) For pain aspirin 600 mg should be given by mouth every three to four hours as needed. If aspirin is not well tolerated by the patient, acetaminophen may be tried at the same dosage and frequency. Medical advice by radio should be obtained for symptoms other than described above or if the symptoms are excessively severe.

NECK PAINS

Pain and stiffness in the back of the neck associated with other signs of general infection as head cold, headache, fever, nausea, and vomiting accompany the onset of several serious diseases. These diseases include cerebrospinal meningitis, poliomyelitis, and tetanus.

In the absence of signs of a generalized infection when only local symptoms are present, a stiff, painful neck usually is due to inflammation of muscles, ligaments, bursae, or nerves of the head and neck.

Wryneck

Wryneck (spasmodic torticollis) is caused by a spasm of muscles of the neck. Contraction of the affected sternomastoid muscle rotates the head to the opposite side and bends the neck to the side of the contracting muscle. A continuing spasm forces the head-neck into a sustained rotated posture. An intermittent spasm causes repeated, jerky movements of the head to one side. The cause of wryneck is unknown, and the condition usually persists for life. Wryneck is sometimes considered related to an underlying psychologic condition. Persons with suspected wryneck should see a physician on reaching port.

Treatment

Heat from hot compresses or a hot water bag should be applied to the painful area of the neck. The area should be massaged gently two or three times daily. For pain, aspirin 600 mg should be given by mouth every three to four hours as needed. If aspirin is not well tolerated by the patient, acetaminophen may be tried at the same dosage and frequency.

Chapter V

Treatment of Diseases

Section H

NEUROLOGICAL and MENTAL DISORDERS

ALCOHOLISM

The Alcohols

THE ALCOHOL FAMILY is made up of many chemical compounds. Ethyl alcohol, the best known member of the group, is the substance that makes fermented and distilled liquors intoxicating. Other alcohols commonly used are methyl alcohol, denatured alcohol, and isopropyl alcohol.

Methyl alcohol, also known as wood alcohol or methanol, is a fuel and has industrial usage as a solvent. Wood alcohol is a poison that *must not be taken internally* because it can cause blindness or death. (See p. 113.)

Isopropyl alcohol is used as a rubbing alcohol and often as a disinfectant. It is poisonous if taken internally.

Denatured alcohol is ethyl alcohol to which other materials (denaturants) have been added to make it unfit for drinking. *For external use only,* it can be applied to the skin as a disinfectant and cooling agent.

Ethyl alcohol (also known as grain alcohol or ethanol) is given special attention in this chapter because it is the active intoxicant of alcoholic beverages. It is a colorless, flammable liquid that is classed as a food because it supplies calories, but has no nutritive value. It acts as an irritant, antiseptic, drying agent, sedative, anesthetic, and hypnotic agent. It is a pain-reliever which, unlike other analgesics such as aspirin, reduces pain by putting the brain to sleep. Ethyl alcohol is considered a drug because of the profound effects it has on the central nervous system. Like barbiturates and narcotics, it causes addiction.

Definitions

Alcoholism is a progressive chronic illness characterized by habitual excessive drinking which interferes with an individual's mental and physical health, and all aspects of his personal life. It is one of four major health problems in the United States, and the number one drug abuse problem. When untreated, alcoholism becomes progressively worse and might eventually result in death.

Alcohol Abuse refers to the isolated or continued habit of drinking in excess of dietary and social customs.

Alcohol addiction is a physiological dependence upon alcohol and there is a pathological craving for it. The body tolerates increasing amounts of alcohol. Withdrawal symptoms begin when the amount of alcohol available to body tissue is reduced in one who is addicted to alcohol.

The *alcoholic* is a person who has the illness of alcoholism. The person has lost the ability to control voluntarily the amount of alcohol consumed. To satisfy his body's craving, the alcoholic's daily consumption grows steadily.

The *problem drinker* is a person who has not lost the ability to control his consumption of alcohol. The use of it, however, frequently harms his health, relations with his family and others, and his job performance.

Alcohol in the Body

Unlike other foods that require slow digestion, alcohol is absorbed rather quickly into the bloodstream, directly through the walls of the stomach and the small intestine. The blood carries it to all body tissues, including the brain where it has an immediate effect. The liver slowly changes the alcohol into carbon dioxide and water. A small amount of it goes out through the lungs, skin, and kidneys. If alcohol is consumed faster than the body can dispose of it, its concentration in the blood increases

and acts as a depressant or anesthetic on the central nervous system.

Initially alcohol seems to produce feelings of stimulation. Alcoholic "numbing" of the judgment center of the brain, which controls our inhibitions and restraints, makes one feel buoyant and exhilarated. Continued drinking on a given occasion increases the percentage of alcohol in the bloodstream. This causes depression of various areas of the brain that affect judgment, emotions, behavior, and physical well-being.

Alcohol abuse generally causes nutritional deficiences and acts as a direct poison. The combination of malnutrition and tissue injury may cause brain damage, heart disease, diabetes, ulcers, cirrhosis of the liver, and muscle weakness.

Sudden death may occur: (1) when the individual has ingested so much alcohol that the brain center which controls breathing and heart action is depressed to a fatal level; (2) when some other depressant drugs, as sleep preparations, are taken along with alcohol; (3) during an accident (one-half of all fatal traffic accidents involve the use of alcohol); or (4) as a result of suicide or murder (many self-inflicted deaths as well as homicides involve the use of alcohol).

Once the user is addicted to alcohol, withdrawal symptoms occur when it is not available to body cells. As alcohol addiction begins, these symptoms may be relatively mild and include hand tremors, anxiety, nausea, and sweating. As dependency increases, so does the severity of the withdrawal syndrome and the need for medical assistance to cope with it.

Management of Patients in Alcoholism

One should think of alcoholism as consisting of three separate conditions: *alcohol intoxication, acute withdrawal state,* and *chronic alcoholism.* Emphasis will be placed mainly on the first two conditions as chronic alcoholism does not lend itself to treatment aboard ship.

Acute Intoxication

Episodes of excessive drinking may be manifested as mild drunkenness or serious drunkenness (stupor or coma).

Mild Intoxication

Mild intoxication usually is self-limiting and its treatment requires only cessation of drinking alcoholic beverages and rest. The victims may show poor control of muscles, poor coordination, double vision, flushing of the face, bloodshot eyes, and vomiting. Behavior varies greatly. It is hard to predict what an intoxicated person will do next. He may cry bitterly, show unexplained happiness, change moods rapidly, or just pass out. Inappropriate behavior, as urinating in public and loud or abusive speech, also is common. Occasionally an intoxicated individual exhibits marked excitement and/or combativeness, and restraints may be needed.

It is impossible to walk off an excess of liquor. Alcohol is metabolized by the body at a constant rate regardless of activity. For example, if a man is needed at once on deck or in the engine room, black coffee, a cold shower, and fruit juice may make him feel better but his reaction time still will be slowed. He will be a wide-awake drunk instead of a sleepy one.

Treatment

For hangover symptoms of jitters, tremulousness, coated tongue, thirst, nausea, and severe headache, the patient should be allowed to remain as quiet as circumstances on the ship will allow. A single dose of an antacid may help the nausea. One or two cups of salted tomato juice and a glass of fruit juice, sipped slowly, also may help. Acetaminophen 600 mg may be given every four hours by mouth for headache, if it can be retained without vomiting.

Serious Intoxication

If a very large amount of an alcoholic beverage is taken in a short period of time, especially if taken on an empty stomach, serious acute intoxication may develop. Symptoms are drowsiness that might progress rapidly to coma; slow snoring breathing; blueness of the face, lips, and fingernail beds; involuntary passage of urine or feces; dilated pupils; and rapid weak pulse.

A suspected alcoholic stupor or coma represents a medical emergency. The signs or symptoms of drunken stupor are much like those of such conditions as insulin shock or diabetic coma (see p. 155 on these two opposite conditions that may cause unconsciousness in diabetics), stroke, poisoning with other drugs, some kinds of food poisoning, and brain injury. A person may have an odor of alcohol on the breath and yet be suffering primarily from a condition unrelated to drinking. The fruity or sweet odor of the breath in *diabetic coma* may be mistaken for alcohol. (Compare columns 6 and 13 of Table 2–2, p. 44.) In diabetic coma, the onset usually is slower than in alcoholism and rapid, deep breathing almost always is present. This distinction is very important because *diabetic coma requires prompt and aggressive treatment.* (See p. 154.) The head should be checked for signs of injury, the pupils of the eyes for equality of size and moderate dilation (in stroke the pupils usually are unequal and nonreactive to light) and the temperature. The patient's clothing or wallet should be checked for identification cards or tags (see p. 46) that might identify medical problems that need special medical attention, as allergies or diabetes. The individual's shipmates should be questioned on whether the patient might have taken drugs, had been injured, or overexposed to fumes or poisons. Personal effects should be checked for drugs if indicated.

Treatment

On the chance that the coma could be due to low blood sugar, as in an *insulin reaction*, an intravenous infusion of dextrose 5% and sodium chloride 0.45% solution should be started while waiting for medical advice by radio. The volume of the IV infusion to be given should be checked among other treatment considerations. If an insulin reaction is suspected and there is no one aboard ship who is trained to administer intravenous infusions, glucagon 1 mg should be given intramuscularly while waiting for medical advice by radio.

If the patient in an alcoholic stupor has not vomited and can be kept awake long enough to swallow, he should be given a large quantity of warm water (500 ml or more) to stimulate vomiting. Tickling the back of the patient's throat with a blunt object such as a spoon will stimulate gagging. The patient's head should be held over a basin in such a position that the person will not aspirate and choke on the vomited matter or have it interfere with breathing. Strong coffee should be given and an ampul of aromatic ammonia crushed and administered by inhalation every 15 minutes as needed. Because warmth is essential, the patient should be put to bed and covered.

The patient's airway should be kept clear by placing him on his side; then on alternate sides frequently to avoid accumulation of secretions. The unconscious patient should not be allowed to sleep on his back, because a deepening of stupor or coma may cause choking on the tongue or vomitus. The condition of the patient should be observed often.

Acute Withdrawal Toxic State

After a prolonged period of heavy drinking, acute withdrawal symptoms usually begin 24 to 48 hours after the intake of alcohol has stopped.

A continuing series of symptoms accompany withdrawal following any cessation of intake of alcohol. They only may be mild as tremor, weakness, sweating, increased reflexes, and gastric upset. However, they may become severe in nature such as severe shaking, convulsions, and progress to the severe alcohol withdrawal syndrome, delirium tremens (DTs).

Impending Delirium Tremens (DTs)

Before a case of DTs is fully developed, often there are a few days of worsening withdrawal symptoms—a warning that DTs are coming. Symptoms may include in various combinations, sweating, flushing, insomnia, elevated temperatures, and odd behavior, which may stop briefly when the victim's attention is directed toward it. Recognition of these symptoms as warnings, followed by prompt treatment, often will prevent a deterioration of the condition and full-blown delirium tremens. *The alcoholic's withdrawal state is a life-threatening emergency.* The value of early recognition and treatment cannot be overemphasized.

Treatment

General supportive care is vital. Because of the risk of convulsions (seizures), the pa-

tient must be observed frequently. He should be protected from extreme heat or cold. Liberal quantities of water, sweetened fruit juice for glucose depletion, and well-salted tomato juice should be offered frequently.

The patient's pulse, blood pressure, and temperature should be taken every four hours. Efforts should be made to allay the patient's fears with reassurance and a careful explanation of procedures. Nightmares, illusions, and hallucinations often are reduced if the patient is placed in a well-lighted room, and in the presence of others rather than in isolation and restraints. If restraints are needed to prevent the patient from hurting himself or others, they should be applied carefully. Thick padding should be placed around the wrists and ankles of the patient and the extremities tied to the side of the bunk. A sheet may be wrapped over the chest, under the arms, and fastened below the bunk. The patient in restraints should be watched carefully to avoid injury.

In treating impending or actual DTs, it is necessary to use medications that will be adequate substitutes to satisfy the body's craving for alcohol. Two such drugs are paraldehyde and diazepam. The first drug of choice is paraldehyde given orally. When withdrawal symptoms are observed, prompt treatment with paraldehyde by mouth should be initiated. It stops the minor symptoms and may be relied upon to prevent the occurrence of the severe withdrawal symptoms of delirium tremens.

Aluminum hydroxide with magnesium hydroxide oral suspension 15 to 30 ml, given just prior to administering the paraldehyde, should help the patient to retain it. Giving the paraldehyde in iced fruit juice may make it more palatable to the patient.

For an adult under 45 years of age paraldehyde 10 ml by mouth should be given every four hours during the first 24 hours, every six hours during the next 24 hours, and finally, single doses at bedtime for two days. *Patients 45 years and over* should receive the paraldehyde every six hours during the first 24 hours.

During the first 24 hours, if there is difficulty in rousing the patient, the next dose of paraldehyde should be withheld and medical advice by radio obtained.

If the patient has *not* completely recovered after 24 hours of treatment with paraldehyde, one should assume that there are complications. The schedule of paraldehyde dosage for the first day's treatment should be continued while an intensive revaluation is initiated.

Diazepam may be used in place of paraldehyde. This drug should be considered if there is a chance that alcohol might be present in the patient's body when the withdrawal symptoms become evident within several hours after the last drink.

Initially, diazepam 10 mg should be given intramuscularly. An intramuscular dose may be repeated in two to four hours, if necessary. Then 5 mg should be given by mouth every four hours, as long as needed. If the patient is restless and cannot sleep, pentobarbital sodium 100 mg may be given by mouth once at bedtime.

Alcoholic Convulsive State (Rum Fits)

Treatment

One of the primary objectives in treating an alcoholic convulsion (seizure) is to prevent the patient from injuring himself or others. He should be placed on his side, tight clothing loosened, and air passages kept open. It is important to see that the patient does not inhale vomitus or fluids into the lungs. To prevent the patient from biting or swallowing his tongue, a gauze-covered tongue depressor should be inserted carefully between the teeth, with the tongue pulled forward, under the tongue depressor. To interrupt a convulsion, diazepam 10 mg should be given carefully and slowly intravenously. If this is not practicable, it should be administered intramuscularly. Medical advice by radio must be sought at once. The treatment outlined for impending DTs (see p. 203) may be followed.

Chronic Alcoholism

The chronic alcoholic usually has a dependence on alcohol. He uses alcohol in larger quantities and at inappropriate times when compared with the people around him. The need or craving for alcoholic drinks may be so strong that he will drink unusual things as shaving lotion or paint remover.

There are varying degrees and patterns of chronic alcoholism. Some alcoholics go on periodic sprees, but between these they drink little or no alcohol. Others drink regularly day by day for long periods. The amount of trouble an alcoholic may cause on a ship varies. If the spree drinker imbibes only when ashore between trips, he may remain an effective seaman. On the other hand, if he has a binge while standing watch, it will be a problem to everyone. Similarly not everyone who drinks regularly, even in large amounts, shows serious signs of drunkenness.

Treatment

Aboard ship all a medical attendant can do for chronic alcoholism is to treat a particular complication as it arises. For serious complications, the patient should be referred for shore care as soon as a convenient port is reached. If the patient is extremely agitated or suicidal, he should be watched carefully.

Regular habits of hygiene, work, eating, recreation, and rest should be encouraged. Chapters of *Alcoholics Anonymous*, found in U.S. ports, provide programs to help these patients.

Convulsions (Seizures)

A convulsion is an involuntary, violent spasmodic contraction, or series of contractions of many muscles. There may be prolonged muscular rigidity or alternating paroxysms and relaxations (jerking movements). Either type may be alarming to watch. A convulsion, like a chill, fever, pain, or constipation, is not a disease but an indication that something is wrong

Convulsions may be part of such diseases and conditions as stroke, chronic alcoholism, poisoning from strychnine and lead, chronic kidney disease, epilepsy, injury (especially fracture of the skull), malaria, neurotic disease, and tetanus.

Treatment

During the seizure, treatment is largely symptomatic and should be aimed at protecting the patient from harming himself. (See Epilepsy, p. 212.) After the convulsion, a careful search should be made for the associated cause, if this is not already known. The patient should be questioned carefully to uncover any leads that may point to any of the diseases or conditions stated previously. If the patient seems to be quite ill or has repeated convulsions, medical advice by radio should be sought.

Delirium

Delirium usually is a temporary mental disturbance characterized by confusion, excitement, seeing imaginary sights or hearing voices (hallucinations), and by various degrees of physical restlessness. Delirium may take the form of a fairly quiet restlessness wherein the patient fidgets and mutters to himself for hours on end; or it may take the form of wild, noisy, and violent actions.

Delirium may be due to mental disease; to poisons that accumulate from certain systemic infections as kidney diseases; or to drug and poison intoxication caused by a variety of agents as lead, carbon monoxide, narcotics, and some medications. Delirium may appear in chronic alcoholism or it may accompany exhaustion, chronic illness, or high fever, and follow severe injury. Delirium may be induced by exposure to a change of environment or inability to adapt to new experiences.

The characteristics of the *low muttering type of delirium* are constant or occasionally disconnected and irrational speech, restless impulses, disturbing dreams, attacks of weeping or excitement, impaired mental and muscular power, involuntary urination and defecation, and frequently, plucking at the bedclothes. When restlessness is present, the patient continually tries to get out of bed, and not infrequently attempts to escape. This type of delirium may be present in all acute infectious fevers, especially in typhoid fever.

In the *violent type of delirium* usually associated with toxic conditions due to uremia, alcoholism, and poisoning by drugs, there is wild maniacal excitement. At different times, the patient may be noisy or quiet, violent or calm. He is difficult to control always and usually is insensible to his surroundings. His speech is rapid and incoherent or irrelevant, eyes open and staring with pupils usually dilated, and face flushed. A homicidal mania may develop suddenly.

Treatment

A delirious patient never should be left unattended. Even when the symptoms appear mild, constant observation is required. Only liquid or injectable medicines should be given. Food or nourishment should be taken slowly at regular intervals. If urination is voluntary, one should make sure that it takes place regularly. If urination does not occur at least once in every eight hours, the fact should be reported promptly in medical consultation by radio. An accurate record should be kept of the patient's condition. Other patients should be prevented from coming near him. Nothing with which the patient might injure himself or others should be accessible to him. The medical attendant always should have at hand the means to restrain a delirious patient quickly.

Treatment should be symptomatic. The case should be reviewed carefully to determine the cause of the delirium. Medical advice by radio should be obtained.

Frequently patients in delirium are so disoriented (unaware of the environment) that they neither feel hunger nor know what to do with food when it is offered to them. This type of individual must be fed and if necessary coaxed to eat. The patient may refuse food entirely and all efforts to encourage eating may fail. If able and willing to feed himself, the food should be cut before giving the tray to him. *Never put knives, forks, and glassware on a mentally disturbed patient's tray.* If possible, food should be served on a paper plate, beverages in a paper cup, and the patient should eat with a spoon.

Patients who are irrational often are not aware of the urge to urinate or to have a bowel movement, so they may soil the bunk. Bedsores develop quickly if the patient is allowed to lie in a wet bunk. If the patient passes only a small amount of dark yellow and odorous urine, he should consume more liquids. If no urine is passed and the bladder is distended, measures should be tried to get the patient to urinate. (See p. 325.)

It may be necessary to restrain the patient. One should try to calm him and explain in simple terms what is going on. Effort should be made repeatedly to reassure him. He never should be left alone, even for a moment. Attendants should be changed as infrequently as possible and only essential visitors should be permitted. Precautions to prevent suicide should be observed. (See Mental Depression, p. 215.) The room should be kept evenly lighted at all times because delirium usually is worse in the dark or in twilight. The source of light should be placed to avoid casting strange shadows.

Medication may be helpful but it must be carefully used. Sedation at times will increase disorientation and excitement. (See Intoxication, p. 202 and DTs, p. 203.)

If both soothing actions and medication fail to quiet the patient, mechanical restraint may have to be used as a last resort. Then minimal force should be applied.

Mechanical restraints may be improvised from bedsheets. In mild cases a top sheet, well-pinned under the mattress at the sides and foot of the bed, will help to control the patient and keep him from leaving his bunk. If this is insufficient, one sheet may be folded or rolled and placed across the patient's legs and fastened to the side rails of the bunk, or beneath the mattress, or to the mattress itself. One or two sheets should be placed across the patient's shoulders. These sheets should be arranged to prevent the patient's leaving the bunk without tying him down too tightly, restricting his circulation, interfering with his respiration, or in any other way injuring him.

A *sideboard* is a simple form of restraint that is the length of the bunk and 18 inches wide. The board should be padded with blankets and secured on the side of the bunk at the head and foot. Its chief value is to prevent the patient from falling out of the bunk.

Leather or cloth cuffs applied to the wrists and ankles may be necessary. The wrists and ankles should be padded with cotton or other soft material before these restraints are applied. The wrists and ankles should be secured to the sides of the bunk in a comfortable position. Care should be taken that the restraints are not so tight they will interfere with circulation. Restraints should be released periodically and the extremities rubbed to stimulate circulation.

A *mummy restraint* sometimes is used to control the entire body while the patient is being transported from one place to another, or while he is receiving a treatment about the head or face. Armpits and groins should be padded with cotton. Except for the head, the body should be wrapped mummy-fashion in a sheet, blanket, or large piece of canvas. Because it immobilizes the entire body, the mummy restraint should be applied only briefly and removed when it is not essential. Other forms of restraint might be used, if necessary.

It should be remembered that mechanical restraints are dangerous, tend to antagonize or irritate the patient, and should be used only when absolutely necessary. These should be applied only with the permission of the Master of the ship. Restraining appliances should not be placed within reach of the patient's fingers or teeth, or where they might cause pressure or discomfort. These devices should not interfere with the patient's breathing. Constant supervision of restrained patients must be maintained.

DRUG ADDICTION

Definitions

Drug Addiction may be defined as the compulsive use of habit-forming drugs.

Drug Dependence is a state of psychological or physical need to continue to use a drug. Certain drugs cause only a psychological dependence, as amphetamines. Other drugs such as narcotics (heroin, codeine, methadone) and barbiturates cause both psychological and physical dependence.

Habituation is the psychological desire to repeat the use of a drug intermittently or continuously for emotional reasons.

Introduction

When drug dependence occurs, both tolerance and withdrawal symptoms can be present. As a person develops tolerance, he requires a larger and larger amount of the drug to produce the same effect. When the use of the addicting drug is stopped abruptly, withdrawal symptoms occur. These vary widely depending on the drug.

Not all character changes related to drug abuse appear detrimental, at least in the initial stages. For example, while using amphetamine a usually bored sleepy person may be more alert and thereby improve his performance. A nervous, high-strung individual on barbiturates may be more cooperative and easier to manage. What must be looked for are not merely changes for the worse, but any sudden changes in behavioral expressions which become routine for an individual. The causal factor may be drug abuse.

Signs which may suggest drug abuse include sudden and dramatic changes in discipline and job performance. Drug abusers also may display unusual degrees of activity or inactivity, and sudden and irrational flare-ups involving strong emotion or temper. Significant changes for the worse in personal appearance may be a cause for concern. Often a drug abuser becomes indifferent to his appearance.

There are other, more specific signs that should arouse suspicions, especially if more than one is exhibited by a single person. Among them are furtive behavior about actions and possessions (fear of discovery); sunglasses worn at inappropriate times and places (to hide dilated or constricted pupils); and long-sleeve garments worn constantly, even on hot days, to hide needlemarks.

Prevention

This section is directed primarily toward emergency first aid for drug addiction and abuse that might occur at sea. However, it is important to stress that steps can be taken long before the emergency occurs to lessen the likelihood of drug abuse ever occurring in the first place.

It is known that heavy drug use frequently stems from boredom and lack of absorbing leisure-time activities. Thus, the Master can take precautions to provide opportunities aboard ship as alternatives to boredom. Among these are group and individual activities that contribute to potential skills and the social and emotional growth of the crew. Also, these may include a variety of recreational and learning experiences that might be provided for crew members during off duty hours. A good ship's library, activities in arts and crafts, or a small woodworking room can be helpful. Film

programs including psychologically oriented films and hobby films, programmed learning courses, language lessons, travel lore, contests, bingo, basic astronomy, expertly guided group discussions, and meditation sessions can contribute toward creating a more lively and involving climate aboard ship.

Drugs of Abuse Classified

Drugs of abuse fall into five main classes: narcotics, depressants, stimulants, hallucinogens, and solvents (as glue).

Narcotics

The drug abuser deeply under the influence of narcotics usually appears lethargic, drowsy, or displays symptoms of deep intoxication. Often the pupils of the eyes are constricted and fail to respond to light.

Some individuals may drink paregoric or cough medicines containing narcotics. The medicinal odor of these preparations often is detectable on the breath. Other narcotic abusers inhale narcotic drugs such as heroin in powder form. Sometimes, traces of this white powder can be seen around the nostrils. Constant inhaling of narcotic drugs makes nostrils red and raw.

For maximal effect narcotics usually are injected directly into a vein. The most common site of this injection is the inner surface of the arm at the elbow. After repeated injections, scar tissue (tracks) develops along the course of such veins. Because of the easy identification of these marks narcotic abusers usually wear long sleeves at odd times. Females sometimes use makeup to cover marks and some males get tattooed at injection sites. When drugs are injected under unsterile conditions, there is a hazard of transmitting hepatitis, malaria and other tropical diseases, and blood poisoning.

The narcotic abuser may be detected by noting the presence of the equipment ("works" or "outfit") used in injecting narcotics. Because anyone injecting drugs must keep the equipment handy, it may be found on his person, or hidden nearby in a locker, washroom, or any place where temporary privacy may be found. The characteristic instruments and accessories consist of a bent spoon or bottle cap, a small ball of cotton, syringe or eyedropper, and a hypodermic needle. All are used in the injection process.

The small ball of cotton usually is kept after use because it retains a small amount of the narcotic that can be extracted, if the abuser is unable to obtain additional drugs. The bent spoon or bottle cap used to heat the narcotic is easily identifiable because it becomes blackened during the heating process.

Treatment of Acute Narcotic Intoxication

Medical advice by radio should be obtained. With all narcotics, including opium, heroin, meperidine, morphine, methadone, and hydromorphone, overdosage produces similar clinical states—depressed respiration being one of the most critical. Severely depressed respiration requires manual or mechanical artificial respiration. (See p. 115.) Even mildly depressed respiration calls for administration of naloxone, a narcotic antagonist.

Naloxone is now the drug of choice for treating acute narcotic intoxication. It is a pure narcotic antagonist with no respiratory depressant effects. (See naloxone hydrochloride injection, p. 284, and the package insert on dosage and frequency.)

Heroin, morphine, and similarly abused short-acting narcotics have a 6 to 12 hour duration of action and the antagonist must be readministered during this time. It is crucial to remember that methadone has a much longer duration of action, 24 to 72 hours. Therefore, a patient with acute methadone intoxication must be observed carefully and treated again as needed with naloxone, every two or three hours for up to three days.

Withdrawal Syndrome

A person with light physical dependence may show few genuine symptoms of withdrawal. Complaints may result from anxiety or from a bid for additional medication. Adolescent addicts rarely show significant evidences of withdrawal. Heavy narcotic addiction may require gradual detoxification, which is not feasible aboard ship. The withdrawal syndrome develops about eight to twelve hours after the last dose. During the first 12 to 24 hours of withdrawal, it may be necessary to administer a low dose of a short-acting nar-

cotic, as 10 mg morphine sulfate intramuscularly once or twice to prevent severe withdrawal symptoms.

Depressants (Including Barbiturates)

Acute intoxication with barbiturates and other central nervous system (CNS) depressants, including chlordiazepoxide, diazepam, glutethimide, and ethchlorvynol resembles acute alcoholic intoxication except that there is no odor of alcohol on the breath. Persons taking depressants may stagger or stumble. The depressant abuser frequently falls into a deep sleep. In general, he lacks interest in activity, is drowsy, and may appear to be disoriented.

Treatment

The treatment for depressants consists mainly of supporting the cardiovascular and respiratory functions. Maintenance of the airway is of crucial importance. Stimulant drugs generally are not effective in restoring normal respiration. Oxygen and intravenous fluids may be needed. If the patient is conscious, gastric lavage will be helpful in removing any unabsorbed drug from the stomach. (See p. 110 on poisoning by central nervous system depressants.) The effects of glutethimide intoxication may persist or recur for several days, despite aggressive management.

Management of Barbiturate Withdrawal Syndrome

When a patient has been diagnosed as physically dependent on a depressant drug of the barbiturate type, the immediate concern is the management of the withdrawal syndrome. This syndrome is very similar to but more life-threatening than narcotic drug withdrawal because of the danger of potentially fatal convulsions. Other serious complications of abrupt withdrawal from barbiturates include hallucinations, delirium, and coma. Close supervision is essential. Medical advice by radio should be obtained.

Aboard ship, probably the optimum that can be achieved is to withdraw gradually the drug of addiction. Dependence on depressants of the barbiturate type is usually a chronic relapsing disorder. Long term treatment is best in a shore-based facility where continued supportive counseling can be maintained with the patient.

Unlike withdrawal from other narcotics, withdrawal from barbiturates and other hypnotic drugs may be associated with cardiovascular collapse and death. Even when withdrawal symptoms are mild, they may signal impending convulsions.

Treatment

Gradual reduction of the dosage of the drug over a period as long as two weeks may be the only pharmacologic treatment needed for patients mildly or moderately addicted to barbituates.

Convulsions, delirium, and high fever should be treated as emergencies. The patient should be given 200 mg of pentobarbital sodium injection intramuscularly at once. Additional doses of 100 mg may be given at hourly intervals until he is asleep, and then as required to maintain sleep for 8 to 12 hours. *Before giving the additional doses, medical advise by radio should be obtained for addiction to barbiturates.*

Stimulants

The behavior of the abuser of stimulants, as amphetamine and related drugs, is characterized by excessive activity. The stimulant abuser is irritable, argumentative, appears extremely nervous, and has difficulty sitting still. In some cases the pupils of the eyes will be dilated even in a bright lighted place.

Amphetamine has a drying effect on the mucous membranes of the mouth and nose with resultant bad breath that has a specific odor. Because of dryness in the mouth, the amphetamine abuser licks his lips to keep them moist. This often results in chapped and reddened lips, which in severe cases may be cracked and raw. Dryness of the mucous membrane in the nose causes the abuser to rub and scratch his nose vigorously and frequently to relieve the itching sensation.

Other observable effects include incessant talking and chain-smoking. The person abusing stimulant drugs often goes for long periods of time without sleeping or eating and usually cannot resist letting others know about his fasting and sleeplessness.

Treatment

The treatment of an overdose from an amphetamine-type stimulant is complex, so medical advice always should be sought by radio. It is important to try to determine if the patient has been abusing barbiturates along with stimulants, as this would influence the treatment required.

Life-threatening toxic doses of stimulants may cause abnormally high body temperatures above 102°F (38.8°C). This should be treated by immersion of the patient's body in cool water. A patient who has ingested an overdose *orally* should be forced to vomit or gastric lavage should be instituted (see p. 110) to remove any unabsorbed drug.

Sedation as diazepam 10 mg may be required orally or by injection; *but this should be administered only upon medical advice by radio.*

Hallucinogens

It is unlikely that persons who use hallucinogenic drugs such as LSD will do so while at work or in other than a recreational time period. Such drugs usually are used in a group situation under special conditions designed to enhance their effect. Persons under the influence of hallucinogens usually sit or recline quietly in a dream or trance-like state. However, the effect of such drugs is not always joyful. On occasion users become fearful and experience a degree of terror which may cause them to attempt to escape from the group or engage in violent action.

Hallucinogenic drugs usually are taken orally. They are found as tablets, capsules, or liquids. Users put drops of the liquid into beverages, on sugar cubes, crackers, or even small paper wads or cloth. It is important to remember that the effects of LSD may recur days or even months after the drug has been taken.

Treatment

Although LSD (lysergic acid diethylamide) is the most commonly used and widely known hallucinogen, others seen frequently include mescaline (the active ingredient of the peyote cactus which originates in Mexico) and psilo-

Table 5–1.   **Narcotics and Other Drugs Commonly Abused—Identification Guide**

Narcotic (Drug) and Slang Name	Physical Symptoms	Look for	Dangers
AMPHETAMINES AND METHAMPHETAMINE (Bennies, Pep Pills, Dexies, Copilots, Wake-ups, Lid Poppers, Hearts, Uppers)	Aggressive behavior, giggling, silliness, rapid speech, confused thinking, no appetite, extreme fatigue, dry mouth, bad breath, shakiness, dilated pupils, sweating, licks lips, rubs and scratches nose excessively, chain smoking, extreme restlessness, irritability, violence, feeling of persecution, abcesses	Pills, tablets, or capsules, of varying colors, chain smoking, syringes	Hallucinations, death from overdose, speeds rate of heart-beat, may cause permanent heart damage or heart attacks loss of weight, addiction, mental derangement, suicidal depression may accompany withdrawal
BARBITURATES (Barbs, Blue Devils, Goof Balls, Candy, Yellow Jackets, Phennies, Peanuts, Blue Heavens, Downers, Red Birds)	Drowsiness, stupor, dullness, slurred speech, drunk appearance, vomiting, sluggish, gloomy, staggers, quarrelsome	Tablets or capsules of varying colors, syringes	Unconsciousness, coma, death from overdose, physiological addiction, convulsions, or death from abrupt withdrawal
BARBITURATE-LIKE DRUGS **Chloral Hydrate,** (Knock-Out Drops, Joy Juice, Peter, Micky Finn (mixed with alcohol))	Similar to Barbiturates	Capsules (blue and white, rust, and red), and syrup	Gastric distress is common. Circulatory collapse may occur.
Benzodiazepines Chlordiazepoxide, Diazepam, Flurazepam and others (Downers)	Similar to Barbiturates	Librium capsules (Green & Black)—Valium Tablets (white 2mg, yellow 5 mg blue 10 mg)—Dalmane capsules (red & yellow)—Other sizes or brands may appear differerently—	
Methaqualone (Luds, Sopors, Qs, the Lovedrug, Quads)	Similar to Barbiturates—also vomiting, hypotension, pulmonary edema	Tablets (White, Green, Pink); Capsules (Light and Dark Blue; Light Green and Dark Green)	Especially dangerous in combination with alcohol
COCAINE (Leaf, Snow, Speedballs)	Muscular twitching, convulsive movements, strong swings of moods, exhilaration, hallucinations, dilated pupils	White odorless powder	Convulsions, death from overdose, feelings of persecution, psychic dependence
HALLUCINOGENS LSD (Acid, Sugar, Big D, Cubes, Trips) DMT (Businessman's High) STP	Severe hallucinations, feelings of detachment, incoherent speech, cold sweaty hands and feet, vomiting, laughing, crying, exhilaration or depression, suicidal or homicidal tendencies, chills, shivering, irregular breathing	Cube sugar with discoloration in center, strong body odor, small tube of liquid	LSD causes suicidal tendencies, unpredictable behavior, brain damage from chronic usage, hallucinations, panic, accidental death, persecution feelings
MARIJUANA (Pot, Grass, Reefers, Locoweed, Mary Jane, Hashish, Tea, Gage, Joints, Sticks, Weed, Muggles, Mooters, Indian Hay, Mu, Griffo, Mohasky, Gigglesmoke, Jive)	Sleepiness, talkative, hilarious mood, enlarged pupils, lack of coordination, craving for sweets, erratic behavior, loss of memory, distortions of time and space, intellectual deterioration	Strong odor of burnt leaves, or rope with characteristic sweetish odor, small seeds in pocket lining, cigarette paper, discolored fingers, pipes	Inducement to take stronger narcotics, anti-social behavior

Table 5-1. **Narcotics and Other Drugs Commonly Abused—Identification Guide** (Continued)

Narcotic (Drug) and Slang Name	Physical Symptoms	Look for	Dangers
NARCOTICS **Heroin** (H, Horse, Scat, Junk, Snow, Stuff, Harry, Joy Powder) **Morphine** (White Stuff, Miss Emma, M, Dreamer)	Stupor, drowsiness, needle marks on body, watery eyes, loss of appetite, bloodstain on shirt sleeve, "on the nod," constricted (small) pupils that do not respond to light, inattentive, slow pulse and respiration	Needle or hypodermic syringe, cotton, tourniquet (string, rope or belt), burnt bottle caps or spoons, glassine envelopes, traces of white powder around nostrils from sniffing or inflamed membranes in nostrils, small capsules containing white powdered substance	Death from overdose, mental deterioration, brain, heart, and liver damage, embolisms, infections from use of dirty needles and equipment
Cough Medicine that contains **Codeine Sulfate** or **Opium** (Schoolboy) Paregoric	From **large doses:** drunk appearance, lack of coordination confusion, excessive itching. **Small doses** exhibit little effect.	Empty bottles of cough medicine or paregoric	Causes addiction
THE VOLATILE SOLVENTS (Model Airplane Glue, Lighter Fluid, Gasoline, Paint Thinner, Many Aerosols, Household and Commercial Fluids)	Violence, drunk appearance dreamy or blank expression, odor of glue or other solvents on breath, excessive nasal secretion, watering of eyes, poor muscular control, delirium, hallucinations	Tubes of glue, glue smears paper or plastic bags, handkerchiefs, empty aerosol cans, lighter fluid containers, gasoline cans	Damage to lung—brain—liver, death from suffocation or choking, anemia

Source: National Institute on Drug Abuse, Public Health Service, U.S. Department of Health, Education, and Welfare

cybin (the active ingredient of a variety of Mexican mushroom). Two synthetic substances, DMT (dimethyltryptamine) and DOM (dimethoxyamphetamine), also known as STP (implying Serenity, Tranquility, and Peace) are abused frequently. When taken in sufficient dosage, any of these substances will produce a temporary state of insanity or "a trip" with illusions (incorrect perception of objects) and hallucinations (a sensory perception without objective stimulus, such as seeing, hearing, feeling, tasting, or smelling something that does not exist). Other abnormal experiences with hallucinogens include a feeling of great excitement and insight, nausea, sweating, tremors, and uncoordination.

Most experienced drug users can control these abnormal feelings and enjoy them. The bad trip that requires skilled help occurs when the user, often inexperienced, suffers a loss of control and is overwhelmed with anxiety, terrifying sights and sounds, delusions of persecution, extreme depression and the belief that he is going out of his mind.

The treatment for a bad trip is basically the talk-down technique. This involves nonmoralizing comforting support from an experienced individual aided by the limitation of external stimuli and having the patient lie down to relax in a quiet darkened area. A tranquilizer such as 10 mg of diazepam by mouth may be used three or four times daily if the talk-down technique is unsuccessful. *These patients never should be left unattended.*

Marihuana Abuse

While marihuana is pharmacologically a hallucinogen, its wide-spread use warrants separate discussion. The user of marihuana (pot) is unlikely to be recognized unless he is heavily under the influence at that time. In the early stages the drug acts as a stimulant and the user may be very animated and appear almost hysterical. Loud and rapid talking with bursts of laughter are common at this stage. In the later stages of the drug's effect, the user may seem to be in a stupor or sleepy.

Marihuana smokers also may be identified by their possession of these cigarettes which often are called sticks, reefers, or joints. A marihuana cigarette often is rolled in a double thickness of brownish or off-white cigarette paper. Smaller than a regular cigarette, with the paper twisted or tucked in on both ends, the marihuana cigarette often contains seeds and stems. Marihuana is greener in color than regular tobacco.

Another clue to the presence of reefers is the way in which they often are smoked. Typically, such smoking occurs in a group situation. The smoke is inhaled deeply and held in the lungs as long as possible. The odor of marihuana is an additional clue to its use. The odor, similar to that of burnt rope, is readily noticeable on the breath and clothing.

Treatment of the Marihuana Abuser

Acute adverse reactions to marihuana are rare. Bad trips usually subside quite rapidly. Prolonged reactions, if they occur at all, usually are seen in the patient who is smoking marihuana for the first time. These prolonged reactions are more likely to occur in unstable personality types. Such severe reactions require treatment with a tranquilizer, as diazepam, administered as in the treatment of hallucinogen reactions (see p. 209.) The more common milder reactions respond to the same talking-down techniques used for LSD and other stronger hallucinogens. Sedation also can be given to allow the patient to "sleep it off."

Solvent Abuse

The glue or solvent sniffer usually retains the odor of the inhaled substance on his breath and clothes. Irritation of the mucous membranes in the mouth and nose may result in excessive nasal secretions. Redness and watering of the eyes often are observed. The user may appear to be intoxicated or lack muscular control. He may complain of double vision, ringing in the ears, vivid dreams, even hallucinations. Drowsiness, stupor, and unconsciousness may follow excessive use of the substance.

Treatment of Acute Intoxication from Solvents

Acute intoxication from the inhalation of solvents is of fairly short duration so treatment rarely is needed. If necessary, the patient should be treated by using the talking-down technique. The patient and others should be protected from possible hostile outbursts. Everyone should avoid whispering or creating other misleading stimuli.

The condition resulting from inhalation of toxic solvents tends to be chronic and resistant to therapy. Laboratory assessment of possible organic damage to bone marrow, liver, kidneys, and the central nervous system is important. The chronic solvent abuser should receive prompt professional medical attention, particularly if signs of toxicity occur.

EPILEPSY
(And Other Convulsive Seizures)

Epilepsy is a chronic nervous disorder characterized by muscular convulsions with partial or complete loss of consciousness. The seizures are brief, recur suddenly at irregular intervals, and usually are followed by several hours of confusion, stupor, or deep sleep. Epilepsy has been called "falling sickness" because the patient falls suddenly and usually makes no effort to protect himself from injury. Epilepsy may vary from mild to severe. In the mild form, there is momentary loss of consciousness or confusion and slight muscular twitching without falling. In the severe form, the patient suddenly falls as if struck by an overwhelming blow.

An epileptic may have a seizure anytime and frequently may have some forewarning of the attack. There will be a brief moment in which to sit or lie down, or otherwise prepare for the seizure. This forewarning or aura may be almost any strange feeling, as an unusual feeling of depression, excitement, pain in the limbs or abdomen, trembling, or a strange odor. From previous experience, the patient will know that these symptoms will be followed almost immediately by a seizure.

Even if this brief forewarning or aura does not occur, the patient suddenly will emit a peculiar cry and fall down. He may strike the floor or any object in his way, cut or bruise himself badly, or break a bone. His body usually becomes stiff and rigid for a short time, during which he stops breathing and becomes blue or purple in the face. This phase of the seizure is followed by generalized spasmodic convulsions of the entire body with jerking of the arms, legs, and head, contortions of the face, and foaming at the mouth. The eyes may roll back and forth, but there is no feeling in them and they can be touched without the patient flinching. He may bite or chew his tongue or cheeks so that froth in the mouth becomes bloodstained. Urination or bowel movements may occur involuntarily.

Usually, after several minutes, the convulsion subsides. The patient may regain consciousness or fall into a deep stuporous sleep that may last for several hours. When he awakes, he may be confused or very grouchy and ill-tempered. He probably will have no recollection of the attack. Occasionally, seizures recur rapidly with fever, rapid pulse, and rapid breathing. This condition, known as status epilepticus, sometimes terminates in death from exhaustion. Otherwise, an epileptic attack seldom is fatal.

It is obvious from the suddenness and nature of the seizures, that epileptics should not be permitted to go aloft. Also, they never should be allowed in the engine room where there are moving parts of machines on which they might fall or other places of potential danger. A person known to be an epileptic generally should be advised not to accept employment at sea.

Treatment

Treatment during the Convulsion—Bystanders should try to prevent the patient from hurting himself and should make him as comfortable as possible. His movements should not be restrained completely, unless he is in danger of falling from a high place or otherwise injuring himself in some unusual manner. To keep him from biting or chewing his tongue, something should be inserted carefully between his teeth, such as a twisted handkerchief or a pencil wrapped in cloth. Hard objects never should be inserted. A coat or pillow should be placed under his head and his threshing legs and arms covered with a blanket to prevent self-injury during the convulsion. Medicines should not be given by mouth. Artificial respiration will not be needed because the phase during which the patient ceases to breathe usually

is very short. After the seizure while dazed, exhausted, or asleep, the patient may be carried or helped to his bunk. Enough bedding should be placed over the patient to keep him comfortably warm. Usually, he will sleep for some time. However, if he is awake and restless he may be given one dose of phenobarbital 60 mg by mouth.

Treatment between Attacks—There is little that can be done at sea to treat epilepsy, except to keep the patient from injuring himself during an attack, and to prevent recurrences by routine use of the patient's prescribed medication.

The severity and frequency of attacks may be reduced by certain medications such as phenobarbital and phenytoin sodium. *Medical advice by radio should be obtained on the dosage of these two medications.* If the patient states that a physician told him he was an epileptic and was placed on phenobarbital and/or other preventive drugs, these medications in the prescribed dosages may be given from the ship's medicine chest during the voyage, if the patient's supply has been depleted.

Treatment of Convulsions Similar to Epilepsy

These usually lack the preceding aura (the beginning of a seizure as recognized by the patient) and have no history of recurrences over a considerable period of time. They may occur in otherwise normal persons as a result of a severe acute illness, brain injury, meningitis, nephritis, insulin injections, high blood pressure, paralytic stroke, brain tumor, toxins, cyanide poisoning, and strychnine poisoning. Such convulsions should be treated as outlined for epilepsy.

MENINGITIS
(Spinal or Cerebrospinal)

Meningitis is an inflammation of the sheath-like membranes (meninges) that cover the brain and spinal cord. Several different organisms may be carried by the blood to the meninges, lodge there, multiply, and eventually cause inflammation (meningitis). The most common forms of this condition are tubercular meningitis, pneumococcal meningitis, gonoccoccal meningitis, staphylococcal meningitis, and meningococcal meningitis.

The symptoms of these forms of meningitis are similar. For emergency diagnosis and treatment at sea, there is no practical need to differentiate among them, except to point out that epidemic cerebrospinal meningitis (meningococcal meningitis) is extremely infectious. Thus one should assume that any form of meningitis is contagious until proven otherwise. *All cases suspected of being meningitis should be handled as though contagious.*

The germ that causes cerebrospinal meningitis usually is present in nose and throat secretions of those suffering from the disease, in carriers who have recovered from it, or those who have been in contact with patients with the disease. The germs are spread directly by person-to-person contact, and indirectly by contact with articles freshly soiled with nose and mouth discharges of patients or carriers. Epidemics of cerebrospinal meningitis (meningococcal) are related to overcrowding and close contacts as those commonly found in barracks, camps, and ships.

About a week after exposure, fever, severe headache, nausea, generalized muscle and joint pains, backache, and rigidity of the neck may develop. Symptoms like those of a common cold may or may not be present. There may be vomiting, irritability, delirium, or convulsions. The patient may become drowsy and difficult to arouse. He may become unconscious. There may or may not be a generalized skin rash— flat, pinhead-sized red spots that have the appearance of bleeding into the skin. These spots may or may not have a small reddish or yellow blister in the center. The patient often lies on his side facing away from the light, with knees drawn up and head thrown back to lessen the painful rigidity of the neck and back.

The most important diagnostic findings for meningitis are (1) fever and prostration, (2) severe headache, and (3) rigidity of the neck. These always are present and a diagnosis cannot be made without them.

Prevention of Spread

The patient should be isolated for at least 14 days after onset of meningitis. All who care for the patient must follow carefully the isolation nursing technique (see p. 321). This includes wearing a gown and mask in the sickroom, and washing the hands each time after giving care.

Crewmen should be advised about the danger of meningitis. They should be told to wash their hands before eating. Also they should cough and sneeze into handkerchiefs to avoid spreading the disease by droplet infection, in case they might have meningitis in an early form before symptoms appear. If possible, the space should be increased between individuals in sleeping quarters. Living and sleeping quarters should be well-ventilated. Chilling, fatigue, and undue mental and physical strain will increase susceptability to the disease and should be avoided, if possible, by those exposed to the infection.

Treatment

Medical advice by radio should be obtained on the treatment of meningitis. 2.4 million units of penicillin G procaine sterile suspension should be given intramuscularly every six hours, if the patient has no history of allergy to the drug. After four days, further medical advice by radio should be requested on whether oral penicillin may be given.

Good nursing care, quiet, and rest in a darkened room are important. It may take persuasion, firmness, and patience to get the patient to take the necessary medicine and fluids when he is irritable, drowsy, or delirious. If the patient cannot swallow whole tablets but is able to take fluids, then the tablets should be crushed, mixed with a little water, and fed to him with a spoon.

If the symptoms are causing severe pain or the rigidity of the back causes a great deal of distress, morphine sulfate 10 mg should be given intramuscularly. For extreme restlessness phenobarbital 30 mg may be given once or twice a day by mouth. It may be necessary to give enemas for constipation.

The amount of urine voided should be measured. Large amounts of water should be given; if equivalent amounts of urine are not being passed, it may be an indication of toxicity or of urine remaining in the bladder. If no urine is voided for 24 hours, the patient will have to be catheterized. (See p. 325.)

MENTAL DEPRESSION

If anyone feels blue or depressed, looks very unhappy, or his actions suggest extreme despondency or depression, the person's condition should not be ignored. The matter should be investigated especially if it involves a normally cheerful person who shows a sudden drastic reversal in attitude or actions. In order to gain his confidence, the patient should be approached in a kindly, tactful manner that will lead into a frank discussion of his problems. Discovery of a serious depression, or even a mild one surely will help the patient and it might avert possible annoyance or tragedy aboard ship.

Four kinds of depressions are described hereafter: mild, severe, stupor, and agitated depression. Common symptoms of each type are listed. There may be other symptoms, and those listed may not be present in every case.

Mild Depression

A person with a mild depression may lack his usual confidence and show increased indecision about what he should do. He may be less talkative and his thinking more difficult and slower than usual. His doubts and fears may be out of place or be more severe than the occasion requires. He may complain of being worried about something which he admits is foolish but he will say, "I just can't get the thought out of my head." He may complain often of malaise, physical weakness, fatigue, headaches, and inability to sleep or eat properly.

The complaints may center on one part of the body as a continually upset stomach or heart palpitation and pain. It often is difficult even for a physician to tell whether such complaints are due to depression or whether they are due to physical illness. The purely mental symptoms of which a depressed patient may complain are very real to him and may suggest a physical illness, both to the patient and to anyone examining him. The evidence should be studied and compared with the symptoms of depression given and with the description of the physical diseases suggested by the evidence as heart trouble, tuberculosis, or high blood pressure. Medical advice by radio may be useful.

Mild depression may be due to some personal problem or misfortune, as illness in the family or concern about money. He may have a guilty conscience about some real or fancied wrong, or he may be in an early stage of some serious mental disease.

Treatment

If the depressed patient's problem is discussed with him, he may get relief. He will need sympathetic understanding, kindly tactful listening, and encouragement from those who are closely associated with him. The attendant should try to relate the present situation with similar difficulties in the patient's past life that he had overcome successfully.

It must be remembered that a depressed mental patient may try to cover up his symptoms by denying that he is depressed or has any personal problem. He may be afraid, confused, or unwilling to share his troubles. One should not try to force the patient to talk, but he should be convinced that the attendant is interested and friendly. The patient's friends or buddies should be advised not to be offended if he seems to be irritable. They should be urged to stay friendly and support him.

It must be remembered that if one is kept busy talking about other things, he will have less time for annoying thoughts. Too much time should not be spent discussing a patient's fears, but their unreality and improbability should be pointed out.

Sometimes a slight change of duties may give the patient new interests, if this can be accomplished. Added duties may renew his confidence in himself; however, too many responsibilities should not be heaped upon him.

The physical complaints of a depressed patient always should be considered. Sometimes merely receiving attention will help to reassure the individual, even if it actually does little physical good.

When port is reached, the patient should be advised to consult a physician and a social service agency, such as United Seamen's Service, Red Cross, or his union's personal service section.

Severe Depression

Succeeding attacks of depression are apt to become increasingly more severe. The patient will not look or act like his usual self. He may slouch about with his head hanging, his facial expression may be set and gloomy, and he will seldom smile or laugh. His whole activity will be slowed down, he may look ill, and may not follow orders. This could be due either to a desire to refuse to do anything or to preoccupation with his problems.

Loss of weight and constipation are common. The patient usually sleeps poorly and wakes early without feeling rested. Sooner or later, such patients become hopeless about their problems and life in general. They develop guilt feelings and needlessly blame themselves for many things they have done or left undone. Besides feeling sinful and unworthy, the severely depressed patient may imagine at times that he or the world is unreal or that he has contracted a loathesome disease.

The patient usually knows where he is, what day it is, and does not see or hear imaginary things. This is useful in distinguishing a simple depression from other mental diseases in which the patient will have hallucinations, see objects that really are not present, hear voices when no one is speaking within his range of hearing, or smell odors that no one else can detect.

Treatment

The emergency treatment of a severe depression is the same no matter what the exact cause may be. Because a depressed patient might attempt suicide, the patient should be with someone else all of the time, if possible. If the patient is able to work, he should be assigned to a job that requires two persons. If sufficiently ill to be admitted to the sickbay, he should not be left in a room by himself. Care should be taken to assure that such observations do not become too obvious or obnoxious to the patient, who may resent them.

Phenobarbital 90 mg by mouth may be given at bedtime if the patient is unable to sleep soundly. This may be repeated once, if necessary. The ship's personnel should be alerted to make sure the patient will eat enough nourishing food.

The patient should be assigned to light duty, if he is able to work at all. He should be encouraged to use his hobbies or be led into spare time occupations. Keeping him busy will reduce the time available to worry about himself. He should not be questioned too closely. Usually he will be in no condition to respond to questions that may be regarded by him as prying and objectionable. Cold or warm showers, one to three times a day, may make the patient feel better, but these should not be forced on him.

Stupor

A severe depression sometimes progresses into a stupor, which may be a symptom of other diseases. The patient may lie awake in bed, but do nothing of his own accord. He may respond very slowly to orders. Mentally dull, he may not know where he is or what day it is. His face will resemble a mask and he can think of little besides death and dying.

Treatment

Medical advice by radio should be obtained without delay for a stuporous patient. Although the patient usually lacks the energy to harm himself, precautions should be taken to prevent suicide. (See Suicide, p. 217.) General supportive nursing care will be needed. The patient may need to be reminded of and assisted with urination, bowel movements, general cleanliness, and eating. The patient may refuse food entirely. Usually this will not be too serious because most ships will reach port before starvation itself becomes a problem. If at all possible, the patient's intake of liquids should not be reduced, especially in hot weather.

Caution—Stupor due to mental depression seldom appears without being preceded by other signs of severe depression. Other causes for stupor always must be suspected. Usually a thorough examination will uncover evidence of poisoning or drug overdose, head injury, or brain disease. At times, a depressed person may become stuporous from a secret suicide attempt.

Agitated Depression

In agitated depression the patient will be restless, sad, fearful, and apprehensive. He will be tense, pace the floor, and wring his hands. He may repeat over and over again, in an explosive manner, such words as "damn." He may become panicky. He may complain that his "brain has rotted," that his "intestines are plugged up," that he "has no heart." He may attempt personal injury, tear his clothes, or try to destroy other articles.

Treatment

Constant reassurance is necessary for agitated depression. The patient can be told that he will be helped, that he is being protected and taken care of, and that things will be all right. Actions and attitudes of those around him can be more important than words. By acting calm, confident, and unhurried, those in attendance will have a good effect on the patient, although he may not seem to be paying attention.

Whenever possible, medical advice by radio should be obtained. Sedation with phenobarbital 90 mg orally four times daily at the direction of a physician may help. Care should be taken to see that the patient actually swallows the medication and does not save it for a suicide attempt. If medication by mouth is refused or if agitation is extreme, diazepam may be given intramuscularly.

Any stimulation should be avoided. The patient should be in a quiet place with one or two friends as attendants and allowed no visitors. (For other details of nursing care, see Delirium, p. 205.) Physical restraint should be avoided, unless there has been or appears to be an immediate and serious danger of a suicide attempt.

SUICIDE PREVENTION

An estimated 75 percent of those who attempt suicide are seriously depressed. Most people who commit suicide had been thinking about it for some time before the act. Many people contemplating suicide do not talk about it, especially the young, elderly, and professional people; but they do go through periods of sleeplessness and general sadness. They may lose their appetite and show a loss of weight. Also they may lose interest in their work, in people, and in activities they once enjoyed.

Another suicidal signal is preparation for death. A person may begin discussing insurance policies or making a will, start giving away prized possessions.

One should take seriously every suicidal threat, comment, or act. Never be afraid to ask the person if he really is thinking about committing suicide. This will not plant the idea in his head. On the contrary, it will relieve him to know that he is being taken seriously.

One should not try to shock or challenge the person by saying, "Oh, go ahead and do it." Such an impatient remark may be hard to hold back if a person has been repeating his threats, or has been bothersome to have around. Such a challenge can be a careless invitation to suicide.

Never try to argue with the individual about whether he should live or die because this argument cannot be won. The only possible position to take is that the person *must* live. Everyone should be willing to listen to what the patient might say. The medical attendant should promise the person that everything possible will be done to keep him alive.

As soon as possible, professional help should be sought. Today there are many drugs that can help greatly to relieve depression. Medical advice by radio always should be obtained.

MENTAL DISORDERS ABOARD SHIP

Many different forms of mental disease have been named and described and each can vary in severity. Even physicians with special training in psychiatry may have difficulty in classifying a particular case. This is one reason why mental illness is discussed in this book under the headings of common symptoms which can be seen by all. (See Delirium, Mental Depressions, Drug Addiction.)

The term "insanity" no longer is used in medicine. In everyday use it refers to speech, thinking, or behavior that is strange or inappropriate. However, the word, "insanity" continues to have social-legal significance. It refers to a person who, because of mental illness, may not be responsible for his actions, may not be able to manage his own affairs, or may be a danger to himself or others.

There are people who do not have a specifically diagnosed mental illness, but cause confusion, extra work, irritation, puzzlement, sorrow, and even danger to those around them.

Naturally enough, these persons do not make good sailors, but due to our present state of medical knowledge and current laws and customs, it is not possible to prevent many of these men from shipping.

In contrast to the sort of person just mentioned, some few persons do have mental diseases, but are skillful and reliable workers at sea. As time goes on, fitness for sea duty may depend less on whether one has some named illness, but more on his actual ability to do a job. For this reason, a careful description of a man's behavior at work, even before any future breakdown, is important to the physician who will examine him later.

There are two other common symptoms of mental disease that may be seen on shipboard. At times, a person will become unusually quiet and withdrawn for no known reason. He may move very slowly or awkwardly, seem dazed or preoccupied, and be unable to carry out instructions or reply to questions. If he speaks, what he says may not have much to do with what is going on around him. He may even sit or lie entirely motionless for long periods, although not really stuporous or in a coma. He may show no interest in food.

The other common symptom of mental disease is an abnormal suspiciousness and irritability. It can be very hard to decide at times whether this person is just a complainer or a loner, or whether he is mentally ill. The distinction is easy if he speaks about hearing the voices of angels or seeing in his room relatives who are long dead. It is not as easy, however, if he speaks about things that could be true, as not getting overtime because his supervisor doesn't like him; or that he is being discriminated against because he belongs to a racial or religious minority.

Treatment

If any of these groups of symptoms for mental disease are serious enough to interfere with a person's work, he should be taken off duty. The person should be observed closely so that he does not harm himself or anyone else. One may learn much by showing an informal friendly interest in such people. Attention should be given to meals, general hygiene, and the bodily comfort of anyone under observation.

A careful record of the person's behavior should be kept for guidance during later diagnosis and treatment.

To calm the patient, phenobarbital, 90 mg by mouth, should be given three times daily. It seldom is wise to force medication because the patient may have strange beliefs about it. For example, he may believe the drug is for the purpose of changing him into a woman or that it is poison.

Medical advice should be obtained by radio. The patient should be examined by a physician at the earliest opportunity.

NEURITIS

Neuritis is a disease of a single nerve, of two or more nerves in separate areas, or of many nerves simultaneously. Usually it is degenerative in nature and rarely is accompanied by inflammation. The disease is characterized by pain and tenderness along the affected nerve area. There may be burning, tingling or numbness, and the area will be sensitive to pressure. When the sciatic nerve, which extends from the buttocks down the back of the thigh to the lower leg, is affected, the condition is *sciatica*. Intense shooting pains on one side of the face is called *facial neuralgia*.

Some causes of neuritis are poor physical condition, chronic local infection as abscessed teeth or diseased tonsils, straining or stretching or other injury to the nerves, pressure on a nerve area from a tumor or overgrowth of bone, and inadequate diet. Neuritis is prominent in beriberi and pellagra, which are "vitamin deficiency" diseases. It may be associated with chronic diseases such as arthritis and diabetes.

Treatment

To determine the underlying cause of neuritis, a complete medical checkup is necessary. Emergency treatment at sea usually is confined to symptoms. The most useful emergency treatment is rest for the affected part and applications of heat. A neuritic arm can be kept at rest in a sling. In severe sciatica the patient must stay in bed.

For severe pain, aspirin or acetaminophen 600 mg and codeine sulfate 30 mg should be given by mouth and repeated every four hours, as necessary. The codeine sulfate should be discontinued and aspirin only given, as soon as the pain is under control. Codeine sulfate should not be continued for more than four days without specific orders from a physician. The patient should get plenty of liquids. A substantial varied diet of easily digested food may help to build up the patient's general health and may improve the neuritic condition, if vitamin deficiency is a contributing cause.

STROKE
(Cerebrovascular Accident)

A stroke occurs when the blood supply to some part of the brain is interrupted. This generally is caused by:

- A blood clot forming in the blood vessel (cerebral thrombosis).

- A rupture of the blood vessel wall (cerebral hemorrhage).

- Obstruction of a cerebral blood vessel by a clot or other material from another part of the vascular system which flows to the brain (cerebral embolism).

- Pressure on a blood vessel, as by a tumor.

A stroke usually occurs suddenly, without warning signs. In more severe cases, there is a rapidly developing loss of consciousness and a flabby, relaxed paralysis of the affected side of the body. Headache, nausea, vomiting, and convulsions may be present. The face usually is flushed but may become pale or ashen. The pupils of the eyes often are unequal in size. The pulse usually is full and rapid and breathing is labored and irregular. The mouth may be drawn to one side and often there is difficulty in speaking and swallowing.

The specific symptoms will vary with the site of the lesion and the extent of brain damage. Mild cases may experience no loss of consciousness and paralysis may be limited to weakness on one side of the body.

The outcome of a stroke will depend upon the extent of brain compression or damage. When fatal, death usually occurs in two to 14 days and seldom at the time of the attack. Most patients with first or second attacks recover, but recurrent attacks are likely. The extent of permanent paralysis will not be determined for at least six months.

Treatment

Good nursing care is essential after a stroke. The patient should be undressed as gently as possible and placed in bed with the trunk of the body, shoulders, and head elevated slightly on pillows. An attendant should be assigned to stay with the patient. Extra care should be taken to prevent the patient from choking on saliva or vomitus. The patient's head should be turned to one side so fluids can flow out of the mouth. Mucus and food debris should be removed from the mouth with a piece of cloth wrapped around a finger. If there is a fever, cold compresses should be applied to the forehead. If the patient is conscious and able to swallow, liquid and soft foods may be given. To prevent bedsores the patient should be kept clean and turned to a different position in bed every three to four hours. Bowel regularity should be maintained.

Medical advice by radio must be obtained, and early evacuation to a hospital should be anticipated. (See Convulsions, p. 212.)

Chapter V

Treatment of Diseases

Section I
RESPIRATORY DISEASES

ALLERGIC REACTIONS

CERTAIN INDIVIDUALS MAY DEVELOP an allergy or hypersensitivity to substances that are harmless to most people. An allergic individual is sensitive to allergens, which are substances that enter the body by being inhaled, swallowed, injected, or by contact with the skin. They may come from bacterial or fungal infections in the body. A manifested allergy may be relatively mild, as a light attack of hay fever or a brief episode of hives; or it may be severe and very serious, as an acute attack of asthma, a stubborn or uncomfortable skin rash, or sudden collapse.

When an allergen reaches a sensitive area of the body, the tissues react irritably or even violently to produce symptoms of allergy. The allergic irritation may occur in almost any organ or tissue of the body with symptoms determined by the location. When the nose and throat are the organs involved, an individual may have sneezing, stuffiness, running nose, and itching of the throat and eyes. The symptoms represent hay fever (allergic rhinitis). If bronchial tissues are affected, there is wheezing, coughing, and difficult breathing (asthma). When the skin is affected, eczema or hives

appear. If the digestive tract is involved, there may be nausea, vomiting, indigestion, abdominal pain, diarrhea, or cramping. An allergic reaction also may affect the brain, causing headache.

Countless substances can cause allergic reactions. A drug such as penicillin is a common cause of drug allergy. An allergy to penicillin may be manifested by hives, skin rash, or swelling of various body parts; or at times, a reaction that resembles serum sickness (malaise, fever, and possibly arthritis occurring about 10 days after the penicillin is given). Drugs which may be associated with allergic reactions include antibiotics, serums, laxatives, sedatives, and tranquilizers. Eczematous dermatitis may result from contact with the skin by metals, dyes, fabrics, resins, drugs, insecticides, industrial chemicals, perfumes, rubber, plastics, and the components of certain plants (as poison ivy or the oil pressed from the shell of the cashew nut).

Serious allergic reactions may occur following bee, wasp, yellowjacket, and hornet stings. Airborne substances which may produce allergy include pollens from weeds, grasses, trees, and plants; house and industrial dusts;

220

mold spores; animal danders (skin and hair shed by domestic or wild animals); feathers found in pillows; kapok; and insecticide sprays or other vapors. In some instances, foods (such as eggs, milk, nuts, wheat, shellfish, chocolate, and fruits) may cause acute or chronic symptoms. There are many other possible allergens, including sunlight, heat, cold, and parasites.

Avoidance of the allergenic substance or substances offers the greatest hope of permanent relief from an allergic disease. In drug allergy, once the diagnosis is suspected or established, the allergenic agent should be stopped and another drug substituted. In allergic contact dermatitis from cashew shell oil, fuel oil, paints, tar, and others, the patient should try to protect his skin from direct and indirect contact with the agents, even if he has to change occupations. Patients allergic to an inhaled substance (as feathers or animal danders) may be unable to avoid them. Airborne pollens are difficult to avoid. A physician may be able to desensitize the patient by a series of injections.

For the temporary relief of asthma, eczema, hay fever, and hives, refer to these conditions elsewhere in the text.

Anaphylactic Shock

Anaphylactic shock is a severe allergic reaction often fatal that produces shock and collapse. It commonly occurs after an injection of a medication such as penicillin. This reaction can occur after contact with almost any allergen. Prevention is best. *Before giving injections or administering any medication, the patient should be asked if ever he had an allergic reaction in the past.* If he did, medical advice by radio should be gotten. A skin rash or other unusual side effect following treatment is a warning to avoid the same medicine in the future.

Treatment

For anaphylactic shock, the patient should be placed in a prone position. The following medications should be administered intramuscularly, immediately: 1:1000 epinephrine hydrochloride injection 0.5 ml, diphenhydramine hydrochloride 50 mg, and hydrocortisone sodium succinate 100 mg. The three medicines

should be given from separate syringes and at different body sites. The epinephrine hydrochloride injection may be repeated in 20 minutes, if the patient's condition remains serious or becomes worse. Obtain medical advice by radio.

ASTHMA

Asthma is characterized by a sudden and widespread narrowing of the smaller air passageways in the lungs. The patient becomes acutely short of breath and a wheezing will be heard during expiration. Most patients have a history of many previous attacks. It is important to differentiate asthma from other causes of shortness of breath, especially that from heart failure.

Extrinsic asthma often is an allergy to pollen, dust, and food, among others, and is common in children. *Intrinsic asthma*, which is due to lung infection, is more common in adults. Asthma often develops for no apparent reason. The disease may be related to emotional upset, climate changes, and minor upper respiratory viral infections. Episodes may start and end suddenly with or without therapy.

Treatment

A bedside vaporizer or turned-on hot shower should be used to humidify the air that is inhaled by the patient with asthma. To offset possible dehydration, the patient should be encouraged to drink plenty of fluids, especially water. More palatable liquids as fruit juices and hot tea may be helpful.

Medications to enlarge the air passageways (bronchodilators), such as ephedrine sulfate 25 mg should be given by mouth every four to six hours. If the patient is unduly nervous or unable to sleep, phenobarbital 15 mg to 30 mg should be given by mouth every four to six hours.

For acute asthmatic episodes, 0.3 ml to 0.5 ml aqueous epinephrine hydrochloride injection 1:1000 should be given *subcutaneously,* and if necessary repeated in 60 minutes.

For an acute asthmatic episode, an aminophylline suppository 500 mg by rectum may be used. Use of a suppository should be restricted to only one or two occasions because repeated usage might cause severe rectal irritation.

Antibiotics may be given in acute asthma, because most adult asthma patients will have a bronchial infection that may or may not be apparent. Medical advice by radio should be obtained as to whether antibiotics are indicated.

If all or some of the above procedures are used, most acute asthma attacks can be treated adequately. (See Bronchitis, p. 223.)

BLEEDING

(Respiratory and Digestive Tracts)

It sometimes is difficult to differentiate between bleeding from the respiratory and digestive tracts. Blood from the nose, throat, or lungs may be swallowed; thereafter, it will have the same appearance in the stool as blood from the digestive tract.

To find the source of blood discharged from either the mouth or rectum, the factors that follow must be considered.

The blood may be bright red, leaving no doubt that it is blood; or it may not look like ordinary blood. If vomited and partly digested, the blood will appear dark and granular like coffee grounds. The vomitus mixed with partly digested food and other stomach contents makes for further confusion. Also, blood may give a stool a black appearance like tar.

There may be much or only a little bleeding. Sputum may be only bloodstreaked, as in some mouth diseases. A teaspoonful or more of bright blood may be coughed up or vomited, if the trouble is farther down the throat, in the lungs, or in the stomach. A pint or more of partly digested material like coffee-grounds may be vomited. Blood in the stool may be so scant that the only means of detection will be by means of the occult blood test materials that are included in the section on *surgical equipment, instruments, and supplies.* (See p. 297.) Such bleeding may be caused by intestinal parasites or gastric ulcer. Or there may be smaller or larger amounts of bright red blood usually from a local disease of the anus or rectum, as piles or a tumor. Digested blood in tarry stools usually occurs in large amounts.

Bleeding from the digestive or respiratory tract usually does not produce pain or other obvious signs or symptoms, except those associated with considerable loss of blood, as faintness, weakness, dizziness, pale moist skin, and rapid thready pulse. Internal bleeding is not uncommon in certain diseases, as stomach ulcer, typhoid fever, cancer, or tuberculosis. Patients suspected of having such diseases should be watched for signs of bleeding. Sometimes in apparently healthy persons, internal bleeding is the first sign of these diseases.

Tables 5–2 and 5–3 list some of the usual characteristics of respiratory and digestive tract bleeding.

The cause of the bleeding will determine treatment. Internal hemorrhage will be indicated by a feeling of faintness, weakness, or dizziness, pale moist skin, and rapid pulse. Such a patient immediately should be placed in bed and kept at absolute rest for several days at least. Sedation by injection should be given to a patient who is mentally disturbed, excited, or restless. Diazepam 5 mg may be given intramuscularly and repeated in four hours, if indicated. If sedation appears to be needed beyond this period of time, medical advice by radio should be obtained.

If the bleeding is from the stomach, the patient should be treated as if he had an ulcer. (See p. 164.)

In all cases of bleeding from the lungs or the gastrointestinal tract, the patient should see a doctor at the next port of call. Unless the bleeding stops promptly, air evacuation may be necessary. Medical advice by radio should be gotten at once.

SHORTNESS OF BREATH
(Dyspnea)

Shortness of breath is not a disease in itself. It may occur normally after exercise, but it may be a symptom of several diseases. The patient may confuse shortness of breath with fatigue, cough, or the production of excess sputum. These conditions must be distinguished from shortness of breath. Usually, the breathing will be rapid and shallow, but patients can feel short of breath with either a rapid or a slow respiratory rate. The normal rate of respiration is 15 to 20 breaths per minute.

Some causes of shortness of breath are chronic heart disease, pneumonia, pleurisy, fever, severe asthma, and emphysema. As a general rule, chronic heart disease usually is associated with fluid (edema) in the legs. Breathlessness in such patients is relieved by sitting or elevation of the head of the bed. Shortness of breath due to lung conditions is not associated with edema.

Treatment

Treatment is directed at the cause of the shortness of breath, most commonly heart or lung disease. Professional medical care generally is required.

BRONCHITIS

Bronchitis is an inflammation of the membrane that lines the bronchial tubes. It should be suspected when a patient coughs, produces sputum, and no obvious cause for these symptoms can be found. A good history and physical examination will help to determine the patient's illness. Without X-ray equipment, adequate evaluation aboard ship may be difficult.

Acute bronchitis

Usually a self-limited disease, acute bronchitis is characterized by the onset of cough and sputum production. This may be due to viruses, bacteria, chemical irritation (smoke, fumes, gases), and in some cases an allergic state (asthmatic bronchitis). The disease frequently begins as a common cold.

Chronic Bronchitis

Chronic bronchitis is present when a cough persists with production of sputum for three months in each of two consecutive years. The principal causes are prolonged irritation of the bronchial mucosa, usually due to heavy cigarette smoking and recurrent bronchial infection.

Bronchitis Due to Viruses

A runny nose and heavy white gelatinous sputum usually are identified with viral bronchitis.

Treatment

The following are recommended: (1) phenylephrine hydrochloride nasal spray should be sprayed into each nostril every four hours;

(2) diphenhydramine hydrochloride* 25 mg may be given by mouth every four to six hours; (3) humidification of air if possible (bedside vaporizer); and (4) for the cough, dextromethorphan hydrobromide with glyceryl guaiacolate syrup may be given, one to two teaspoonfuls every three or four hours.

Bronchitis Due to Bacteria

A bacterial infection can complicate viral bronchitis. It usually is associated with heavy cigarette smoking, emphysema, or chronic bronchitis. A runny nose usually is not present and the sputum almost always is yellow and thick.

Treatment

Before giving any medication, the patient should be asked if he is allergic to it.

The treatment consists of (1) humidification of air (bedside vaporizer or turned-on hot shower); (2) for the cough dextromethorphan hydrobromide with glyceryl guaiacolate syrup may be given, one teaspoonful every three to four hours; and (3) for fever, aspirin 600 mg by mouth every three or four hours as needed. If aspirin is not well tolerated by the patient, acetaminophen may be tried at the same dosage and frequency. Antibiotic treatment usually is indicated. Ampicillin 250 mg should be given by mouth four times daily. If the patient is sensitive to penicillin, erythromycin 500 mg or tetracycline 500 mg should be given by mouth four times daily.

Antibiotic therapy should be continued until the sputum is normal in volume and appearance. *If antibiotic therapy seems indicated beyond ten days, medical advice by radio should be obtained.*

Bronchitis Due to Irritation

Treatment

The patient should be removed from the source of the irritation. The patient and others who enter his room should not be allowed to smoke. In severe smoke inhalation, oxygen therapy is helpful.

---

*Because diphenhydramine hydrochloride may cause drowsiness or dizziness, the patient should be excused from working at heights or close to moving machinery, while taking the medication.

Table 5-2
Bleeding from the Mouth

Color and Appearance	Amount and Method	Most likely Source	Cause	Remarks on Treatment
Bright red	Blood-streaked sputum	Local: From mouth tissues, gums, throat, back of nose	Pyorrhea, cold in head, laryngitis, pharyngitis	Mouthwash or other symptomatic treatment. See dentist at first port of call.
Bright red	*Coughed up (teaspoonful or more)	Lungs	Tuberculosis of lung, cancer	Symptomatic treatment (see below). See doctor at first port of call.
Bright red	In sputum or phlegm: Coughed up, frothy, bubbly, pink or red	Lungs	Heart disease	Symptomatic treatment (see Heart Disease). See doctor at first port of call.
Brown (like prune juice)	In phlegm: Coughed up (½ to 1 teaspoonful)	Lungs	Pneumonia	See Pneumonia.
Bright red	Vomited (cupful or more)	Stomach	Hemorrhage from ulcer, cancer, ruptured vessel. Probably very recent or still continuing	Symptomatic. Use icebag.
Dark brown (like coffee-grounds)	Vomited (usually considerable in amount; one pint or more)	Stomach (old blood, mixed with partly digested food)	Stomach or duodenal disease, or blood swallowed after extraction of tooth. Bleeding probably occurred 2 or 3 hours previously, and has stopped or lessened in amount	Ulcer, cancer.

*Coughed-up blood may result from a paroxysm of coughing or it may come from the back of the throat without any great amount of coughing, until the blood actually is in the mouth.

Table 5-3
Blood in Stools

Color and Appearance	Amount and Method	Most likely Source	Cause	Remarks on Treatment
Bright red	Streaked feces	Lower end of digestive tract: hemorrhoids, anal fissure	Constipation (hard fecal matter that injures mucous membrane), local injuries, fissures, piles, cancer	If present with every stool and not reduced by cathartics which soften stools, see doctor at first port of call.
Bright red	Teaspoonful or more	Lower end of digestive tract	Ulcer or tumor of rectum, ulcerative colitis, dysentery, typhoid	See doctor at first port of call.
Tarry	Abundant	Upper part of digestive tract	Stomach or duodenal ulcer; gastritis; liver; kidney or heart disease; typhoid; dysentery; tumor; cancer	Symptomatic treatment. See doctor at first port of call.

Bronchitis Due to Allergy

Allergenic bronchitis occurs to individuals with a history of asthma, wheezing, or prior respiratory infections (asthmatic bronchitis).

Treatment

If the patient is wheezing, a bronchodilator such as ephedrine sulfate 25 mg may be given by mouth four times daily. If this causes undue nervousness or inability to sleep, phenobarbital 15 mg may be given by mouth at the same time. Oral intake of fluids, especially water should be encouraged.

COLDS
(Common Cold, Coryza, Rhinitis)

Few illnesses cause so much loss of working time and personal discomfort as the common head cold. Its symptoms are familiar: runny nose, red and watery eyes, malaise, aching muscles, chilliness, and often a sore scratchy throat and cough. A cold lowers a person's resistance to other diseases and permits secondary infections. Symptoms of a cold may precede many communicable diseases, so medical attendants should watch carefully for other symptoms of these diseases. Diphtheria, measles, and septic sore throat may start as a cold. A cold may lead to bronchitis, pneumonia, and middle ear disease.

Treatment

Unless symptoms develop that indicate a more serious disease, the treatment for colds should be symptomatic. The patient should be kept in bed until the temperature is normal and he feels reasonably able to function. Aspirin 600 mg should be given by mouth every three or four hours to help relieve the symptoms. If aspirin is not well tolerated by the patient, acetaminophen may be tried at the same dosage and frequency. Phenylephrine hydrochloride 0.25% nasal spray may be used every four hours for two or three days. An antihistamine as diphenhydramine hydrochloride 25 mg may be given by mouth every four to six hours, as needed. Because the diphenhydramine hydrochloride may cause drowsiness or dizziness, the patient should be excused from working at heights or near moving machinery, while taking the medication.

The patient should force fluids as water and fruit juices. He should be advised to blow his nose gently to avoid forcing infectious material into the sinuses and middle ear. When symptoms subside for 24 hours, the patient should get out of bed but restrict activities for a day or two before returning to full duty.

COUGH

Coughing is a sudden forceful expulsion of air from the lungs usually in a series of efforts. Although annoying, a cough helps to get rid of phlegm (sputum) that builds up in air passages.

Coughs are productive or non-productive (dry). The sputum may be purulent (with pus), copious or scanty, thick or thin and fluid, clear or frothy, odorless or foul-smelling, blood-streaked or frankly bloody. A cough may be acute or chronic, occasional or persistent, slight or severe, painful or painless.

Coughing is not a disease in itself but a symptom. An acute cough usually is caused by an infection of the upper respiratory system. A productive cough that lasts for more than three months frequently means that the patient is suffering from chronic bronchitis, even though he does not recognize that he is ill until he becomes short of breath. Because of cigarette smoking and air pollution, thousands of people become victims of chronic bronchitis and eventually emphysema. Chronic cough with fever suggests more serious conditions, such as tuberculosis, pneumonia, or even carcinoma of the lung. Chronic cough without fever may indicate heart disease, bronchial asthma, or bronchiectasis (infection and degeneration of the air passages).

The following generalities may be helpful:

Simple bronchitis usually follows a viral infection or "cold" that is accompanied sometimes by a sore throat, a raw heavy feeling behind the breastbone, and a dry cough that changes into a productive cough.

Pleurisy is manifested by a severe pain in the chest wall that is aggravated by deep breathing.

Asthma occurs in allergic individuals, usually starting at a young age in a family with a history of hay fever, hives, or asthma. It is detected by a wheezing sound during breathing, more pronounced on exhaling than inhaling.

With *pneumonia,* usually there is fever, often a productive cough with pus or sputum, and pain in the chest.

Tuberculosis of the lungs may be associated with slight but prolonged cough. Fatigue may be an early symptom, followed by sweats and loss of weight.

Cancer of the lung has become alarmingly frequent in persons who have been heavy smokers (a pack of cigarettes a day for twenty years or so). Early diagnosis of cancer is difficult but cough, spitting blood, persistent fever, or a weight loss may be early warnings.

When a cough accompanies an acute illness, especially when there is fever, the medical attendant should obtain a good history from the patient. After examining the patient and his sputum, the medical attendant should decide on the most likely cause of the illness and prepare a carefully worded request to *obtain medical advice by radio.*

Treatment

The cough due to a cold and viral bronchitis is treated symptomatically with aspirin, phenylephrine hydrochloride 0.25% nasal spray, and humidifiers as described under Bronchitis. For a cough, one 5 ml teaspoonful dextromethorphan hydrobromide with glyceryl guaiacolate syrup should be given every four hours as needed.

For treatment of a cough due to pneumonia, pleurisy, asthma, and tuberculosis, see the appropriate headings.

As a hygienic measure, the patient should be given disposable tissues to cover his mouth when coughing. All used tissues should be put into a paper bag for appropriate disposal. Antihistamines are not indicated.

Specific treatment should be directed to the cause of the illness. The patient's pulse, temperature, and rate and depth of respiration should be noted.

See Asthma, p. 221; Bronchitis, p. 223; Pneumonia p. 229; Pleurisy, p. 229; and Tuberculosis, p. 231.

HAY FEVER

Hay fever is a common allergy that affects the upper respiratory tract. Generally caused by pollen, it is a seasonal disease that is prevalent in the spring, late summer, and fall. Symptoms resemble those of an aggravated head cold as congestion of nose and eyes, sneezing and asthma. (See Asthma, p. 221.) An attack may last from four to six weeks during which the patient may lose a lot of weight.

Treatment

At sea, the treatment is entirely symptomatic. Patients with hay fever usually are familiar with the symptoms and with the effects of their various remedies. Usually they do not have to go to bed or stop their regular work. More severe symptoms may be treated with diphenhydramine hydrochloride 25 mg by mouth four times a day. Because the medication may induce drowsiness as a side effect, all precision work, potentially hazardous work, or standing watch should be curtailed for the patient.

HOARSENESS (Laryngitis)

This is a harsh, discordant, grating quality imparted to the voice by an abnormal condition of the larynx (voice box) or other part of the throat. Usually it is due to laryngitis, an acute or chronic inflammation of the larynx.

In *acute laryngitis* usually there is a barking cough. The hoarseness may result in complete loss of the voice for a few hours or days. Local irritation prompts frequent efforts to clear the throat. Acute laryngitis may be caused by exposure, dust and other irritants, mouth breathing, excessive smoking, overindulgence in alcohol, acute infectious disease, or an intense emotional upset.

Chronic laryngitis stems from repeated attacks of acute laryngitis, chronic disorders of nose and throat, mouth breathing, dental disease, tuberculosis or cancer of the throat, asthma, hay fever, overuse of the voice, and excessive use of alcohol or tobacco.

Treatment

In acute laryngitis with fever, chills, and toxicity, an antibiotic may be indicated. *Always make sure the patient is not allergic to the medication.* Before administering an antibiotic, medical advice by radio should be obtained. If there is any sign of airway obstruction, medical advice by radio should be sought immediately. Cool vapor or steam inhalation is recommended with complete voice rest.

If a patient is *not* feverish, and has lost his voice from shouting or other abuse, he should rest his voice and avoid irritants such as smoking. If the hoarseness persists, patients should seek medical advice at their earliest convenience to make sure that cancer is not the cause.

HYPERVENTILATION SYNDROME
(Anxiety Attacks)

The hyperventilation syndrome is characterized by abnormally prolonged, rapid, and deep breathing. It is one of the commonest non-disabling conditions seen in routine medical practice. The patient may feel very sick, tired and apprehensive, with a pounding heart and labored breathing. Fear arising from these symptoms may produce a feeling of serious illness or impending death in the patient.

A patient who possesses three or more of the following symptoms may be suffering a hyperventilation attack:

- A feeling in the top of the head that is hard to describe.
- Dizziness or lightheadedness.
- Blurring of vision.
- Dryness or bitterness of the mouth.
- Tingling of the hands or around the mouth.
- Tightness or a "lump" in the throat.
- Shortness of breath.
- Pounding of the heart.
- A feeling of great tiredness or weakness.
- A feeling of being in a dream.
- Drawing-up of the hands at the wrist and knuckles, but with straight fingers in severe attacks only.
- Fainting.

Treatment

Reassurance of the patient is the most important treatment for hyperventilation. Resting in a quiet place for a few minutes often helps. Breathing into a paper or plastic bag may assist the hysterical patient who is continually hyperventilating. Breathing at a maximal depth until satisfactory respiration is achieved may assist the type which is characterized by deep, sighing respirations. In cases that are hard to manage, diazepam 5 mg may be given by mouth twice a day for several days. If these measures are not successful, some other condition either alone or accompanying anxiety may be present. Care must be taken to see that a more dangerous condition is not overlooked. *Medical advice by radio should be obtained.*

INFLUENZA (Flu)

Influenza is an acute, infectious, respiratory disease caused by a virus. Early symptoms resemble those of an acute cold in the head. However, headache and aching or pain in the small of the back, joints, and bones are much more severe than with a common cold.

During an influenza epidemic, there is no mistaking these symptoms. However, when cases occur singly or in small groups, differentiating between influenza and the common cold, acute laryngitis, acute bronchitis, and the onset of communicable and other acute diseases is difficult, if not impossible. Influenza usually is thought of in terms of epidemics. The severity of the symptoms of epidemic influenza vary greatly. The symptoms may be so mild that few people realize they are in the midst of a potentially dangerous epidemic. During other epidemics, the disease may be complicated by pneumonia which should be suspected if the patient develops symptoms such as dyspnea (breathing difficulty), cyanosis (bluish skin), or rales (abnormal sounds that accompany breathing). A stethoscope should be used to check the chest area for rales. Other common complications of influenza are pleurisy, kidney disease, and middle ear disease.

Treatment

Influenza is a serious highly contagious disease. Prevention of the spread of the disease is an important part of treatment. *Get medical advice by radio.* The disease may be spread by coughing, sneezing, and other methods of direct contact. The patient suspected of having influenza should be isolated from other crewmen not having similar symptoms. The principles of isolation nursing should be observed.

In epidemics, the following procedures must be carried out: The temperature of all crew members should be taken twice a day, morning and evening. A person with a fever should be put at absolute bed rest and kept there until the temperature has been normal for 24 hours.

For constipation, 30 ml of milk of magnesia should be given nightly.

For pain, aspirin 600 mg should be given by mouth every three to four hours as needed. If aspirin is not well tolerated by the patient, acetaminophen may be tried at the same dosage and frequency.

In isolated cases, influenza with mild symptoms should be treated as for the common cold (see p. 225) or any acute fever with signs of upper respiratory irritation.

Prevention

Influenza vaccines now are available that help to prevent the disease in a majority of cases, if taken early enough. Flu vaccine is most effective if it is administered one to six months before the influenza virus attacks, and if the viral strain used in the vaccine is exactly the same as the epidemic strain.

In a year when an influenza epidemic is possible, seamen should contact a U.S. Public Health Service facility or a local health department for advice about getting the correct vaccine. Prompt immunization is in order for high risk groups—as the chronically ill, heart patients, those aged 65 and over, among others.

The virus used to make the vaccine is grown in eggs. Thus, anyone with a known allergy to eggs should receive the vaccine only under special medical supervision.

NASAL CONGESTION

The acute form of nasal congestion generally is associated with the common cold, sinus infection, hay fever, or the early stages of many diseases that start with symptoms resembling those of the common cold.

Chronic nasal congestion often is associated with anatomic defects, as a deviated septum, enlarged turbinates, or unusually small nasal openings.

Treatment

To open the nasal passages phenylephrine hydrochloride nasal spray 0.25% should be used every four hours, as needed. The nasal spray should *not* be used for more than three consecutive days. For minimal congestion, no treatment may be needed. Warm steam inhalations several times daily for five to ten minutes may be used.

NOSEBLEED (Epistaxis)

Usually bleeding from the nose has local causes but it may be a warning of a serious condition elsewhere in the body.

Some local causes are direct violence as from a blow, deviation of the septum, chronic nasal infection that produces areas of diseased mucous membrane, acute colds in the head, enlarged adenoids, enlarged blood vessels similar to varicose veins, tumors, syphilis, atrophic rhinitis (characterized by foul breath), foreign bodies, and fracture of the base of the skull.

Some underlying systemic causes of nosebleed are high blood pressure, some forms of kidney and liver disease, extremes of heat and cold, overindulgence in alcoholic beverages, heart disease, and abnormal blood coagulation.

Treatment

Most nosebleeds can be stopped by simple compression of the nose. The thumb and forefinger should be gently but firmly placed on each side of the lower end of the nose and pressed together. The patient should sit upright in a chair with head bent forward. Steady pressure should be applied for at least 10 minutes and repeated, if necessary. There should be no movement while pressure is applied to the nose in order to forestall possible additional damage to the bleeding vessel. The patient should be reassured.

If bleeding persists after repeating the procedure several times, the patient's nose should be blown gently to remove clots. Then the nose should be sprayed several times with phenylephrine hydrochloride 0.25% nasal solution. The nose should be packed with strips of petrolatum gauze cut about a half inch in width. First, the lower portion of the nose should be packed and the gauze worked upward. *After the packing is completed, the attendant should make sure that both ends of the gauze protrude from the nose.* The pack should remain in the nose for at least 24 hours and the patient should rest in bed. External pressure may be applied to the nose when the pack is in place. There may be some discharge of blood and serum while the pack is in place.

If all these measures fail, medical advice by radio should be obtained, especially if the patient is elderly.

PLEURISY

Pleurisy is inflammation of the pleural membranes that line the chest cavity and surround the lungs. The disease may follow any condition that lowers the person's ability to resist infection. Often it is associated with bronchitis, pneumonia, and tuberculosis.

The onset of pleurisy usually is sudden with a cough and a sharp stabbing pain in the chest that is aggravated by breathing or coughing. If the pleura over the diaphragm are affected, rather than the pleura at the side of the lung next to the chest wall, the pain may appear as an abdominal pain possibly associated with muscle spasms and tenderness of the abdomen. It may resemble the pain caused by abdominal conditions such as gallstone colic or stomach disease. Chills and fever usually are associated with pleurisy.

Simple pleurisy should not last long. However, if the symptoms are severe, complications may be likely. The most common complication is the collection of fluid in the space between the two layers of pleurae. Fluid in this space may press against the lung and interfere with the entry of air into the organ, causing shortness of breath. In some cases pus forms in this space (empyema). A pulmonary embolism (blood clot in the lung) also can cause a pleurisy-like pain, often accompanied by blood in the sputum.

Treatment

A patient suspected of having pleurisy always should be checked for possible pneu-

monia. The patient should be kept in bed as long as he has active symptoms and fever. For pain, aspirin 600 mg should be given by mouth every three to four hours as needed. If aspirin is not well tolerated by the patient, acetaminophen may be tried at the same dosage and frequency.

If pain is not controlled by aspirin or acetaminophen alone, oral codeine sulfate 30 mg may be given along with either of these medications every three to four hours for the first 24 to 48 hours. *Medical advice by radio should be obtained on the repeated use of codeine sulfate.*

After two or three days, if the patient does not seem to be getting better, medical advice by radio again should be obtained.

PNEUMONIA

Pneumonia is an inflammation of the terminal air sacs of the lungs and the small bronchioles leading into them. (See Fig. 1-20.) Next to bronchitis, it is the most common acute infectious disease of the lungs.

Symptoms of pneumonia are fever, chills, pain in the chest, a fast rate of breathing, and dark brown sputum (like prune juice). Pneumonia may begin in association with another disease, or it may start as a separate and distinct illness. In the first situation, it may occur as a complication of a common cold, bronchitis, serious injury, an operation, or other illness. It may be indicated by the sudden exaggeration of the symptoms of the associated disease, in addition to the usual symptoms of pneumonia. As a separate and distinct illness, pneumonia may develop suddenly without any marked symptoms of serious illness.

Treatment

Medical advice by radio should be obtained on the medication suggested below. The best possible general care must be given to a pneumonia patient. His strength must be conserved and he should be kept as comfortable and quiet as possible. He should be urged to force fluids, especially water, with lemonade, weak tea, or fruit juice. His convalescence should be a gradual return to normal activity. He should not return to work until checked by a physician.

Although not highly contagious, pneumonia is transmissible to others, so the patient should be kept in a room by himself. A paper handkerchief or toilet paper always should be used to cover the cough or catch the expectoration. The contaminated handkerchief should be burned or appropriately disposed. The general principles of *isolation technique* should be observed (see p. 321).

Penicillin, which is the drug of choice of most suspected cases of pneumonia, usually shortens the illness, reduces symptoms, and is lifesaving in the most serious types of disease. The patient should be given penicillin V potassium 1000 mg (four 250 mg tablets) by mouth every six hours for the first day; then 500 mg by mouth every six hours for at least five days. Some types of pneumonia do not respond to penicillin but will respond to other antibiotics. If the pneumonia is not responding to penicillin or the patient is allergic to penicillin, tetracycline 500 mg should be given by mouth every six hours.

For pain, aspirin 600 mg should be given by mouth every three to four hours as needed. If aspirin is not well tolerated by the patient, acetaminophen may be tried at the same dosage and frequency. The patient should rest in bed. To avoid chest congestion, he should be encouraged to take several deep breaths every hour and to expectorate.

SINUSITIS
(Sinus Trouble or Inflammation)

During head colds or other respiratory infections, various microorganisms may pass from the nose into one or another of the sinuses, through the small opening that connects these bone cavities with the nose. When the sinuses become infected and the mucous membrane is inflamed, the condition is called *sinusitis*. When the inflammation plugs the openings that ordinarily drain the sinuses, secretions will accumulate in the sinuses causing pressure and possibly fever. (The areas of pain in sinusitis are shown in Fig. 1–7.)

Sinusitis may be a temporary condition. As the sinus infection clears, the blocked secretions drain and the swollen mucous membrane will shrink to normal. Frequently, however, the sinusitis becomes chronic, wherein there will be more or less continuous local pain or discomfort, tenderness on pressure over the affected sinus area, and a mild discharge from the nose.

Treatment

For an acute sinus attack with severe pain and fever, the patient should be put to bed and treated as described for a Common Cold (See p. 225.) To help relieve discomfort or pain, hot, moist compresses or a hot water bag should be applied over the forehead, nose, and cheeks. Unless symptoms develop that indicate a serious disease, the treatment is symptomatic and anti-infectives such as antibiotics are inadvisable.

If sinusitis continues or recurs frequently, the patient should be advised to consult a physician at the first convenient port.

SORE THROAT

A common complaint, sore throat may be only local or it may be part of a serious illness. Laryngitis (inflammation of the voice box), tonsillitis (inflammation of the tonsils), and an abscess in the tissues of the tonsillar area are examples of localized throat conditions. Diphtheritic and streptococcal sore throat are examples with marked systemic effects. Streptococcal sore throat resembles scarlet fever but differs clinically in the absence of a skin rash.

Pharyngitis and tonsillitis are common causes of sore throat and frequently accompany an ordinary head cold. Pharyngitis may result from excessive use of the voice; too much tobacco or alcohol, or mouth breathing.

Pharyngitis may be part of an acute disease, such as influenza, scarlet fever or measles. If caused by a streptococcus, the resulting "strep" or septic sore throat may be very sore, with high fever and prostration.

Tonsillitis may lead to an abscess of the tonsil. This condition is indicated by swelling on one side of the back of the throat, great pain, and difficulty in opening the mouth and in swallowing. These symptoms are relieved immediately when the abscess breaks, which reduces pressure and pus drains into the throat.

To inspect the throat, a good light should be used with a tongue depressor (or the handle of a spoon) to hold the tongue down. Views will be needed of the tonsils to the right and left, and of the back wall of the pharynx. If the tonsils are reddened, irritated-looking and enlarged, tonsillitis or pharyngitis is present. Small sores on the tonsils will indicate only a simple tonsillitis. If the sores are covered with a grayish membrane and are difficult to swab off, the condition may be diphtheria. If a tonsil is greatly swollen and red, it may contain pus and the condition may be a peritonsillar abscess.

Sore throat often begins with fever, malaise, headache, muscle pains, and a slight chill or chilly feeling. The throat feels sore, particularly on swallowing. Within a few hours the tonsils and throat are swollen, red, and the tongue is coated. If inflammation progresses sufficiently, swallowing will be difficult.

If a peritonsillar abscess develops, the pain will be acute and knifelike on the affected side.

If the infection is a "strep" throat, fever and prostration will be severe and the patient will be very sick.

Treatment

For simple tonsillitis or sore throat, gargling with warm saltwater (a teaspoonful to a pint) every three hours may be all that is needed. Smoking should not be permitted. The patient with fever should be on bed rest. An ice bag or cold compress applied to the neck may be comforting, as will be pieces of cracked ice for the patient to suck. For pain, aspirin 600 mg should be given by mouth every three to four hours as needed. If aspirin is not well tolerated by the patient, acetaminophen may be tried at the same dosage and frequency. Liquids should be given freely. A liquid or soft diet is allowed.

For a suspected "strep" throat, an initial dose of penicillin V potassium 500 mg should be given by mouth followed by 250 mg every six hours for ten days. If the patient is suspected of being allergic to penicillin, oral erythromycin 250 mg should be given every six hours for the full ten day course. *Medical advice by radio should be obtained before the patient is given antibiotics.*

TUBERCULOSIS (TB, Consumption)

This infectious disease is caused by the tubercle bacillus. Although the lung (pulmonary) disease is the most common, TB bacteria may attack other tissues in the body: bones, joints, glands, or kidneys. Unlike most contagious diseases, tuberculosis usually takes considerable time to develop, often involving repeated, close, and prolonged exposures to a patient with the active disease. A healthy body usually is able to control the tubercle bacilli, unless the invasion is overwhelming or the disease resistance is low from chronic alcoholism, poor nutrition, or another weakening condition.

The pulmonary form of the disease is spread most often by coughing and sneezing.

A person may have tuberculosis for a long time before it is detected. Symptoms may consist of nothing more than a persistent cough, slight loss of weight, night sweats, and a continual "all-in" or "tired-out" feeling that persists when there is no good reason for it. More definitive signs pointing to tuberculosis are a cough that persists for more than a month, raising sputum with each cough, spitting of a teaspoonful or more of blood, persistent or recurring pains in the chest, and afternoon rises in temperature.

When he reaches a convenient port, a seaman with one or more of these warning signs should see a physician.

Treatment

Every effort should be made to prevent a man who has active tuberculosis from going to sea. He is a risk to the crew's health as well as his own. At sea, anyone with definitive signs of tuberculosis must be isolated if he is coughing and raising sputum.

The treatment of tuberculosis by medications usually will not be started at sea. This is not emergency treatment.

To prevent spread, the patient should spit into disposable tissues. The patient should hold disposable tissues over his mouth and nose when coughing or sneezing and place them into a paper bag. Used cups and paper bags should be disposed of in an appropriate sanitary manner. (See Isolation Technique, p. 321.)

The medical attendant should follow good nursing isolation techniques. The patient's bed-clothes, eating utensils, and personal clothing should be handled in the usual way without special procedures.

Tuberculosis Control

A tuberculosis control program has three objectives: (1) to keep diseased individuals from signing-on the vessel, (2) to locate those who may have developed the disease while aboard ship and initiate treatment, and (3) to give preventive treatment to persons at high risk of developing the active disease. The first objective can be achieved by periodic, thorough physical examinations that include chest X-rays and tuberculin skin testing.

To locate those who might have developed active tuberculosis, when in port a chest X-ray should be taken and a medical evaluation requested if a crew member develops symptoms of a chest cold that persist for more than two weeks.

Also, when any active disease is discovered, an intensive study should be made to detect a possible spread among close associates of the patient and others in prolonged contact with him. Such persons are regarded as contacts and are considered at risk of the disease. The tuberculin skin test is a major tool in detecting incipient tuberculosis. Those with positive tuberculin reactions should have a chest X-ray taken. If the chest X-ray shows no disease, preventive treatment with isoniazid may be prescribed.

Chapter V
Treatment of Diseases

Section J
DISEASES OF THE SKIN

RASHES OF SUDDEN ONSET

A VARIETY OF DISORDERS may show a generalized rash, or a local rash that spreads rapidly to become generalized. These can be very frightening, both because of the explosive onset and the widespread involvement. The patient may have several other symptoms as generalized itching, chills, fever, muscle aches, and joint pains. However, a patient may feel perfectly fine and still be totally covered with skin lesions. Such patients should be isolated until the cause is determined because a generalized rash can be due to a contagious infection.

Some of these generalized rashes may be clinically typical and easy to recognize if the examiner is familiar with the disease. At times, it is impossible to differentiate among some of these diseases. *Generalized rashes of sudden onset usually are due either to an allergic reaction or to an infection.* Often an infection is treated with medicines to which a patient may show an allergic reaction, as a rash.

Allergic reactions, can be secondary to any foreign material introduced into the body, either by mouth, by injection, or by inhalation. (See Allergic Reactions, p. 220.) Potentially offending agents to be considered include: all oral or injectable medications, as antibiotics, tranquilizers, analgesics, mood-altering drugs, insulin; many foods, as nuts and shellfish; and inhalants (fumes from paints or solvents, marijuana, smoke). The rash can begin at any time within minutes to a few weeks after being exposed to the offending agent.

The clinical picture may vary widely, the most typical appearance being that of a red rash with some parts elevated and others flat. A vivid red color is distinctive when present. This clinical picture usually is not associated with lesions within the mouth. Less commonly, such eruptions may look like an eczematous dermatitis, (see Eczema, p. 237), hives, bull's-eye-like lesions, or blisters of all sizes. Unless the rash has been present for a long time, lymph nodes usually are not enlarged.

Many infections commonly viral in origin appear as generalized rashes. In general, viral exanthems (diffuse skin rashes caused by viral infections) are associated with a preceding illness. The rashes can follow an upper respiratory infection, as cough, runny nose, and sore throat; or gastrointestinal symptoms, as abdominal pains, vomiting, and diarrhea. These viral exanthems may be "nonspecific," and not conform to any typical clinical picture, or "specific," as the characteristic viral infections of measles, German measles, chickenpox, or smallpox. (See descriptions of other specific viral diseases.)

Most generalized rashes caused by infections come under the category of *non-specific viral exanthems*. These rashes usually start in the head and neck area and gradually move down to cover the rest of the body. The surface of the lesions is smooth and scales are not formed. If associated with an upper respiratory illness, the lymph glands in the neck may be tender and enlarged. Also, the tongue may seem smooth and red, and red dots often can be seen on the roof of the mouth. The entire rash may last five to ten days.

Other rashes from generalized infections may result from scarlet fever, Rocky Mountain spotted fever, the secondary stage of syphilis, and pityriasis rosea:

• *Scarlet fever* usually follows a strep throat bacterial infection. The skin assumes a diffuse pink color, which feels like fine sandpaper to the touch. As the rash resolves, the skin peels.

• *Rocky Mountain spotted fever* begins about the wrists and ankles with hive-like lesions that rapidly assume a purple color in the center. Patients are toxic, with severe headache and high temperatures.

• Although *secondary syphilis* may be generalized, the individual lesions remain discrete, and almost never blend with one another. The lesions are round to oval patches which may

have a surface scale on top. The palms and soles are characteristically involved. The lymph glands are typically enlarged and if itching occurs, it is very mild.

• *Pityriasis rosea* may be of viral origin, although its cause is not definitely known. The skin lesions may look exactly like those of secondary syphilis described above. However, lymph nodes are not enlarged, the palms and soles are not involved, and itching, which usually is present, may be severe at times. Pityriasis rosea may begin with a single large round patch before the rest of the rash appears. The rash spontaneously disappears in one or two months.

SKIN INFECTIONS (Pyodermas)

Bacterial infections of the skin (pyodermas) differ from each other in location and in the depth and severity of skin involvement. Some of these conditions are associated with poor hygiene or tend to occur in individuals with lowered body resistance due to a chronic condition. Any person with recurrent skin infections should be referred to a physician for a complete physical examination and a laboratory study. The milder forms of pyoderma, as folliculitis (see p. 238), may be precipitated by exposure to skin irritants, as industrial oils and solvents. The pustules and small cystic lesions of acne may resemble some of the pyodermas. Trauma to the skin from cuts, abrasions, or insect bites also may predispose an individual to skin infection.

CONTACT DERMATITIS

Reactions of the skin to external agents may be due to a reaction to harsh chemicals; or an allergy to poison ivy, foods, or drugs. These reactions may occur on the first exposure to the substance or not until the exposure has continued for a long period of time. In addition to chemicals as hydrazine, other contactants that may be encountered at sea include shoes, metals, cleaning agents, cashew nut shell oil, fuel or other oils, and solvents, among others. The location of the involved skin often is a clue to discovering the correct offending agent.

As in eczema, itching nearly always is present, and the eruption may occur in either an acute or a chronic form. *Acute contact dermatitis* exhibits redness, swelling, and blisters. The blisters may vary from pinhead size to inches in diameter. The blister fluid is clear and straw-colored, which on drying crusts where the intact blisters originally were present. If the blister fluid assumes the color and consistency of pus, this may represent a secondary bacterial infection. *Chronic low-grade contact dermatitis* may appear as only slight redness and scaling with some scratch marks or superficial cracks (fissures) in the skin. (See Fig. 5-1.)

Treatment

The patient should be removed from the area where contact occurred with the offending agent. For itching, diphenhydramine hydrochloride 25 mg should be given by mouth four times a day. Because this medication may induce drowsiness as a side effect, all precision work, potentially hazardous work, or standing watch should be curtailed for the patient. Cool compresses of aluminum acetate solution (two powder packets to 500 ml of water) should be applied to the area. (See Eczema, p. 237.) During the acute stage calamine lotion should be used after the compresses. This latter treatment will speed the drying of the blisters. When the lesions begin to subside, the calamine lotion may be replaced by hydrocortisone ointment 1%, rubbed sparingly three times daily into the affected areas. If there is secondary bacterial infection, it should be treated as described under Eczema.

Chronic contact dermatitis without blisters should be treated with small quantities of hydrocortisone ointment 1% well-rubbed into the affected areas three times a day. White petrolatum should be applied as necessary to keep the involved skin well lubricated.

Severe contact dermatitis with massive swelling or widespread involvement may be treated in the acute stage with baths to which a cup of oatmeal or cornstarch has been added. Large doses of diphenhydramine hydrochloride may be needed for symptomatic relief. Because this medication may produce drowsiness as a

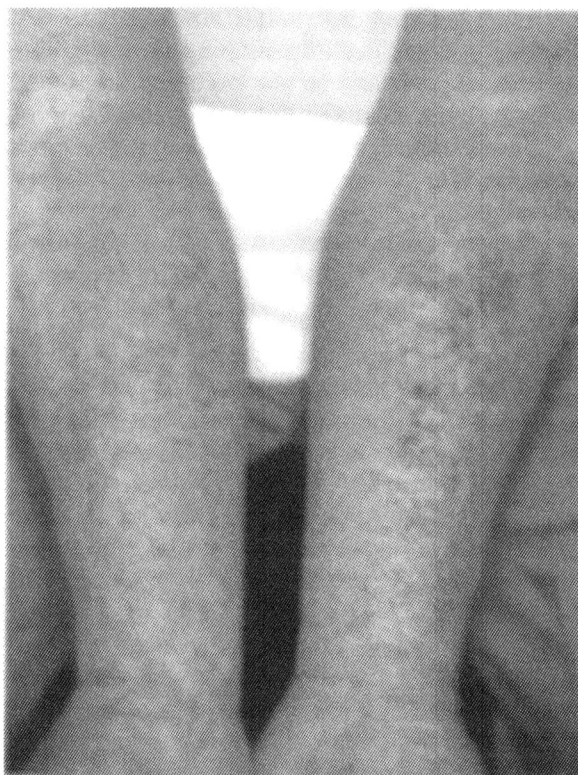

Fig. 5–1. Contact dermatitis.

side effect, the patient should avoid or curtail precision work, potentially hazardous work, or standing watch. To control inflammation and swelling until the patient can be transferred to a medical facility, it may be necessary to give hydrocortisone sodium succinate 100 mg by intramuscular injection. *Medical advice by radio should be obtained* to determine the dose of diphenhydramine hydrochloride and the need for the hydrocortisone sodium succinate by intramuscular injection. Prompt evacuation to a medical facility may be indicated.

BOILS (Furuncles) and CARBUNCLES

Whereas folliculitis (see p. 238) resembles small pimples around hair follicles, boils and carbuncles show deeper and more severe skin involvement. A *furuncle or boil* is a localized, painful, red swelling of skin and deeper tissue around one follicle. As the lesion progresses, it tends to point at the surface and discharge pus when heat is applied in the form of hot compresses. A *carbuncle* is a similar process involving several hair follicles with several draining points. Both furuncles and carbuncles are painful and may be accompanied by tender swollen glands near the site of infection. Fever, chills, and other signs of serious generalized infection will be present if septicemia (blood poisoning) is a complication. The degree of generalized involvement with serious symptoms depends on the affected individual's ability to fight the infection.

As with any inflammation, white blood cells accumulate in the infected area and ingest the bacteria. Sometimes the white cells kill off the bacteria early in the development of a pimple or boil and the inflammation subsides without coming to a head. If the white cells are somewhat less successful, a wall of success-fully-resisting body cells is built up around the boil. The tissue in the center of the boil then breaks down, and together with the bacteria and white blood cells form the yellowish-white center or core of the boil. This dead matter may be absorbed if the pimple or boil is small or it may break through the skin and discharge itself. Boils at this early stage *never* should be squeezed or drained as this may interfere with the body's ability to resist the infection and cause bacteria to enter the blood-stream. *The boil may be opened by the attendant only after it comes to a head.*

Treatment

The same treatment applies to both boils and carbuncles although the latter are considered more serious infections. Initially, when the lesion appears as a red hard swelling, hot water compresses made from clean white washcloths or torn white sheets should be applied to the involved skin areas for 15 minutes. Hot saline solution (two level teaspoonfuls of table salt to 1000 ml of water) can be used for the compresses. The temperature of the compresses should *not* be so hot that they burn the patient's skin. If the compresses cannot be handled comfortably by the attendant, then they are too hot for the patient. Bacitracin ointment should be applied to the lesions following the compresses.

When the boil comes to a head with a white spot at the center, it may be incised and drained. First the skin should be cleansed with rubbing alcohol. Then, the tip of a sterile

knife blade or needle should be inserted into the white center of the boil so that pus is discharged. As long as there is drainage of pus, skin lesions should be covered loosely with sterile gauze squares. Otherwise the lesions may be left open to the air.

Folliculitis, boils, or carbuncles on or around the nose, nostrils, and on the lips should *not* be opened, except by a physician. There is always the danger of extension of the infection to the brain with serious consequences, even death. These lesions should be allowed to discharge spontaneously.

In addition to local therapy, treatment with systemic antibiotics should be given for boils if local treatment fails, the lesions are multiple or large, or there is associated fever. Treatment with systemic antibiotics is recommended for all cases of carbuncles; even if single these are serious infections, which are difficult to cure with topical therapy. Erythromycin 500 mg should be given by mouth four times daily for ten days. If the patient has systemic symptoms such as malaise, nausea, or fever, he should be on bed rest along with ample fluid intake. For pain, aspirin 600 mg should be given by mouth every three to four hours as needed. If aspirin is not well tolerated by the patient, acetaminophen may be tried at the same dosage and frequency.

CELLULITIS

Cellulitis is another infection of the skin and deeper underlying tissue caused by staphylococci, streptococci, and occasionally other bacteria. It often begins after a wound injury to the skin followed by redness, swelling, and tenderness of the area. The margins of skin involvement are flat and usually ill-defined. Cellulitis has a tendency to spread and may involve lymphatic vessels resulting in red streaking of an area which sometimes precedes septicemia (blood poisoning). In severe cellulitis, signs of systemic infection such as malaise, chills, and fever are present.

Treatment

Treatment for cellulitis includes bed rest, elevation of the affected part, and warm soaks four or five times daily, for 15 to 30 minute periods. Antibacterial therapy for ten days should be given as outlined previously for carbuncles.

ECZEMA (Atopic Dermatitis)

Eczema is a common, noncommunicable inflammation of the skin, usually seen in individuals with a personal or family history of eczema, asthma, or hay fever. It occurs most commonly in children and adolescents, but may persist or become reactivated in adults. Factors that provoke eczema include infections, emotional stress, and allergic reactions.

Patients with eczema invariably complain of itching that at times may be severe. Changes on the skin may be either acute or chronic. Acute changes (seen more often in children) usually begin with redness and oozing that result in moist and crusted lesions. Itching leads to scratching so that scratch marks and secondary bacterial infection are common. Although eczema may affect any part or all of the body, favored sites include the wrists, front of elbows, and back of knees.

As the eczema becomes more chronic, the skin becomes thickened and leathery, with darkening in color of the affected areas, and the itching and scratch marks persisting. Secondary infection also may complicate chronic eczema.

Treatment

It is very important to reduce the itching. This can be accomplished by giving diphenhydramine hydrochloride 25 to 75 mg by mouth every four to six hours, as needed. Because this medication may induce drowsiness as a side effect, all precision work, potentially hazardous work, or standing watch should be curtailed for the patient. At bedtime the dose of diphenhydramine hydrochloride should be increased to 100 mg to help induce sleep and reduce itching.

During the acute stage, oozing can be suppressed with compresses made by soaking clean soft cloths in cool aluminum acetate solution (two powder packets to 500 ml of water) and applying them for 15 minutes three times daily. To help relieve the inflammation, hydrocortisone ointment 1% should be applied sparingly and rubbed in well after each compressing. When oozing subsides and in chronic eczema,

hydrocortisone ointment can be continued for persistent redness and itchiness. A hand and body cream may be applied.

When mild secondary infection is present, bacitracin ointment can be applied three times daily in addition to the above topical treatment. More severe infection usually requires treatment with erythromycin 250 mg by mouth four times daily for ten days. Medical advice by radio should be obtained.

HAND ECZEMA
(Chronic Hand Dermatitis)

Hand eczema is mentioned separately because it often shows up as a localized form of an eczematous dermatitis. It can exhibit the same clinical appearance despite having a wide variety of causes. It may be the only manifestation of eczema, contact dermatitis, or even an allergy to an inflammation elsewhere, especially a fungal infection (ringworm, athlete's foot) of the bottom of the feet. Seemingly insignificant but frequent exposures to soaps and detergents or chronic immersion in water alone may result in a chronic hand dermatitis. Interference with performance of duties may result.

Acute changes usually are absent and itching may be mild or absent. Often the hands are reddened slightly, scaly, and may have deep, painful fissures.

Treatment

If possible, for hand eczema the patient should be removed from the source of irritation. Hydrocortisone ointment 1% should be applied sparingly and thoroughly rubbed in four to six times a day. When the need for treatment with hydrocortisone ointment lessens, white petrolatum should be applied so that the hand will be kept lubricated at all times.

ERYSIPELAS (St. Anthony's Fire)

The term erysipelas comes from two Greek words meaning red skin. The infection is a type of superficial cellulitis caused by specific bacteria (streptococci). There is marked involvement of lymphatic vessels. Erysipelas may develop in skin injured by scratches, abrasions, or other wounds, and in apparently normal skin by the seeding of bacteria usually from the nose or upper respiratory tract. Most often the onset is sudden with chills, fever, headache, occasional nausea and vomiting, rapid pulse, and a typical local skin inflammation usually on the face (especially nose and cheeks). However, erysipelas may appear on other parts of the body usually when related to wound injury. The affected skin area is painful, red, hot, and swollen. Unlike cellulitis, the lesion has a sharply defined elevated advancing border. The surface of the patch is at first smooth and shiny and later becomes covered with small blisters.

Treatment

Prompt treatment of erysipelas is necessary because the disease can lead to serious complications as abcesses, even death.

Initially for the infection, 500 mg penicillin V potassium should be given by mouth on an empty stomach, followed by 250 mg also by mouth every six hours for ten days. If the patient is allergic to penicillin, erythromycin 500 mg can be given by mouth every six hours for four days, followed by 250 mg every six hours for six more days.

Local treatment of the inflamed area consists of continuous warm soaks of saline solution (two level teaspoonfuls of table salt to 1000 ml of water) applied for 20 minutes at a time to the involved area every three to four hours.

FOLLICULITIS

Folliculitis is a superficial infection around the hair follicles usually caused by staphylococci strains of pus-forming bacteria. It is seen as redness around single or multiple hair follicles with progression to small red bumps within which pus develops. In addition to the face, especially the beard area, most often the extensor aspects of the body are involved, as the front of the legs and backs of arms.

Treatment

Treatment of folliculitis includes cleansing of the involved areas several times daily with a surgical detergent such as povidone-iodine. Skin irritants, as chemicals and oils, and friction from tightly fitting clothing should be avoided. Bacitracin ointment may be applied two or three times daily. However, as ointments are sometimes poorly tolerated, a drying lotion such as calamine lotion may be beneficial. Pricking the individual pustules with a sterile needle may hasten the clearing of lesions.

If the folliculitis is extensive or gives evidence of being resistant, treatment with a systemic antibiotic is indicated. Erythromycin 250 mg by mouth every six hours for ten days may be used.

HEAT RASH (Prickly Heat, Miliaria)

During hot humid weather heat rash may occur at sea. The rash will appear during any activity that produces sweating while exposed to heat (as in the engine room) or during a feverish illness while confined to bed. Although noncontagious, it may occur in multiple individuals if all were exposed to the same precipitating environment. The problem is caused by a blockage of the sweat glands.

Itching usually is present and may vary from mild to severe. The rash occurs mainly on the trunk and neck, but may be seen on any body area where constant friction or pressure play a role. The lesions consist of blotchy redness with tiny bumps and small blisters. A more mild asymptomatic form may occur in which very small clear blisters are the only lesions, similar to the tiny bubbles seen just before a sunburn peels.

Treatment

Most important for heat rash is removal of the patient as soon as possible from the offending environment to a cool dry location. Frequent soothing baths made with one cupful of cornstarch to a tub of water is helpful, followed by a rubdown with rubbing alcohol, and when dry, an application of talc. Application of various creams or ointments should be avoided as this might aggravate the condition. Severe itching can be suppressed with diphenhydramine hydrochloride 50 mg by mouth every four to six hours. Because this medication may produce drowsiness as a side effect, precision work, potentially hazardous work, or standing watch should be curtailed while the patient is receiving the medication.

HERPES SIMPLEX TYPE 1
(Cold Sores or Fever Blisters and
Herpes Keratitis)

Herpes simplex type 1 is an acute viral infection of the face that may occur on any area of the skin or mucous membranes. Once the initial episode occurs, it is presumed that the virus remains in a dormant state in the infected area and may be reactivated by a variety of excitants (as fever, trauma, exposure to sunlight, menstruation, or stress). Herpes simplex type 1 lesions most commonly occur on the lips, as cold sores or fever blisters. Also, it causes *ophthalmic herpes keratitis* (see p. 145), an eye infection that is responsible for several thousand cases of blindness annually in the United States.

Involvement of the genitalia is also seen with increasing frequency because of orogenital sexual activity. (The next section refers to herpes simplex type 2 that infects the genitals.) Because of the contagiousness of the disorder, direct contact (sexual or nonsexual) easily can transfer the infection to another person.

The eruption often is accompanied by an itching or burning sensation localized to the area of involvement. The infection appears the same whether localized on the lips or elsewhere. The lesions either begin singly or as a cluster of clear blisters, surrounded by a halo of redness. The blisters become cloudy, often developing a central dimple, ulcerate within 48 hours, and eventually crust-over before healing. Lesions in moist areas, as the mouth, tend to lose the roofs of the blisters, leaving shallow circular erosions that crust and heal. Lymph glands nearest the infection may react by becoming swollen and tender.

Herpes simplex sometimes is found on the fingers. When caring for patients with cold sores or fever blisters, attendants are cautioned to wear rubber gloves to protect the fingers from direct contact with lesions and possible infection by the type 1 virus.

Treatment

There are no medications known now that can cure recurrent herpes simplex infections. For symptomatic relief, compressing is recommended for the infected area, using a washcloth soaked in aluminum acetate solution (two packets to 500 ml of water) for 15 minute periods four times daily. Between periods of compressing, the lesions should be dabbed with 70% of rubbing alcohol to help the blisters clear up more quickly. On reaching shore, the patient should consult a physician.

HERPES SIMPLEX TYPE 2
(Genital Organs)

Genital herpes is a venereal disease caused by the herpes simplex type 2 virus. It was estimated to be the second most prevalent form of VD in the United States in 1976. (See p. 248.)

HERPES ZOSTER (Shingles)

Shingles is an acute viral infection caused by the same virus that causes chickenpox. The disease probably can be contracted by exposure to a patient with either shingles or chickenpox. The infection involves only one cranial or spinal nerve on one side of the body. This gives rise to two prominent characteristics of this disease: (1) because nerves are involved, the patient often experiences localized itching and/or severe pain; and (2) because only one nerve root is involved, skin lesions appear only in the areas supplied by the one nerve. Therefore, lesions occur in a very localized segmental distribution on only one side of the body. The occurrence of shingles of the eye or tissues around the eye is a serious problem that requires early medical attention. Occasionally, herpes zoster may become generalized, recognizable by the appearance of blisters disseminated widely on the skin surface. This complication requires evacuation of the patient to a medical facility.

Pain usually is present. It may be severe enough to mimic acute abdominal colic or even a heart attack. As in herpes simplex, clear blisters crop up in groups that become cloudy, then dimpled, and finally crust before healing. The blistered areas are surrounded by a halo of redness. The rash may take several weeks to clear completely, but the pain may persist for months longer.

Treatment

Depending on the patient's response to severe pain, codeine sulfate 30 mg or 60 mg should be given by mouth for shingles. *The attendant should obtain medical advice by radio to continue this medication.* Localized care should include cool compresses of aluminum acetate solution (mix two packets to 500 ml of water) applied for a 15 minute period four times daily. After drying, the entire involved area should be covered with calamine lotion. Also, secondary local bacterial infections should be treated with bacitracin ointment applied four times daily.

HIVES
(Urticaria, Welts, Angio Edema)

Hives are a common problem that result from allergy to a large number of agents. These agents may be either internal or external. Examples of internal causes include infections as hepatitis and mononucleosis; dental abcess; drugs as aspirin, barbituates, antibiotics, and narcotics; foods as shellfish, eggs, strawberries, and nuts; and anxiety states. External agents include insects, jellyfish, and rarely certain chemicals.

Individual lesions of hives usually last for several hours, but new lesions may come and go for a week or longer after a single exposure to the causative agent. Occasionally, hives may persist for months or years if the cause cannot be found.

Hives can occur anywhere on the body and are typically itchy. They show suddenly as pink or white slightly raised bumps, varying in size from a matchhead to large areas of the body. The lesions have a smooth surface and do not develop scales, crusts, or blisters. (See Fig. 5-2.)

In addition to typical hives, swelling may occur on certain body areas, as the hands, feet, lips, or face. Swelling that occurs inside the mouth may obstruct breathing so emergency medical care will be required.

Treatment

A diligent search for the offending agent is necessary, or continued exposure may result in persistent hives. Diphenhydramine hydrochloride, 25 to 75 mg depending on severity and patient response, should be given by mouth every four to six hours to help suppress the

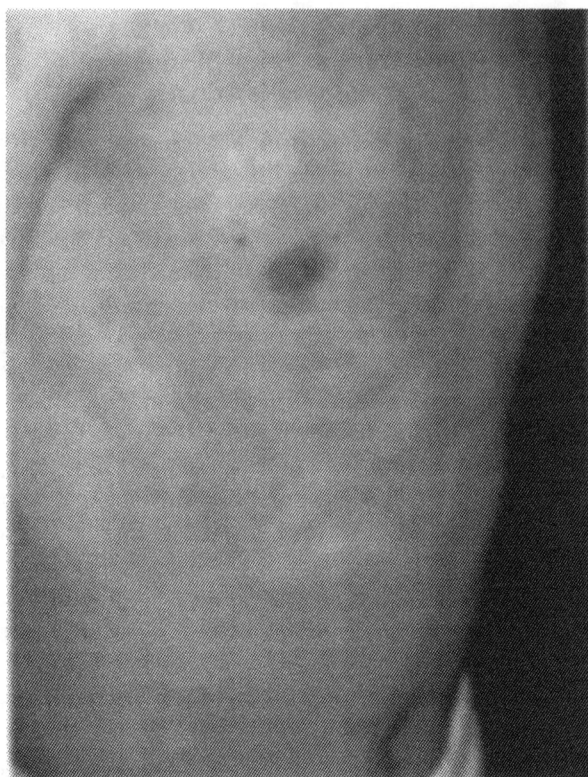

Fig. 5–2. Hives (urticaria).

itching and shorten the course of illness. Drowsiness may result as a side effect of diphenhydramine hydrochloride, so the patient should be excused from standing watch, or doing precision work or potentially hazardous work while receiving the medication.

Severe reactions or oral involvement may require 0.3 to 0.5 ml epinephrine hydrochloride injection 1:1000 to be administered subcutaneously. (See Anaphylactic Reaction, p. 221.)

IMPETIGO

Impetigo is a highly contagious superficial skin infection caused by staphylococcal and streptococcal bacteria. Lesions begin as small red patches which develop blisters on the surface. The blisters may not be noticed, as they quickly rupture and form honey-colored crusts or scabs. As the condition progresses, healing may occur in the center with a surrounding crust that may resemble a ringworm. Because impetigo occurs more commonly on the face or extremities of the body, it may complicate pre-existing skin conditions as eczema or insect bites. If the lesions of impetigo are severe or widespread, generalized symptoms of malaise, fever, and chills may occur.

Untreated impetigo runs a chronic course with new lesions occurring over a period of many weeks. Usually there are no serious complications. Occasionally certain types of bacteria are present that can lead to serious kidney disease. Thus prompt treatment is necessary for all cases of impetigo.

Treatment

Cleanliness is of utmost importance for impetigo. Strict isolation of a patient should be followed until the lesions begin to heal.

The crusts should be removed gently by washing three or four times daily with povidone-iodine cleanser. This should be followed with compresses of warm aluminum acetate solution (mix two packets with 500 ml of water). Once the crusts are removed, bacitracin ointment should be applied after each compressing. If the patient is not allergic, systemic antibiotic treatment should be given with oral penicillin V potassium 250 mg four times daily for a 10 day course. For a patient allergic to penicillin, erythromycin 250 mg should be given by mouth four times daily for 10 days.

If there are systemic symptoms as fever and chills, the patient should be placed at bed rest with ample fluid intake. Aspirin 600 mg should be given by mouth every three to four hours as needed. If aspirin is not well tolerated by the patient, acetaminophen may be tried at the same dosage and frequency.

LICE INFESTATION (Pediculosis)

The head louse, body louse, and pubic louse are three types of small sucking insects that infest man. All three types cause severe skin irritation and itching. Scratching permits germs responsible for impetigo, boils, and carbuncles to invade the body. This secondary bacterial infection is a frequent complication and must be treated in addition to the pediculosis (louse infestation). (See Skin Infections, p. 234.) Poor personal hygiene, unclean clothes or bed linens, and direct contact with an infested person or his belongings favor infestation with lice.

Head Louse Infestation (Pediculosis Capitis)

It usually is difficult to see *Pediculus humanus capitis*, the louse responsible for infestation of the hairy regions of the head. More frequently one finds the eggs or nits that appear as small gray or white sacs firmly attached to scalp hairs. These lice usually stay on the head but may wander to infest other hairy parts.

Treatment

After a bath or shower that includes a shampoo, a thin layer of gamma benzene hexachloride cream 1% should be applied to the entire scalp and left on overnight for about 12 hours. Care should be taken to keep the cream out of the eyes. The patient should shampoo again the following morning. Then a fine-toothed comb should be used to dislodge the nits from the hair. An infested individual should not allow others to use his comb or wear his hat.

Body Louse Infestation (Pediculosis Corporis)

Body lice are a problem because they may transmit diseases such as typhus fever and relapsing fever. These lice (*Pediculus humanus corporis*) usually are not seen on the body as they live in the seams of clothing and attach to the body only when they are feeding. Nits appearing as small grey or white sacs also are seen in the seams of clothing. On examination of the patient the attendant will see scratch marks and bite marks which appear as tiny punctures with encircling redness. Lesions are located mostly on areas where the clothing comes in close contact with the skin, as the shoulders, chest, around the waist, and buttocks.

Treatment

For body lice the infested individual should bathe thoroughly and apply a thin layer of 1% gamma benzene hexachloride cream to the entire body, taking care to avoid getting it into the eyes. Sixty grams (about two ounces) of the medication may be required to cover the body entirely. After leaving the medication on for 24 hours, the patient again should bathe thoroughly and be provided with fresh clothes and bed linens. Clothes may be decontaminated

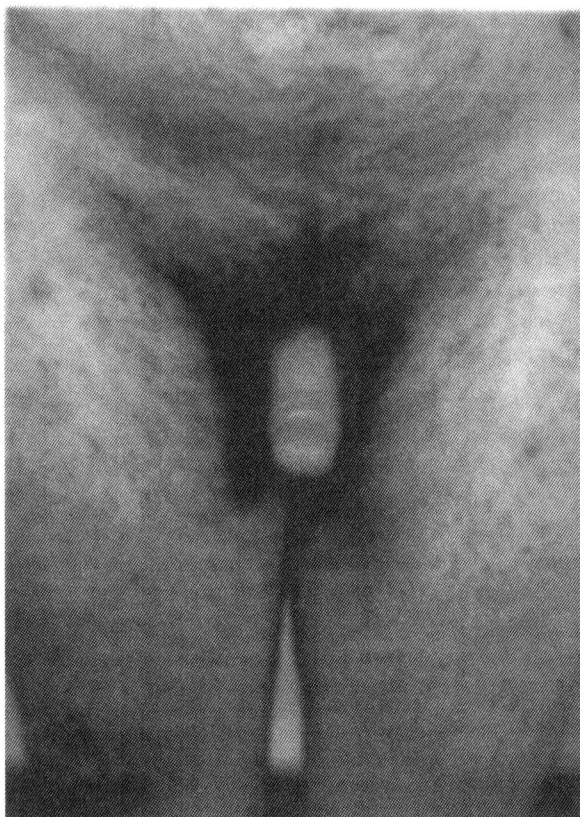

Fig. 5–3. Pubic Louse (*Pediculosis pubis*).

by dry cleaning or by boiling. Preventing re-infestation may be difficult in crowded quarters. A mass delousing may be carried out by blowing 1% malathion (premium grade) powder under the clothing and by treating the garments with steam under pressure.

Pubic Louse Infestation (Pediculosis Pubis)

Pubic lice often are called crab lice because of their flattened crab-like shape. Although *Phthirus pubis* (crab louse species) usually infests the coarse hairs of the pubic region, they may be found on the lower abdomen, in the armpits, on the chest of a hairy individual, and even in the eyebrows. This type of pediculosis may be transmitted by sexual intercourse, or from contact with toilet seats, clothing, and bedclothes. (See Fig. 5–3.)

On examination of the patient, one usually sees the pale blue–gray bite marks on the skin, or the eggs appearing as gray or white sacs attached to the skin at the base of the pubic hairs. The crab lice are almost transparent and difficult to detect.

Treatment

To eliminate pubic lice and their nits, the infested individual should bathe thoroughly and apply a thin layer of 1% gamma benzene hexachloride cream to the pubic area and other parts involved. After leaving the medication on for 24 hours, the patient again should bathe thoroughly and be provided with fresh clothes and bed linens. The medication never should be applied about the eyelids or eyelashes. Appropriate measures to decontaminate clothing and living quarters, toilets, and bunks should be carried out as described under body louse.

PARONYCHIA
(Infection of the Nail Fold)

A paronychia is an infection of a nail fold, usually on a finger, marked by redness, pain, and swelling that leads to a discharge of pus. The acute paronychias of sudden onset usually are caused by bacteria such as staphylococci or streptococci that enter a small cut or scratch around the nail. The chronic paronychias more commonly are caused by a yeast (*Candida*) infection that tends to occur in individuals, as dishwashers who immerse their hands in water for long periods of time.

Treatment

Paronychia infections should be treated with warm soaks of aluminum acetate solution (using two packets to 500 ml of water) for 20 minutes three to four times daily. Incision and drainage is indicated when the lesion points to discharge pus, as with boils. (See p. 235.) An antibiotic ointment such as bacitracin should be applied between soaks. If fever or swollen painful glands are present in the armpits, systemic antibiotic treatment with erythromycin 250 mg by mouth four times daily for seven to ten days should be given. Care should be taken to avoid injury to the affected finger and to prevent unnecessary or prolonged contact with water or other liquids. If the paronychia does not respond to the above measures and becomes chronic, the patient should be referred to a skin clinic for more specific therapy when on shore leave. Dishwashers and other food service workers should be excused from food preparation until the lesions have healed.

RINGWORM FUNGI
(Dermatophytoses)

Ringworm fungi or dermatophytes are plant organisms that grow in the uppermost layer of the skin and cause infections of the skin, hair, and nails. The clinical picture of ringworm varies widely and depends both on the part of the body affected and the causative fungus. The presence of secondary bacterial infection or the development of an allergic reaction to the fungus may further modify the clinical appearance. Almost everyone is exposed to these fungi at some time or another. However, actual infection is uncommon and is influenced by many factors as: geographic area; local climatic conditions favoring fungal growth as warmth, moisture, and darkness; injury or trauma to the skin; individual predisposition; and the presence of other medical conditions which may lower resistance.

Many other skin diseases resemble ringworm. The exact diagnosis is made by identifying the fungus under the microscope and/or growing it in culture.

Treatment

Treatment of ringworm fungus consists of simple local therapy which may be given until an exact diagnosis can be made in port by a physician who will prescribe further treatment.

Ringworm of Scalp (Tinea Capitis)

Ringworm of the scalp is more commonly seen in children. Lesions occur as round, scaly patches showing hairs broken off close to the base, and sometimes black dots. The *inflammatory type*, which shows varying degrees of swelling, redness, and pustules, usually heals with considerable scarring and permanent hair loss.

Favus is another type of ringworm of the scalp, sometimes showing a honeycomb-like crusting with a mousy odor. It is common in some countries, especially in eastern Europe and western Asia. Seamen going ashore in these areas should avoid close contact with persons who appear to have scalp disease.

Treatment

Until the patient with ringworm of the scalp can be seen by a physician, local therapy should be given. The scalp should be shampooed daily. The infected hairs should be clipped closely and properly disposed of. The scissors may be sterilized by boiling. A topical antifungal preparation as benzoic and salicylic acids ointment should be applied two or three times daily to the entire scalp, especially the involved areas. In cases of marked inflammation and crusting with pustules, lukewarm compresses with aluminum acetate solution (using two packets to 500 ml of water) should be applied for 15 minutes three times daily. For any secondary bacterial infection or pustular scalp disease, antibiotic therapy should be prescribed as erythromycin 250 mg by mouth four times daily for ten days.

Ringworm of Nails (Onychomycosis)

This ringworm condition involves toenails more often than fingernails. Initially there is a white or yellow discoloration along the lateral margins of the nails. The nails become progressively more discolored, elevated, thickened, and fragmented.

Treatment

Onychomycosis is very difficult to treat. Local therapy of limited usefulness may be given with 1% tolnaftate solution applied sparingly two or three times daily until the patient sees a physician. The nails should be kept closely trimmed.

Ringworm of Bearded Area (Tinea Barbae) or Barber's Itch

Lesions may resemble those in ringworm of the body or scalp. There may be round scaly plaques that tend to clear centrally, or more inflammatory lesions with redness, pustules, and broken-off hairs.

Treatment

For barber's itch topical therapy with benzoic and salicylic acids ointment, or 1% tolnaftate solution three times daily may be given until the patient sees a physician. In more acute cases with considerable crusting, wet compresses with aluminum acetate solution (two packets to 500 ml of water) should be applied several times daily.

If there is much pus and crusting, or if the patient has systemic signs of secondary bacterial infection with fever and malaise, treatment should be given with erythromycin 250 mg by mouth four times daily for seven days or according to medical advice by radio. Proper hygiene includes washing the face and other involved areas once or twice daily with liquid povidone-iodine cleanser or similar surgical soap. A person with barber's itch should not permit anyone to use his shaving materials.

Ringworm of Groin (Tinea Cruris) and Armpits

This common condition seen in one or both groin areas is aggravated by sweating, increased temperature, friction from rubbing of the legs, or tightly fitting clothing. Lesions appear as red or brown scaly plaques with sharply outlined borders often showing small red bumps or blisters.

Treatment

In acute cases there may be considerable weeping from the lesions, so cool compresses with aluminum acetate solution (two packets to 500 ml of water) should be applied for 15

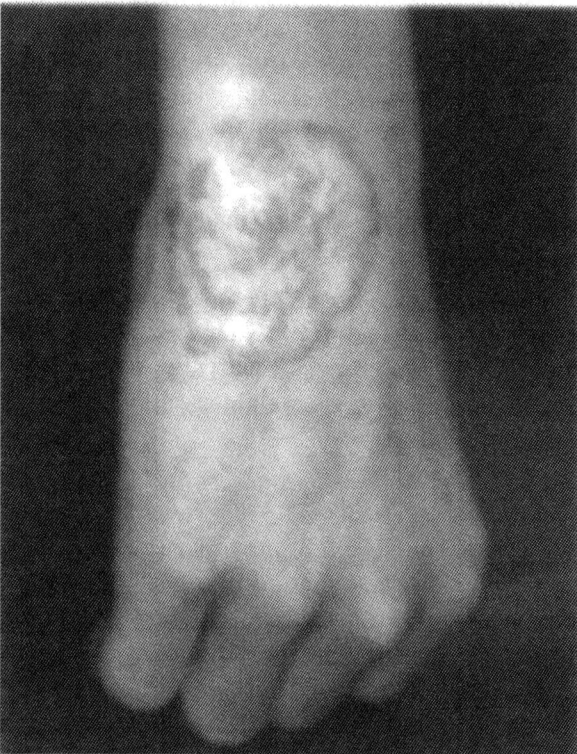

Fig. 5–4. Ringworm (Tinea corporis).

minutes three or four times daily. When the acute inflammation has subsided, the area should be treated three times daily with 1% tolnaftate powder. A yeast infection caused by *Candida* may resemble tinea cruris but will not respond to tolnaftate. (See p. 233.) While in port, the patient should be referred to a physician for specific treatment.

Ringworm of General Body Surface (Tinea Corporis)

Tinea Corporis which involves the trunk and upper extremities is not common in temperate climates. It occurs as one to several large or small round scaly plaques on the body, often showing minute blisters on the surface. (See Fig. 5–4.) The lesions tend to show central clearing with extension at the margins. This condition sometimes can be spread from the infected fur of dogs or cats to man.

Treatment

Until the patient can see a physician, local therapy is of limited usefulness. Benzoic and salicylic acids ointment or 1% tolnaftate solution may be applied sparingly to the body area three times daily.

Ringworm of Feet (Tinea Pedis) or Athlete's Foot

Ringworm of the feet is a very common condition which usually begins in the webs of toes especially between the fourth and little toe. One or both feet may be affected. The involved skin areas show redness with moist whitish scaling, often with cracks or fissures and raw areas. The condition may spread onto the soles and appear as red patches with scaling and deep-seated blisters.

Treatment

In all cases of ringworm it is important after bathing to dry the feet thoroughly especially between the toes. In mild cases, 1% tolnaftate solution should be applied sparingly two to three times daily and tolnaftate powder 1% sprinkled into the socks. If possible, the patient should wear open-toed sandals with thin socks or preferably no socks.

In more acute ringworm conditions where there is considerable swelling, redness and weeping, the feet should be soaked in cool aluminum acetate solution (using two packets to 500 ml of water) for 15 minutes followed by the application of bacitracin ointment three times daily. If cellulitis is a complication, this should be treated with erythromycin 250 mg by mouth four times a day for five days. When the acute inflammation has subsided, then local therapy with 1% tolnaftate solution or powder may be applied as discussed previously.

Occasionally sensitivity of a section of the skin may be a reaction to a distant focal infection. These reactions often are manifested by small red bumps or blisters on the hands. Fungi are not present in these lesions which subside with treatment of the primary condition.

SCABIES (The Itch)

This highly contagious skin disease is caused by the female mite which burrows into the skin to deposit her eggs. In several days the eggs hatch and the cycle is repeated. Symptoms are severe itching that is worse at night. Scabies is transmitted by close contact with an affected individual or by contaminated bed linens. The characteristic skin finding is the burrow which appears as a short thread-like gray line under the skin. Burrows may not always be evident but scratch marks, scabs, small blisters or red bumps commonly are seen. Lesions tend to occur on the finger webs, wrists, armpits, genitalia, lower buttocks, nipples, umbilicus, but not on the face.

Treatment

For the intense itching of scabies, diphenhydramine hydrochloride 50 mg by mouth should be given three times daily as necessary. Because of possible side effects, as drowsiness or dizziness, a patient receiving diphenhydramine should be excused from working at heights or in the vicinity of dangerous machinery. The patient should take a hot shower with gentle scrubbing to remove any scabs from all involved areas. Then gamma benzene hexachloride cream 1% should be applied in a thin layer to the entire body below the neck. After 24 hours the patient should bathe again, put on clean clothing, and change bed linens. If necessary, one repeat application may be given in four days. The clothing previously worn and all bed linens should be washed. All contacts should be given prophylactic treatment or be checked for the disease at intervals.

Chapter V

Treatment
of
Diseases

Section K

VENEREAL DISEASES

INTRODUCTION

THESE COMMUNICABLE DISEASES, spread chiefly by sexual contact, are listed in order of estimated prevalence: gonorrhea, herpes simplex, syphilis, chancroid, lymphogranuloma venereum, and granuloma inguinale. The greatest number of new infections occurs among young adults. Herpes simplex of the genitals is being seen with increasing frequency today. This increase may be due to self-infection or to greater orogenital sexual activity.

PREVENTION

The best way to escape venereal infection is to abstain from promiscuous sexual intercourse. Many prostitutes have several venereal diseases at the same time—as syphilis with gonorrhea, and either one or both with herpes. Anyone who has sexual relations with casual contacts is more likely to become infected with a venereal disease.

Next to avoidance of promiscuous sexual contacts, protection of the male's penis with a condom during intercourse and careful cleansing afterward are the safest methods of escaping infection. A supply of condoms should be available aboard ship. The condom or rubber is a thin elastic covering that forms a protective sheath over the penis. If properly used, it should prevent infection during intercourse, unless the point of contact with an infective lesion is beyond the area covered by the condom. The condom should be of good quality and new. To prevent tearing or puncturing, the condom should be kept in its original container until used. It should not be kept days or weeks in an inside pocket because body heat and sweat may cause deterioration.

The condom comes rolled or should be rolled before use. It must be placed over the penis before sexual contact. The tip of the condom should be held to form a pocket to receive the ejaculate. The rest of the condom is then unrolled to cover the entire penis. As soon as the male has an orgasm, the penis should be withdrawn from the vagina before it softens, because the condom may loosen and expose the penis to infection. The condom is removed by grasping at the open end with the fingers and pulling it down quickly so that it comes off inside out. The condom should be discarded without further handling because it may contain infectious material. *The man should urinate at once, and immediately wash the genitalia, lower abdomen, and thighs with soap and water* before any bacteria penetrate the skin. The longer that washing is delayed, the less good it will do.

VD IN THE HOMOSEXUAL AND BISEXUAL

In some areas of the United States, there is a high incidence of syphilis among male homosexuals. When examining a homosexual suspected of syphilis, the area surrounding the anus and anal canal must be examined for chancres. The mouth also should be examined closely. (See Fig. 5–5.)

There is a higher incidence of pharyngeal gonorrhea in individuals who practice orogenital sex. Therefore, individuals with homosexual contacts should have a culture made from the pharynx and the rectal area after reaching port.

Treating and interviewing individuals with homosexual contacts must be done in a non-threatening, non-demeaning, and calm fashion.

GONORRHEA (Clap)

Gonorrhea is the most prevalent of the venereal diseases. The infection is caused by the gonococcus bacterium. The usual onset from the time of infection to appearance of symptoms or signs (incubation period) is from two to 14 days after exposure, with an average of three to five days. However, the incubation period may be delayed up to a month. The disease is more easily identified in males than females. Because up to 80 percent of females have no symptoms, a large reservoir of untreated gonorrhea exists. The ordinary symptoms in the male include sudden onset of pain or burning on urination, urgent and frequent urination, and the presence of a white or yellow discharge from the urethra. With these symptoms, a presumptive diagnosis of gonorrhea may be made. A more accurate diagnosis is possible by examining Gram-stained smears of the discharge under the microscope. The organisms appear Gram-negative and occur both inside and outside the white blood cells.

Treatment

If the ship is not more than a day or two from port, it is advisable for the medical attendant to withhold antibiotic treatment for uncomplicated gonorrhea. Instead, the patient should be referred to a physician in port for diagnostic tests and treatment. A crewman

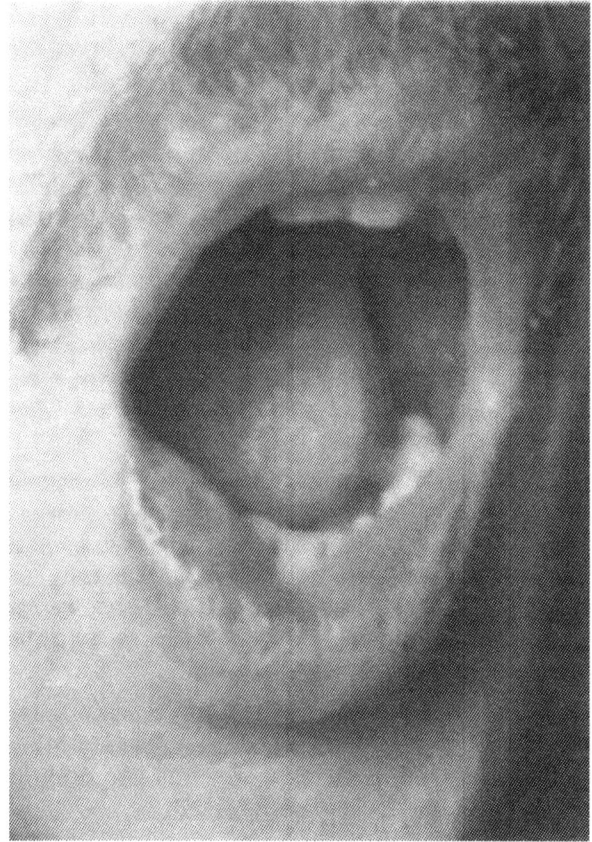

Fig. 5–5. Primary syphilis of the lip.

known to have been exposed to gonorrhea should receive the same treatment as those who have a proven gonorrhea infection.

If the patient is to be treated aboard ship, medical advice by radio should be obtained. For both women and men, the drug of choice is pencillin G procaine in large doses by injection. The patient first should receive one gram of probenecid by mouth. Thirty minutes later, a total of 4.8 million units of penicillin G procaine sterile suspension should be divided into at least two doses and administered intramuscularly at different sites of the buttocks.

An acceptable alternate penicillin treatment for both women and men is ampicillin 3.5 grams (14 capsules of 250 mg) with one gram of probenecid, both administered by mouth at the same time.

When the patient is allergic to penicillin, ampicillin, probenecid, or has had a previous anaphylactic reaction, tetracycline should be given by mouth. The treatment would be tetracycline hydrochloride 1.5 grams (six capsules or tablets of 250 mg) as the first dose, followed by 500 mg four times a day for four days, for a total dosage of nine grams.

All gonorrhea patients who are treated with any drug other than the recommended dosage schedule of procaine penicillin, should have a blood test for syphilis once a month for four months. *If this testing would not be practical, the patient must receive a course of tetracycline hydrochloride or penicillin therapy, which also is adequate to cure syphilis. (See p. 249.) More than one venereal disease may occur together, which may necessitate other or additional treatment.*

Patients who are treated for gonorrhea should have follow-up tests for the disease. From men, follow-up urethral specimens should be obtained seven days after completion of treatment. From women, cervical and rectal specimens should be obtained seven to 14 days after completion of treatment.

Complications of gonorrhea include inflammation of the prostate gland, swollen testicles, urethral stricture, sterility, swollen and painful joints, meningitis and endocarditis.

If the testicles become swollen, the patient should be placed on bed rest with the scrotum supported by a folded towel between the thighs or an adhesive plaster support. An ice bag covered with a towel should be applied. For pain, aspirin 600 mg should be given by mouth every three or four hours as needed. If aspirin is not well tolerated by the patient, acetaminophen may be tried at the same dosage and frequency.

HERPES SIMPLEX TYPE 2
(Male and Female Genitals)

Genital herpes is a sexually transmitted venereal infection that is caused by a virus called *herpes simplex*. Most herpes infections of the genital organs are caused by the type 2 herpes simplex virus. Herpes facial infections (as cold sores and fever blisters on the lips) are usually caused by the type 1 herpes simplex virus. Herpes types 1 and 2 are antigenically different types. Although type 1 usually occurs on the face and type 2 on the genitals, at least 10% of each type are occurring on the other site. This is due in part to an increase in oro-genital activity. In 1976, herpes simplex of the genitals was estimated to be the second most prevalent venereal disease, after gonorrhea.

Genital herpes usually appears as a number of small blisters on the penis, the lips of the vagina, around the anus, or on the thighs and buttocks. The fluid-filled blisters usually are painful, although they only may tingle. Within a day or two the blisters break, leaving open sores that take one to six weeks to heal. Lymph glands near the infection may react by becoming swollen and tender. In most cases a doctor can diagnose herpes by the appearance of the lesions. Occasionally other tests may be used to confirm the diagnosis.

Genital herpes, like fever blisters, can be recurrent. After the sores are healed, the virus remains dormant in the body for a period of time. Weeks or months later, there may be a recurrence of the active infection. Recurrent attacks tend to be less severe than the initial attack, to heal more quickly, and to become less frequent with time.

Treatment

Like the common cold, which also is caused by a virus, there is no cure for genital herpes type 2 infections. However, there are things that can be done to help relieve the symptoms, promote healing of the lesions, and prevent secondary infection from other microorganisms. One of the best of these is a hot bath. Soaking in a tub or sitz bath as hot as the patient can tolerate for 15 to 20 minutes, two or three times daily, will help lessen pain and promote healing of the lesions. If the sores are irritated by urination, a little petroleum jelly applied on them will help. Cotton underwear should be worn because nylon underwear and pantyhose can trap moisture and prevent healing.

To help relieve the symptoms, aspirin 600 mg may be given by mouth every three or four hours as needed. If aspirin is not well tolerated by the patient, acetaminophen may be tried at the same dosage and frequency.

Precautions

While treating the herpes symptoms, a careful watch should be kept for the presence of other venereal diseases. On shore, serologic tests for syphilis may be performed.

The attendant should not palpate any genital lesion without a rubber glove on the hand. Direct contact with herpes lesions may possibly infect the fingers with herpes type 2 virus.

Because genital herpes can be transmitted by sexual intercourse, people with herpes should not have sexual intercourse until the lesions have healed completely. Because it is not known if someone with herpes is infectious after the lesions have healed, it would be a good idea to use a condom at other times to prevent giving herpes to a noninfected partner.

A baby born to a woman with an active genital herpes infection is at risk of being infected. Herpes infections in the newborn can be serious. Therefore, a pregnant woman who has had genital herpes always should tell her doctor.

There is evidence that a woman with genital herpes is at greater risk of developing cancer of the cervix, although not all women with herpes will develop cancer. It is important for a woman with genital herpes to have a Papanicalaou (Pap) test every six months. Cancer of the cervix is curable, if it is discovered early.

SYPHILIS

Syphilis is a venereal disease caused by the spirochete *Treponema pallidum.* Although it can penetrate ordinary skin through small cuts or abrasions, the spirochete can enter unbroken, moist mucous membranes of the genitalia and mouth. Most syphilitic infections are contracted and transmitted through sexual contact. The early stages of syphilis usually are painless and cause little disability. The lesions may heal without treatment and the disease can lie dormant in the body for several years. In the late stages syphilis can cause serious damage to the brain and spinal cord that may result in insanity and paralysis. The disease can damage the heart valves leading to heart failure; and it can affect other organs in the body, as the eyes and liver. Once the damage is done, it cannot be reversed by treatment.

The first stage, primary syphilis, is characterized by the presence of a chancre at the point where the germs entered the body. There is a delay of ten days to three months after contact, before the onset of any visible sign of the infection. Following the appearance of the initial syphilitic chancre, there is an additional delay of one to four weeks before the serologic (blood) test for syphilis will become positive. The typical syphilitic chancre will occur on or about the genitalia. (See Fig. 5–6.) However, a chancre may occur anywhere on the body where there has been contact with an infective lesion. Such lesions usually are single, but may number more than one. Lesions often are smooth and clean-looking on the surface. Sometimes the lesion ulcerates and leaves a reddish sore with the base of the ulcer covered by a yellow or grayish exudate. Unless there is secondary infection with pus-forming organisms, the syphilitic chancre will be painless even when touched or manipulated by the examiner. The lesion has a characteristic firmness when felt between the thumb and forefinger.

Often there will be one or more rubbery, hard, painless, enlarged lymph nodes in one or both groins, or in other regions if the chancre is extragenital. In the presence of a secondary infection, the node may be tender. Accurate diagnosis requires the use of a microscope to demonstrate the organisms by the dark-field examination technique. These lesions will heal

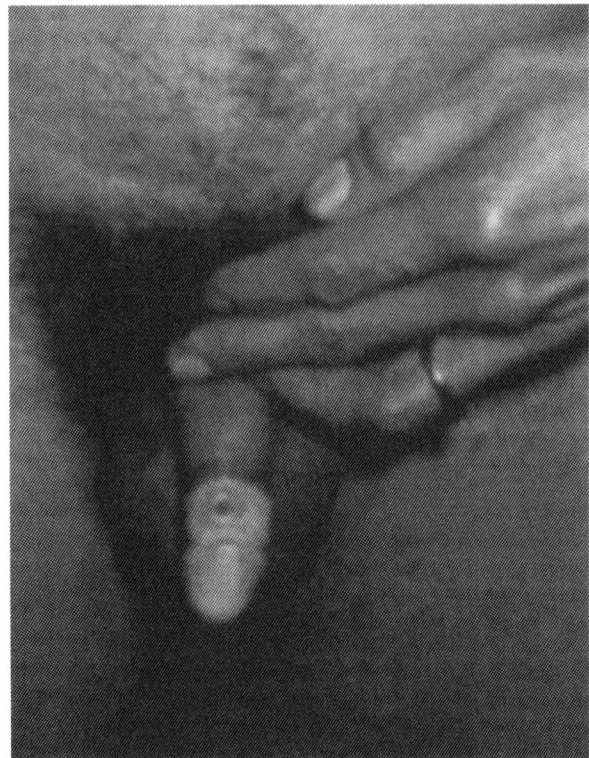

Fig. 5–6. Penile ulcer, syphilis chancre.

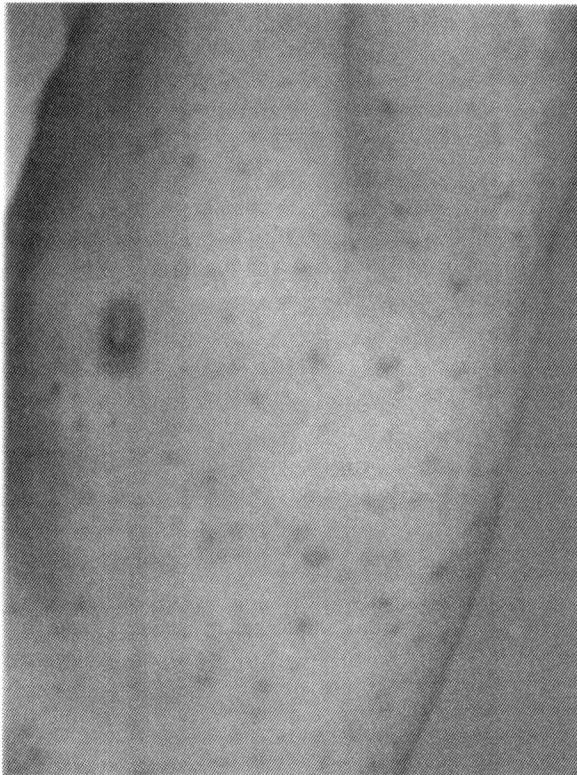

Fig. 5–7. Secondary syphilis.

spontaneously, usually within six weeks. In the chancre stage, the disease is highly contagious.

No local or systemic treatment should be applied or given if the patient can be brought to a medical facility within a reasonable time. The local application of antibiotics or antiseptics is especially distressing to a physician because these usually nullify the diagnostic value of the dark-field examination.

The secondary stage of syphilis usually develops in about six to eight weeks after the appearance of the primary chancre. In fact, the primary syphilitic chancre still may be present at the time of onset of the secondary stage. However, the secondary stage may be the first manifestation occurring some 10 to 14 weeks after the infecting contact. The most consistent feature of secondary syphilis is a nonitching skin rash which may be generalized in the form of small flat or slightly elevated bumps; or it may be localized on the palms, soles, or genital areas. (See Fig. 5–7.) Lesions on the genitalia often are eroded. Mouth ulcers or flat whitish mucous patches also are typical of secondary syphilis. A less frequently encountered sign in-

cludes patchy loss of scalp hair. Patients with secondary syphilis may complain of malaise (not feeling well), headache, sore throat, and a low-grade fever. The presence of these symptoms plus a generalized rash, a rash involving the palms and soles that does not itch, and is associated with enlarged small lymph nodes in the neck, armpits, and groin, should arouse suspicion of secondary syphilis. It should be noted that moist lesions of secondary syphilis are teeming with spirochetes and thus are highly infectious. The diagnosis is confirmed by dark-field examination of the lesions and a blood test for syphilis, which is nearly always positive in this stage of the disease.

The symptoms of the second stage, like those of the first stage disappear without treatment when the disease is in the latent (hiding) stage. However, about 25 percent of such patients will undergo one or more relapses into the secondary stage.

Late symptomatic or tertiary syphilis follows the secondary stage. A quiescent period up to 20 years may pass before the onset of symptoms and signs of the third and final stage. The end result of this last stage of untreated syphilis is destruction of various organs, especially the heart and nervous system. Patients should be advised to cooperate with the physician and accept the indicated treatment. A spinal tap may be important to determine accurately the stage of the disease so that adequate therapy can be administered.

Treatment

If a patient develops syphilis while at sea without a physician in attendance, he should be advised to obtain medical care when the ship reaches port. Patients with suspected infectious syphilis should be kept isolated from other members of the crew. Primary chancres should be cleansed daily with soap and water, and the affected area soaked with normal saline solution (two level teaspoonfuls of table salt to 1000 ml of water) for 20 minutes, four times a day. *Any patient with a generalized rash should be considered possibly infectious until a definitive diagnosis is made.*

To treat the infection, the drug of choice is benzathine penicillin G for a total dosage of 7.2 million units. Single injections of 2.4 million units should be given intramuscularly every five days (a total of three injections over a ten-day period). Alternately penicillin G procaine sterile suspension may be given intramuscularly in daily doses of 1.2 million units for ten days, for a total dosage of 12 million units. If the patient is sensitive or allergic to penicillins, then erythromycin or tetracycline are alternate drugs. Either of these drugs may be administered in oral doses of 500 mg, four times a day for 20 days, for a total dosage of 40 grams. In the absence of a penicillin allergy, penicillin is the drug of choice because its effectiveness in the late stages of syphilis has been proven.

About 50 percent of patients with early infectious syphilis, when treated with penicillin, will manifest the Jarisch-Herxheimer reaction, usually within six to 12 hours after the first injection. This reaction is characterized by fever, chills, joint aches, increased swelling of the primary lesion(s), or increased prominence of the secondary rash. Occasionally, a patient who is on the verge of secondary syphilis will develop lesions of secondary syphilis during the Jarisch-Herxheimer reaction. This reaction is caused by the rapid destruction of the syphilis organisms and is mentioned only because it is likely to be confused with an allergic penicillin reaction. Aspirin is sufficient treatment. This reaction does not occur after subsequent doses of penicillin.

CHANCROID (Soft Chancre)

Chancroid, almost always acquired during sexual intercourse, is caused by a small acid-fast gram-negative bacillus *Haemophilus ducreyi.*

Females may harbor this infection without any clinical evidence, so the disease most often is identified in sexually promiscuous uncircumcised males. The incubation period (the time following the infecting contact to the initial appearance of symptoms) is short, varying from one to 12 days, usually averaging three to five days.

It is important to know that chancroid and syphilis may be acquired from a single exposure. Chancroid, which has a shorter incubation period, will appear first; therefore the possibility of a primary syphilis infection existing at the same time must be considered. The initial chancroid lesion usually appears as a small inflammatory bump, which soon forms a blister or pustule that rapidly breaks down to form a very painful ulcer. Because of the tendency toward self-inoculation, multiple satellite lesions develop on opposing skin surfaces, or on areas adjacent to the first lesion.

In the male, the commonest sites of involvement include the tip of the prepuce (foreskin), the inner prepuce, the groove proximal to the glans (head), shaft, and lastly the base of the penis.

In the female, the lesions are characteristically on the external genitalia. As opposed to syphilis, chancroid lesions are more often multiple than single. The lesions usually remain small, shallow to punched-out and round to oval with a red, elevated, ragged border. The base has a granular appearance and usually is covered with a grayish-yellow dirty-appearing, foul-smelling discharge. Typically, the lesions are soft and lack the characteristic hardness of the syphilitic chancre; they are extremely tender to the touch and may bleed easily when manipulated. Inguinal lymph node enlargement may occur in approximately 50 percent of cases, following the appearance of the primary lesion by about one to two weeks.

The chancroidal bubo usually occurs on one side as a single inflamed mass with symptoms and signs that mimic the primary lesions, as tenderness with warmth and redness of the overlying skin. These buboes tend to become soft and may rupture through the skin surface leaving a drainage sinus tract. It should be noted that chancroid is a local infection which usually is not associated with constitutional symptoms. The presence of multiple, painfully tender, not hard genital ulcers, with or without a bubo and without systemic symptoms suggests a diagnosis of chancroid. Laboratory confirmation of the clinical diagnosis usually is dependent upon identifying the Gram-negative organisms on stained smears.

Treatment

Chancroid should be treated by cleansing the ulcers with soap and water once daily, and soaking the lesions in normal saline solution (two level teaspoonfuls of table salt to 1000 ml of water) for 20 minutes four times a day. If the patient is not allergic to sulfonamide drugs, sulfisoxazole may be administered orally in a dose of 1000 mg four times a day until the lesions are healed (usually about two weeks). Sulfisoxazole may be administered without masking incubating syphilis or interfering with further laboratory diagnosis of concomitant syphilis. Patients with a bubo should be put to bed with an ice bag applied to the painful mass for the first two days, or until the discomfort is lessened. Thereafter, the recovery time may be shortened by the application of a hot water bottle to the inguinal region.

Occasionally, sulfonamide-resistant strains of chancroid are encountered. These usually respond to oral therapy with tetracycline hydrochloride 500 mg four times a day. *If the latter drug is administered, the patient must receive a course of tetracycline or penicillin therapy which also is adequate to cure syphilis.* (See p. 249.) Before initiating a course of tetracycline or penicillin as therapy for chancroid, medical advice by radio should be obtained. This is necessary because the patient might be incubating syphilis or have a mixed infection of chancroid and syphilis.

LYMPHOGRANULOMA VENEREUM
(LGV, Lymphopathia Venereum)

LGV is a systemic disease of venereal origin caused by a virus-like organism. The infectious agent is a *Bedsonia* organism (*Chlamydia*) closely related to that of psittacosis. The disease clinically is recognized more commonly in males. Subclinical or inapparent infections, or an asymptomatic carrier state have been described in females. After a variable incubation

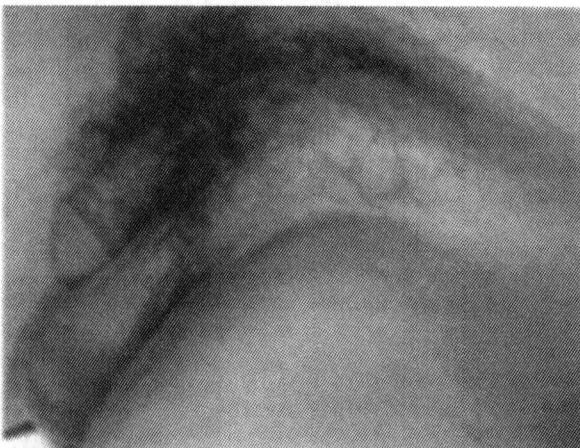

Fig. 5–8. Lymphogranuloma venereum.

period averaging one to four weeks, the appearance of a small painless genital lesion has been described in fewer than 25 percent of cases. The lesion usually is an inconspicuous bump, blister, or shallow ulcer that heals within a few days and typically goes unnoticed by the patient. The earliest clinical signs are fever up to 103°F (39.4°C), chills, headache, malaise (not feeling well), coughing, and pain in the muscles and joints. Shortly after the onset of these symptoms, the patient becomes aware of a painful swelling in one or both groin areas. (See Fig. 5–8.) The swelling occurs in one groin in approximately two-thirds of cases.

The inguinal bubo is common in males. Early in the course of regional node involvement, one can feel one or more enlarged discrete movable tender nodes. These eventually become matted together giving rise to an oval-shaped mass. Because of the involvement of lymph nodes both above and below the inguinal ligament, the mass may be compressed or divided by the inguinal ligament. This produces a characteristic grooved appearance with the long axis of the inflamed elliptical mass running parallel to the groin-fold. As the disease progresses, some of these matted nodes undergo softening. Because there are nodes in different stages of evolution, the mass becomes large and lobulated with alternating areas of softening and hardness. The overlying skin becomes swollen, sometimes bluish-red in color and fixed to the underlying mass. When pus forms and breakdown occurs, multiple fistulous tracts may open to the skin surface. Other symptoms less commonly found include lower abdominal pain and diarrhea due to involvement of nodes in the pelvis and around the rectum.

In brief, the patient with LGV appears as an acutely ill individual with no residual primary genital lesion, but with a painful, tender, firm, oval-shaped inguinal mass. The pain is exaggerated when walking due to the pressure by the inguinal ligament. Some relief may be obtained by walking bent over. Unless one suspects LGV, there is great temptation to diagnose a patient with these symptoms and signs as one suffering from a confined inguinal hernia. Such patients have been known to have been subjected to unnecessary surgery.

At sea, the diagnosis of LGV must rest on the appearance of the lesions and the other symptoms. On reaching port a skin test (Frei test) and a blood test (complement fixation) should be made to lend support to any LGV diagnosis. When one makes a bedside diagnosis of LGV, appropriate treatment should be instituted.

Treatment

Bed rest is essential for a patient with LGV because continued activity will prolong the inflammatory process, discomfort, and period of recovery. An ice bag should be applied to the inguinal region for the first two or three days of treatment to help relieve local discomfort, tenderness, and warmth. Thereafter, local application of continuous heat from a hot water bottle will get rid of the inflammation. A bubo that can be moved back and forth should have any pus withdrawn through the intact skin using an 18 gauge needle and a 20 ml or larger syringe. *However, the withdrawal of pus should not be attempted except on medical advice by radio.* Systemic drug therapy should be started in the form of sulfisoxazole 1000 mg four times a day (every six hours).

If the elevated temperature returns to normal within three or four days after the initiation of systemic drug therapy, this will support the LGV diagnosis. Drug therapy should be continued until there is no evident decrease in the size of the involved lymph nodes. The duration of treatment in most cases rerequires 30 to 50 days. Often, small firm areas of scar tissue under the skin persist indefinitely where lymph node areas were involved.

An occasional patient may appear to respond poorly to sulfonamide drugs. If the patient still runs a fever, and his discomfort has not lessened or the bubo decreased in size after seven to ten days of such therapy, tetracycline hydrochloride should be substituted in doses of 500 mg orally four times a day. The tetracycline should be continued for one or two weeks, or longer according to medical advice received by radio. *Milk and antacids should be avoided when taking tetracycline because they inactivate the drug.* LGV patients who receive tetracycline should have a follow-up blood test (serological test) for syphilis every one or two months for at least six months. This will help to detect any incubating syphilis which may be masked temporarily by the antibiotic.

GRANULOMA INGUINALE (Donovanosis)

Granuloma inguinale is a chronic infectious bacterial disease of the skin, mucous membranes, and subcutaneous tissues. The causative organism is *Calymmatobacterium granulomatis.* The disease is most prevalent among dark-skinned races and usually involves the genital, inguinal, or perianal regions showing no tendency to heal spontaneously. However, it is the least contagious and least frequently encountered of the veneral disease discussed in this book.

The incubation period is reported to vary from several days to several months. The earliest lesion occurs painlessly on the external genitalia as a firm, flat-topped bump or a small, soft, pale red nodule under the skin. The surface becomes soft giving rise to a painless ulcer with a typical elevated soft bright pink velvety granular base that bleeds easily. As the disease progresses, the lesions become painful or itchy. The initial lesion enlarges in diameter and new lesions may grow together, as they develop. Other lesions are spread through secondary infection of adjacent or opposing skin surfaces. Small lesions have a button-like appearance, are sharply defined, and are covered by a red velvety surface of granulation tissue. As the lesions enlarge, they form an irregular snake-like outline. Their advancing borders have distinctive rolled edges with glazed, beefy red granulations piling onto the bordering surface of uninvolved skin. Although localized swellings or abscesses may develop in the inguinal regions, swollen lymph nodes are not characteristic of this disease. Secondary infection of the lesions with other bacteria is quite common. This may give rise to acute inflammation, local tissue destruction, and scarring. Laboratory diagnosis is possible by examining smears or biopsy specimens under the microscope.

Treatment

The use of saline solution (two level teaspoonfuls of table salt to 1000 ml of water) soaks or compresses three or four times a day will help in the local treatment of oozing or secondarily infected skin lesions of granuloma inguinale. For the infection, tetracycline hydrochloride 500 mg should be given by mouth four times a day for three to six weeks. Because relapses have been reported after an apparent cure, the treatment should be continued for at least two weeks after the ulcers have healed. In longstanding cases, the disease may require as many as 12 weeks of therapy.

URETHRITIS (Non-specific)

Non-specific urethritis denotes a symptomatic urethritis (inflammation of the urethra) in which the causative organism or organisms cannot be determined. This urethritis is not due to gonorrhea, trichomonas, candida, or any other of the common agents. The disease is thought to be venereally transmitted. The incubation period usually is seven to 20 days. Symptoms are pain on urination and a scant watery discharge.

Treatment

For non-specific urethritis, tetracycline hydrochloride 500 mg should be given by mouth four times a day for one week. Patients with urethritis who receive tetracycline should have a follow-up test (serological test) for syphilis every one or two months for at least six months. This will help to detect any incubating syphilis which may be masked temporarily by the antibiotic.

PRECAUTIONS
for VD Patients and Medical Attendants

If there is a sore on the penis or a discharge from the urethra, a clean gauze dressing should be kept on the penis and the dressing changed frequently. The penis should be washed thoroughly with soap and water, then dried.

The hands should be washed thoroughly with soap and water after touching the penis and after handling gauze, bandages, or underwear that has come in contact with open sores. Extra care should be taken never to touch the eyes after handling material that may be contaminated with gonorrheal pus. Gonorrhea of the eyes, easily acquired and difficult to treat at sea, may cause permanent impairment of vision, even total blindness.

Gauze, cotton sponges, or other disposable material soiled with discharges of pus should be burned, or wrapped for other disposal, so they will not be touched or handled by others.

All items used by patients during the highly contagious second stage of syphilis, which is marked by fever, mouth sores, and skin rash, should be laundered, boiled, or chemically disinfected. This applies to underwear, bed linen, towels, eating utensils, bedpans, and urinals.

For Patients Ashore

The patient should protect himself from reinfection or cross-infection. Sex contacts should be avoided. The patient should guard others from his infection. He should not have sexual relations until his physician advises that it is safe to do so.

If the patient wants to marry, he should ask the doctor's advice on when the marriage may be lawful. In many States couples wishing to marry are required by law to have a blood test before they can get a marriage license, to make sure they are free from active venereal infection. This law is intended to prevent the spread of infection between spouses and from an infected mother to her unborn children.

The syphilis spirochete can pass into an unborn child from an infected mother. Unless treated, the child may be born dead, live only a short time, or become sickly, deformed, or feebleminded. However, if a syphilitic woman is given proper treatment before the fifth month of her pregnancy, nine times out of ten, she will give birth to a normal noninfected child. That is why every expectant mother, whether there is reason to suspect infection or not, should have a blood test as soon as she knows she is pregnant.

Patients should protect others from chance infection. Although VD seldom is spread except by direct sex contact, a patient should take extra care to keep from spreading it indirectly. Until the doctor states a patient is no longer infectious, he should put forth extra effort to practice good personal hygiene, as follows:

• Use only his own toilet articles (as towels, washcloth).

• Avoid kissing.

• Do not swap bites of food, lend his pipe, or share cigarettes.

• Do not sleep with others.

• Do not soil toilet seats with his discharges.

• Wash his hands thoroughly with soap and water after using the toilet.

• Take hygienic precautions with soiled dressings(see p. 325).

Chapter VI

Sickbay and the Medicine Chest

THE SICKBAY

THE NEED FOR A HOSPITAL aboard certain merchant vessels of the United States was established by Acts of Congress as contained in the Statute, Title 46, United States Code, Section 660–1, and implementing regulations. This hospital space, commonly referred to as the "sickbay," serves as both hospital and dispensary.

SHIP'S MEDICINE CHEST

The need for a supply of medicines for certain merchant vessels of the United States was established by Acts of Congress as contained in the Statute, Title 46, United States Code, Section 666, and implementing regulations. The term *Ship's Medicine Chest*, refers to the pharmaceuticals, surgical supplies and equipment, and other chemicals that are stored in the sickbay or a locked compartment of reserved storage space in the ship's general storeroom. The medicine chest of olden times (see figure, p. vii) was designed to be moved from a wrecked ship, or taken ashore to be refilled by an apothecary.* Today the medicine chest is a permanent part of the sickbay area of the vessel.

By statutory authority,† the space aboard merchant vessels for the sickbay must have not less than 120 cubic feet and not less than 16 square feet (floor space) for each seaman lodged therein. All fixtures chosen should offer the maximum useable area in shelf space and drawers (not too deep or shallow) for the floor space they occupy. The fixtures should be of

---

* It is interesting to note that Section 8 of a Federal Act for the Government and Regulation of Seamen in the Merchant Service, approved July 20, 1790, stated: "That every ship or vessel belonging to a citizen of the United States, of the burthen of one hundred and fifty tons or upwards, navigated by ten or more persons in the whole and bound on a voyage without the limits of the United States, shall be provided with a *chest of medicines*, put up by some apothecary of known reputation, and accompanied by directions for administering the same; and the said medicines shall be examined by the same or other apothecary once at least in every year, and supplied with fresh medicine in the place of such as shall have been used or spoiled . . ." (Source: Williams, R.C. *The United States Public Health Service, 1798–1950.* Published by the Commissioned Officers Association of the USPHS, p. 28, 1951.)

† 46 U.S.C. 660–1.

resistant stainless steel, or other easily cleaned material that humidity will not damage.

There should be adequate cabinet and drawer space to provide separate storage space for different groups of pharmaceuticals, such as *internal* medications, *external* drug preparations, *poisons*, and *controlled substances* (requiring greater security). Also, a refrigerator should be available, not necessarily in the sickbay, for medications that require storage in a cool or cold place. To avoid confusion, the equipment, instruments, and surgical supplies should be stored in space separate from those holding pharmaceuticals.

Cabinets should be large enough to hold a "working quantity" of the recommended pharmaceuticals, p. 257+, and surgical equipment, instruments and supplies, p. 294+. They should permit orderly and convenient storage. All standup medication containers should be arranged alphabetically, preferably by generic name, with the labels clearly visible. Adequate lighting should be provided.

Narcotics, stimulants, and sedatives in Schedule II of the Controlled Substances Act (see Appendix D) should be kept in the Master's safe. All other controlled substances should be kept in a locked compartment except paraldehyde, which requires refrigeration.

The shelves of the medicine cabinet should be equipped with guardrails, dividers, or other devices; and drawers should have catches to prevent bottles and other items from falling or moving when the ship rolls and pitches. Also, it has been suggested that the cabinet(s) be attached to the bulkhead at a right angle to the keel of the vessel, which may prevent items from falling off the shelves.

Immediately after use, the medications and surgical supplies should be returned to their proper places. Medicines never should be put into the medicine cabinet in an open unlabeled glass, cup, or other container. If the content of a container is not known for certain, it should be destroyed. Sterile packages of such items as gauze compresses, syringes and needles should not be opened until just before use. If bottles, boxes, and packages of items are scattered on shelves or in drawers, it will be difficult to find specific items when needed. Disorder possibly can lead to serious error in the selection of a medication.

The crew or passengers taking prescribed medications for chronic ailments should be advised to bring aboard a supply adequate for the voyage.

Generally the shipping company will delegate the immediate responsibility for the ship's sickbay and the *medicine chest* to a deck or staff officer who is trained in fundamental medical techniques. This officer should be the only person (except the Master) to have a key to the sickbay, to the *medicine chest*, and the locker where reserve medicines are stored. This officer should be responsible solely to the Master for the sickbay and medical supplies. A duplicate set of sickbay keys should be in the Master's safe, or other secure place.

PHARMACEUTICAL PREPARATIONS

Use of the Table of Pharmaceutical Preparations

It is assumed that the officer who has the responsibility for the care and treatment of seamen, aboard a merchant vessel in either the A or B categories (described below), will have had training in the administration and use of the recommended pharmaceutical preparations.

Column A of Table 6–1 shows the minimum number of packaged items (figures in UNIT column) recommended for oceangoing merchant vessels without a doctor aboard. The quantities of medications are based on an estimated four-month inventory for a crew complement of 25 to 40 persons.

Column B of Table 6–1 gives the minimum number of packaged items recommended to be carried aboard merchant vessels engaged in trade solely in coastal, Great Lakes, and nearby foreign ports, and not more than 12 hours away from a port of call. The quantities of medications are based on an estimated four-month inventory for a crew complement of approximately 25 persons.

Column C of Table 6–1 gives the minimum number of packaged items recommended for fishing boats or private craft which normally do not carry more than 15 persons, and are never more than a few days from home port, or only a few hours from a port of call.

Table 6–1

Pharmaceutical Preparations Recommended for the Ship's Medicine Chest

Item No.	Description of Item	Unit	Quantities A	B	C	Notes
1.	Acetaminophen Tablets, 300 mg, 100s	bot.	5	3	3	
2.	Acetazolamide Tablets, 250 mg, 100s	bot.	1	—	—	
3.	Alcohol, Rubbing (70% isopropyl alcohol or equivalent), 480 ml	bot.	6	2	2	
4.	Alkaline Aromatic Solution Tablets, 100s	bot.	2	1	—	
5.	Aluminum Acetate Powder, Packets, 2.2 g, for making equivalent Aluminum Acetate Solution (Burow's), 12s	box	2	—	—	
6.	Aluminum Hydroxide Gel, with Magnesium Hydroxide or Magnesium Trisilicate, Oral Suspension, 360 ml	bot.	6	—	—	
7.	Aluminum Hydroxide, with Magnesium Hydroxide or Magnesium Trisilicate, Chewable Tablets, 100s	bot.	10	3	3	
8.	Aminophylline Suppository, Rectal, 500 mg, 12s	box	2	1	—	Refrigerate.
9.	Ammonia, Aromatic Inhalant, Crushable Ampuls, 0.3 or 0.4 ml, 12s	box	2	1	1	Refrigeration Preferable
10.	Ampicillin Capsules, 250 mg, 100s	bot.	3	1	—	
11.	Amyl Nitrite Inhalant, Crushable Ampul, 0.3 ml, 12s	box	1	1	—	Refrigerate.
12.	Aspirin Tablets, 300 mg, 100s	bot.	6	2	2	
13.	Atropine Sulfate Injection 0.4 or 0.5 mg/ml, 20 ml Vial	each	6	—	—	
14.	Bacitracin Ointment, Topical, 500 units/g, 30g Tube	each	6	2	—	
15.	Belladonna Tincture, 30 ml Dropper Bottle	bot.	2	1	—	
16.	Benzoic and Salicylic Acids Ointment, 30 g Tube	each	2	1	—	
17.	Benzoin Tincture, Compound, 120 ml	bot.	1	1	—	
18.	Calamine Lotion, Plain, 120 ml	bot.	8	1	1	
19.	Calcium Gluconate Injection 10%, 10 ml Ampul, 10s	box	1	—	—	
20.	Charcoal, Activated, Powder, 120 g	bot.	1	1	1	
21.	Chlorinated Lime, 340 g can	each	12	3	—	
22.	Chloroquine Phosphate Tablets, 250 mg, 100s	bot.	1	—	—	
23.	Clove Oil, 20 ml	bot.	1	1	1	

Table 6–1 (Continued)
Pharmaceutical Preparations Recommended for the Ship's Medicine Chest

Item No.	Description of Item	Unit	Quantities A	B	C	Notes
24.	Codeine Sulfate Tablets, 30 mg, 100s	bot.	1	1	—	C–II: Controlled Substance, Schedule II.
25.	Cyclizine Hydrochloride Tablets, 50 mg, 100s	bot.	4	1	1	
26.	Dextran Injection 6% and Sodium Chloride 0.9%, 500 ml, with Administration Set	bot.	6	—	—	
27.	Dextromethorphan Hydrobromide Syrup 15 mg/5 ml, with Glyceryl Guaiacolate, 120 ml	bot.	12	4	4	
28.	Dextrose 5% and Sodium Chloride 0.45%, Injection, 1000 ml	bot.	6	—	—	Administration sets should be obtained from the same manufacturer as the intravenous solution.
29.	Dextrose Injection 50%, 50 ml, Ampul	each	4	1	—	
30.	Diazepam Injection, 5 mg/ml, 2 ml Ampul or Disposable Syringe	each	20	—	—	C–IV: Controlled Substance, Schedule IV.
31.	Diazepam Tablets, 5 mg, 100s	bot	2	1	—	C–IV: Controlled Substance, Schedule IV.
32.	Digoxin Tablets, 0.25 mg, 100s	bot.	1	—	—	
33.	Diphenhydramine Hydrochloride Capsules, 25 mg, 100s	bot.	2	1	1	
34.	Diphenhydramine Hydrochloride Injection, 50 mg/ml, 1 ml, Disposable Cartridge or Syringe, 10s	pkg.	5	1	—	
35.	Diphenoxylate Hydrochloride 2.5 mg with Atropine Sulfate 0.025 mg Tablets, 100s	bot.	1	1	—	C–V: Controlled Substance, Schedule V.
36.	Disinfectant–Detergent, General Purpose, Concentrate, Phenolic Synthetic Type, 480 ml	bot.	6	2	2	
37.	Ephedrine Sulfate Capsules, 25 mg, 100s	bot.	1	—	—	
38.	Epinephrine Hydrochloride Injection 1:1000, 1 ml Disposable Cartridge or Syringe, 10s	pkg.	2	1	1	
39.	Erythromycin Tablets, 250 mg, 100s	bot.	2	—	—	

Table 6–1 (Continued)
Pharmaceutical Preparations Recommended for the Ship's Medicine Chest

Item No.	Description of Item	Unit	Quantities			Notes
			A	B	C	
40.	Ethyl Chloride, Spray Bottle, 100 g	bot.	2	1	1	
41.	Eyewash or Eye Irrigating Solution, Isotonic, Sterile, in Plastic Squeeze Bottle, 120 ml.	bot.	6	1	1	
42.	Fluorescein Sodium Ophthalmic Strip, Sterile, 200s	pkg.	1	—	—	
43.	Furosemide Tablets, 40 mg, 100s	bot.	1	—	—	
44.	Gamma Benzene Hexachloride Cream 1%, 60 g Tube	each	12	2	—	
45.	Glucagon for Injection 1 mg, with Diluent, Vial	pkg.	6	—	—	
46.	Hand and Body Lotion, Cream Type, 240 ml	bot.	8	2	2	
47.	Hemorrhoidal Suppositories, 12s	box	6	1	1	Regfrigeration Preferable
48.	Homatropine Hydrobromide Eye Drops 5%, 5 ml Dropper Bottle	bot.	1	—	—	
49.	Hydrocortisone-Neomycin-Polymyxin B Ear Drops, 5 ml Dropper Bottle	bot.	8	—	—	
50.	Hydrocortisone Ointment 1%, 30 g Tube with Rectal Tip	each	6	2	2	
51.	Hydrocortisone Sodium Succinate for Injection, 100 mg Vial	each	5	—	—	
52.	Hydrogen Peroxide Solution 3%, 120 ml	bot.	6	2	—	
53.	Insect Repellent, as Diethyltoluamide Solution, 60 ml	bot.	12	4	4	
54.	Insulin Injection (Regular Insulin) U–100, 10 ml Vial	each	3	1	—	Refrigerate.
55.	Ipecac Syrup, 30 ml	bot.	4	1	1	
56.	Kaolin Mixture with Pectin, 240 ml	bot.	6	2	2	
57.	Lactated Ringer's Injection, 1000 ml	bot.	6	—	—	Administration sets should be obtained from the same manufacturer as the intravenous solution.
58.	Lidocaine Hydrochloride Injection 1%, 2 ml Ampul	each	12	—	—	
59.	Lubricating Jelly, 5 g Tube	each	48	6	—	
60.	Magnesium Sulfate, 454 g	bot.	1	—	—	

Table 6-1 (Continued)
Pharmaceutical Preparations Recommended for the Ship's Medicine Chest

Item No.	Description of Item	Unit	A	B	C	Notes
61.	Menthol Ointment, Compound, 30 g Tube	each	12	4	4	
62.	Meperidine Hydrochloride Injection 50 mg/ml, 1 ml Disposable Cartridge or Syringe, 10s	pkg.	2	—	—	C–II: Controlled Substance, Schedule II.
63.	Metaraminol Bitartrate, Injection, 10 mg/ml, 1 ml Ampul	each	10	—	—	
64.	Milk of Magnesia, 480 ml	bot.	8	2	2	
65.	Mineral Oil (Liquid Petrolatum), 480 ml	bot.	1	1	—	
66.	Morphine Sulfate Injection 10 mg/ml, 1ml Disposable Cartridge or Syringe, 10s	pkg.	2	1	—	C–II: Controlled Substance, Schedule II.
67.	Naloxone Hydrochloride Injection 0.4 mg/ml, 1 ml Ampul	each	6	—	—	
68.	Nitroglycerin Tablets, 0.4 mg, 100s	bot.	2	1	1	Keep container tightly closed. Store at controlled temperature, 59°F to 86°F (15°C to 30°C)
69.	Oxygen, Size E Tank	each	2	1	—	
70.	Paraldehyde, 30 ml	bot.	6	2	—	C–III: Controlled Substance, Schedule III. Refrigerate.
71.	Penicillin G Procaine, Sterile Suspension, Injection 600,000 units/ml, 1 ml Disposable Cartridge or Syringe, 10s	pkg.	2	1	—	Refrigerate.
72.	Penicillin G Procaine, Sterile Suspension, Injection, 2,400,000 units/4 ml Disposable Syringe	each	12	—	—	Refrigerate.
73.	Penicillin V Potassium Tablets, 250 mg, 100s	bot.	3	1	—	
74.	Pentobarbital Sodium Capsules, 50 mg, 100s	bot.	3	1	—	C–II: Controlled Substance, Schedule II.
75.	Pentobarbital Sodium Injection 50 mg/ml, 2 ml Ampul, 10s	pkg.	1	—	—	C–II: Controlled Substance, Schedule II.
76.	Petrolatum, White, 60 g Tube	each	6	2	2	
77.	Phenobarbital Tablets, 30 mg, 100s	bot.	3	1	—	C–IV: Controlled Substance, Schedule IV.

Table 6–1 (Continued)
Pharmaceutical Preparations Recommended for the Ship's Medicine Chest

Item No.	Description of Item	Unit	Quantities			Notes
			A	B	C	
78.	Phenylephrine Hydrochloride Nasal Spray 0.25%, 15 ml Spray Bottle	bot.	12	4	4	
79.	Phenytoin Sodium Capsules, 100 mg, 100s (formerly Diphenylhydantoin Sodium)	bot.	2	1	—	
80.	Pilocarpine Hydrochloride Eye Drops 2%, 15 ml Dropper Bottle	bot.	2	1	—	
81.	Polymyxin B-Neomycin-Bacitracin Eye Ointment, 4 g Tube	each	6	2	—	
82.	Polymyxin B-Neomycin-Gramicidin Eye Drops, 10 ml Dropper Bottle	bot.	3	1	—	
83.	Povidone-Iodine Skin Cleanser Liquid, 120 ml	bot.	6	2	2	
84.	Povidone-Iodine Solution, 1% Available Iodine, 240 ml	bot.	4	1	1	
85.	Prednisolone Sodium Phosphate Eye Drops 1%, 5 ml Dropper Bottle	bot.	1	—	—	
86.	Probenecid Tablets, 500 mg, 100s	bot.	1	—	—	
87.	Proparacaine Hydrochloride Eye Drops 0.5%, 15 ml Dropper Bottle	bot.	1	—	—	Refrigerate.
88.	Pyrimethamine Tablets, 25 mg, 100s	bot.	1	—	—	
89.	Quinine Sulfate Tablets, 300 mg, 100s	bot.	3	—	—	
90.	Sodium Bicarbonate Injection, 3.75 g (44.6 mEq), 50 ml Ampul	each	3	—	—	
91.	Sodium Bicarbonate Powder, 454 g	bot.	1	1	1	
92.	Sodium Biphosphate and Sodium Phosphate Solution for Enema, Squeeze bottle with Rectal Tip, 135 ml	bot.	12	2	—	
93.	Sodium Chloride Injection 0.9%, 1000 ml	bot.	6	2	—	Administration sets should be obtained from the same manufacturer as the intravenous solution.
94.	Sodium Chloride Tablets, 1 g, 1000s	bot.	2	1	1	
95.	Sulfadiazine Silver Cream 1%, 400 g jar	each	2	—	—	
96.	Sulfisoxazole Tablets, 500 mg, 100s	bot.	6	2	—	
97.	Sunscreen Preparation (see p. 291)	pkg.	a sufficient quantity			
98.	Talc (Talcum Powder), 120 g Can	each	6	3	3	

Table 6–1 (Continued)
Pharmaceutical Preparations Recommended for the Ship's Medicine Chest

| Item No. | Description of Item | Unit | Quantities | | | Notes |
			A	B	C	
99.	Tetanus Immune Human Globulin, 250 Units, Disposable Syringe	each	10	—	—	Refrigerate.
100.	Tetanus Toxoid, Adsorbed, Single Dose, Disposable Syringe	each	10	—	—	Refrigerate.
101.	Tetracycline Hydrochloride Capsules, 250 mg, 100s	bot.	3	1	—	
102.	Tolnaftate Powder, 1%, 45 g	box	12	3	3	
103.	Tolnaftate Solution, 1%, 10 ml Plastic Squeeze Bottle	bot.	6	2	2	
104.	Whisky, Medicinal, 480 ml	bot.	2	1	1	
105.	Zinc Oxide Paste, 30 g Tube	each	12	3	3	

Generic Names of Drug Products with Corresponding Brand Names*

Many medications are available commercially under one or more brand or proprietary names. *References to medications in this text are by their generic or nonproprietary names.* To minimize confusion or the possibility of error, it is strongly recommended that everyone, both ashore and aboard merchant vessels, refer to a medication by its *generic name.*

For reference and procurement purposes, an alphabetical listing of drug products by generic names with corresponding brand or proprietary names (each followed by its manufacturer) is provided hereafter. It should be noted that many products listed also are marketed commercially under their generic names by various manufacturers.

Acetaminophen Tablets 300 mg or 325 mg

Acetagesic (Kay Pharmacal)
Amphenol (O'Neal, Jones & Feldman)
Anapap (Fellows Medical Mfg.)
Apadon (Elder)
Apamide (Dome)
APAP (Ulmer)
Bandigesic (Acid-Eze)
Capital (Carnrick)
Dapa (Ferndale)
Dimindol (Blueline)
Dularin (Dooner)
Febridol (Amid)
Febrinol (Vitarine)
Fendon (American Pharmaceutical Co.)
Menalgesia (Clapp)
Napap (Robinson)
Nebs (Eaton)
Pyrapap (Savage)
SK-APAP (Smith Kline & French)
Tapar (Parke-Davis)
Temlo (Hyrex-Key Pharmaceuticals)
Tem-Pain (Carroll)
Tempra (Mead)
Tylenol (McNeil)
Valadol (Squibb)

Acetazolamide Tablets, 250 mg

Diamox (Lederle)

---

* The Drug Products Information File (DPIF) was used as the primary reference for multiple-source drug products. DPIF is a computer-processable data base on commercially available drug products that was developed and is maintained under copyright by the American Society of Hospital Pharmacists (ASHP), 4630 Montgomery Ave., Washington, D.C. 20014.

Listing of proprietary names for drug products is for information only and is not intended to be comprehensive. Inclusion of any proprietary name is not intended as an endorsement of the drug product or its manufacturer, either by ASHP or the U.S. Public Health Service.

Inclusion of any drugs for which patent or trademark rights exist shall not be deemed, and is not intended as a grant of, or authority to exercise, any right or privilege protected by such patent or trademark.

Aluminum Acetate Solution
(Burow's Solution)
Domeboro Powder Packets (Dome) (for making equivalent aluminum acetate solution)

Aluminum Hydroxide with Magnesium
Hydroxide Oral Suspension and Tablets*
Acid-Eze (Acid-Eze Company)
Alphagel (Medical Specialties)
Aludrox (Wyeth)
Alu-Mag (Premo)
Alurex (Rexall)
Creamalin (Winthrop)
Delcid (Merrell)
Gelumina Plus (American Pharmaceutical Co.)
Kamadrox Jel (Elder)
Kudrox (Kremers-Urban)
Maalox (Rorer)
Medagel (Medical Specialties)
WinGel (Winthrop)

Aluminum Hydroxide with Magnesium
Trisilicate Oral Suspension and Tablets*
A-M-T (Wyeth)
Co-Lu-Gel M-T (Ulmer)
Gelusil (Warner-Chilcott)
Malcogel (Upjohn)
Tricreamalate (Winthrop)
Trilox (Blueline)
Trisogel (Lilly)

Ampicillin (or Ampicillin Trihydrate)
Capsule 250 mg
Acillin (ICN Pharmaceuticals)
Alpen (Lederle)
Amcill (Parke-Davis)
Ampi-Co (Coastal)
Omnipen (Wyeth)
Pen-A (Pfizer)
Penbritin (Ayerst)
Pensyn (Upjohn)
Polycillin (Bristol)
Principen 250 (Squibb)
QIDamp (Mallinckrodt)
SK-Ampicillin (Smith Kline & French)
Supen (Reid-Provident Lab.)
Totacillin (Beecham)

* All dosage forms may not be available in all listed brands.

Chloroquine Phosphate Tablet 250 mg
Aralen (Winthrop)

Cyclizine Hydrochloride Tablet 50 mg
Marezine (Burroughs-Wellcome)

Dextran, High Molecular Weight, Injection 6%
with Sodium Chloride 0.9%, 500 ml
Dextran 75 (Abbott)
Dextran 70 (Cutter)
Gentran 75 (Travenol)
Macrodex 70 (Pharmacia)

Dextromethorphan Hydrobromide Syrup with
Glyceryl Guaiacolate
2/G-DM (Dow)
Expectran-DM (Ross)
Gylate-D (Medical Specialties)
Glycotuss-DM (Vale)
Queltuss (Westerfield)
Robitussin-DM (Robins)
Sorbase Cough Syrup (Fort David)

Diazepam Tablet 5 mg and Injection
Valium (Roche)

Digoxin Tablet 0.25 mg
Lanoxin (Burroughs-Wellcome)

Diphenhydramine Hydrochloride Capsule
25 mg and Injection*
Bax (McKesson)
Benadryl (Parke-Davis)
Rohydra (Robinson)

Diphenoxylate Hydrochloride with
Atropine Sulfate Tablet
Lomotil (Searle)

Epinephrine Hydrochloride Injection 1:1000
Adrenalin (Parke-Davis)

Erythromycin (or Erythromycin Stearate)
Tablet 250 mg
Bristamycin (Bristol)
E-Mycin (Upjohn)
Erypar (Parke-Davis)
Erythrocin (Abbott)
Ilotycin (Lilly)
Kesso-mycin (McKesson)
Robimycin (Robins)
RP-mycin (Reid-Provident)

Eye Irrigating Solution, Isotonic, Sterile
Blinx (Barnes-Hind)
Dacriose (Smith, Miller & Patch)
Eye-Stream (Alcon)
Neo-Flo (Professional Pharmacal)

Furosemide Tablet 40 mg
Lasix (Hoechst)

Gamma Benzene Hydrochloride Cream 1%
Kwell (Reed-Carnrick)

Hydrocortisone–Neomycin–Polymyxin B,
Ear Drops
Cortisporin (Burroughs-Wellcome)

Hydrocortisone Sodium Succinate for
Injection 100 mg
Solu-Cortef (Upjohn)

Jelly, Lubricating, Sterile
K-Y (Johnson & Johnson)
Lubafax (Burroughs-Wellcome)

Kaolin Mixture with Pectin
Kao-Con (Upjohn)
Kaoparin (McKesson)
Kaopectate (Upjohn)
Ka-Pek (American Pharmaceutical Co.)
Keotin (Blueline)
Paocin (Beecham)
Pargel (Parke-Davis)
Pektamalt (Warren-Teed)
Tourista (Rexall)

Lidocaine Hydrochloride Injection 1%
Xylocaine Hydrochloride (Astra)

Meperidine Hydrochloride Injection
Demerol Hydrochloride (Winthrop)

Metaraminol Bitartrate Injection
Aramine (Merck Sharp & Dohme)

Naloxone Hydrochloride Injection
Narcan (Endo)

Penicillin G, Procaine, Sterile Suspension
Injection
Crysticillin A.S. (Squibb)
Diurnal-Penicillin (Upjohn)
Duracillin A.S. (Lilly)
Pentids-P A.S. (Squibb)
Pfizerpen-A.S. (Pfizer)
Wycillin Suspension (Wyeth)

Penicillin V Potassium Tablet 250 mg
Betapen VK (Bristol)
Compocillin-VK (Ross)
Dowpen VK (Dow)
Kesso-Pen VK (McKesson)
Ledercillin VK (Lederle)
Penapar VK (Parke-Davis)
Pen-Vee K (Wyeth)
Pfizerpen VK (Pfizer)
QIDpen VK (Mallinckrodt)
Robicillin VK (Robins)
Ro-Cillin VK (Rowell)
SK-Penicillin VK (Smith Kline & French)
Uticillin VK (Upjohn)
V-Cillin K (Lilly)
Veetids (Squibb)

Pentobarbital Sodium Capsule
50 mg and Injection
Nembutal Sodium (Abbott)

Phenobarbital Tablet 30 mg
Luminal (Winthrop)

Phenylephrine Hydrochloride
Nasal Spray 0.25%
Alconefrin 25 (Webcon)
Biomydrin (Warner-Chilcott)
Coryban-D Nasal Spray (Roerig)
Isohalant Improved (Elder)
Isophrin Hydrochloride (Riker)
Neo-Synephrine Hydrochloride (Winthrop)
Sinarest Nasal Spray (Pharmacraft)
Synasal (Texas Pharmacal)

Phenytoin Sodium Capsule, 100 mg, 100s
(formerly Diphenylhydantoin sodium;
renamed in 1975)
Dilantin Sodium (Parke-Davis)
Kessodanten (McKesson)

Pilocarpine Hydrochloride Eye (Ophthalmic)
Drops 2%
Almocarpine 2% (Ayerst)
Mi-Pilo 2% (Barnes-Hind)
Isopto Carpine 2% (Alcon)
Pilocar 2% (Smith, Miller & Patch)

Polymyxin B-Neomycin-Bacitracin Eye
(Ophthalmic) Ointment
Mycitracin Ophthalmic Ointment (Upjohn)
Neo-Polycin Ophthalmic Ointment (Dow)
Neosporin Ophthalmic Ointment (Burroughs-
   Wellcome)

Ophthel (Elder)
Polyspectrin Ophthalmic Ointment (Allergan)
Pyocidin Ophthalmic Ointment (Smith, Miller
& Patch)

*Polymyxin B-Neomycin-Gramicidin Eye
(Ophthalmic) Drops*
Neo-Polycin Ophthalmic Solution (Dow)
Neosporin Ophthalmic Solution (Burroughs-
Wellcome)

*Povidone-Iodine Solution, Surgical Scrub
and Skin Cleanser*
Betadine (Purdue-Frederick)
Isodine (Blair)
Ultradine (Ulmer Pharmacal)

*Prednisolone Sodium Phosphate Eye
(Ophthalmic) Drops 1%*
Inflamase Forte (Smith, Miller & Patch)

Probenecid Tablet 500 mg
Benemid (Merck Sharp & Dohme)

*Proparacaine Hydrochloride Eye
(Ophthalmic) Drops 0.5%*
Alcaine (Alcon)
Ophthaine (Squibb)
Ophthetic (Allergan)

Pyrimethamine Tablet 25 mg
Daraprim (Burroughs-Wellcome)

*Sodium Biphosphate and Sodium Phosphate
Solution for Enema*
Enemeez (Armour)
Fleet Enema (Fleet)
Travad Enema (Baxter)

Sulfadiazine Silver Cream, 1%
Silvadene (Marion Labs.)

Sulfisoxazole Tablet 500 mg
Gantrisin (Roche)
SK-Soxazole (Smith Kline & French)
Sodizole (First Texas Pharmaceuticals)
Sosol (McKesson)
Soxomide (Upjohn)

Tetanus Immune Human Globulin, 250 units
Ar-Tet (Armour)
Gamatet (Hollister-Stier)
Gamulin T (Dow)

Homo-Tet (Savage)
Hu-Tet (Hyland)
Hyper-Tet (Cutter)
Immu-Tetanus (Parke-Davis)
Pro-Tet (Lederle)
T-I-Gammagee (Merck Sharp & Dohme)

*Tetracycline Hydrochloride
Capsule/Tablet 250mg*
Achromycin V (Lederle)
Amtet (Amid)
Bristacycline (Bristol)
Centet-250 (Central)
Cyclopar (Parke-Davis)
Fed-Mycin (Federal Pharmacal)
G-Mycin (Coast)
Kesso-Tetra (McKesson)
Maytrex (Mayrand)
Paltet (Palmedico)
Panmycin Hydrochloride (Upjohn)
Piracaps (Tutag)
QIDtet (Mallinckrodt)
Retet (Reid-Provident)
Robitet '250' Hydrochloride (Robins)
Ro-Cycline 250 (Rowell)
Sarocycline (Saron)
SK-Tetracycline (Smith Kline & French)
Sumycin '250' Hydrochloride (Squibb)
Tetrachel (Rachelle)
Tetracyn (Pfizer)

Tolnaftate Powder 1% and Solution 1%
Tinactin (Schering)

Inspection of Pharmaceutical Preparations

To help assure the best possible medical treatment at sea, careful attention must be given to procuring and storing medications for the sickbay. The *Federal Food, Drug, and Cosmetic Act* provides that each new drug approved for marketing must be both safe and effective for the conditions of use as described by the manufacturer on the label and the accompanying package insert (see p. 266). The continued safety and effectiveness of drug products, however, depends upon their natural stability, the expertise of the manufacturer or packager, and the conditions of storage.

The person delegated the responsibility for the contents of the medicine chest aboard ship should be alert for signs of deterioration or contamination that could make a medication unfit for use.

For tablets or capsules, some of the signs of deterioration are crystal formation on the surface; cracking or splitting of the coating; seepage of liquid from the capsule; color change, mottling effect; or unusual odor.

In a liquid medication (including injections), the signs of deterioration may be discoloration; precipitation or crystal formation in a solution that ought to be clear; caking or clumping of suspensions (failure to disperse uniformly); separation of emulsions into layers; and turbidity (cloudiness) which may indicate contamination by bacterial or fungal growth.

In ointments or creams, the signs of deterioration may be reduced volume (shrinkage due to evaporation of moisture from creams); separation of ingredients; discoloration; crystal formation on the surface; and leakage from tubes due to corrosive action of the ingredients on the container.

Although information is presented in this chapter about the physical signs of deterioration of medications aboard ocean vessels, which can render them unfit for use, it is important that periodic inspections be made by a pharmacist. Changes may occur in medications, which to a pharmacist are predictable, even though not physically apparent. It is recommended that such inspections be performed annually.

Procurement of Pharmaceutical Preparations

The following should be observed to help assure that the medications when purchased will meet appropriate standards at the time of use:

• Purchase medications in the manufacturer's package, whenever possible.

• Procure medications in the smallest practicable size, such as aspirin tablets 300 mg in containers of 100s, rather than 1000s. Also, capsules, tablets, and other dosage forms should be obtained in individually packaged and labeled doses when available.

• Date all medication containers upon receipt.

• Place the new stock behind the old stock on the shelf for proper rotation of supplies.

• Establish an arbitrary maximum shelf life for packages not having an expiration date,

such as five years, after which the stock will be destroyed and replaced.

• When medications are first received, read carefully all labels on containers to assure that the vendor has not made an error in supplying the kind and strength of medication requested.

Federal Labeling Regulations

Medications should be procured only from reliable drug vendors, whose products meet in full the Federal regulations that relate to the selling of medications. A repackaged medication (taken from the manufacturer's original package by a local vendor) must meet the same labeling requirements as the manufacturer's package.

Under Federal label regulations for medications, there are two categories of drugs: (1) those medications which require a prescription before they can be dispensed (*prescription legend* drugs); and (2) those which can be bought without a prescription (*over-the-counter* drugs). A *prescription legend* drug carries the following statement on the container's label: *CAUTION: FEDERAL LAW PROHIBITS DISPENSING WITHOUT A PRESCRIPTION* A more detailed discussion of the differences between the labeling requirements of the two groups of drugs follows.

Prescription Legend Drugs: These drugs require medical supervision for safe use and may not be purchased by the lay public without a doctor's prescription. Such drugs are judged by the Food and Drug Administration to be dangerous for a layman to use in self-medication. The label(s) on a container of a medication in this group usually cannot include all the detailed directions and cautions that would be needed to use the drug safely and effectively. This additional prescribing information, by regulation, is usually printed by the manufacturer and included with the medication as a *package insert*. Aboard ship this *package insert* should be retained for reference, preferably attached to the medication's container, until all the medication is used.

Aside from the package insert, labels affixed to containers of prescription legend drugs must include, as a minimum:

• The manufacturer's brand or trade name, if there is one.

• The non-proprietary (generic) or official name corresponding to the trade name of the drug, or of its active ingredients.

• The quantity or proportion of each active ingredient.

• The name and address of the manufacturer, packer, or distributor.

• The net amount of the drug in the package.

• The lot or control number.

• The expiration date, if any.

• The recommended storage temperature. When none is specified, the drug should be stored at controlled room temperature 59° F to 86° F (15° C to 30° C).

• Labels for drugs subject to the Controlled Substances Act and manufactured after May 1, 1971 carry one of the following symbols in the right-hand corner of the principal label: C-I, C-II, C-III, C-IV, or C-V. These drug products include most narcotics, depressants, and stimulants. (See Merchant Vessels and Controlled Substances, p. 439, for additional information.)

Over-the-counter Drugs: These drugs, which include such medications as aspirin tablets and milk of magnesia, are considered to be safe and effective for self-treatment when used according to the labeled directions. They can be purchased without a doctor's prescription order.

All over-the-counter drugs must bear a seven-point label. The seven points to be included are:

• The name of the product.

• The name and address of the manufacturer, packer, or distributor.

• The net contents of the package.

• The established name, quantity, and proportion of all active ingredients.

• The name of any habit-forming drug in the preparation.

• Cautions and warnings needed for the protection of the user.

• Adequate directions for safe and effective use.

Care should be exercised when purchasing medications to assure that only adequately labeled medications, as discussed above, are received. A packager, who identifies only casually the name of a medication on the container's label, is supplying a potentially dangerous product, and increasing the potential for accidental misuse or poisoning.

Storage of Pharmaceutical Preparations

As previously noted, and repeated here for emphasis, poor storage conditions can accelerate markedly the deterioration of medications to the point where they are not fully active, or in some instances, toxic. A program of *stock rotation* should be carried out, that is *first in, first used.*

The shelf life of drug products frequently is determined by Federal regulations. When such a product has a limited shelf life, it will be shown as an expiration date on the container's label. However, to help insure potency and safety of medications with no expiration date on the container's label, the shipping company should establish a policy on maximum shelf life. A reasonable policy might be that all drug products not carrying an expiration date be replaced every five years. It is recommended that a loose-leaf notebook be kept in the medicine chest in which a page would be allotted in sequence for each month for the next six years. On receipt each drug product would be logged-in with its replacement date on the page designated for the month it would be replaced. This not only will facilitate identifying those items that should be replaced when the vessel is in port but will minimize the possibility of not replacing an outdated item.

Medications must be stored at the proper temperature and protected against excessive humidity and light if they are to remain potent during their recommended shelf life. Labels on drug containers give the temperature at which the drug preparation should be stored when other than controlled room temperature, 59° F to 86° F (15° C to 30° C), is required.

Deterioration usually is hastened by excessive heat, freezing, sunlight, and exposure to the atmosphere. All bottles should be kept tightly closed.

Storage Temperature

Official temperature definitions for drug storage are published in the United States Pharmacopeia (USP).

The following definitions apply:

COLD—Any temperature not exceeding 46° Fahrenheit (F) or 8° Centigrade (C). A *refrigerator* is a cold place in which the temperature is held between 36° F and 46° F (2° C and 8° C).

COOL—Any temperature between 46° F and 59° F (8° C and 15° C). Note: an article for which storage in a cool place is indicated may, alternatively, be stored in a refrigerator.

CONTROLLED ROOM TEMPERATURE—A temperature maintained thermostatically between 59° F and 86° F (15° C and 30° C).

EXCESSIVE HEAT—Any temperature above 104°F (40°C).

PROTECT FROM FREEZING—The container's label bears a notice to protect from freezing, when, in addition to the risk of breakage of the container, unintentional freezing subjects a product to loss of strength or potency, or to destructive alteration of the dosage form.

Rational Use of Medications

There is a widespread belief by the general public that any discomfort, physical or mental, can be eliminated by swallowing, injecting, or applying medications. This helps to account for the fact that the many medications available today are much overused or misused. One concerned with the use and administration of medications, such as the medical attendant aboard ship, should realize that no drug is completely harmless to everyone whether it be aspirin or a lifesaving antibiotic. Thus medication only should be considered for therapy after a careful evaluation of the patient's injury or illness.

Although the development of modern pharmaceutical products has contributed significantly to the high level of medical care available today, drugs must be prescribed, dispensed, and administered with respect for their often powerful physiological actions. This is true of "over-the-counter" home remedies as well as the "prescription legend" drugs. Volumes have been written about the hazards involved in the use and misuse of drugs, and only a relatively brief summary of the subject can be presented here. Prior to using any drug, persons responsible for handling medications aboard ship should be thoroughly familiar with the information included in this book on pp. 271+. In addition, other available information sources, such as a package insert, should be consulted. Also, the Master or medical attendant generally should *seek medical advice by radio before using a prescription legend drug.* Most unfavorable reactions to drug therapy can be prevented by careful, knowledgeable use.

This book includes discussions of various treatment methods as well as descriptive information on a variety of medications. However, it is very important to note that many different factors affect the treatment of each individual patient. These include age, sex, size and physical condition of the patient, in addition to certain characteristics of the illness or injury. Thus, the treatment methods as well as the uses and dosages of medications noted in THE SHIP'S MEDICINE CHEST AND MEDICAL AID AT SEA should be viewed as guidelines rather than definitive directions for use in all cases.

Dosage and Frequency of Use

The mechanisms by which many drugs are absorbed, used, and removed from the body may be affected significantly by age and body weight. This is particularly important to consider when treating infants and small children and, in some cases, the elderly. This book does not provide recommended pediatric dosages. Either the package insert, some other authoritative reference source, or medical advice by radio should be consulted before administering a drug to a child. For some particularly potent drugs and for many anti-infective agents, recommended dosage may be specified in relation to the patient's weight (such as 10 mg/kg). In order to arrive at the correct dose, determine the patient's weight as closely as possible, convert to kilogram, if necessary (see Chart p. 301) and then calculate the dose.

Once the correct drug and dosage have been determined for a patient, it is important that the therapy be continued for the proper length of time. Administering a drug for too long a period subjects the patient to unnecessary risks of toxicity or other adverse reactions. Insufficient therapy, however, is a more frequent problem, particularly when the patient is administering his own medication. The patient may begin to feel better and reduce the dose or discontinue taking the medication without the underlying condition being corrected. This often is seen in the case of anti-infective drugs where too early discontinuation of therapy may lead to a relapse—sometimes more serious than the original condition. Patients with chronic conditions including heart disease and diabetes also may do themselves a great deal of harm by altering their drug therapy without medical advice. The person responsible for medical care aboard ship should see that all individuals taking medication, whether prescribed before or during the voyage, comply with the prescribed regimen. Crewmembers on long-term therapy should be instructed to bring aboard enough medication to last the entire voyage. The ship's Master should try to provide needed drugs in the event that a patient's personal supply is depleted, contaminated, or lost.

The timing of a medication's administration is frequently an important factor in its effectiveness. With many drugs, particularly the anti-infectives, it is necessary to maintain a rather constant concentration of the drug in the bloodstream. This is achieved best by administering the drug at uniform intervals, such as every six hours around the clock, if necessary. Generally, the severity of the patient's condition and the dosage instructions provided in the monograph or literature accompanying the drug will dictate the optimum frequency of administration. For some drugs, again including many of the anti-infectives, it is advisable to avoid taking the drug at mealtimes. Such recommendations should be followed as closely as possible for best results.

Hazards Involved in the Use of Medications

Persons responsible for the use of medications aboard ship should be aware of the various types of adverse reactions which might result from therapy. These may be categorized basically as *side effects, extension effects (or toxicities)*, and *interactions*.* The reader is cautioned that only a brief review of these very complex issues can be presented here, and the drug literature and/or medical advice by radio should be consulted if unforeseen problems in therapy occur.

Side effects are drug-induced reactions which differ pharmacologically from the main effects for which the drug is administered. Side effects may be mild or severe, and they always should be considered when prescribing or administering a drug. One frequently encountered side effect is drowsiness. It may be produced to a greater or lesser degree in some patients by several pharmacological classes of medications, such as an antihistamine taken to treat an allergy. Patients on such a drug should not, for example, operate machinery or stand watch while taking the drug. A commonly troublesome side effect of treatment with some antibiotics is diarrhea or rectal itching due to direct irritation of the gastrointestinal tract or to overgrowth of intestinal microorganisms. Hives (urticaria) is another frequent adverse reaction to anti-infectives. The irritation of the stomach lining produced by aspirin, to some extent in nearly all patients, is another example of a possibly serious side effect of a drug which is mistakenly considered to be harmless.

Extension effects or toxicities of drugs involve problems of the *degree* of a patient's reaction to a drug. These include reactions resulting from accumulation of abnormal quantities of the drug in the body due to kidney, liver, or other malfunction; overdosage (too large a dose taken accidentally or intentionally); hypersensitivity or allergy (a stronger than normal reactivity); and idiosyncrasy (an unusual sensitivity). Frequently these undesirable drug reactions can be foreseen and prevented with a careful history, noting *any* past drug allergies or reactions, and physical examination. At other times, however, especially the unusual hypersensitivity or idiosyncratic reactions are very difficult or impossible to forsee.

---

* A detailed discussion of this subject may be found in: Martin, Eric W.: *Hazards of Medication*, J. B. Lippincott Company, Philadelphia, 1971.

This is one of the main reasons why *no medications should be prescribed, administered or taken indiscriminately.* Particular care should be exercised aboard ship, because a reaction which could be managed quite easily in a hospital or doctor's office may be much more difficult to handle at sea. No medication should be administered until one is satisfied that the patient is not allergic to it.

Antibiotics (particularly the penicillins) are noted for producing hypersensitivity reactions, although many other drugs may have a similar effect in susceptible individuals. The degree of reaction may vary from slight itching or hives to anaphylactic shock, circulatory and respiratory collapse, and death. It is important to note that a slight hypersensitivity reaction after one exposure to a drug may be followed by a much more severe reaction to a subsequent exposure to the same or a related drug. Although some persons have been successfully treated with a drug to which they have reported previous reactions, it is best not to take any chances aboard ship. Avoid giving a patient any drug to which he feels he may be allergic. Further, all individuals responsible for shipboard medical care should be prepared to treat drug hypersensitivity reactions (anaphylactic shock), if they should occur. (See p. 221.)

Drug overdosage or the erratic following of a prescribed regimen may present a problem with some patients aboard ship. If a patient is suspected of not complying with the prescribed drug regimen, another individual, such as the medical attendant, should thoroughly counsel the patient and take such steps as may be indicated to see that the regimen is followed.

Interactions of medications with other drugs and with foods are now recognized as an important factor to be considered in initiating and maintaining effective therapy. Before administering additional medications aboard ship, one must be aware of all the drugs that a patient may be taking (either prescription drugs obtained elsewhere or over-the-counter remedies). Although certain conditions are treated more effectively by a combination of two or more drugs, it is *incorrect* to assume that this is always, or even frequently, true. As more is learned about the very complex interactions between different drugs and the human body,

the importance of avoiding the use of unnecessary drugs is being recognized. It is well documented that the incidence of adverse drug reactions rises sharply as the number of different drugs a patient is taking increases. An example of a particularly serious drug-drug interaction is the dangerous (and occasionally fatal) combination of two or more central nervous system (CNS) depressants. A tranquilizer such as chlorpromazine in combination with a sedative such as pentobarbital, or a narcotic analgesic such as meperidine in combination with a tranquilizer such as diazepam, may produce stupor, coma, cardiac and/or respiratory arrest. *It also is important to remember that ethyl alcohol is a central nervous system depressant, and in conjunction with other CNS depressants including those listed above, death may result following only moderate alcohol intake. It is best to advise any patient taking drugs to exercise moderation or, ideally, abstinence in consumption of alcoholic beverages.* In addition to the enhanced CNS depression which might result, alcohol may react with a number of other drugs to produce nausea, vomiting, and other unfavorable manifestations.

Drugs frequently interact with foods, lessening or completely negating the desired pharmacological action. Calcium-containing foods including milk, as well as many commercial antacid products, hinder the absorption of orally administered tetracycline. Some drugs, including most antibiotics, should be administered on an empty stomach (one hour before or two hours after eating) for best effect. Other drugs, including aspirin-containing analgesics, are best given with food or milk to decrease the chance of gastrointestinal irritation. The package insert accompanying a drug product lists the most significant of the known drug and/or food interactions and specifies the recommended administration routes and intervals. These recommendations should be followed closely for optimum therapeutic results.

Used with knowledge and care, medications can be lifesaving, but used irrationally, they may do irreparable harm. Persons responsible for administering medical care aboard ship should learn as much as possible about the drugs which they use, and seek medical advice by radio whenever they are in doubt. In this way, their patients will receive sound drug therapy which will do much to improve overall care.

Pharmaceutical Preparations: Uses, Adult Dosage, and Cautions

Pertinent information (monographs), that relates to *use, adult dosage* and *caution,* has been prepared on each medication recommended for merchant vessels. The monographs are arranged alphabetically by the product's generic or non-proprietary name. Many of the brand or proprietary names for these products are listed on pp. 262-265.

1. Acetaminophen Tablets, 300 mg

USE: For headache and mild to moderate pain in muscles and joints. When fever accompanies pain, its antipyretic action is useful. It does not cause gastric irritation or bleeding or, in usual dosage, lengthen the blood clotting time. It may be used for patients allergic to aspirin.

ADULT DOSAGE: Two 300 mg tablets every four hours; total daily dose should not exceed eight 300 mg tablets.

CAUTION: Do *not* give repeatedly over an extended period of time to patients with anemia or with heart, lung, kidney, or liver disease. Skin reactions may occur in a few individuals.

2. Acetazolamide Tablets, 250 mg

USE: Acetazolamide, usually categorized as a diuretic, is useful in a number of conditions requiring control of body fluid secretions. It is recommended for shipboard use for the emergency treatment of acute congestive glaucoma.

ADULT DOSAGE: Medical advice should be obtained to help confirm the diagnosis of acute glaucoma, and plans should be made to provide care by an eye specialist. In the meantime, acetazolamide may be administered to lower the intraocular pressure in an oral dosage of 250 mg every 4 to 6 hours.

3. Alcohol, Rubbing (70% isopropyl alcohol or equivalent)

USE: As an antiseptic for "degerming" the skin prior to injecting medications and other surgical procedures. For disinfecting the hands, rub the skin gently but thoroughly for three minutes with gauze or cloth soaked with the alcohol. Used as a rubbing compound, it produces a mild redness and a burning sensation and evaporates from the skin with a cooling effect. It irritates mucosa and open cuts.

If heat sterilization is not available, instruments such as knives, scissors, and syringes may be disinfected by soaking them in 70% isopropyl alcohol for 20 minutes, *but add one-fourth teaspoonful of sodium bicarbonate as a corrosion inhibitor. Do not leave stainless steel instruments in it for long periods because they may rust or corrode.* This procedure is effective against vegetative forms of bacteria but not against spores. Germicidal activity of isopropyl alcohol is greater than that of ethyl alcohol.

CAUTION: Never give internally. Signs and symptoms of poisoning by isopropyl alcohol and ethyl alcohol are similar, except that gastritis with pain, nausea, and vomiting is greater with isopropyl alcohol. Medical advice by radio should be obtained when isopropyl alcohol ingestion is suspected.

4. Alkaline Aromatic Solution Tablets

USE: These tablets, when dissolved in the proper amount of water, make a mild, soothing solution for use as a mouthwash, or as a gargle for sore throat. Dissolve one or two tablets in a half glass of warm water (follow directions on package), and use as a gargle or mouthwash every two hours, or as indicated.

5. Aluminum Acetate Powder, Packets, 2.2 g, for making equivalent aluminum acetate solution (Burow's Solution)

USE: A solution/mixture, prepared from a powder pack as indicated on the carton, is used as a soothing, astringent wet dressing for inflamed or "weeping" areas of skin. It is an effective, simple remedy for inflamed areas of the skin due to insect bites, poison ivy, or certain fungal infections such as athlete's foot (acute dermatophytosis).

ADULT DOSAGE: Mix one or two packets in 500 ml of water as directed on the package for specific conditions, or as directed by a physician. Do *not* strain or filter. It is applied in the form of wet compresses to the affected areas, or to fixed dressings. Also, it may be used as a soak in acute conditions of the hands or feet affected with contact eczema or athlete's foot.

CAUTION: Keep away from the eyes. For external use only.

6. Aluminum Hydroxide Gel, with Magnesium Hydroxide or Magnesium Trisilicate, Oral Suspension

USE: In treating gastric hyperacidity and peptic ulcer. It generally promotes healing and relieves pain. Neutralizes hydrochloric acid in the stomach without producing an alkaline reaction or disturbing normal electrolyte balance.

ADULT DOSAGE: 10 ml every two to four hours after meals and at bedtime. Dose and frequency depend on severity of symptoms and relief obtained. The dose range is 5 to 30 ml per administration.

CAUTION: Moderate constipation or diarrhea may occur. It should *not* be administered simultaneously with other drugs, such as tetracycline hydrochloride and barbiturates, because it might interfere with their absorption.

7. Aluminum Hydroxide, with Magnesium Hydroxide or Magnesium Trisilicate, Chewable Tablets

USE: Same as for the oral suspension; however, somewhat less effective.

ADULT DOSAGE: One or two tablets, chewed thoroughly before swallowing, every two to four hours after meals and at bedtime.

CAUTION: Same as for the oral suspension.

8. Aminophylline Suppository, Rectal, 500 mg

USE: To assist breathing in patients who have bronchial asthma, asthmatic bronchitis, pulmonary emphysema, and certain types of heart failure. Wheezing is usually an indication for use.

ADULT DOSAGE: Insert one 500 mg suppository rectally. This dose may be repeated in eight to twelve hours. The total dose should not exceed 1 g (2 suppositories) in 24 hours.

CAUTION: Store in a refrigerator 36° F to 46° F (2° C to 8° C) to prevent deterioration. Because the drug also is a diuretic, increased

urination probably will occur following administration. Remove any wrapping before inserting the suppository.

9. Ammonia, Aromatic Inhalant, Crushable Ampul, 0.3 or 0.4 ml

USE: As an irritating stimulant for faintness, collapse, or weakness, particularly that following minor emotional upsets; and for failing circulation or respiration. Indirectly results in an increase in respiration and blood pressure. The ampuls, wrapped in gauze and cotton, can be crushed readily with the fingers.

ADULT DOSAGE: Administer by inhalation. Crush one ampul in a handkerchief or gauze and hold under the patient's nose and mouth.

CAUTION: Although inhalation of large concentrations of ammonia is harmful to the lungs, adverse effects are not to be expected from normal use of this preparation. Do *not* use if patient's face is flushed (red).

10. Ampicillin Capsules, 250 mg

USE: (1) For uncomplicated gonorrhea and (2) for other susceptible infections. *Give only on radio advice from a physician.*

ADULT DOSAGE: (1) For the treatment of uncomplicated gonorrhea, as an alternative to procaine penicillin injection. For the male and female, a total of 3.5 grams (fourteen 250 mg capsules) are administered simultaneously with 1 gram (two 500 mg tablets) of Probenecid, all in one single dose. (2) Recommended for susceptible infections of Gram-negative bacteria and Gram-positive bacteria. The usual dosage is one to two 250 mg capsules/tablets four times a day.

CAUTION: Ampicillin, chemically quite similar to penicillin, can cause the same types of allergic reactions, such as anaphylactic reaction and skin rash. *Persons allergic to penicillin should be assumed to be allergic to ampicillin.* Before administering, determine from the patient, if possible, whether he is allergic to either penicillin or ampicillin. Allergic (anaphylactic) reactions can be severe to fatal. If the patient is allergic to the drug, medical advice by radio should be obtained for an alternative anti-infective treatment. When reactions occur, discontinue ampicillin, and give emergency treatment. (See anaphylactic reactions p. 221).

Ampicillin may produce other side effects such as nausea, vomiting, or diarrhea.

11. Amyl Nitrite Inhalant, Crushable Ampul, 0.3 ml

USE: (1) For acute attack of angina pectoris. Its effect appears in about 30 seconds and lasts about three minutes, sufficient duration for the majority of angina attacks. (2) As an initial antidote for cyanide gas poisoning.

ADULT DOSAGE: For pain, crush one ampul in a handkerchief or gauze. Hold the crushed ampul under the nose and mouth long enough for the patient to breathe several times while in a sitting position. For use in the initial treatment of cyanide poisoning. (See Chapter III, p. 112.)

CAUTION: More likely to produce headache and a rapid drop in blood pressure than nitroglycerin given under the tongue. Also, reflex rapidity of heart action is more pronounced than with nitroglycerin.

12. Aspirin Tablets, 300 mg

USE: (1) To relieve aches and pains in acute infectious diseases, such as influenza, the common cold, and sinusitis. (2) To relieve headache, neuralgia, muscular aching, joint pains and fever.

ADULT DOSAGE: For headache, one or two 300 mg tablets, repeated in four hours, if necessary. For joint pains and aches, and pains associated with neuralgia, colds and other diseases, two tablets repeated every four hours, as needed. For severe pain not relieved by aspirin alone, two tablets administered with one tablet of codeine sulfate 30 mg may be indicated.

CAUTION: Some individuals are sensitive to aspirin. Small doses may cause swelling of the eyelids, nose, lips, tongue, or the entire face; and also may cause a hive-like rash, dizziness, and nausea. In some persons this sensitivity is very severe. These individuals usually know that aspirin can cause them to have a reaction and that they should not take the drug. Individuals sensitive to aspirin frequently are subject to hay fever, asthma, or hives. In such

individuals, acetaminophen should be considered as an alternative to treat mild pain.

Gastrointestinal disturbances (dyspepsia, nausea, vomiting, and concealed bleeding) sometimes occur, especially with prolonged administration of aspirin. These effects can be diminished by taking the drug with milk or food. Aspirin should be avoided by persons taking oral anticoagulant drugs.

For poisoning by aspirin, see p. 114.

13. Atropine Sulfate Injection, 0.4 to 0.5 mg/ml

USE: Injectable atropine sulfate is included for use as an antidote in the treatment of poisoning by insecticides containing organophosphate or carbamate chemicals as part of their formulation. These chemicals are found most commonly in pesticides such as Parathion®, Diazinon®, and Sevin®. (See Poisonings, p. 114.)

ADULT DOSAGE: If it is determined that one of the above poisons is involved, atropine sulfate should be administered at once to prevent coma, cyanosis, or convulsions. In organophosphate or carbamate poisoning, two (2) to four (4) mg should be given intramuscularly at once, followed by two (2) mg every 15 to 60 minutes, until the skin is flushed and dry, or mild rapid pulse occurs. *If cyanosis occurs, oxygen also should be administered.*

CAUTION: The above doses that are needed to counteract the poison result in dry, flushed or warm skin, dryness of the mouth, rapid pulse, and rapid breathing. These symptoms may lead to restlessness, hallucinations, disorientation; then depression, medullary paralysis, and death.

14. Bacitracin Ointment, Topical, 500 units/g

USE: For local treatment of skin infections caused by susceptible bacteria. *Not* to be used on large open wounds or on a "weeping" area.

ADULT DOSAGE: Apply a thin layer twice daily, after cleaning the area with mild soap and water.

CAUTION: Hypersensitivity reactions occur rarely.

15. Belladonna Tincture

USE: To relieve recurring spasm of the gastrointestinal tract.

ADULT DOSAGE: The medication should be given three times a day. Begin with a dose of 20 drops in a half glass of water. If necessary, increase each dose by one drop until relief is obtained without disturbing side effects, such as difficulty of vision, dizziness, increase in the pulse rate, and dryness of the mouth. When these symptoms appear, the dose should be lowered by two or three drops, or to a level just below that causing the symptoms.

CAUTION: Contraindicated in angle-closure glaucoma. Patients with glaucoma should use belladonna or atropine only on medical advice.

NOTE: Thirty drops are about equal to 0.6 ml of the tincture, or 0.2 mg of atropine sulfate (the active ingredient).

16. Benzoic and Salicylic Acids Ointment (Whitfield's Ointment)

USE: This ointment may be useful in treating fungal infections of the skin. When applied to skin, it causes the upper layers of the skin to peel off (keratolysis). This action along with a mild antifungal effect helps in the treatment of the infection.

ADULT DOSAGE: The ointment should be applied once or twice daily to the involved area.

CAUTION: External use only. Its use should be discontinued, if irritation or redness occurs.

17. Benzoin Tincture, Compound

USE: (1) For bedsores, and fissures or cracks of the lips.
(2) To protect the skin when extensive taping with adhesive is done.

ADULT DOSAGE: (1) and (2) Apply to the skin as needed.

18. Calamine Lotion, Plain

USE: For relieving itching or irritated skin, heat rash, hives, and ivy poisoning. Shake the bottle well. Wet a pad of cotton with the lotion and pat it on the affected area.

CAUTION: Do not use on open or "weeping" sores unless directed by a physician.

19. Calcium Gluconate Injection, 10%

USE: This injectable medication is intended primarily to be used in case of poisoning by oxalic acid or sodium fluoride. (See p. 111 and p. 114.) These poisonings may cause a depletion of the calcium content of the blood resulting in convulsions (tetany). Calcium gluconate injection acts by restoring needed calcium to the blood.

ADULT DOSAGE: Two to 10 ml of the 10% solution of calcium gluconate should be administered intravenously very slowly until convulsions stop.

CAUTION: Administer with great care and discontinue when the convulsions are brought under control. Overdosage will seriously affect the heart and may result in such symptoms as weakness, depression, loss of appetite, nausea, and vomiting.

20. Charcoal, Activated, Powder

USE: In the initial treatment of most poisonings (because of its property to adsorb many poisons).

ADULT DOSAGE: 10 g (two tablespoonfuls). Mix the powder with water prior to administration. Repeat if the patient vomits.
NOTE: Activated charcoal is a general antidote. It should not be used in place of the antidote specific for a poison when the specific antidote is available. (See text on treatment of poisoning, p. 108.)

21. Chlorinated Lime

USE: As a disinfectant and deodorant for feces, urine, glass, and earthenware. (Not for disinfecting metal instruments or rubber articles.) It is sprinkled liberally over the substance to be disinfected, mixed thoroughly (if indicated) by stirring with a wooden tongue depressor or other suitable implement, and allowed to stand for at least one hour. A small amount of water may be added to facilitate mixing, if necessary.

CAUTION: Open container cautiously away from face and eyes. Replace lid immediately after use to prevent loss of chlorine. Chlorinated lime loses much of its activity, even with careful storage, in a year. Keep separated from internal medications.

22. Chloroquine Phosphate Tablets, 250 mg

USE: To prevent and treat malaria. When a ship is in a known malarial area, obtain medical advice from a physician on prophylactic measures effective in that region.

ADULT DOSAGE: (1) Suppressive (preventive) treatment schedule: begin treatment with chloroquine phosphate two weeks before entering a malarial port. Continue the drug four weeks after the last exposure. The dosage will be 500 mg (two tablets) by mouth once weekly on the same day of each week. Pyrimethamine 25 mg (one tablet) by mouth should be given concurrently with the chloroquine phosphate dose. (2) For acute attack: initially give a dose of 1 g (four tablets) of chloroquine phosphate; then six hours later give 500 mg (two tablets); then two tablets daily on the next two days.

CAUTION: Do not administer to pregnant women or patients with psoriasis or porphyria. Use with caution in patients with liver disease.

Side effects while taking the small weekly suppressive dose are relatively mild and infrequent, and consist mainly of itching and stomach discomfort. When given more frequently to treat acute malaria, the drug may cause headache, eye disturbances, itching, and stomach discomfort with nausea or diarrhea. The drug has caused retinitis, blindness, abnormal condition of the blood (blood dyscrasia), and other serious untoward effects when administered for prolonged periods of time.

23. Clove Oil

USE: For the relief of toothache when there is a cavity in the tooth. If possible, dry the cavity with cotton wrapped on a toothpick and then pack it with a piece of cotton that has been dipped in oil of cloves. This procedure may be repeated as often as necessary. Because clove oil has an irritating effect on tissues, use extra care to avoid contacting surrounding gum or other mouth areas.

24. Codeine Sulfate Tablets, 30 mg

USE: (1) To relieve pain, often to supplement the action of non-narcotic analgesics such as aspirin. It is less constipating, less addicting, produces less respiratory depression, and causes less nausea and vomiting than morphine. (2) To relieve coughing.

ADULT DOSAGE: (1) For persistent and severe pain, give one or two 30 mg tablets by

mouth. This dose may be repeated after two hours if necessary; but do not give additional doses less than four hours apart. Discontinue codeine sulfate as soon as pain lessens enough to be relieved by aspirin. A combination of one 30 mg tablet of codeine sulfate and two 300 mg aspirin tablets is more effective than codeine sulfate alone for pain. (2) For the persistent and severe coughing accompanying severe respiratory infections, give half a 30 mg tablet as often as every two hours, if necessary. This time interval should be lengthened as soon as the cough is controlled. Codeine sulfate should be discontinued if the cough can be relieved by other agents.

CAUTION: Codeine sulfate is an addicting drug but has less addiction liability than morphine or meperidine. It may produce nausea, vomiting, constipation, and dizziness.

WARNING: Schedule II Controlled Substance. Keep in the Master's safe. An exact record of its use must be kept.

25. Cyclizine Hydrochloride Tablets, 50 mg

USE: To prevent and treat seasickness (motion sickness).

ADULT DOSAGE: Give one 50 mg tablet 30 minutes before sailing or before rough weather, if seasickness is expected. Continue giving one tablet three times a day before meals during period of actual or potential seasickness.

CAUTION: May cause some drowsiness and dryness of the mouth. Patients exhibiting drowsiness while receiving cyclizine hydrochloride should *not* be allowed to operate complicated machinery or stand watch.

26. Dextran Injection 6% and Sodium Chloride 0.9%, 500 ml

USE: To expand plasma volume and maintain blood pressure in the emergency treatment of shock caused by a loss of blood. Dextran should be purchased in a package which includes an administration set. *Give on radio advice of a physician.*

ADULT DOSAGE: 500 ml infused intravenously at the rate of 20 to 40 ml per minute, so that the entire amount is given over a period of 15 to 30 minutes. Repeated injections may be given when necessary, if blood or its derivatives are not available. Total amount administered should not exceed 20 ml per kilogram of body weight during the first 24 hours.

CAUTION: Blood is preferred over plasma or dextran in the treatment of shock associated with bleeding and severe burns. Hypersensitivity reactions (rash, itching, nasal congestion, difficult breathing, tightness of the chest, and mild hypotension) are the primary side effects observed. However, the incidence is low and the reactions generally mild. Do not allow the bottle to drain completely of fluid, in order to prevent air from entering the patient's vein.

27. Dextromethorphan Hydrobromide Syrup 15 mg/5 ml, with Glyceryl Guaiacolate

USE: For relieving or preventing cough. This preparation is particularly useful for relatively severe coughs which are persistent and distressing to the patient.

ADULT DOSAGE: Give one 5 ml teaspoonful every six to eight hours. It will be more effective if given at regular intervals, rather than at times the patient is distressed by coughing. For cough, dextromethorphan hydrobromide is generally as effective as codeine sulfate.

CAUTION: Adverse reactions are mild and infrequent, and include slight drowsiness, nausea, and dizziness. If cough persists, obtain medical advice by radio.

28. Dextrose 5% and Sodium Chloride 0.45% Injection, 1000 ml

USE: Intravenously, (1) to provide calories for energy, (2) to replace water in dehydrated patients, (3) to replace chloride and sodium loss, (4) to increase the blood volume in shock or hemorrhage. *Give on radio advice of a physician.*

ADULT DOSAGE: Administered intravenously. One has to adjust dosage for the patient and condition being treated. Most intravenous solutions should not be administered at a faster rate than 500 ml per hour, except in emergency situations.

CAUTION: Careful sterile procedures must be followed. Do not administer unless solution is clear and free of particles. The patient must be checked frequently while it is being administered. Do not allow the bottle to drain completely of fluid, in order to prevent air from entering the patient's vein.

29. Dextrose Injection, 50%, 50 ml

USE: Intravenously, for insulin shock (reaction) when the patient is unable to take carbohydrates by mouth. *Give on radio advice of a physician.*

ADULT DOSAGE: Quantity administered and dilution (if any) must be adjusted for the patient and condition being treated. Administer slowly intravenously, taking care that none of the concentrated solution is injected into tissue surrounding the vein, where it may cause tissue damage.

CAUTION: Sterile procedures must be followed. Do not administer unless solution is clear and free of particles. If a glass ampul is used, particular care should be taken to assure that the solution is not contaminated as the ampul is opened and the medication removed.

30. Diazepam Injection, 5 mg/ml, 2 ml

USE: (1) For treatment of severe agitation, including acute alcohol withdrawal states and convulsions; (2) this medication may be useful for shivering due to generalized hypothermia, see p. 339; and (3) for controlling convulsions (seizures), see p. 204.

ADULT DOSAGE: Usual dosage is from 2 to 10 mg, which may be repeated once in one to four hours, depending upon the response and the severity of the condition.

CAUTION: The injection should be given only on medical advice. Intravenous injection is *not* recommended, as this route of administration causes a very rapid therapeutic effect and side effects which may lead to respiratory arrest.

Overdosage leads to fatigue, drowsiness, diminished reflexes, dizziness, mental confusion, and coma. It should not be given with sedative/hypnotic preparations or narcotics, as it may intensify sedation. Side effects with normal dosages may include dryness of the mouth, subnormal body temperature, fever, slurred speech, or visual disturbances in very few persons. The dosage should be adjusted or discontinued if these symptoms occur.

The drug should be given with extreme caution to persons prone to drug abuse.

WARNING: Controlled Substance, Schedule IV. Keep an exact record of its use. Store in a locked cabinet.

31. Diazepam Tablets, 5 mg

USE: (1) For treatment of common anxiety and tension; (2) for management of agitation during alcohol withdrawal; and (3) it may be of some value for the relief of "backache" caused by skeletal muscle spasms.

ADULT DOSAGE: Varies from 2 to 10 mg, two to four times a day, depending upon the condition being treated.

CAUTION: Overdosage leads to fatigue, drowsiness, light headedness, diminished reflexes, dizziness, mental confusion, and coma. Patients exhibiting drowsiness should *not* be allowed to work complicated machinery or stand watch. Diazepam should *not* be given with barbiturates or similar sedative/hypnotic preparations, or with narcotics.

Side effects from normal dosages may include dryness of the mouth, subnormal body temperature, fever, slurred speech or visual disturbances. The dosage should be adjusted or discontinued if these symptoms occur.

The drug should be given with extreme caution to persons prone to drug abuse. Long-term use of larger than therapeutic doses may result in psychic and physical dependence.

WARNING: Controlled Substance, Schedule IV. Keep an exact record of its use. Store in a locked cabinet.

32. Digoxin Tablets, 0.25 mg

USE: Digoxin is most commonly used in the treatment of congestive heart failure. It is anticipated that the only need for digoxin aboard ship is for the patients who run out of their personal supplies of this medication.

ADULT DOSAGE: The usual dosage is 0.25 mg to 0.50 mg once daily. The patient should start on the dosage previously prescribed by his physician. This medication requires individual dosage adjustment with careful clinical monitoring of cardiac function, until correct cardiac response is obtained.

CAUTION: Patients taking digoxin who exhibit symptoms such as vomiting, nausea, or loss of appetite probably are exhibiting early signs of overdosage and toxicity. A slow pulse (60 per minute or below) also indicates overdose. Should any of these signs occur, the dosage should be reduced or stopped for at least a day.

33. Diphenhydramine Hydrochloride Capsules, 25 mg

USE: (1) To relieve the symptoms of skin rash (urticaria), hay fever and other allergic disorders—but *not* for the treatment of bronchial asthma; (2) to relieve the itching of insect bites and skin inflammations; and (3) to prevent motion sickness.

ADULT DOSAGE: One 25 mg capsule up to four times a day.

CAUTION: Principal side reactions: drowsiness, dizziness, and gastrointestinal upset. *Patients exhibiting drowsiness should not be allowed to operate complicated machinery or stand watch.*

34. Diphenhydramine Hydrochloride Injection, 50 mg/ml, 1 ml

USE: Same as for diphenhydramine hydrochloride capsules, and in addition the supportive treatment of anaphylactic (severe allergic) reactions.

ADULT DOSAGE: Intravenous or deep intramuscular, 10 mg to 50 mg every three hours for severe symptoms (maximum daily dosage, 400 mg).

CAUTION: Doses of 100 mg or more, given by injection to patients with hypertension or cardiac disease, may seriously elevate the blood pressure and accelerate the heart rate. Subcutaneous injection should be avoided because of pain and irritation.

35. Diphenoxylate Hydrochloride 2.5 mg with Atropine Sulfate 0.025 mg, Tablets

USE: This preparation is nonspecific and useful only for the symptomatic treatment of diarrhea. It frequently is effective in diarrhea associated with inflammation or irritation of the gastrointestinal tract, food poisoning, and drug-induced diarrhea.

NOTE: This preparation has advantages over paregoric (camphorated tincture of opium), in that it has low bulk and is relatively free of addicting properties.

ADULT DOSAGE: Give 2 tablets, 3 or 4 times daily, until symptoms are controlled; then reduce dosage for maintenance as required. *If symptoms are not controlled in 24 to 48 hours, obtain medical advice by radio on alternative treatment.*

CAUTION: Do *not* exceed recommended dosage. These tablets contain a subtherapeutic quantity of atropine sulfate to discourage deliberate overdosage. In high dosage the effects of atropine may interfere with the desired constipating effect of diphenoxylate.

Side effects of diphenoxylate may include nausea, vomiting, abdominal cramps, drowsiness, dizziness, skin rash, and insomnia.

WARNING: This is a Schedule V Controlled Substance. Keep an exact record of its use. Store in a locked cabinet.

36. Disinfectant-Detergent, General Purpose, Concentrate, Phenolic Synthetic Type

USE: As an all-purpose disinfectant (in appropriate dilutions) for the sickbay or a patient's quarters. Examples of use: to disinfect bed linens, clothing, towels, surgical dressings, glassware, dishes, bedpans, urinals, lavatories, toilet seats, and bowls. Other uses include the disinfection of rubber goods, and surgical and dental instruments. Remove all blood, dirt, and exudate before soaking items in the disinfectant solution.

CAUTION: Poisonous and caustic in its concentrated form. Do not use on humans or other living animals. Store separately from internal medications.

Many brands have similar effectiveness. Purchase only products labeled with complete directions for dilution and use. Directions vary with the brand. Follow carefully directions on the container in preparing the disinfectant for use.

37. Ephedrine Sulfate Capsules, 25 mg

USE: (1) To relieve difficult breathing in asthma; (2) to prevent asthmatic attacks in chronic cases (effects appear from 30 to 60 minutes after administration); and (3) to relieve nasal congestion in hay fever and severe head colds.

ADULT DOSAGE: One 25 mg capsule four times a day. If ephedrine is used for several days, phenobarbital may be indicated to overcome its stimulant effects (one phenobarbital 30 mg tablet up to three times a day).

CAUTION: Adverse effects include tremors, heart palpitation, mental anxiety, insomnia, and headache. It should *not* be given to patients with chronic heart disease, high blood pressure, diabetes, or hyperthyroidism. It may cause urinary retention in older men.

38. Epinephrine Hydrochloride Injection, 1:1000, 1 ml

USE: (1) For acute asthma attacks, severe reactions to penicillin, aspirin, insect bites; (2) for cardiac or circulatory failure; and (3) employed topically, to check bleeding.

ADULT DOSAGE: By subcutaneous or intramuscular injection, 0.3 ml of 1:1000 solution, every two hours as necessary. The usual dosage range is 0.1 to 0.5 ml.

CAUTION: Epinephrine may cause anxiety, heart palpitation, and headache. Excessive doses can cause acute hypertension and irregular heartbeat. *Except in life-threatening situations,* it should *not* be administered to patients with hypertension, diabetes, hyperthyroidism, and heart disease.

39. Erythromycin Tablets, 250 mg

USE: For a variety of susceptible infections. Give this antibiotic only when medical advice from a physician has been received by radio. It may be useful for patients allergic to penicillin, and for some infections resistant to penicillin.

ADULT DOSAGE: One 250 mg tablet, four times a day (for serious infections dosage may be increased to two 250 mg tablets, four times a day); and continued for 48 hours or more *after* symptoms have subsided.

CAUTION: Occasionally, a skin rash may develop which will require that the drug be discontinued. If the drug is discontinued due to a sensitivity reaction, *medical advice by radio should be obtained on alternate therapy.* Sometimes abdominal discomfort, cramping, or nausea and vomiting may occur; these complaints usually diminish as therapy continues.

40. Ethyl Chloride Spray

USE: As a local anesthetic by freezing the surface of the skin in minor operative procedures, such as incision of carbuncles and furuncles, and removal of localized growths. Its use in surgical procedures is limited because the anesthetic effect is very short; thawing of frozen tissue is painful; and freezing may injure cells, decrease resistance to infections, and delay healing.

It is of limited value in alleviating pain associated with frostbite, burns, and insect stings.

ADULT DOSAGE: Applied topically as a spray, dosage varies with the procedure and the patient's response. Use the smallest dose needed to produce the desired effect. Hold the container about 12 inches from the area being treated and direct the spray downward until a light frosting appears.

Rapid vaporization produces freezing of superficial tissues. Insensitivity of peripheral nerve endings (local anesthesia) usually is maintained up to one minute.

CAUTION: Highly flammable with potential for explosion. Do not use in areas where ignition may occur. *Smoking must be prohibited.* Do *not* apply to broken skin or mucous membranes. Cover adjacent skin with petrolatum to protect against tissue sloughing.

Avoid inhalation because deep general anesthesia followed by death has been reported.

41. Eyewash or Eye Irrigating Solution, Isotonic, Sterile

USE: For irrigating or flushing the eye to wash away foreign particles, mucous secretions, and fluorescein dye used in diagnosis.

DIRECTIONS: Point the tip of the applicator downward toward the eye and gently squeeze the plastic bottle to irrigate. Use generously.

NOTE: The use of a sterile isotonic irrigating solution for the eyes is definitely superior to the use of an eyecup with a non-sterile solution, because it eliminates the chance of infection from either the eyecup or the solution.

CAUTION: Keep the container tightly closed. Do not touch the dispensing tip to the eye or any surface because this may contaminate the solution.

42. Fluorescein Sodium Ophthalmic Strips, Sterile

USE: For the detection of lesions or small foreign bodies embedded in the cornea of the eyeball. Damaged corneal tissue absorbs the dye and the wound (lesion) appears greenish or yellowish.

DOSAGE AND ADMINISTRATION: Anesthetize the eye with one drop of proparacaine hydrochloride eye drops 0.5%. Remove the fluorescein strip from the sterile wrapper without touching the dyed end. Moisten the dyed end with sterile eye irrigating solution. Lift the upper eyelid and touch the dyed tip of the strip to the outside corner of the eye; allow the dye to flow across the eye.

CAUTION: Before using the strip, if the eye is dry, instill a drop of sterile eyewash solution.

43. Furosemide Tablets, 40 mg

USE: Furosemide is a *potent* short-acting diuretic. It is indicated in the treatment of excess body fluid (edema) associated with congestive heart failure, cirrhosis of the liver, or certain kidney diseases. For the treatment of hypertension (high blood pressure), it may be used, either alone or in combination with other drugs.

DOSAGE: The usual oral adult dosage is 40 mg to 80 mg as a single dose in the morning, for two to four consecutive days each week, followed by a drug-free period. However, the dosage will vary weekly, depending upon the patient's condition.

CAUTION: *This drug should be used only after getting medical advice by radio. If excessive doses are administered, there is a rapid loss of sodium, potassium, and calcium electrolytes, in addition to water. This rapid depletion is one of the principal undesired side effects of usage;* others are dermatitis, nausea, vomiting, and diarrhea. The excessive loss of electrolytes usually is indicated by weakness, dizziness, lethargy, leg cramps, vomiting, and/or mental confusion. Should any of these conditions develop during treatment with the drug, it should be discontinued or its dosage adjusted downward.

The drug is contraindicated in women of childbearing age.

44. Gamma Benzene Hexachloride Cream, 1%

USE: For infestations of scabies, lice, and chiggers. A single application usually eliminates the parasites; but a second application is sometimes necessary.

ADULT DOSAGE: After a bath or shower, apply a thin layer directly to the involved skin and hair (but not to the face). Keep it on the skin for 12 to 24 hours, depending on the infestation. Then the patient should bathe or shower thoroughly and put on clean clothes. The bed linen should be changed. If the first application is not successful, a second application may be made after four days. *Clothing and bed linen should be boiled to prevent reinfection.* Instructions on the package should be read and followed carefully.

CAUTION: It is irritating to mucous membranes and should *not* come in contact with the eyes. If accidental contact occurs with the eyes, flush with sterile irrigating solution. Prolonged and repeated applications should be avoided, as there may be absorption through the skin.

45. Glucagon for Injection, 1 mg

USE: The primary use of glucagon is for emergency treatment of patients with severe insulin shock (hypoglycemic reactions) caused by insulin overdosage. It should be used when no one aboard is trained to administer dextrose injection intravenously. It results in a smooth, gradual termination of the patient's coma in 5 to 20 minutes. The drug is useful only if liver glycogen is available. It is of little or no value in starvation, adrenal insufficiency, or chronic hypoglycemia.

ADULT DOSAGE: Glucagon usually is administered subcutaneously or intramuscularly. It may be given intravenously, but this route is not recommended in treatment of patients aboard ship. Glucagon injection is prepared by adding 1 ml of the supplied diluent to the vial of freeze-dried glucagon powder. The usual dose is from 0.5 mg to 1.0 mg, repeated once or twice at twenty-minute intervals, depending upon the depth and duration of the coma. As soon as the patient wakens, carbohydrates, such as candy, should be given orally to prevent secondary hypoglycemic reactions. Failure of the patient to respond within 20 minutes after the second injection necessitates immediate intravenous administration of dextrose.

CAUTION: In emergency situations where low blood sugar only is suspected but not established, glucagon should *not* be substituted for intravenous dextrose.

STORAGE: Follow the directions on the package insert.

46. Hand and Body Lotion (Cream Type)

USE: As a general purpose emollient and protectant for the skin. It may be used by the medical attendant following frequent hand washing. It may also be used as a general body or back rubbing lotion for patients. A bland unscented or very mildly scented lotion should be selected for this purpose.

CAUTION: Hand and body lotions may become contaminated during use, particularly if the lotion contacting the skin is permitted to flow back into the bottle. Containers of lotion should be used by only one person at a time, and destroyed after use by any patient with a communicable disease.

47. Hemorrhoidal Suppositories

USE: For temporary relief of itching, burning, and soreness from hemorrhoids (piles). It soothes inflamed hemorrhoids. The patient should avoid straining on the stool, heavy lifting, coughing, and excessive sneezing. Control constipation (so that straining should not be necessary) with *mild* laxatives. Warm baths may help.

ADULT DOSAGE: Remove the wrapper and insert one suppository as deeply as possible into the rectum in the morning, at bedtime, and immediately after each bowel movement.

CAUTION: Keep refrigerated. If the suppository is soft, hold it under cold water before removing the foil wrapper. Do *not* use if there is bleeding from the rectum. Discontinue use if any of the following occurs: eye pain, rapid pulse, blurring of vision, or dizziness. Use less often if dryness of the mouth occurs.

48. *Homatropine Hydrobromide Eye Drops, 5%*

USE: Homatropine hydrobromide 5% solution is used to dilate the pupil. It causes cycloplegia (paralysis of the ciliary muscle of the eye) and mydriasis (dilation of the pupil). It may be prescribed in the treatment of inflammation of the cornea or the iris.

ADULT DOSAGE: To produce cycloplegia, one drop is instilled into the eye only as often as directed by a physician. Before using, medical advice by radio should be obtained.

CAUTION: Because vision is impaired for several hours after use, caution must be exercised in the assignment of tasks such as operation of machinery or reading gauges.

49. *Hydrocortisone-Neomycin-Polymyxin B Ear Drops*

USE: (1) For local bactericidal action against infections caused by sensitive organisms; and (2) to reduce inflammation, pain, and itching. It is used only for infections of the external ear and external ear canal. After the ear has been cleansed and carefully dried, the medication may be instilled into the canal, or applied to the external surface of the infected ear.

ADULT DOSAGE: Three or four drops instilled three times a day; or a cotton wick may be kept moist with the medication.

CAUTION: Its use is inadvisable in persons with herpes simplex, chickenpox, tuberculosis, and fungal or acute pus-forming infections. *Medical advice by radio should be sought before using on persons* with perforated eardrum, chronic infection of the middle ear, or before continuing treatment beyond a seven day period.

50. *Hydrocortisone Ointment, 1%*

USE: For temporary relief of certain skin disorders, common rashes, inflamed skin, and disorders causing itching and discomfort. It may be used for temporary relief of itching, burning, and soreness from hemorrhoids (piles).

ADULT DOSAGE: Apply a thin film to the affected skin two to four times a day. Apply sparingly and with gentle rubbing. Clean the skin before each use.

WARNING: Do not apply to the eyes. Do not use for extended periods of time without a physician's order. Discontinue use if the condition gets worse.

51. *Hydrocortisone Sodium Succinate for Injection, 100 mg*

USE: *Use on medical advice only,* for: (1) severe shock—large doses combined with standard methods of combating shock help restore blood pressure and circulation; (2) acute allergic reactions—after epinephrine (or other substances that elevate blood pressure) to combat severe asthma, drug reactions, and anaphylactic reactions (such as penicillin reactions); and (3) to control life-threatening inflammation of the lungs after a patient has inhaled vomitus (aspiration pneumonitis).

ADULT DOSAGE AND ADMINISTRATION: Dosage depends on type and severity of the condition. The dose may be as low as 20 mg per day to suppress inflammation, or as high as 2.5 g or more in severe shock. Administer intramuscularly or intravenously. Before using, medical advice by radio should be obtained.

CAUTION: Not for patients with ulcerated corneas, acute psychoses, or a history of active or inactive tuberculosis, except in special life-threatening situations. *Use with caution* in patients with a history of stomach ulcers, and in patients suffering from infections.

52. *Hydrogen Peroxide Solution, 3%*

USE: Its inclusion in the recommended list of pharmaceutical preparations is primarily to utilize the oxygen produced in the adjunct treatment of trench mouth (Vincent's Infection).

ADULT DOSAGE: As a mouth rinse, dilute with equal parts of water and use several times per day, especially after meals. The patient should be told to swish it vigorously in the mouth, then to expectorate.

CAUTION: Its use in wounds should be limited to the initial cleaning, as it is irritating to tissues and may interfere with healing. It should *never* be instilled in a closed body cavity from which the gas formed has no free egress. Keep tightly closed in a cool place. Because it readily loses oxygen on storage, it should be replaced at frequent intervals, at least every six months.

53. Insect Repellent (Diethyltoluamide) Solution

USE: To repel mosquitoes, chiggers, flies, and other biting insects. It can be used on clothing or the skin, protecting for up to eight hours. Shake several drops into the palm of one hand and after rubbing the hands together, apply to the exposed skin and clothes at points where insects are likely to bite through, such as over the shoulder blades, ankles, knees, and hips.

54. Insulin Injection (Regular Insulin) U-100 (100 Units per ml)

USE: For treating diabetic acidosis or coma; and in combination with intermediate or long-acting insulins, to give better control of blood sugar levels after breakfast, dinner, or during the night.

ADULT DOSAGE: There is no average dose. Because it has a short duration of action (5 to 8 hours), and several doses are required daily for diabetic control, regular insulin seldom is used to treat a well-controlled diabetic. Other insulin preparations, such as isophane insulin suspension (NPH), with a longer duration of action are used. Insulin preparations usually are given by injection under the skin. Insulin injection (regular insulin) is the only form of insulin which may be administered intravenously. Therefore, it is used in the treatment of emergency situations such as diabetic acidosis and diabetic coma. *If these conditions are suspected, obtain medical advice by radio on the intravenous use of insulin injection.*

CAUTION: Keep under refrigeration, but not frozen. *In case of an overdose, give the patient fruit juices or candy, and obtain medical advice by radio.* (See Diabetes, p. 154.)

55. Ipecac Syrup

USE: To cause vomiting in cases of poisoning.

ADULT DOSAGE: Give the patient 15 ml by mouth followed by one or two glasses of water. Vomiting should start within half an hour. If vomiting does not occur in 30 minutes, the dose may be repeated once.

WARNING: Do *not* use ipecac syrup if a patient has taken a corrosive acid, lye, or any solvent like mineral spirits or gasoline. (See p. 108.) *In any case of poisoning, medical advice by radio should be obtained immediately.*

56. Kaolin Mixture With Pectin

USE AND ADULT DOSAGE: For simple diarrhea give four 15 ml tablespoonfuls as the first dose, then two 15 ml tablespoonfuls after each loose stool, or every four hours. If no relief is obtained with this treatment in 12 hours, medical advice by radio should be obtained.

Because commercial products from different sources vary somewhat in strength, dosage instructions in the package insert should be given precedence over the above.

57. Lactated Ringer's Injection

USE: For (1) replacing body salts and fluids due to excessive bleeding, vomiting, or diarrhea; and (2) substituting for whole blood or plasma when these are not available. *Get medical advice by radio before administering this intravenous fluid.*

ADULT DOSAGE: Amount depends on the condition of the patient. The usual amount administered is 2000 to 3000 ml per 24-hour period.

CAUTION: As with any injection, careful sterile procedures should be observed. Do *not* administer any intravenous solution unless it is clear and free of particles. To keep air from entering the vein, which could result in a fatal air embolism, do *not* allow the bottle to drain completely.

58. Lidocaine Hydrochloride Injection, 1%

USE: (1) As a local anesthetic in minor surgical procedures; (2) a topical anesthetic on broken skin and mucous membranes; (3)

for ventricular premature beats; and (4) for rapid heart action (tachycardia).

ADULT DOSAGE: The dosage varies with the procedure and the response of the patient. The smallest dose needed to produce the desired effect should be used (see package insert). As a local anesthetic, inject slowly and with frequent aspiration to guard against intravascular injection.

CAUTION: The 2 ml ampul contains no preservative; therefore, *discard the unused contents immediately. Obtain medical advice by radio,* before using for the above cardiac indications (3) and (4).

59. Lubricating Jelly

USE: A lubricant for insertion of rectal thermometers, catheters, appliances or surgical instruments.

60. Magnesium Sulfate (Epsom Salt)

USE: (1) As a quick-acting laxative; and (2) as an external hot wet dressing.

ADULT DOSAGE: (1) For constipation, dissolve one tablespoonful in ¼ glass of water (ice water or orange juice is preferred) and give before breakfast; and (2) for hot wet dressings and soaks in the treatment of bruises, sprains, and swollen joints, mix 1 pound with 1 pint of hot water and apply compresses moistened with the heated solution for 20 minutes every two hours. Keep the solution hot. Use two compresses, applied alternately; this permits relatively continuous application of heat. *Take care not to make the solution too hot.* It should be just hot enough to permit handling without discomfort. An alternative method is to soak the injured part for 20 minutes in a basin filled with the heated solution; repeat every two hours until the pain is relieved.

CAUTION: Never give magnesium sulfate or any other cathartic to a patient with abdominal pain without first consulting a doctor by radio. The patient may have appendicitis which can be seriously aggravated by a laxative.

61. Menthol Ointment, Compound

USE: To relieve muscle pain. While not as effective as the application of heat, the compound does provide some psychological benefit to the patient. When it is rubbed into the skin at the site of the discomfort, it produces a sensation of penetration and warmth.

ADULT DOSAGE: Apply a small amount over the painful area and gently rub into the skin three or four times daily.

CAUTION: Keep away from the eyes, mucous membranes, and irritated or inflamed skin. Heat, from a hot water bottle, heating pads, or hot packs, is a better means of relieving muscle pain. Do *not* apply heat on top of this compound.

62. Meperidine Hydrochloride Injection, 50 mg/ml, 1 ml

USE: For the relief of all types of moderately severe to severe pain. Usually effective within 20 minutes. The effect lasts for three to five hours. In general, it has all of the uses of morphine.

ADULT DOSAGE: The usual adult dose by intramuscular injection is 50 mg to 100 mg. This dose may be repeated in three to four hours.

CAUTION: Administer only when medical advice has been obtained by radio. Because it is potentially addictive, do not use this drug for long periods of time. The patient should be switched to a nonnarcotic analgesic as soon as possible. Dizziness and drowsiness are the most common side effects; therefore, patients should be warned against operating machinery, or unnecessarily exposing themselves to hazards. Meperidine depresses respiration to the same degree as morphine. *See cautions under morphine sulfate.* Meperidine should be used with caution in situations where the use of morphine sulfate entails a risk.

WARNING: This drug is a Schedule II Controlled Substance. Keep locked in the Master's safe. An exact record of its use must be kept.

63. Metaraminol Bitartrate Injection, 10 mg/ml, 1 ml

USE: To restore blood pressure that may have fallen seriously due to trauma, shock, hemorrhage (excessive bleeding), certain infectious diseases, or adverse reactions to drugs. *Before use, obtain medical advice by radio.*

ADULT DOSAGE: Most commonly 5 mg administered subcutaneously, or intramuscularly. In the emergency treatment of severe shock, inject intravenously, with subsequent intramuscular or subcutaneous doses as required. Effects appear within one or two minutes following intravenous administration, in approximately ten minutes following intramuscular injection, and in five to 20 minutes following subcutaneous injection. The duration of action varies from 20 minutes to one hour, or longer. The interval between doses depends largely on the patient's response, but should never be less than 10 minutes; this prevents a cumulative effect.

CAUTION: Overdosage may produce a sustained elevation of blood pressure and severe headache. Use with extreme caution in patients with overactive thyroid, high blood pressure, heart disease, or diabetes.

64. Milk of Magnesia

USE: As an antacid or laxative. To relieve (1) heartburn and sour stomach (when given in small doses); and (2) as a laxative (when larger doses are given).

ADULT DOSAGE: For sour stomach and heartburn, give one 5 ml teaspoonful in one-fourth glass of water, up to four times a day. For constipation, give from one to two 15 ml tablespoonfuls daily as needed.

CAUTION: Never give milk of magnesia or any other cathartic to a patient with abdominal pain, without first consulting a doctor. The patient may have appendicitis which can be aggravated by a laxative.

65. Mineral Oil (Liquid Petrolatum)

USE: Mineral oil (liquid petrolatum) is used as a skin emollient or protective agent. Also, it may be used to help remove ointments or creams from treated skin areas.

It may be indicated by mouth after ingestion of certain poisons, including alkalis (see p. 108).

ADULT DOSAGE: Apply liberally over areas of the skin.

CAUTION: It should *not* be used as a laxative as it may cause a depletion of oil soluble vitamins (A, D, E, and K) from the body.

66. Morphine Sulfate Injection, 10 mg/ml, 1 ml

USE: For severe pain not relieved by other analgesics. *Obtain medical advice by radio prior to use.* Discontinue as soon as the pain can be relieved by other drugs that can be given orally and are less addicting.

ADULT DOSAGE: For the relief of severe pain following injuries or burns, and severe pain of sudden origin in the abdomen or chest, give 10 mg intramuscularly. If the pain is unrelieved, or if it recurs soon after the first dose, a second dose of 10 mg intramuscularly may be given one hour or more later. Give third and subsequent doses, *if necessary*, at intervals of at least four hours—not sooner. If the patient is to be transferred within four hours after receiving morphine, note the time and dosage on a tag securely tied to the front part of the patient's clothing.

CAUTION: An addicting drug. Do not repeat the injection unless ordered by a physician.

NEVER GIVE MORPHINE:
1) when the respiratory rate has slowed to less than 12 breaths per minute;
2) when breathing is difficult and the lips and skin are blue;
3) when mental dullness, unconsciousness, or coma are present, especially after head injury; and
4) for any uses other than herein recommended, except on the order of a physician.

WARNING: Morphine sulfate is a Schedule II Controlled Substance. Keep an exact record of its use. Keep stock locked in the Master's safe.

67. Naloxone Hydrochloride Injection, 0.4 mg/ml, 1 ml

USE: For the *emergency treatment* of respiratory depression resulting from the administration of narcotics, as morphine and meperidine. Also indicated for the detection of suspected acute *narcotic overdosage.*

ADULT DOSAGE: May be given by subcutaneous, intramuscular, or intravenous injection. The intravenous route of administration is recommended for emergency situations. The usual dose is 0.4 mg, repeated every two or three minutes until a favorable response is achieved. If *no* improvement is noted after two or three doses, another cause of the depression should be suspected.

Obtain medical advice by radio on whether use of naloxone is indicated.

CAUTION: The use of naloxone does not preclude the use of other resuscitative measures when indicated, such as the maintenance of an adequate airway, artificial respiration, and cardiac massage. Naloxone is *not* effective in the treatment of respiratory depression caused by non-narcotic drugs, such as alcoholic beverages, hypnotics such as pentobarbital and phenobarbital, and paraldehyde.

68. Nitroglycerin Tablets, 0.4 mg

USE: For an acute attack of angina pectoris.

ADULT DOSAGE: One 0.4 mg (1/150 grain) tablet dissolved under the tongue (sublingually) at the onset of chest pain usually provides complete relief in one to three minutes. Flushing of the face or a throbbing headache may appear. The drug may be given hourly up to several times a day without harm. The person should sit when taking the drug.

CAUTION: A volatile substance. Tablets lose potency upon exposure to air, excessive heat, or moisture. Keep bottle tightly capped and in a relatively cool place. Store tablets in original glass bottle only; do not transfer to another container. If the container is opened during a voyage, replace it with a new lot on returning to home port.

69. Oxygen

USE: To make up for lack of oxygen in blood and tissues, the signs and symptoms of which are cyanosis (bluish color to skin and nail beds); dyspnea (rapid, shallow breathing); rapid, thready pulse, and restlessness. Oxygen may be indicated for respiratory diseases, cardiac diseases, poisoning from gases, massive hemorrhage, and shock.

ADULT DOSAGE: The usual adult dose is six to eight liters per minute by mask; and five to six liters per minute by nasal catheter.

CAUTION: Only trained personnel should administer oxygen. *Use of oxygen presents an explosion hazard.* In the immediate area, do not allow any smoking; nor open flames; nor electrical devices; nor flammable liquids (such as alcohol and ether); nor any device that may cause a spark or is combustible.

70. Paraldehyde

USE: Primarily for alcohol withdrawal symptoms (impending delirium tremens). The drug has a pungent, disagreeable taste which may be improved somewhat by giving it to the patient with chipped ice or with cold drinks such as juice or milk.

ADULT DOSAGE: For oral use, see Impending Delirium Tremens, p. 205.

CAUTION: It is *not* recommended to be used by injection. Never use paraldehyde that is brownish or has a sharp odor of vinegar. Store in a refrigerator in tight, light-resistant containers. *Discard the unused contents of any container that has been opened for more than 24 hours.*

WARNING: This medication is a Controlled Substance that is in Schedule III. Keep an exact record of its use.

71. Penicillin G, Procaine, Sterile Suspension, Injection, 600,000 units/ml, 1 ml

USE AND ADULT DOSAGE: For susceptible infections. For general information on the indications for use of this antibiotic preparation, see the package insert. Dosage varies with the disease being treated. Prior to administering, it, obtain medical advice by radio.

ADMINISTRATION: By deep intramuscular injection, which will yield adequate blood levels for 12 to 24 hours for most susceptible organisms. Preferred injection site is in the inner aspect of the upper outer quadrant of the buttock. For repeated injections, alternate buttocks. Before injecting, pull back on the syringe plunger to make sure that the needle point does not lie within a blood vessel. If blood appears, remove the needle and discard syringe and needle. Prepare a new dose and repeat the procedure in another site.

CAUTION: Penicillin preparations should not be used in patients with known hypersensitivity to the drug. If administered to these patients, a severe allergic (anaphylactic) reaction may occur rapidly and could result in death. *Before administering any penicillin preparation, if possible, determine if the patient is allergic to penicillin.* Should the patient be allergic to the drug, medical advice by radio should be obtained for an alternative anti-infective treatment.

In all cases where a penicillin injection preparation is being given, epinephrine hydrochloride injection 1:1000 should be at hand, ready for immediate administration in case of a severe anaphylactic reaction. (See treatment for anaphylactic reaction, p. 221.)

72. Penicillin G, Procaine, Sterile Suspension, Injection, 2,400,000 units/4 ml

USE AND ADULT DOSAGE: For uncomplicated gonorrhea in the male or female, 4.8 million units of Procaine Penicillin, Aqueous Suspension, divided into at least *two doses*, is injected intramuscularly at different sites. This dose should be accompanied by 1 gram (two 500 mg tablets) of oral Probenecid, preferably given at least 30 minutes prior to the penicillin injections. Give on radio advice of a physician.

ADMINISTRATION: By deep intramuscular injection. The preferred injection site is the inner aspect of the upper outer quadrant of a buttock. Before injecting, pull back on the syringe plunger to make sure that the needle point does not lie within a blood vessel. If blood appears, remove the needle and discard syringe and needle. Prepare a new dose and repeat the procedure in another site.

CAUTION: Penicillin preparations should not be used in patients with known hypersensitivity to the drug. If administered to these patients a severe allergic (anaphylactic) reaction may occur rapidly that could result in death. *Before administering any penicillin preparation, if possible, determine if the patient is allergic to penicillin.* Should the patient be allergic to the drug, obtain medical advice by radio for an alternative anti-infective treatment.

In all cases where a penicillin injection preparation is being given, epinephrine hydrochloride injection 1:1000 should be at hand, ready for immediate administration in case of a severe anaphylactic reaction. (See treatment for anaphylactic reaction, p. 221.)

73. Penicillin V Potassium Tablets, 250 mg

USE: For susceptible infections. Give on medical advice by radio.

ADULT DOSAGE: Usually, an initial dose of two 250 mg tablets should be given by mouth followed by one 250 mg tablet every six hours.

CAUTION: Penicillin preparations should *not* be used in patients with known hypersensitivity to the drug. If administered to these patients a severe allergic (anaphylactic) reaction may occur rapidly and could result in death. *Before administering any penicillin preparation, if possible, determine if the patient is allergic to penicillin.* Should the patient have a history of sensitivity to any penicillin or has other known or suspected allergies, obtain medical advice by radio for an alternative anti-infective treatment.

If an anaphylactic reaction does occur, prompt treatment is needed. (See treatment for an anaphylactic reaction, p. 221.)

74. Pentobarbital Sodium Capsules, 50 mg

USE: (1) Primarily for promoting sleep in extreme insomnia or stress; and (2) for the emergency control of convulsions in tetanus and epilepsy.

ADULT DOSAGE: Two 50 mg capsules at bedtime for sleep. Do not exceed 200 mg per dose, or 500 mg in divided doses, in a 24-hour period.

CAUTION: *This drug is habit-forming and may be addicting, if taken regularly for a long time.* Some neurotic persons attempt to accumulate a supply of this drug (or other Controlled Substance) by hiding the dose they have been given to swallow. Subsequently, with the intent of achieving a feeling of well-being, or with suicidal intent, they may take an overdose. Make certain that this sedative is taken only when the medical attendant is present.

WARNING: A Schedule II Controlled Substance. Keep locked in the Master's safe. Keep an exact record of its use.

75. Pentobarbital Sodium Injection, 50 mg/1 ml, 2 ml

USE: Pentobarbital Sodium injection produces a rapid short-acting sedative-hypnotic effect in the treatment of conditions where immediate sedation is needed, including extreme excitement, mania, or acute convulsive disorders.

ADULT DOSAGE: Pentobarbital sodium injection usually is given intramuscularly, but may be given intravenously slowly for control of acute convulsions. As a hypnotic, the adult dose initially is 150 mg *by the intramuscular route. It should be used only on medical advice by radio.* No more than 250 mg totally should be injected in any one site because of possible tissue irritation.

The adult dose for a convulsion should be 100 mg *given slowly intravenously. It should be used by this route only on medical advice by radio.*

CAUTION: Overdose results in respiratory depression and/or weak heartbeat. Oxygen should be administered when overdosage is suspected.

WARNING: A Schedule II Controlled Substance. Keep locked in the Master's safe. Keep an exact record of its use.

76. Petrolatum, White (White Petroleum Jelly)

USE: As a bland and neutral protective dressing. Apply to minor burns, abrasions, or dry skin.

77. Phenobarbital Tablets, 30 mg

USE: (1) For relatively prolonged sedation, as in some anxiety and tension states, hypertension, heart disease, and gastrointestinal disorders; and (2) for controlling the seizures of epilepsy.

ADULT DOSAGE: As a sedative, one 30 mg tablet, one to four times daily. For sleep, 90 mg at bedtime. For controlling convulsive seizures, the dose of phenobarbital must be adjusted to determine the smallest effective dose. The average range for an adult is between 50 and 120 mg daily, although much higher doses may be required for short periods of time.

CAUTION: Excessive doses of this long-acting barbiturate may lead to drowsiness and lethargy. It may alter the effectiveness of other drugs.

WARNING: A Schedule IV Controlled Substance. Keep locked in a cabinet in the sickbay. Keep an exact record of its use.

78. Phenylephrine Hydrochloride Nasal Spray, 0.25%

USE: Phenylephrine hydrochloride nasal spray is used to relieve nasal stuffiness due to allergy, hay fever, or the common cold.

ADULT DOSAGE: Tilt the head back and spray each nostril twice, every three or four hours.

CAUTION: Do not use for longer than three days. Never allow more than one person to use the same spray bottle.

79. Phenytoin Sodium Capsules, 100 mg (Formerly Diphenylhydantoin Sodium; renamed in 1975)

USE: To prevent or reduce the severity and frequency of epileptic seizures (especially grand mal and psychomotor). It is used often with phenobarbital or other anticonvulsant agents.

ADULT DOSAGE: One 100 mg capsule, three times a day, after meals or with snacks (to prevent stomach upset). Response to the drug may not begin for a week or more; take proper precautions in case of seizures during that interval.

CAUTION: Side effects include failure of muscular coordination, difficulty of vision, skin eruptions, swelling of the gums, and gastrointestinal upset. Reactions frequently are mild and do not interfere with therapy, if dosage is adjusted properly. However, more severe reactions that involve the liver and bone marrow can occur.

80. Pilocarpine Hydrochloride Eye Drops, 2%

USE: For the management of glaucoma. (See Glaucoma, p. 143.) Pilocarpine hydrochloride eyedrops constrict the pupil. It is anticipated that the need for this medication aboard the ship will be for a patient who has run out of his own supply of the medication.

ADULT DOSAGE: For glaucoma, two drops in the eye every six hours daily, or as prescribed.

CAUTION: To prevent contamination of the medication during administration, keep the tip of the eye dropper or the dropper container from touching any part of the eye or surrounding areas.

81. Polymyxin B-Neomycin-Bacitracin Eye Ointment

USE: (1) For superficial eye infections, inflammation of the eyelids and tear sacs; and (2) for the prevention of eye infection when an injury renders the eye or adjacent area vulnerable to infection. This eye ointment frequently is used in conjunction with polymyxin B-neomycin-gramicidin eye drops for treatment at night.

If the eye infection does not improve in 24 hours, medical advice by radio should be obtained.

ADULT DOSAGE: When used alone (without the drops), apply approximately one-half inch on the inside of the lower eyelid every three to four hours. (See Fig. 315.) If used in conjunction with the above-mentioned eye drops, apply only at bedtime.

CAUTION: Prevent the tip of the eye ointment tube from touching the eyelid or surrounding areas (thus preventing contamination of the medication). The ointment should be used for a limited period of time only, because prolonged use may result in overgrowth of nonsusceptible organisms, including fungi. Persons who are allergic to any of the components of the preparation should not be treated with this medication.

82. Polymyxin B-Neomycin-Gramicidin Eye Drops

USE: (1) For superficial eye infections, and inflammation of the eyelids and tear sacs; and (2) for the prevention of eye infection, when an injury renders the eye or adjacent area vulnerable to infection.

If the eye infection does not improve in 24 hours, medical advice by radio should be obtained for possible alternative therapy.

ADULT DOSAGE: The dosage and frequency will vary depending on the severity of the infection. The suggested dosage is one or two drops, two to four times daily, used in conjunction with the polymyxin B-neomycin-bacitracin eye ointment applied at bedtime. In acute infections, initial therapy should be one or two drops every 15 to 30 minutes, reducing the frequency as the infection is controlled.

CAUTION: To prevent contamination of the medication, keep the tip of the eyedropper or dropper container from touching any part of the eye or surrounding areas. Prolonged use may result in an overgrowth of nonsusceptible pathogenic organisms, including fungi; so the eyedrops should be used only for a limited period of time. This medication should not be used by persons who are allergic to any of its components.

83. Povidone-Iodine Skin Cleanser, Liquid

USE: For use whenever a germicidal, cleansing action is required. May be used by sickbay personnel for preoperative and postoperative scrubbing and washing, as a skin degerming agent for preparing the patient's skin, and for preventing and treating acute inflammatory skin infections. This product forms a rich lather which is readily water washable from skin and natural fabrics.

ADULT DOSAGE: Wet the skin and apply a sufficient amount of the cleanser to work up a rich lather. Allow the lather to remain a few minutes and rinse the area with clean water. Repeat this process two to three times a day as needed.

CAUTION: For external use only. If ingested, see Poisoning, p. 108, for treatment.

84. Povidone-Iodine Solution, 1%

USE: As a topical antiseptic* or germicidal solution applied on the skin or mucous membranes to prevent and control susceptible skin infections, certain infections of the mouth and scalp, and for preoperative preparation of the skin.

This preparation retains the nonselective, broad range of germicidal (microbicidal) action of iodine, without the undesirable features in-

---

* An antiseptic stops or inhibits the growth of pathogenic organisms without necessarily killing them.

herent in tincture of iodine. Unlike the tincture of iodine, it can be bandaged or taped without fear of "burning" the skin area.

ADULT DOSAGE: Apply full strength as often as needed to the skin or mucosal lesions by painting, swabbing, or as a wet soak. This solution does not cause stinging or irritation when applied.

CAUTION: For external use only. Local hypersensitivity reactions occur rarely; these are noted primarily in individuals who are sensitive to iodine.

If povidone-iodine is ingested, see poisoning, p. 108, for treatment.

86. Prednisolone Sodium Phosphate Eye Drops, 1%

USE: Use only after receiving medical advice from a physician by radio. For emergency use in the event of injury to the eye or eyelid, resulting from a thermal or chemical burn. First the eye should be examined for injury to the cornea with the aid of fluorescein dye. (See Fluorescein Sodium Ophthalmic strips, p. 279.)

ADULT DOSAGE: Initially, place one or two drops in the eye every hour during the day, and every two hours during the night, until improvement occurs. Thereafter, one or two drops, two to four times daily, for a limited period of time.

CAUTION: Several times a day the eyelids should be opened widely with the fingers to prevent scars forming between the eyelid and the white of the eye.

These eye drops are contraindicated in the treatment of infectious conditions such as tuberculosis, fungal, viral (herpes simplex), and pus forming infections of the cornea and eyelid. *Repeated use in the eye for prolonged periods can result in cataract formation and increased intraocular pressure.*

Again, this preparation should be used only after medical advice by radio has been obtained. Advice given should include the number of days it is to be administered.

86. Probenecid Tablets, 500 mg

USE: As an adjunct to intensive therapy with penicillin G, with ampicillin, and a number of other penicillins, for prolonging the effective blood concentration of these drugs. Also, it is used to promote the elimination of uric acid in the treatment of gout and gouty arthritis.

Probenecid is included in the standard list of medications because it is used with injectable or oral penicillins in the treatment of uncomplicated gonorrhea.

ADULT DOSAGE: Generally, one 500 mg tablet, two to four times a day. For its use in the treatment of uncomplicated gonorrhea, see *drug monographs on use of either penicillin G procaine, sterile suspension, injection, 2,400,000 units or ampicillin capsules, 250 mg.*

CAUTION: Probenecid is well-tolerated, but occasional patients may experience nausea. Rarely, sensitivity may result in a skin rash.

87. Proparacaine Hydrochloride Eye Drops, 0.5%

USE: To produce surface anesthesia of the eye, if necessary, for removal of a foreign body. This drug has a rapid onset (within 20 seconds), but short duration of action (about 15 minutes).

ADULT DOSAGE: One or two drops instilled two or three minutes before beginning the procedure.

WARNING: Because the solution discolors when exposed to warm temperatures, it should be kept in the refrigerator. *Replace open bottles at the start of each voyage.* Check unopened bottles for discoloration. Do *not* use a discolored (brownish) solution. The patient should be warned *not* to rub the eye for at least 30 minutes after instilling, as it may injure the cornea of the eye.

88. Pyrimethamine Tablets, 25 mg

USE: In conjunction with chloroquine for suppressive prophylaxis of malaria in areas where *Plasmodium malariae* parasites are not resistant to it. Pyrimethamine also may be used in conjunction with other antimalarial agents (as quinine) against *Plasmodium falciparum,* a malarial parasite.

ADULT DOSAGE: For malaria prophylaxis, with chloroquine phosphate, one 25 mg tablet once weekly on the same day of each week. Obtain medical advice by radio before starting any member of the crew on this medication.

CAUTION: Side effects from the recommended dose are few, but toxicity increases substantially with larger doses. Loss of appetite, nausea, vomiting, and suppression of blood cell formation occur with larger doses over a prolonged period.

89. Quinine Sulfate Tablets, 300 mg

USE: In the treatment of acute attacks of malaria (except resistant *P. falciparum*). Quinine sulfate is *not* administered to prevent infection but to keep the *Plasmodium* parasite in check so that clinical symptoms do not develop. When the drug is stopped, the symptoms of the disease may reappear. Combination of quinine sulfate with pyrimethamine may be effective in reducing recurrences of *Plasmodium falciparum* infections. *Obtain medical advice by radio, before initiating treatment.*

ADULT DOSAGE: For acute malarial attacks, two 300 mg tablets every eight hours, for 10 to 12 days. For infections caused by *Plasmodium falciparum* (resistant to chloroquine), a combination of quinine and pyrimethamine 50 mg, daily for three days, may be used to prevent recurrences.

CAUTION: Quinine sulfate may produce toxic symptoms, such as ringing in the ears, or a sensation of fullness in the head. Larger doses may cause hearing difficulty or deafness. There may be severe headache, flushed skin, disturbed vision, profuse sweating, abdominal pain, nausea, vomiting, diarrhea, delirium, convulsions, and collapse.

90. Sodium Bicarbonate Injection, 3.75 g [44.6 milliequivalent (mEq)], 50 ml Ampul

USE: This injectable form of sodium bicarbonate is used to combat acute metabolic acidosis that may develop in uncontrolled diabetes or following cardiac arrest. It should be used only after medical advice from a physician has been received by radio. For more details, consult the package insert accompanying the container.

ADULT DOSAGE: The dosage and method of administration will be determined by the physician being contacted for medical advice.

CAUTION: The potentially large amounts of sodium being given with bicarbonate require

that caution be exercised in the use of sodium bicarbonate in patients with congestive heart failure.

The addition of sodium bicarbonate to infusions containing calcium salts (such as Lactated Ringer's Injection) should be avoided. A haze may result (showing an incompatibility) from the sodium bicarbonate-calcium admixture.

91. Sodium Bicarbonate Powder (Baking Soda)

USE AND ADULT DOSAGE: For symptomatic relief of insect bites and stings. Make a soothing paste by adding a small amount of water to the powder and apply to the affected area.

Weak solutions are used frequently as irrigants and washes.

CAUTION: Do *not* use as an antacid for heartburn or sour stomach. "Bicarb" has little merit as a gastric antacid; the duration of action is brief and excessive use may produce metabolic alkalosis.

92. Sodium Biphosphate and Sodium Phosphate Solution for Enema

USE: When a cleansing enema is indicated, or to assist in eliminating fecal impactions.

ADULT DOSAGE AND ADMINISTRATION: The rectal unit is ready for use. Remove the cover, gently insert the prelubricated tube into the rectum, and squeeze out the contents of the plastic bottle (135 ml or 4½ fluid ounces). The preferred position to administer an enema is to have the patient lie on his left side with knees flexed, or in the knee-chest position. This position should be maintained until a strong impulse to defecate is felt, usually within two to five minutes.

CAUTION: This should *not* be used in the presence of abdominal pain, nausea, vomiting, cardiac disease, severe dehydration, or debility.

93. Sodium Chloride Injection, 0.9%, 100 ml

USE: Intravenously, (1) to replace chloride and sodium loss that occurs in extensive vomiting or diarrhea; (2) to maintain the extracellular fluid; and (3) as a diluent for injection of other drugs. *Obtain medical advice by radio before administering.*

ADULT DOSAGE: Depends on patient's condition. Generally, from 1500 to 3000 ml may be given over 24 hours. Do not give intravenous solutions at a faster rate than 500 ml per hour, except on medical advice by radio.

CAUTION: As with any injection, sterile procedures should be observed. Do not administer any intravenous solution unless it is clear and free of particles. Watch the solution carefully while it is being administered. Do *not* allow the bottle to drain completely of fluid, in order to keep air from entering the patient's vein.

94. Sodium Chloride Tablets, 1 g

USE: To help avoid heat exhaustion, heatstroke, or heat cramps, by replenishing body salts lost through excessive perspiration.

ADULT DOSAGE: Depends on the amount of perspiration. For profuse sweating, give one tablet with a full glass of water, every four hours during working hours. If weather is hot but perspiration is not excessive, give one tablet with a full glass of water, every eight hours while awake. (See p. 105.)

95. Sulfadiazine Silver Cream, 1%

USE: To aid in the prevention and treatment of infection in second- and third-degree burns. *In all cases of severe burns, pain and shock should be controlled and medical advice by radio sought immediately.*

ADULT DOSAGE: Sulfadiazine silver, 1% cream should be applied to cleansed burned areas once or twice daily to a thickness of approximately one-sixteenth inch, using a sterile gloved hand. Burned areas should be covered with the cream at all times, and dressings usually are not required. Treatment with sulfadiazine silver cream should be continued as long as there is a possibility of infection or until the patient can be evacuated, unless a significant adverse reaction occurs.

CAUTION: Local or systemic adverse reactions to the drug may occur. Pain, burning, or itching following application of sulfadiazine silver cream have been most frequently reported. Medical advice by radio should be sought to

determine whether the drug should be discontinued.

96. Sulfisoxazole Tablets 500 mg

USE: To treat susceptible infections, primarily of the urinary tract.

ADULT DOSAGE: Usually, eight 500 mg tablets (4 g) for the first dose, then two 500 mg tablets four times a day, until the temperature has been normal for at least 48 hours. *Use only after medical advice by radio has been obtained, and in the dosage recommended.* Give each dose with a full glass of water.

CAUTION: Toxic reactions, which rarely occur, include skin rashes, itching, fever, nausea, vomiting, headache, dizziness, mental depressions, moderate to extreme reduction in the amount of urine, blood in the urine, and jaundice. If any of these appear, *stop the drug* and seek medical advice by radio as to alternate therapy.

97. Sunscreen Preparations

USE: Use of a sunscreen preparation blocks out varying degrees of ultraviolet solar radiation, which causes sunburn. Prolonged or excessive exposure to the sun without protection may cause wrinkling and damage to the skin, which can lead to solar keratoses and skin cancer.

No sunscreen preparation is totally effective. The most effective way to avoid injury from the sun is to cover the exposed skin with appropriate clothing. However, where there is exposure to the sun's rays, either directly or by reflection from the water, an effective sunscreening preparation should be applied to exposed skin prior to and during daylight periods of strong sunlight.

There are a number of effective sunscreening preparations commercially available. Thus, no specific preparation is recommended. It is important, when considering a preparation for use, to know the sunscreening ingredient and its effectiveness in the formulation.

An *alcoholic* solution of para-aminobenzoic acid (PABA) or its esters (salts), such as a formulation of 5% PABA in an alcoholic solution (50% to 70%), is one of the most effective sunscreening formulations. The group of chemicals, benzophenones, also are effective sunscreens.

ADULT DOSAGE: Sunscreening preparations should be applied according to the directions on the container's label.

CAUTION: On some individuals, the chemicals in sunscreen preparations may cause burning and redness in the area of application. If this occurs, the preparation should be discontinued immediately.

98. Talc (Talcum Powder)

USE: As a skin lubricant and protectant, and as a dusting powder for such skin irritations as chafing and prickly heat.

CAUTION: Do not use as a lubricant for hands or gloves at the time of surgery. Any talc entering surgical incisions, wounds, or certain body cavities may cause a granuloma formation.

99. Tetanus Immune Human Globulin, 250 units

USE: To provide passive immunity to tetanus in a patient who has sustained a potentially contaminated wound, and is lacking active immunization (with adsorbed tetanus toxoid).

ADULT DOSAGE: For passive immunization, 250 units by *intramuscular* injection only.

If active immunization with adsorbed tetanus toxoid cannot be established, give a dose of *tetanus immune human globulin,* and a reinforcing (booster) dose of 0.5 ml *adsorbed tetanus toxoid* at the same time in a different extremity with a separate syringe.

If the patient has received a booster dose or full basic series within the past 12 months, do not give either the toxoid or the tetanus immune human globulin.

CAUTION: Side effects following intramuscular administration are infrequent, mild, and usually confined to the injection area. Although systemic reactions are rare, epinephrine hydrochloride 1:1000 should be available for immediate use.

Store at 35.6° F to 46.4° F (2° C to 8° C) and avoid freezing.

100. Tetanus Toxoid, Adsorbed

USE: For active immunization against tetanus.

ADULT DOSAGE: For primary immunization of adults and children over six years of age, three doses (see package insert for amount of each dose) are required. These are injected intramuscularly into the lateral aspect of the upper arm. The second dose is given four to six weeks after the first; and the third dose, six months to one year after the second. Thereafter, the recommended dose is administered every ten years.

In wound management it is not necessary to give booster injections more often than every five years. If a dose is given as a part of wound management, the next routine dose to maintain ability to react promptly to a booster injection of Tetanus Toxoid will not be needed for another ten years.

CAUTION: Store in the refrigerator, but avoid freezing. This preparation should *not* be used for the protection of an exposed person who has not been actively immunized previously against tetanus, nor for the treatment of a patient who has tetanus. Severe reactions to the toxoids are rare; some local soreness and redness may persist for two or three days. Epinephrine hydrochloride injection 1:1000 always should be available for use in case of an anaphylactic reaction.

101. Tetracycline Hydrochloride Capsules,* 250 mg

USE: For susceptible infections; *to be given after receiving medical advice by radio.*

ADULT DOSAGE: Usually, one 250 mg capsule every six hours. In severe illness, increase to two 250 mg capsules every six hours.

Because food interferes with absorption of tetracycline, the drug should not be given orally less than one hour before meals, or sooner than two hours after meals. Tetracycline should not be administered with milk, or calcium-containing foods. Antacids containing aluminum, magnesium, or calcium also will impair absorption of tetracycline from the gastrointestinal tract, and should not be given with tetracycline.

CAUTION: Prolonged therapy may result in superinfection of the colon with non-susceptible

---

* Some brands are available in tablet dosage form.

bacteria and yeast. The drug may produce loss of appetite, nausea, vomiting, bulky loose stools, and diarrhea in some patients.

102. Tolnaftate Powder, 1%

USE: For topical treatment of a number of acute and chronic fungal infections of the skin. It is specific for the treatment of ringworm, athlete's foot, and susceptible fungal infections of the groin and inner surfaces of the thighs.

The powder can be used advantageously in conjunction with the solution on naturally moist skin areas where drying may enhance the therapeutic response. The powder is of particular value, following complete remission, in maintaining this state or in reducing the risk of infection.

ADULT DOSAGE: A small quantity of the powder is dusted on the fungal infections and the surrounding areas. The powder should be spread evenly over the areas by light rubbing.

Using the powder in conjunction with the solution is an effective means of treating athlete's foot. The solution is applied to the fungal lesions and the powder is dusted lightly into the shoes. To avoid reinfection, the dusting of the shoes should be continued for several weeks after an apparent cure.

CAUTION: If the patient shows no improvement after three weeks, or if evidence of irritation or sensitivity develops, or if lesions become worse after use of the drug, treatment should be discontinued. Then medical advice by radio should be obtained on further treatment.

103. Tolnaftate Solution, 1%

USE: For topical treatment of a number of acute and chronic fungal infections of the skin. It is specific for the treatment of ringworm, athlete's foot, and susceptible fungal infections of the groin and inner surfaces of the thighs.

The tolnaftate powder (see above) can be used advantageously in conjunction with tolnaftate solution on naturally moist skin areas where drying may enhance the therapeutic response.

ADULT DOSAGE: Apply one or two drops (only a small quantity required) and rub well into lesions twice daily for two or three weeks.

CAUTION: Treatment with tolnaftate should be discontinued if the patient shows no improvement after three weeks. If there is evidence of irritation or sensitivity, or if the lesions become worse, discontinue use of the drug. Then medical advice by radio should be obtained about further treatment.

104. Whisky, Medicinal

USE: As a mild sedative or tranquilizing agent.

As a specific treatment in methyl (wood) alcohol poisoning.

ADULT DOSAGE: Depending upon the patient's condition and tolerance, 15 ml to 60 ml may be administered as a single oral dose, either straight or diluted with water or juice.

CAUTION: Whisky and all other alcoholic beverages are central nervous system depressants. They should be administered *with great caution* to patients who are mentally depressed or who are taking other drugs. *Many patients do not understand the importance of these precautions and deaths have occurred as a result.* This is an area in which the medical attendant can play a vitally important educational role.

105. Zinc Oxide Paste (Lassar's Plain Zinc Paste)

USE: A nontoxic, protective, water insoluble, mildly astringent, and antiseptic paste employed in a large variety of diseases and irritations of the skin. Zinc oxide paste differs from zinc oxide ointment in that it is somewhat more protective.

DOSAGE: Apply as needed in a thin layer to skin areas to be treated or protected from sunlight or weather.

SURGICAL EQUIPMENT, INSTRUMENTS, AND SUPPLIES

Use of the Table of Surgical Equipment, Instruments, and Supplies

It is assumed that the officer aboard a merchant vessel, in either the A or B categories described below, who has the responsibility for the care and treatment of seamen, will have had training in the administration and use of the recommended items.

Column A of Table 6–2 shows the minimum number of items (figures in UNIT column) recommended for oceangoing merchant vessels, without a doctor aboard. The quantities are based on an estimated four-month inventory for a crew complement of 25 to 40 persons.

Column B of Table 6–2 gives the minimum number of items recommended to be carried aboard merchant vessels engaged in trade solely in coastal, Great Lakes, and nearby foreign ports, and not more than 12 hours away from a port of call. The quantities are based on an estimated four-month inventory for a crew complement of approximately 25 persons.

Column C of Table 6–2 presents the minimum number of items recommended for fishing boats or private craft which normally do not carry more than 15 persons, and are never more than a few days from home port, or a few hours from a port of call.

Table 6–2

Surgical Equipment, Instruments, and Supplies Recommended for the Ship's Medicine Chest

Description of Item	Unit	Quantities			Notes
		A	B	C	
Equipment					
Basin, emesis, kidney shape	each	1	1	–	
Basin, wash, with rim	each	1	1	–	
Bedpan	each	1	1	–	
Board, spine, long	each	1	1	1	
Cane, with rubber tip	each	1	1	–	
Crutch, adjustable, wood, with rubber tips	pair	1	–	–	
Cushion, crutch, sponge rubber, arm	each	2	–	–	
Heating pad, electric, waterproof, AC/DC	each	1	–	–	
Hot water/ice bag, rubber, stopperless type	each	1	1	–	
Litter, Stokes	each	1	1	–	
Oxygen unit, portable, with size E oxygen cylinder, adult face mask, regulator, tubing, wrench, instruction books (all in self-contained carrying case)	each	2	1	1	
Refrigerator, about 3.2 cu ft capacity, with inside thermometer, cyclamatic automatic defrosting, to operate on ship's electrical current, and fitted with a lock	each	1	1	–	
Restraining equipment					Restraints may be improvised from bedsheets. (See pp. 205–6.)
Cuffs, leather or cloth	pair	2	1	–	
Mummy restraint	each	1	1	–	
Sideboard	each	2	2	–	
Resuscitator, hand-operated, with excess pressure relief device, inlet check valve w/nipple for optional connection to low pressure oxygen line	each	1	1	1	Consists of a compressible bag with a check valve, storage bag/grommets, adult face mask, and a non-rebreathing valve.

Table 6–2 (continued)

Surgical Equipment, Instruments, and Supplies Recommended for the Ship's Medicine Chest

Description of Item	Unit	Quantities			Notes
		A	B	C	
Equipment (continued)					
Scales, adult, weighing, clinical, 300 pound capacity	each	1	–	–	
Sphygmomanometer, aneroid, 300 mm scale, hand type, complete in case	each	1	1	1	Unit for taking blood pressure.
Splint, Hare traction	each	1	–	–	
Splints, inflatable, arm, for above/below elbow, assorted sizes, 6s	pkg.	1	1	1	
Splints, inflatable, leg, for above/below knee, assorted sizes, 6s	pkg.	1	1	1	
Splints, finger, aluminum padded, assorted sizes, 6s	pkg.	1	1	1	
Sterilizer, steam pressure type, for dressings and instruments	each	1	–	–	Should be of a type with a drying phase
Stethoscope, disc-diaphragm type	each	1	1	1	
Stretcher (litter), folding, rigid pole	each	1	–	–	
Thermometer, bath	each	2	–	–	
Tray, with cover, for small instrument sterilization	each	1	–	–	To be a component of the sterilizer; must fit inside sterilizer compartment
Urinal, male	each	2	–	–	
Receptacle, with pedal-operated lid, 12 liter (4 gal)	each	1	–	–	
Instruments					
Airway, pharyngeal, plastic, adult and child sizes	each	2	1	1	
Blade, surgical knife, detachable, small tang, no. 10, sterile 6s	pkg.	1	1	–	
Blade, surgical knife, detachable small tang, no. 11, sterile, 6s	pkg.	1	1	–	
Blade, surgical knife, detachable small tang, no. 15, sterile 6s	pkg.	1	1	–	
Forceps, dressing, bayonet-shaped, Adson, 7⅛ inch	each	1	1	1	
Forceps, hemostat, curved, Halstead, mosquito, 5 inch	each	2	–	–	
Forceps, hemostat, straight, Halstead mosquito, 5-inch	each	2	–	–	
Forceps, hemostat, curved, Kelly, 5½-inch	each	2	–	–	
Forceps, splinter, tweezers, 3½-inch	each	1	1	1	
Handle, knife (scalpel), #3	each	2	1	–	For detachable surgical knife blades
Scissors, bandage, Lister, angular, one point sharp, one point blunt, 7¼-inch	each	3	1	1	

Table 6–2 (continued)
Surgical Equipment, Instruments, and Supplies Recommended for the Ship's Medicine Chest

Description of Item	Unit	Quantities A	B	C	Notes
Supplies					
Adhesive tape, surgical, 2 inches by 5 yards	roll	6	1	1	
Adhesive tape, surgical, porous, hypoallergenic, 2 inches by 10 yards	roll	2	1	–	For use on patients allergic to regular adhesive tape.
Administration set, intravenous, with butterfly hub needle, 19-gauge x 1½-inch, sterile, disposable (IV Set)	each	6	1	–	Procure from the same manufacturer that supplies the intravenous fluids.
Applicators, wood, cotton tipped ends, sterile, ¹⁄₁₂ inch by 6 inches, 2s	pkg.	25	25	25	
Bandage, cotton, elastic, rubberless, 4 inches by 5½ yards, roll, 12s	box	1	–	–	
Bandage, cotton, elastic, rubberless, 3 inches by 5½ yards, roll, 12s	box	1	½	½	
Bandage, cotton, elastic, rubberless, 2 inches by 5½ yards, roll, 12s	box	1	½	½	
Bandage, gauze, roller, sterile 1 inch by 10 two ply, clinging, two safety pins, 12s	pkg.	1	1	1	Elastic gauze bandage similar to Kling® bandage
Bandage, absorbent, adhesive, ¾ inch by 3 inches, 100s	box	2	1	1	Absorbent bandage with adhesive similar to Band-aids®
Forceps, splinter, tweezers, 3½-inch yards, 12s	box	1	1	1	
Bandage, gauze, roller, sterile, 3 inches by 10 yards	each	6	3	3	
Bag, mortuary transfer, leakproof (see mortuary transfer bag, leakproof)	each	2	–	–	
Bandage, muslin, triangular, folded, with two safety pins, 37 inches by 52 inches	each	2	1	1	May be used as a sling or as a general bandage wrap.
Bottle, vial, amber, 9 dram, glass or plastic, for capsules or tablets, 72s	box	1	–	–	Gummed labels should be procured and kept with these bottles.
Catheter, double eye, pointed, Robinson, sterile, disposable:					
6 French	each	1	1	–	For urinary catheterization. 6- and 8 French can be used for pharyngeal suction.
8 French	each	1	1	–	
10 French	each	1	1	–	
12 French	each	1	1	–	
14 French	each	1	1	–	
16 French	each	1	1	–	

Table 6–1(Continued)
Pharmaceutical Preparations Recommended for the Ship's Medicine Chest

Item No.	Description of Item	Unit	Quantities			Notes
			A	B	C	
	Supplies (continued)					
	Catheterization tray, sterile, disposable, regular type: a 14 French straight catheter, sterile gloves, small forceps, cotton balls, lubricant, antiseptic solution, underpad and drape, specimen container and label	each	3	1	–	
	Catheter, urethral, balloon, round tip, self-retaining, double eye, modified Foley, sterile, 5 ml bag:					
	14 French	each	1	–	–	
	20 French	each	1	–	–	
	Catheterization tray, sterile, disposable, retention type: with 5 ml bag, 16 French Foley catheter, sterile gloves, small forceps, cotton balls, lubricant, antiseptic solution, 10 ml syringe with 9 ml sterile water, underpad and drape, specimen container and label	each	2	1	–	
	Clinical record chart, pad	pad	1	1	–	
	Collar, cervical, with strap	each	1	–	–	
	Cotton, absorbent, sterile, 115 g	pkg.	3	1	1	
	Finger cots, rubber assorted sizes, 12s	box	1	1	1	
	Flashlight (penlight type), with replacement batteries	each	1	1	1	
	Gauze, petrolatum, 6 inches by 36 inches, sterile, 6s	box	2	1	1	
	Gauze, bandage, tubular ⅞-inch by 5 yards, rolled, with applicator	roll	1	1	1	Covering bandage for fingers and toes.
	Gloves, surgical, sterile, disposable, large size (size no. 7½ or 8), 12s (pair)	box	1	–	–	
	Gowns, surgical, disposable	each	50	–	–	
	Hammer, reflex testing, 8-inch	each	1	–	–	
	Masks, face, disposable, 100s	box	2	–	–	
	Medicine cup, (waxed paper or plastic), 30 ml, graduated, disposable, 100s	box	1	1	1	
	Mortuary transfer bag, leakproof	each	2	–	–	
	Needle holder, suture, Hegar-Mayo 5½ inch	each	2	–	–	
	Needle, hypodermic, 18 gauge, 2-inch, sterile, 6s	pkg.	6	–	–	
	Needle, hypodermic, 25 gauge, ½-inch sterile, 6s	pkg.	6	1	–	
	Occult blood detection tablet, with 60 filter papers, 60s	pkg.	1	–	–	For detection of occult blood in feces or sputum.
	Orangewood Sticks, 25s	pkg.	1	1	1	
	Otoscope, battery type, with aural and nasal speculum	each	1	–	–	Maintain replacement lamps and batteries.

Table 6–2 (continued)
Surgical Equipment, Instruments, and Supplies Recommended for the Ship's Medicine Chest

Description of Item	Unit	Quantities			Notes
		A	B	C	
Supplies (continued)					
Pad, abdominal, sterile combined dressing, gauze, 8 inches by 7½ inches, individually sealed	each	6	3	3	
Pad, cotton, eye, sterile, individually sealed, 12s	pkg.	1	1	1	
Pad, non-adherent sterile dressing, non-woven cotton and rayon fabric with perforated plastic cover, individually sealed, 3 inches by 4 inches, 100s	pkg.	1	1	1	Similar to Telfa® type gauze pads. Dry dressing material for wounds.
Safety pins, rustless, assorted sizes, 50s	card	1	1	1	
Scrub brush, hand	each	2	2	1	
Sheath, rubber (condoms) 3s	pkg.	a sufficient quantity			
Sheet, waterproofing, 45 inches by 72 inches	each	2	1	1	
Skin closure, adhesive, surgical, sterile (butterfly closure), ¼-inch, 25s	pkg.	4	1	1	To close wounds in place of sutures when feasible.
Sponge (pad), isopropyl alcohol impregnated, sterile, individually sealed in plastic foil, nonwoven, cotton or rayon, 1½-inch by 2 inches, 100s	pkg.	1	1	1	For preparation of the skin prior to injections.
Sponge, surgical, sterile, eight ply, gauze, 4 inches by 4 inches, in sealed envelopes, 200s	pkg.	1	¼	¼	
Sponge, surgical, sterile, eight ply, gauze, 2 inches by 2 inches, in sealed envelopes, 200s	pkg.	1	¼	¼	
Suture, tapered, ½ circle nontraumatic needle, 1⅛ inch, absorbable, nonboilable, 27 inches long, size 00, sterile, individually sealed, 12s	pkg.	1	–	–	
Suture armed, ½ circle, 1-inch nontraumatic needle, nonabsorbable, silk, braided, 18 inches long, size 000, sterile, individually sealed, 12s	pkg.	2	1	–	
Suture, armed, ⅜-circle, 11/16-inch needle, 000 size, sterile, absorbable, individually sealed, 12s	pkg.	1	–	–	
Suture, armed, nonabsorbable, polyester, ⅜-circle, ½-inch needle with nontraumatic point, size 5-0, sterile, sealed, 12s	pkg.	1	–	–	
Suture removal kit, containing: suture removing forceps, sterile, and suture removal scissors, sterile	kit	1	–	–	

Table 6–2 (continued)
Surgical Equipment, Instruments, and Supplies Recommended for the Ship's Medicine Chest

Description of Item	Unit	Quantities			Notes
		A	B	C	
Supplies (continued)					
Syringe, ear and nose, rubber, 90 ml (3-ounce)	each	2	1	1	
Syringe, glass, 120 ml (4 ounce) complete with removable rubber bulb and tip	each	4	1	1	
Syringe, hypodermic, insulin, 100 units/ml, 1 ml, ¾-inch 25 gauge needle affixed, sterile, disposable, sealed	each	24	6	1	
Syringe, hypodermic, Luer, 2 ml, 25 gauge ¾-inch needle affixed, sterile, disposable, individually sealed	each	24	6	1	
Syringe, hypodermic, Luer, 5 ml, 21 gauge 1½-inch needle affixed, sterile, disposable, sealed	each	12	1	1	
Syringe, Luer, general lavage, large tip with metal syringe adapter, 50 ml	each	2	1	1	
Syringe, cartridge holder for injectable medications	each	2	1	–	To be used with a drug unit dose system (a closed injection system such as Tubex®
Test strip and color chart combined (urinary blood, glucose, ketone, protein, bilirubin, and pH), 100s	bot.	1	1	1	Similar to Bili-Labstix®
Test tablets, kit, glucose (reducing sugar) in urine, individually sealed, 36s	pkg.	3	–	–	Similar to Clinitest® tablets.
Tissues, facial	box	6	3	3	
Thermometer, clinical, fever, combination oral-rectal (stubby type)	each	6	2	2	
Tourniquet, non-pneumatic, blood-taking type, composed of gum rubber with velcro type fastener	each	1	1	1	
Tongue depressors, wood, 100s	box	1	¼	¼	
Towels, paper, sterile, disposable, individually wrapped, 12s	pkg.	2	1	–	
Towels, surgical, cotton, 12s	pkg.	1	–	–	
Tube, stomach, with funnel	each	2	1	–	For stomach lavage in case of poisoning.
Urine collection bag, with tubing, sterile, disposable	each	2	1	–	
Visual chart, "Snellen" type	each	1	–	–	For eye examination.
Wrapping material, autoclave	pkg.	1	–	–	For wrapping instruments and dressings for sterilization.
Wrapping (sealing) tape, ½-inch by 60 yards, sterilization indicator	roll	1	–	–	See preceding entry.

Procurement and Storage of Surgical Equipment, Instruments, and Supplies

The kinds of surgical equipment, instruments, and supplies and quantities that are recommended to be maintained on board vessels are shown in table 6-2. These items will be either reusable or disposable, sterile or non-sterile.

Where commercially available, packaged sterile disposable supplies and equipment should be procured, especially disposable needles, syringes, medicine cups, dressing and suture trays, catheter trays, enema preparations, and surgical gloves. It is now generally recognized that the incidence of hepatitis and many other infections has been decreased through the use of commercially packaged sterile disposables. When items are processed and sterilized aboard ship, there is always the danger that they will be inadequately sterilized, and their use could possibly result in adding an infection to an already ill patient.

Commercially packaged and presterilized disposables are protected by inner and outer envelopes which are mechanically sealed. This type of packaging prevents biological contaminants from gaining access to the interior; so sterility will be maintained for as long as the package remains intact. However, assurance that the item is "sterile" is only one aspect of commercial packaging. Other advantages are: clear instructions on the package prevent misunderstanding and encourage proper use; packages can be opened easily without breaking asepsis; and often, the package wrapping can serve as a sterile field.

The contents of unopened or intact sterile disposable packages should remain sterile until opened. However, to be assured that the contents have not deteriorated, *they should be replaced at least every five (5) years or on the expiration date, whichever occurs first.*

In purchasing supplies, whether reusable or disposable, it is important to know the approximate usage of the article to avoid either overstocking or understocking. When receiving surgical supplies, to insure rotation of stock, it is important that new items be placed on shelves *in back of or under those on hand.* This procedure will help assure that the oldest supplies will be used first.

Sterilizing Surgical Equipment, Instruments, and Supplies

Should it be necessary to process and sterilize reusable (nondisposable) supplies, equipment or instruments, only persons who have been fully trained in sterilization techniques and procedures should be assigned to this activity. To a significant extent, the knowledge and integrity of the people who do the work determine the quality and safety of the finished product.

When it is necessary to prepackage and sterilize reusable items for future use, the following factors should be kept in mind. Under normal conditions of clean storage, items enclosed in wrapping material suitable for sterilization by steam under pressure, and sterilized correctly, can be depended upon to remain sterile for at least 30 days. This also applies to articles placed in autoclavable plastic coverings with effective closures. Changes in atmospheric conditions surrounding the packages, deterioration of the wrapping material, and rough handling of the packages are contributing factors to possible contamination.

If a great number of these prepackaged sterile supplies have not been used by the end of 30 days, an effort should be made to reduce the need for resterilization by decreasing the sterile inventory of the unused articles. Before resterilization, all components of the package including the wrapper, must be completely reprocessed.

Table 6–3
WEIGHTS AND MEASURES WITH APPROXIMATE EQUIVALENTS

Selected Metric System Units with Approximate Equivalents* in Other Systems

Metric Weights

1 kilogram (kg), 1000 grams	= 2.2 pounds (lb) Avoirdupois
1 gram (g or Gm), 1000 milligrams	= 15 grains (gr)
1 milligram (mg), 0.001 gram	= 1/60 grain
1 microgram (mcg), 0.001 milligram	= 1/60,000 grain

Note: Care must be continually exercised to not misinterpret the abbreviation "g" for "gr" as, dosage-wise, one gram (g) is 15 times as potent as one grain (gr).

Metric Liquid Measures

1 liter (l), 1000 milliliters	= 32 fluid ounces (fl. oz)
1 milliliter (ml)	= 16 minims (min)

Note: A milliliter (ml) is the approximate equivalent of one cubic centimeter (cc).

Household Measures and Approximate Equivalents

240 ml	=	tumblerful or cup	=	8 fluid ounces
120 ml	=	teacup	=	4 fluid ounces
60 ml	=	wineglass	=	2 fluid ounces
15 ml	=	tablespoonful	=	3 fluid drams
8 ml	=	dessertspoonful	=	2 fluid drams
5 ml	=	teaspoonful	=	1 fluid dram

Note: In most cases, the modern household containers have been found to *average* 25% greater capacity than the theoretical quantities shown above.

---

* More than one approximate equivalent may be customary and acceptable when conversion is necessary

Selected Apothecary and Avoirdupois Systems Units with Approximate Equivalents in the Metric System

Apothecary Weights	*Metric System Equivalents*
1 ounce, 480 grains	= 30 grams
1 dram, 60 grains	= 4 grams
1 grain	= 60 or 65 milligrams

Apothecary Liquid Measures

1 quart (qt), 32 fluidounces	= 1,000 milliliters (ml)
1 pint (pt), 16 fluidounces	= 500 ml
1 fluid ounce (fl oz)	= 30 ml
1 fluid dram, 60 minims	= 4 ml
1 minim	= 0.065 ml

Avoirdupois Weights

1 pound (lb)	= 454 grams
1 oz	= 28.35 grams

Selected Metric System Lengths with Approximate English Equivalents

1 meter (m)	= 39.37 inches
1 centimeter (cm)	= 0.4 inch
1 millimeter (mm)	= 0.04 inch

Selected English System Lengths with Approximate Metric Equivalents

1 yard (yd)	= 0.9 meter
1 foot (ft)	= 0.3 meter
1 inch (in)	= 2.5 centimeters

---

between systems, such as Metric to Apothecary. Some examples of this are as follows: *one* grain may be expressed in the Metric System either as 60 mg or 65 mg; *one and one-half* (1½) grains as either 90 mg or 100 mg; and *five* grains as either 300 mg or 325 mg.

Chapter VII

General Nursing Care

INTRODUCTION

THE FOLLOWING MATERIAL is concerned with procedures which can be done at sea either in the sickbay or in the patient's cabin.

The persons responsible for patient care and observation should have a genuine interest in the total welfare of the patient. The attendant to the patient not only should be observant, but should listen to what the patient has to say. The patient's complaints may give a clue to what is wrong.

SICKBAY

The seaman's cabin generally is used as sick quarters. However, the sickbay should be ready at all times for occupancy. It should be used only for care of the sick or injured. Basic supplies and equipment should be stored in the room and placed in cupboards, not on open shelves. Excess personal articles should be stowed in drawers or lockers.

Admission to Sickbay

The patient's history, physical examination, and type and extent of the injury or illness will determine the course of action. In life-threatening emergencies, treatment should be started immediately. When initiating care of a patient, this procedure should be followed:

• Take the patient's temperature, blood pressure, and pulse. Note if the pulse is thready, weak, rapid, or irregular.

• Observe the kind of respirations, whether shallow, labored, or stertorous (snore-like).

• Note whether there are any visible signs of injury or illness, such as skin lesions, abnormal swelling, or discoloration of the skin.

• Start treatment. (In a dire emergency, as in hemorrhage, or when breathing has stopped, treatment should start without delay.)

• Information on the patient should be recorded in the *Medical Logbook*. This should include the patient's vital signs, complaints, symptoms, and the attendant's observations. *The record is a legal document that should be kept carefully and accurately.*

• If the patient is admitted to the sickbay, an accurate list should be made of clothing, personal belongings, and valuables. Valuables should be secured under lock and key.

VITAL SIGNS

Vital signs are those measures of body-functioning which indicate how effectively the body is carrying out the essential activities of living. These measures include the following:

- Temperature
- Pulse
- Respiration
- Blood pressure
- Level of consciousness

Temperature

Temperature is the balance between the heat produced and the heat lost by the body. Body temperature is measured by a clinical thermometer, which has a column of mercury that will not fall of its own accord, but must be forcibly shaken down. The mouth, the most convenient place of taking a temperature, should not be used if the patient recently had hot or cold drinks or food. An oral temperature never must be taken when the mouth is dry, parched, or inflamed; or when the patient is restless, delirious, unconscious, or irrational. Also, an oral temperature should not be taken if the patient is a young child or infant as there is danger of biting, breaking the thermometer, and swallowing the glass and mercury.

Taking Temperature

See Table 7–3 (p. 319) for instructions on cleaning and sterilizing thermometers.

ORAL METHOD: When taking an oral (mouth) temperature, this procedure should be followed:

- Shake the column of mercury in the thermometer down to read about 96°F (35.5°C).
- Place the mercury end of the thermometer under the tongue and instruct the patient to keep his lips tightly closed but not to bite the thermometer with his teeth. The bulb of mercury should touch the base of the tongue.
- Leave the thermometer in the patient's mouth for three minutes before removing and reading it.
- The normal mouth temperature is 98.6°F (37°C).

RECTAL METHOD: Although a rectal temperature is the most accurate, the method is used chiefly when the conditions previously mentioned make the oral method impractical, or when a high degree of accuracy is required. A thermometer used for taking a rectal temperature has a short blunt mercury tip to prevent injury to the rectum.

When taking a rectal temperature, this procedure should be followed:

- Lubricate the mercury tip of the rectal thermometer with a lubricating jelly.
- Insert the thermometer about 1½ inches into the rectum.
- Hold the thermometer in place for three minutes.
- Wipe the thermometer free of the lubricating jelly, going from the top of the thermometer toward the mercury before attempting to read it.
- 99.6°F (37.5°C) is the normal body temperature by rectum.

AXILLARY METHOD: The least accurate temperature reading is from the axilla (armpit) area, because the temperature of the surface of the body is being measured. When taking an axillary temperature, this procedure should be followed:

- Make sure that the patient's armpit is dry.
- Place the bulb of the thermometer in the center of the patient's dried axilla, with the opposite end slanting toward the body.
- For seven minutes, keep the patient's arm close to his body to hold the thermometer in place.
- 97.6°F (36.4°C) is the normal axillary (armpit) temperature.

Reading a Thermometer

Clinical thermometers can be calibrated to the Fahrenheit (F) scale or the Centigrade (C) scale. The Fahrenheit thermometer usually ranges from 92°F to 108°F, while the Centigrade ranges from 35.5°C to 41°C. Comparable readings of the Fahrenheit and Centigrade Scales can be seen in Table 7–1.

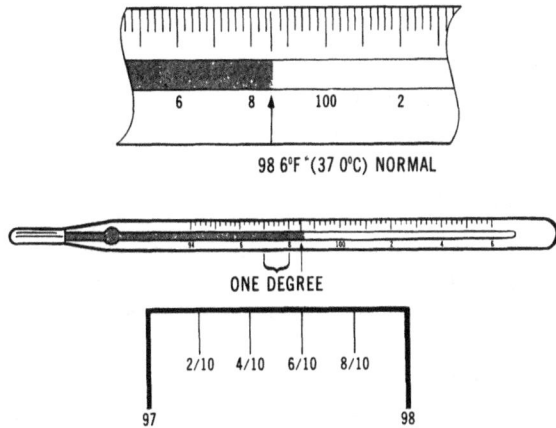

Fig. 7–1. Thermometer calibration.

Table 7–1

Comparable Readings—Fahrenheit and Centigrade Scales

Fahrenheit (F)		Centigrade (C)
108° }	Usually Fatal	{ 42.2°
107		41.7
106 }	Critical Condition	41.1
105		40.6
104		40.0
102 }	High Fever	39.4
103		38.9
101		38.3
100 }	Moderate Fever	37.8
99		37.2
98.6 }	Healthy (Normal) Temperature in Mouth	{ 37.0
98		36.7
97		36.1
96 }	Subnormal Temperature	35.6
95		35.0

Notice the scale (calibrations) on the thermometer shown in Fig. 7–1. The space between each long line on the scale designates one degree. There are four short lines between each of the long lines which divide the degree into fifths. Each fifth designates two-tenths (0.2) of a degree. On the Fahrenheit thermometer between the 98-degree and 99-degree lines, there is a long line marked with an arrow that indicates the normal oral body temperature of 98.6°F or 37°C.

When reading a thermometer, this procedure should be followed:

• Hold the thermometer horizontally so that the numbers are on the bottom and the lines (calibration) at the top.

• Hold the thermometer at eye-level and rotate the thermometer slowly between the thumb and index finger.

• Observe the area between the lines and the numbers until the mercury is seen. Notice where the mercury ends.

• Rotate the thermometer to see which number is closest to the end of the column of mercury. Then rotate the thermometer slightly to see how many lines the mercury extends past that whole number.

• The temperature reading is the digit (whole number) marked by the long line, plus two-tenths, four-tenths, six-tenths, or eight-tenths of a degree. (See Fig. 7–2.)

• After reading and recording the temperature, shake the mercury down by holding the thermometer firmly between the thumb and index finger, at the end that does not contain the mercury. Flick the wrist with quick, short, jerking movements. After reading, the thermometer should be washed in a lukewarm (water) solution, rinsed well, and wiped with an alcohol sponge before it is used again. If an ill patient with an elevated temperature is kept under continuous observation, the same thermometer should be used throughout the episode.

The Pulse

The pulse is the alternate contraction and expansion of an artery, corresponding to the heartbeat.

The purse rate is taken most easily at the wrist. When taking a pulse rate, this procedure should be followed:

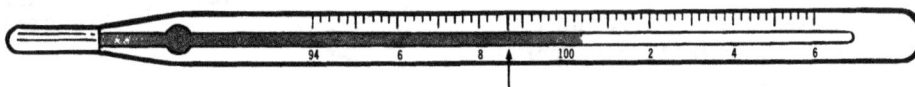

Fig. 7–2. Sample thermometer reading.

• Place the middle fingertip over the artery on the thumb side of the patient's wrist.

• Move your finger until the pulsebeat is located and exert enough pressure to make the pulse distinct, but not blotted out.

• *Never* use your thumb because it has a pulse that might be confused with that of the patient.

• When the pulse is felt plainly, count the beats for one minute.

• Record the character of the beat whether strong or feeble, rapid or slow, and regular or irregular. (See Table 7–2 for normal pulse rates and terms.)

Table 7–2

Normal Pulse Rate

60–70	Men
70–80	Women
80–90	Children over seven years
80–120	Children from one to seven years
110–130	Infants

Pulse Classified in Adults

60 & below	Slow or subnormal
60–80	Normal (men, women)
80–100	Moderate increase
100–120	Quick
120–140	Rapid
140 & above	Running (hard to count)

The pulse is slower when the patient is at rest and increases with exercise or other activity, as after a heavy meal or during a fever. If the pulsebeat cannot be located at the wrist, it can be counted at the temple, just in front of either ear.

Respiration

Respiration is the inhaling of air and the exhaling of gases (or air) from the lungs. A respiration is one breath taken-in and one breathed-out.

The normal respiratory rate, usually between 14 and 20 per minute, will vary under certain conditions. Exercise, activity, and fever as a rule will increase the rate. When a person is at rest, the rate will decrease. It is more important to observe the *kind of respirations*

than to count the number; for example, shallow, labored, stertorous (snore-like) breathing. It is best to observe or count respirations when the patient is unaware of it.

Blood Pressure (B/P)

Blood pressure readings are obtained by using a sphygmomanometer (see Figs. 7–3a and 7–3b) and a stethoscope to measure the force exerted by the blood on an artery in the arm. This procedure is one requiring accuracy and skill that are acquired through practice.

Blood pressure varies in the healthy person due to many factors. Emotional and physical activity have an effect on the blood pressure. During periods of physical rest and freedom from emotional excitement, the pressure will be lowered. Age in itself will be a factor in elevating blood pressure.

An injury or internal bleeding can result in a great loss of blood, which causes a lowered blood pressure. Shock is marked by a dangerous drop in B/P.

Blood pressure is expressed in millimeters of mercury. The *systolic pressure* (as the heart beats or contracts) is recorded above a line and the *diastolic pressure* (as the heart rests) is recorded below the line. In the blood pressure recording 120/80: the *systolic pressure* is 120 and the *diastolic pressure* is 80. These are within normal range. A slight variation from this value is insignificant.

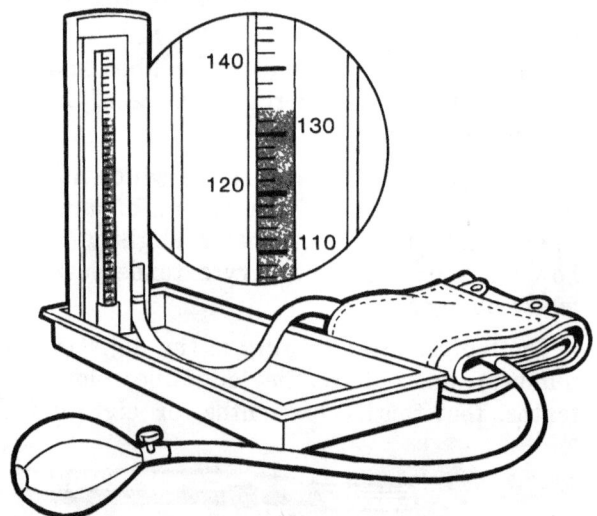

Fig. 7–3a. Sphygmomanometer, mercury (box type), for taking blood pressure.

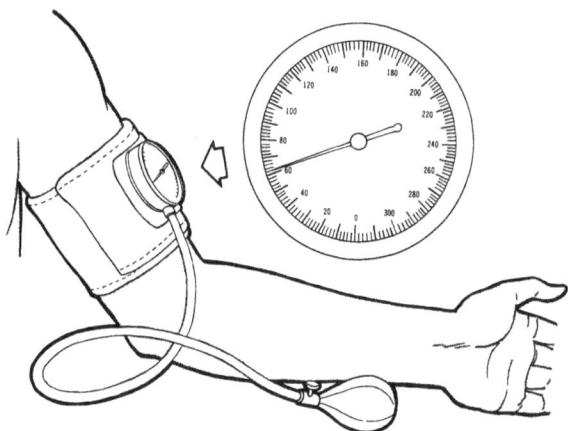

Fig. 7–3b. Sphygmomanometer, aneroid (dial type), for taking blood pressure.

When taking a blood pressure, the patient should lie or sit with the arm supported that is to be used. Measurements may be made in either arm. When taking a blood pressure, this procedure should be followed:

• Explain the procedure to the patient to prevent excitement and anxiety.

• Place the cuff around the patient's arm, above the elbow. (See Fig. 7–4.) Check to see that the valve on the bulb has been fully closed (turned clockwise).

• Before inflating the cuff with air, find the arterial pulse on the inner side of the bend of the elbow.

• Keep fingers on this pulse and inflate the cuff by pumping on the rubber bulb until the pulse disappears.

• Place the earpieces of the stethoscope in the ear (with the earpieces directed up) and position the disc of the stethoscope over the space where the pulse was felt.

• Hold the disc of the stethoscope snugly in position over the pulse with one hand, while pumping the cuff with the other.

• Pump the cuff until the mercury on the scale of the mercury apparatus, or the needle on the gauge of the aneroid apparatus, is about 30 points above the systolic pressure that was obtained previously, by noting when the arterial pulse was felt to disappear.

• Loosen the valve slightly and permit the pressure to drop *slowly* while listening carefully for the sound of the blood pressure. Soon a definite beat will be heard, but it will be quite faint. If this beat is missed or if there is a question as to the reading where it started, the valve should be tightened again, pumped again once more, and one should listen for the sound. The number at which the first sound is heard is the *systolic pressure*. This number should be recorded.

• Continue slowly to deflate the cuff until the last sound is heard. The reading at which the sound disappeared is the *diastolic pressure*.

• Open the valve completely and allow the cuff to deflate.

If there is difficulty obtaining the blood pressure reading, it may be due to the valve being opened too much, causing the pressure to drop too rapidly; or the attendant might have expected a louder sound through the stethoscope.

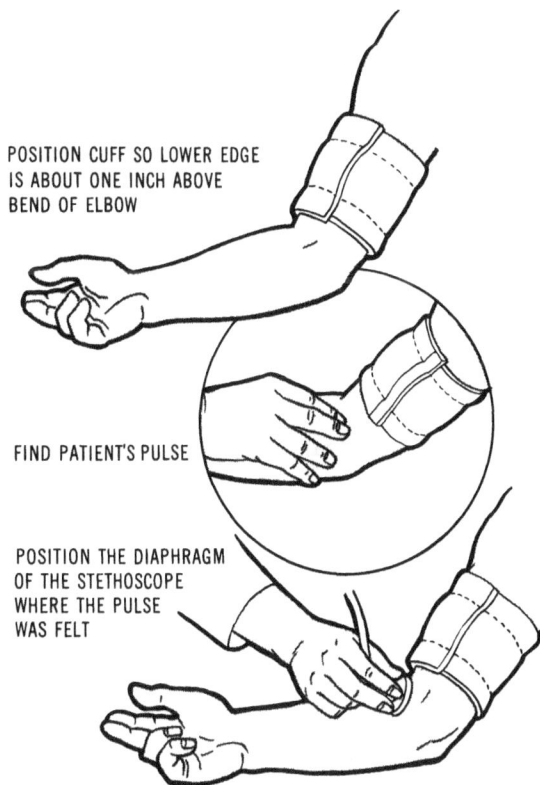

POSITION CUFF SO LOWER EDGE IS ABOUT ONE INCH ABOVE BEND OF ELBOW

FIND PATIENT'S PULSE

POSITION THE DIAPHRAGM OF THE STETHOSCOPE WHERE THE PULSE WAS FELT

Fig. 7–4. Taking blood pressure—position of cuff and stethoscope on patient's arm.

Levels of Consciousness

Consciousness is controlled by the brain and the involuntary nervous system. There are four levels of consciousness: alertness, restlessness, stupor, and coma.

The alert patient is well aware of what is going on and reacts appropriately to the factors in the environment. Facilities to supply his body needs will be requested, such as a urinal or bedpan, medication for pain, or a drink of water.

The restless patient is extremely sensitive to the factors in the environment, and exaggerates them. The patient may scream with moderate pain. He may call for the urinal, but is unable to wait until it arrives. He wants constant attention, and moves about in bed continuously and thrashes from side to side.

The stuporous patient lies quietly in bed, seems to be sleeping and requests nothing. Even when awakened, there is a quick return to a sleeplike state which makes feeding difficult. The patient may be incontinent, exhibiting involuntary loss of urine or feces.

The degree of stupor is determined by the stimuli required to awaken the patient. If awakened by a voice, the level of consciousness would be described as light stupor. If awakened only by pressure, such as tapping him lightly on the side of the face or by applying pressure over the eyelids, the level would be described as deep stupor.

The patient in a coma lies quietly in a bed, appears to be sleeping, and cannot be awakened. The patient will not ask for a drink or urinal, he cannot swallow, and may be incontinent or may retain urine. Pressure over the eyelids, strong sensations, or calling by name will not awaken the patient.

What Levels of Consciousness Mean

The alert patient is one whose brain is functioning adequately.

The restless patient's brain is extremely active in its attempt to meet the body's needs. Restlessness often is observed in the following patients:

• Anyone frightened, worried, or in pain because the brain is hyperactive in preparing the body to fight or flee.

• Anyone hemorrhaging, because the brain is receiving a lessened or inadequate blood supply.

• Those with a head injury or brain tumor, if the increased pressure on the brain is cutting off the blood supply to a part of the brain.

• A person who has suffered a heart attack, because the weakened heart is not pumping enough blood around the body and to the brain.

• Those in shock, when blood pressure is so low that there is insufficient force to pump blood to the brain.

Restlessness is an early sign of the preceding conditions. When the brain is unable to correct the conditions that cause restlessness, it will be followed quickly by stupor, coma, and death.

Observation of the level of consciousness means that an attempt is made to awaken the sleeping patient regardless of whether it is in the middle of the day or night, so it can be observed whether he really is sleeping, or whether he is in a stupor or coma.

CARE OF BED PATIENT

A patient who is unable to maintain his own personal hygiene must be aided totally or partially. Personal hygiene includes care of the mouth, teeth, skin, and hair.

Oral Hygiene

Teeth should be brushed by the patient, if possible. Care should be taken to protect the bed during the procedure.

If it is necessary to brush the patient's teeth, this procedure should be followed:

• Remove the pillow and turn the patient's head to the side toward the attendant.

• Place a towel under the side of the head and chin to protect the bedding.

• Brush the patient's teeth, then have him rinse his mouth with water and expectorate into an emesis (kidney) basin. Teeth should be brushed after meals, at bedtime, or as often as necessary.

Removable dentures are best cleaned when brushed under tepid water. They should be cleaned at least twice daily. Dentures should be removed from unconscious or confused patients and placed in a container filled with water.

Bed Bath

If able, the patient should take his own shower or tub bath. If this is not possible, he should complete as much of his bath as he can. The room should be warm and free of drafts. If the patient needs assistance to bathe, a bath blanket should be placed over the top linen. When bathing a patient, this procedure should be followed:

• Wash the patient's face, neck, and ears; then dry.
• Wash the patient's arms, giving special attention to the axilla (armpit). Rinse well and dry.
• Next wash the patient's legs and back, including the area around the anus.
• Have the patient wash the genitalia, if able.
• Change the water as often as necessary.
• Give the patient clean pajamas and bed linen.

Bedmaking

The most important part of making the patient's bed is to have it smooth and free of wrinkles. This means the bedclothes under the patient must be pulled tight, and be anchored well under the mattress to keep them tight. Pillows should be used for comfort, support, and to maintain correct body posture. Top covers should be lightweight and adequately warm. They should be long enough to cover the patient's shoulders and provide adequate toe space. The covers should be fastened securely at the bottom of the bed.

To protect the mattress, a waterproof sheet may be placed lengthwise across the middle of the bed, on top of the bottom sheet, and firmly tucked-in on both sides. The drawsheet, placed over the waterproof sheet, also should be tucked-in firmly on both sides to ensure a smooth bed. A drawsheet may be made by placing an ordinary sheet lengthwise across the middle of the bed. Replacing a soiled drawsheet is less fatiguing to the patient than having the full bottom sheet changed.

SUTURING

Ordinarily, the advice to the attendant regarding suturing of wounds would be—DO NOT ATTEMPT IT. However, if many days are to elapse before the patient can be seen by a physician, the attendant should be knowledgeable in the various suture procedures and materials. Suturing is a skill that must be learned through doing, under supervision. There are many complications that can occur if suturing is performed by an inexperienced person. Only under extreme circumstances should suturing be attempted unless the attendant has had specific training in wound closure. It would be more appropriate to use adhesive butterfly strips when possible. (See p. 62.)

Before discussing the method of suturing, some of the *contraindications* to wound closing should be delineated:

1. If there is reddening and edema of the wound margins, established infection manifested by discharge of pus, persistent fever or toxemia— *do not close the wound.* If these signs are minimal, the wound should be allowed to "clean up." This process may be hastened by warm, sterile water dressings or irrigations with sterile water or saline.

2. If the wound is a large gaping one of soft tissue, *leave it unsutured,* for it is certain to contain myriads of bacteria and suturing would prevent the drainage of the pus that would develop. Delayed primary closure is performed, preferably within three to seven days after injury, upon the indication of a healthy appearance of the wound. Healthy muscle tissue which is viable (capable of living) is evident by its color, consistency, blood supply, and contractility. Muscle which is dead or dying is comparatively dark, mushy, and often malodorous. It does not contract when pinched nor does it bleed when cut. If this type of tissue is evident, make every effort to bring the patient under the care of a physician. The wound should be lightly packed with vaseline gauze and dry sterile gauze which has been fluffed with forceps.

3. If the wound is deep, consider the support of the surrounding tissue and if there is not enough support to bring the deep fascia together, *do not suture the surface* because dead

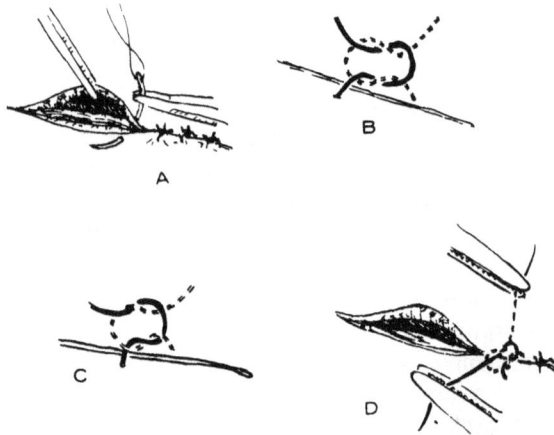

Fig. 7–5., 7–6. Technique of suturing a wound.
A, Method of passing interrupted sutures;
B, Tying a nonslip, square knot;
C, Tying a granny knot which will slip;
D, Suturing a wound with interrupted, square-knot-sutures.

(hollow) space will be created below. In this type of wound which is generally gaping, muscles, tendons, and nerves most probably will be involved. Only a surgeon should attempt this type of wound closure for reconstructive surgery becomes necessary if it is incorrectly done.

If the wound is relatively small, shallow, freshly incurred, free from dirt, foreign bodies, and signs of infection, the attendant should take steps to close it if a physician's services cannot be anticipated within a few hours.

Materials for Closing a Wound

There are several different materials used for closing wounds. Sutures may be divided into two classes—absorbable and nonabsorbable. *Absorbable sutures* are absorbed by the tissue fluids and are usually used in the deeper layers of the wound. In this class are plain catgut or chromicized catgut (treated so as to be absorbed more slowly than plain gut). Nonabsorbable sutures are not absorbed by body tissues and are usually used to close the skin, although in some techniques for hernia and fracture repairs they are used beneath the surface. They consist chiefly of silk, cotton, and synthetic material (dermol, nylon, etc.), or stainless steel wire. In case of emergency, ordinary sewing thread may be used after it has been boiled or autoclaved.

Needles used in suturing are either round or cutting, straight or curved. They vary in length and thickness, also in shape for different types of suturing. In suturing the skin, the cutting type is usually preferred; a round type is usually used for deep sutures or when suturing near blood vessels.

Preparation of Materials and Patient

All instruments to be used should be checked and be sterile, appropriate sterile suture material selected, a good light provided and the position of the patient on the table planned so that access to the wound will be unhampered. The wound should be cleansed with povidone iodine skin cleanser and sterile dressings. Sterile drapes should be used if they are available; if not, the area surrounding the wound should be covered with sterile material such as towels and only that part of the anatomy left exposed which is to be sutured.

The attendant should scrub his hands and forearms with soap and water for 15 minutes, clean his fingernails thoroughly, and dry with a sterile towel. He should then put on sterile gloves. See p. 320+.

Some type of anethesia will ordinarily be necessary during the process of closing the wound. Using a sterile syringe and needle, inject lidocaine hydrochloride injection, 1% into the prepared skin just back from the raw wound edges. (See pp. 282 and 312.)

Technique for Suturing

The outline of the wound should be carefully studied so that when the suturing actually starts the corresponding parts may be accurately apposed. Puckering, due to faulty apposition of edges, places undue tension on the tissues and creates an unsightly scar which may interfere with the function of the part.

The suture needle should enter the skin from $1/4$ to $1/2$-inch from the edge of the wound, depending upon the amount of tension which will be placed on the wound edges (the greater the length and depth of the wound—the greater the tension necessary). Then arc under the opposite edge and reenter the surface at the same distance from the edge, i.e., $1/4$ to $1/2$-inch. The suture is then tied, using a square knot, with just enough tension to bring the wound edges together gently, after which the ends are cut $1/2$-inch from the knot. The remaining stitches are inserted in the same manner as described above and, depending upon the amount of suture tension on the wound edges, at a distance of ½ to ¾ of an inch apart. (See Fig. 7–5.)

Care must be used to handle the tissues as delicately as possible to reduce additional injury upon tissue already damaged.

Suture Removal—All skin sutures are usually left in place from five to seven days, depending upon the location and amount of tension upon the wound edges. They must be removed aseptically to prevent infection being implanted along the wound tract. This is done by pulling one edge of the thread taut with a pair of sterile tweezers and cutting the thread with sterile scissors or knife point between the place where the thread is grasped and where it enters the skin. It should be cut below that portion originally exposed to the surface, by pulling rather firmly and upward with the thumb forceps. The thread is then removed by pulling gently on the part held by the tweezers. In this way the air-exposed and likely contaminated thread is not pulled through the tissues.

ADMINISTERING MEDICATIONS

Safe Effective Procedures

The hands should be washed before any medication is prepared. Before administering a medication, the patient should be asked about any known allergy to it.

In administering medications, the label on the container should be checked three times: (1) when the bottle is taken off the shelf, (2) before any medication is removed from the container, and (3) when the bottle is replaced on the shelf.

Before administering any medications, the attendant should know the therapeutic action, side effects, cautions, and contraindications to the drug. The attendant should have read the drug monographs. (See p. 271+.) The package insert also is a good source of information about the drug.

The following points should be remembered when administering medicines:

Always give medicine on time.

Read the label three times before giving medication (see above).

Record the date and time of day, name of the medicine, the amount given, and the route of administration. Do not record these until the drug actually has been taken.

A suitable container such as a disposable medicine cup should be used to administer capsules, tablets, and liquids. Capsules and tablets should be poured into the bottle cap, then placed into the container. Solid medications should not be contaminated by placing them in the dispenser's hands.

Medications to be given more than once a day should be spaced at a reasonable interval. For example, four times a day: at 0800—1200—1600—2000. Antibiotics, if ordered four times a day, should be administered every six hours: at 2400—0600—1200—1800. This is done to help maintain an adequate level of the antibiotic in the system at all times.

Medications ordered before meals should be given one-half hour before the meal. Medications administered to induce sleep usually are given 30 minutes before sleep is desired. One should be careful in administering hypnotics to avoid having the patient asleep when he should be awake.

Cough syrups should not be diluted. Water should not be given for 15 minutes after any cough syrup because it will diminish the soothing effect of the medication.

Routes for Administering Medications

Oral

The easiest and generally the safest and most desirable way to administer a medication is by the oral route. Generally, absorption into the bloodstream begins to reach a therapeutic level in about 30 to 90 minutes and lasts four to six hours, depending on the characteristics of the drug and the formulation. Taking the medication on an empty stomach usually will cause more rapid absorption than when taken after a meal.

Tablets or capsules are swallowed more easily by most persons if placed on the back of the tongue, then washed down with a suitable fluid (usually water).

Sublingual

Many soluble drugs are absorbed readily when placed in contact with the sublingual mucosa under the tongue. Substances that may be destroyed by the digestive juices, or those urgently needed for self-administration as soluble nitroglycerin tablets, may be given this way.

Rectal

Drugs may be given by rectum as liquids or suppositories. Generally, drugs administered by rectum for a systemic effect are absorbed erratically and only should be used as an alternative route.

Vaginal

Most medication by the vaginal route is for local effect and the drug used may be in the form of a suppository, powder, gel, foam, or vaginal douche. A medication may be given by this route for a systemic effect because absorption does occur through the vaginal mucosa; but this usually is not a route of choice.

Intranasal

Drugs may be given intranasally for either local or systemic action. Nose drops or sprays as phenylephrine usually are applied to the nasal mucosa for their vasoconstrictive effect.

Subcutaneous (Under the Skin)

Small quantities of fluid medication can be injected easily subcutaneously. This route is used when rapid absorption is desired, when the patient cannot or will not swallow a drug, is vomiting, or the action of the medication would be destroyed by secretions of the stomach or intestine. The usual sites of subcutaneous injections are the extensor surfaces of the upper arms, the back, and the lateral aspects of the thighs. The maximum effect of the injection usually occurs in about 30 minutes.

When giving a subcutaneous injection, this procedure should be followed:

- Assemble the equipment
  Disposable syringe
  Disposable 25-gauge, one-half inch needle
  Medication
  Prepackaged alcohol sponges

- If the medication is in a multiple-dose vial, clean the rubber diaphragm on the vial with a prepackaged alcohol sponge. If the medication is in an ampul, which has been previously filed (colored band), remove the top of the glass

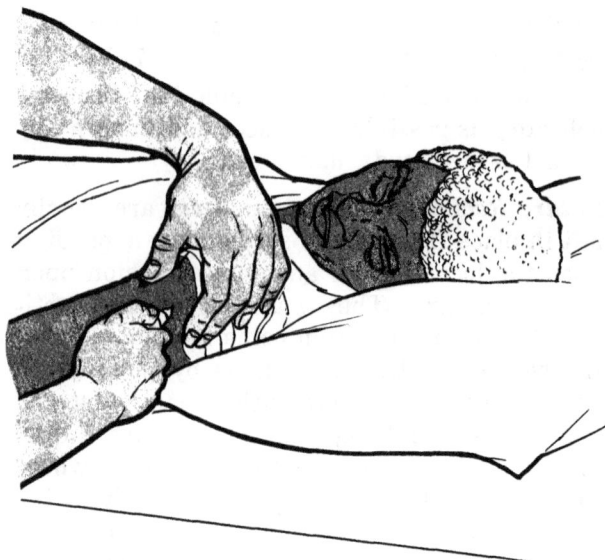

Fig. 7–7. Site of a subcutaneous injection.

ampul by wrapping a piece of gauze around the top part and break it off. If the ampul does not have a colored band, file the neck of the ampul and then break off the top.

- Remove the guard from the needle without touching the needle. If the medication is in a vial, inject into the vial an amount of air equal to the amount of drug to be withdrawn to help facilitate withdrawal of the medication. Withdraw the correct amount of medication. Point the needle up and expel any air in the syringe.

- Select an area on either arm, just below the shoulder on the outer aspect, and cleanse the skin with a prepackaged alcohol sponge. (See Fig. 7–7.)

- Grasp the skin between the thumb and forefinger, and firmly and quickly insert the needle at the prescribed angle. (See Fig. 7–8.) Draw back gently on the plunger. If no blood appears

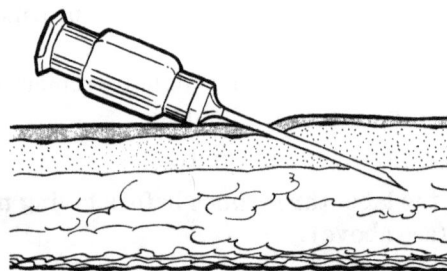

Fig. 7–8. Subcutaneous injection.

in the syringe, inject the medication and withdraw the needle. If blood appears, redo the procedure at a new site with sterile equipment.

• Rub the site of injection with an alcohol sponge.

• Replace the needle in the needle guard, and break the needle and the tip of the syringe.

• Discard the used equipment.

Intramuscular (Into a Muscle)

Because of the relative vascularity of muscle, medications injected intramuscularly (IM) are absorbed more quickly than those given subcutaneously. A maximum effect is obtained in about 15 minutes. Also, this route may be used when a medication irritates the subcutaneous tissue or to obtain prolonged action, as in the injection of aqueous procaine penicillin.

When giving an intramuscular injection, this procedure should be followed:

• Assemble the equipment

    Disposable syringe

    Disposable needle, 1½-inch length, 20- or 22-gauge, depending upon the thickness (viscosity) of the medication

    Medication

    Prepackaged alcohol sponges

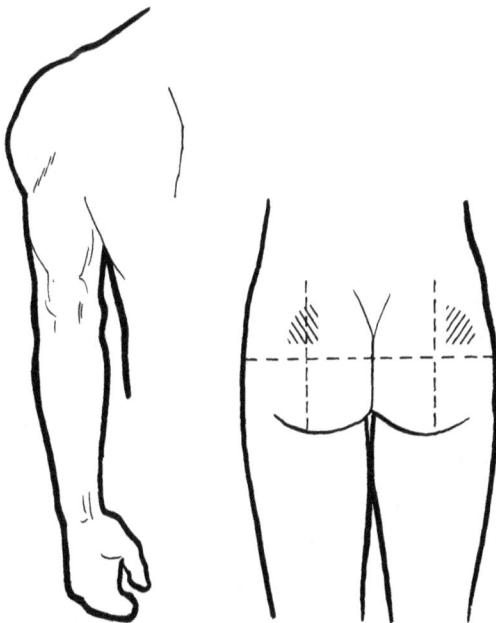

Fig. 7–9. Sites of an intramuscular injection.

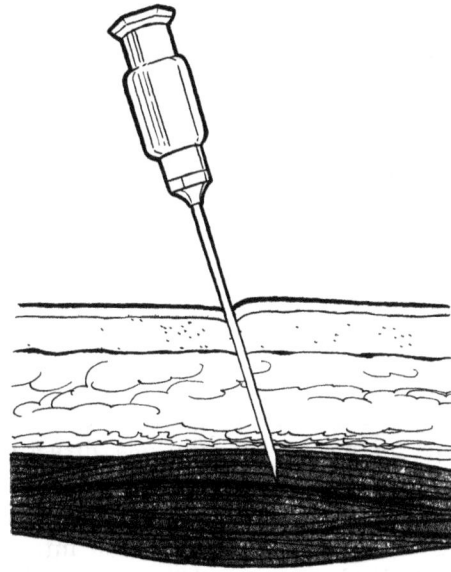

Fig. 7–10. Intramuscular injection.

• If the medication is in a multidose vial, clean the rubber diaphragm on the vial with a prepackaged alcohol sponge. If the medication is in an ampul which has been previously filed (colored band), remove the top of the glass ampul by wrapping a piece of gauze around the top part and break it off. If the ampul does not have a colored band around it, score the neck of the ampul with the enclosed file.

• Remove the guard from the needle without touching the needle. If the medication is in a vial, inject into the vial an amount of air equal to the amount of drug to be withdrawn to help facilitate withdrawal of the medication. Withdraw the correct amount of medication. Expel any air from the syringe.

• Select a site for the injection. The preferred site is in the outer upper quadrant of either buttock. If the buttocks can't be used, the anterior-lateral aspect of either thigh or the upper third of the outer side of the upper arm (deltoid muscle) can be used. (See Fig. 7–9.)

• If the buttock is the injection site, stretch the skin with the thumb and forefinger and insert the needle at a right angle to the skin, deeply enough to penetrate the subcutaneous fat and enter the muscle. (See Fig. 7–10.) If the upper arm is the injection site, compress the tissue between thumb and the forefinger and direct the needle in a straight course.

• Draw back on the plunger of the syringe. If no blood appears, insert the medication and withdraw the needle. If blood appears, repeat the procedure at another site using new sterile equipment.

• Rub the site of the injection with an alcohol sponge.

• Replace the needle in the needle guard and break the needle and the tip of the syringe.

• Dispose of the used equipment.

Intravenous (IV)

Intravenous administration refers to the introduction of sterile solutions directly into a vein. (See Fig. 7–11.) Giving a large quantity of solution is referred to as an *infusion*.

Injection of sterile medication into a vein is indicated when rapid absorption and action is desired. An infusion of a sterile solution is started when fluids cannot be taken by mouth.

Veins of the inner aspect of the elbow generally are used for the administration of intravenous solutions. These veins are easy to reach, tend to be quite superficial, are fairly large, and are well supported by muscular and connective tissue.

Veins on the back of the hand and at the ankle sometimes are used, but they are more difficult to enter and tend to roll easily.

Either arm may be used for intravenous therapy. If the patient is right-handed and both arms appear to be equally usable, the left arm is selected usually so that the right arm is free for the patient's use.

Always make sure that sterile technique is used when a vein is being entered. When per-

forming an intravenous infusion, this procedure should be followed:

• Assemble equipment.

    Container of parenteral fluid or IV solution

    Administration set

    Needle (20- or 21-gauge, 1½ inch or 2 inches)

    Prepackaged alcohol sponges

    Tourniquet

    Stand for IV container

    Arm board

• Remove the protective covering and the rubber diaphragm from the solution's bottle.

• Remove the administration set from the package. Remove the protective cover from the spike, and insert the spike into the administration site of the bottle.

• Remove the protective cover from the end of the administration set. Invert the bottle so that the solution flows into the drip chamber and through the tubing.

• When the tubing is completely full of solution, close the slide clamp.

• Place the needle onto the end of the tubing, being careful to maintain aseptic technique. (Some administration sets come with the needle already attached.)

• Place the standard for the IV container in a convenient position near the bed.

• Cut several pieces of one-half inch tape.

• Place the patient's arm on a board with a tourniquet under the arm, about 1½ inches above the intended site of entry. Secure the arm to the board with a bandage.

• Apply the tourniquet about two inches above the site of the infusion and direct the ends away from the site of the injection.

• Ask the patient to open and close his fist. Observe and palpate for a suitable vein.

• Cleanse the skin thoroughly with an alcohol sponge at and around the site of the injection.

• Use the thumb to retract down on the vein and the soft tissue about two inches below the intended site of injection.

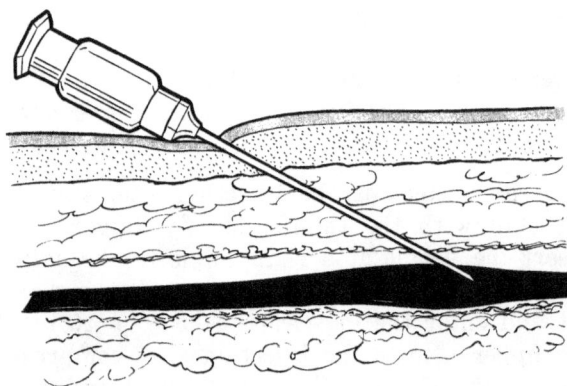

Fig. 7–11. Intravenous injection.

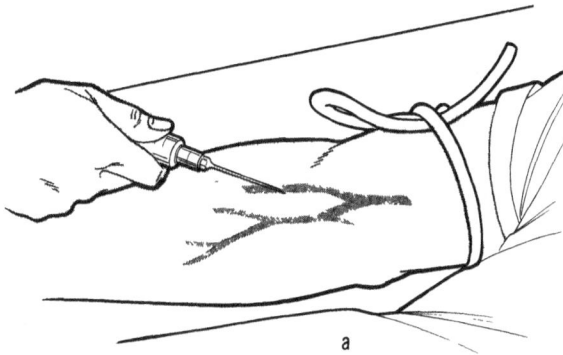

Fig. 7–12a. Site of an intravenous injection.

• Hold the needle at a 45° angle with the bevel up in line with the vein (see Fig. 7–12a) and directly alongside the wall of the vein at a point about one-half inch away from the intended site of venipuncture. Allow the fluid to enter the needle and drip out. (*This will remove all the air from the tubing, in order to prevent an air embolism.*) Then, clamp the tube and proceed.

• Insert the needle through the skin, lower the angle of the needle until nearly parallel with the skin, following the same course as the vein, and insert it into the vein.

• When blood comes back through the needle, open the pinch clamp and insert the needle three-fourth inch to one inch further into the vein.

• Release the tourniquet.

• Open the clamp on the infusion tube.

• Tape the needle securely in place. (See Fig. 7–12b.)

• *Regulate the rate of flow (drops per minute) carefully.* Observe at frequent intervals to pre-

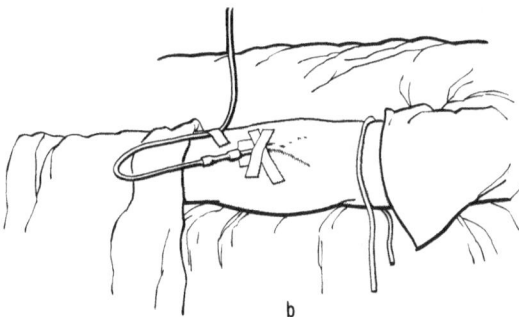

Fig. 7–12b. Intravenous injection procedure.

vent variance in flow and to see that it is stopped before all the solution is administered (*to prevent air from entering the vein*). The number of drops per ml will vary with different administration sets. This information will be found on the administration set packaging. For example, if the set delivered 15 drops per ml, and it is desired that 1000 ml of solution be administered in a five hour period, the rate of flow would be about 50 drops per minute.

• Anchor the arm on an armboard.

• Observe frequently the site of the infusion to detect puffiness of tissue (indicating swelling from infiltration of the solution into the tissues). *If present, discontinue the intravenous infusion and restart in another vein, using another sterile needle.*

Eye Medications

The eye is a delicate organ, highly susceptible to infection and injury. Although the eye is never free of microorganisms, the secretions of the conjunctiva have a protective action against many that cause disease. For the maximum safety of the patient, equipment used and solutions and ointments introduced into the conjunctival sac (inside of eyelids) should be sterile.

Because direct application should not be made onto the sensitive cornea, medications intended to act upon the eye or the eyelids should be instilled onto the lower conjunctival sac.

Exposing Lower Conjunctival Sac

When exposing the conjunctival sac to administer eye medications, this procedure should be followed:

• Have the patient look up.

• Place a thumb near the margin of the lower lid, immediately below the eyelashes.

• Exert pressure downward over the bony prominence of the cheek.

• As the lower lid is pulled down and away from the eyeball, the conjunctival sac is exposed.

Instilling Eye Drops

Sterile eye drops are supplied in either a plastic bottle fitted with a device which will

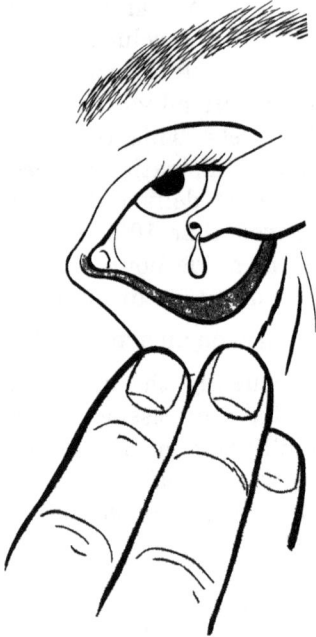

Fig. 7–13. Instilling eye drops.

dispense drops when inverted and squeezed, or in a bottle fitted with a sterile dropper. It is recommended that this procedure be followed to administer eye drops:

• The person administering the drops should wash his hands prior to instillation of the eye drops. If the patient's eyes are discharging, sterilized cotton balls should be in readiness to cleanse the discharge from the lids. The cotton balls should be moistened with sterile ophthalmic irrigating solution, or sterile sodium chloride solution 0.9% warmed to about 100°F (37.7°C). Several absorbent tissues also should be kept in readiness.

• Cleanse the discharge, using the moist cotton balls, by wiping the eyelids from the inner to the outer side. Use a new cotton ball for each stroke. If no discharge is present, this step (and the cotton balls) may be omitted. CAUTION: *Never use dry cotton on the eye.*
• Hold the dropping device over the lower eyelid, parallel to the eye but with the dispensing hand resting upon the patient's forehead, so that the dropping device is elevated at about a 45° angle over the lower lid. (See Fig. 7–13.)

• Take absorbent tissue in the other hand and gently draw down the lower lid by placing fingers on the cheek.

• Be sure that the patient is looking up.

• Drop the prescribed number of drops into the pocket formed by the lower lid. Do not allow the dropping device to touch any part of the eye.

• Do not allow drops to fall directly onto the cornea of the eyeball because of the danger of possible injury to it or because of any unpleasant sensation it may create.

• Instruct the patient to close his eye gently and rotate the eyeball to spread the medication evenly. CAUTION—*Use only sterile medication prepared for eye use.* Prior to use, check for an expiration date on the labels.

Application of Eye Ointment

Before application of an ointment, the eyelids and the eyelashes should be cleansed of any discharge, as previously described under "instillation of eyedrops." When applying ointment to the eye, this procedure should be followed:

• Hold the tube in an almost horizontal position to control the quantity of ointment applied and to minimize the chance of touching the eyeball or the conjunctiva with the tip. (See Fig. 7–14.) One-half inch of the ointment should be extruded from the eye ointment tube and dis-

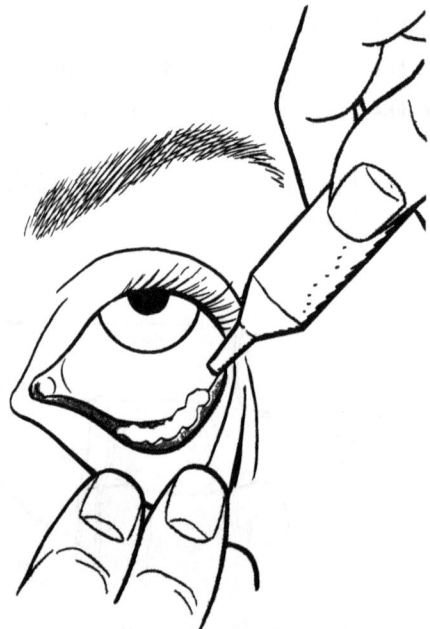

Fig. 7–14. Application of eye ointment.

tributed in the lower conjunctival sac, after exposing the inner surface of the lower lid (by applying two fingers to the cheek).

• Following the application, instruct the patient to close the eyelids and move the eyes. This will spread the ointment under the lid and over the surface of the eyeball.

Conjunctival Irrigation

A sterile ophthalmic isotonic irrigating solution in a disposable "squeeze" bottle should be used for irrigation. The following procedure should be followed:

• Cleanse any discharge from the eye, as previously described under "instillation of eye drops."

Separate the eyelids, and gently squeezing the bottle of irrigating solution, direct the flow from inner to outer canthus (corner of the eye). Use only sufficient force to cause a continuous flow of the solution.

• Wipe the cheeks with a towel or absorbent tissue.

Ear Medications

To prevent discomfort, medications for the ear should be warmed before instilling them. Do *not* overheat. Eardrops can be instilled best if the patient lies on his side with the ear uppermost to be treated. Before instilling eardrops, it may be necessary to use a cotton-tipped applicator to remove secretions from the external ear.

When administering eardrops, this procedure should be followed:

• Straighten the ear canal by gently pulling the earlobe upward and backward for adults; downward and backward for infants and small children.

• Hold the tip of the dropper or inverted dropper-bottle at the opening of the ear and instill a few drops of the medication. Do not insert the dropper or the dropper-bottle into the ear canal.

• Tell the patient to remain in this position for a few minutes to allow the medication to remain in contact with the surfaces of the canal and to prevent leakage of drops from the ear.

• Place a small amount of cotton loosely into the ear canal to keep the medication from draining out.

• Instruct the patient to remove the cotton anytime after five minutes.

INFECTION CONTROL

Asepsis

Asepsis is the absence of disease-producing microorganisms called pathogens. Asepsis generally is divided into two descriptive forms: *medical asepsis* and *surgical asepsis*. Concepts of medical and surgical asepsis, as used in this book, are based on the following definitions.

Medical Asepsis

Medical asepsis refers to practices which attempt to reduce the number of disease-producing microorganisms and hinder their transfer from one person or place to another. The reason for observing medical aseptic practices is that the environment always has disease-producing microorganisms which in some individuals and under certain circumstances can cause illness. Therefore, reducing the number of germs and hindering their transfer will increase the safety of the environment. Any number of methods may be used to help achieve this aim: washing, boiling, sterilization, and disinfection are a few examples. If the patient and all those caring for him practice the precautionary measures intended to maintain medical asepsis, the potential will be lessened to spread the patient's disease to others aboard ship; and the patient will be protected against infection by a new organism.

To maintain medical asepsis, the following points should be remembered:

• Wash the hands after every contact with the patient, and with equipment and supplies used in caring for him.

• Provide disposable wipes. When he coughs or sneezes, instruct the patient to cover his mouth and nose, and to turn his head away from others.

• Provide the patient with the necessary articles to wash his hands after using the urinal or bedpan.

• All disposable articles taken from an infected patient's room should be placed in a double bag and sealed, using a strong adhesive tape. Infectious articles should be autoclaved or burned.

Surgical Asepsis

The term surgical asepsis is used to describe the techniques that protect the patient against infection. These techniques range from the complex technical ritual that is essential in the operating room, to the use of sterile dressings on minor wounds.

It is recognized that the skin is the first line of defense against microbial invasion. Therefore, in the handling of any wound (any break in the skin), the use of a sterile technique is mandatory. Hands should be washed and scrubbed thoroughly (see Handwashing, p. 319). Modification of this technique is acceptable in situations in which the chance of infection is reduced. Therefore, it is safe to eliminate gloves when doing minor dressings or giving injections. However, when doing minor dressings, sterile pick-up forceps should be used to handle sterile dressings.

To maintain surgical asepsis, the following points should be remembered:

• Sterile forceps may be used to handle sterile equipment and supplies.

• Sterile rubber gloves are put on after the hands are thoroughly scrubbed and dried (see p. 320).

• Only sterile articles should be placed on a sterile field.

• Do not allow sterile instruments or dressings to come in contact with anything but the wound.

• Avoid undue talking when treating wounds. Germs in the spray from the nose and throat can contaminate the materials and the wound itself.

• Avoid leaning across sterile materials or across an open wound. Lint or dust from a person's clothing can contaminate materials and the wound.

Disinfection and Sterilization

It is assumed that the ship's officer who is responsible for the sickbay and the care of the sick and injured will have had prior training on the application and effectiveness of various methods for disinfection and sterilization. Thus, the information on disinfection and sterilization given here is brief but should serve as a useful reference. *Presterilized disposable surgical supplies and instruments should be used whenever possible to reduce the need for sterilization or disinfection aboard ship.*

The terms *sterilization* and *disinfection* have precise meanings and should be used appropriately in considering methods for preparing equipment, instruments, and surgical supplies. By *sterilization* is meant the complete destruction or removal of all forms of microbial life. This usually is accomplished by steam under pressure (autoclaving). *Disinfection* is the reduction of disease-producing microorganisms (generally including nonresistant spores), usually by chemical germicides or boiling water.

Some agents for disinfection or sterilization are listed in the *key* that accompanies the table on p. 319.

Where an autoclave (steam under pressure) is not available, or in those instances where disinfection is an acceptable method, the actual disinfection procedure and disinfectant to be used should be selected by the shipping company. The shipping company should consider the hazards of specific types of contamination to be encountered, as well as the scope of medical services provided, and the physical facilities aboard ship.

All objects or surfaces must be cleaned thoroughly prior to use of specific methods of sterilization or disinfection. The use of a liquid disinfectant for instruments, and rubber or polyethylene tubing that come in direct contact with patients, should be followed by flushing or rinsing with sterile distilled water and drying. *Whenever there is a choice, sterilization by steam under pressure (autoclaving) is preferable to disinfection.*

In the table that follows, specific recommendations are grouped by types of objects to be disinfected or sterilized, and by contaminating organisms. The *letters of the alphabet* designate specific procedures that are acceptable in each situation. It should be noted that certain agents tend to cause some materials to corrode or rust.

Table 7-3
DISINFECTION AND STERILIZATION

Objects	Disinfectant	Exposure

Smooth, hard surfaced objects:
  nondietary area
  dietary area
	Aqueous phenolic solution at recommended use dilution.
	Sodium hypocholorite 100 ppm available chlorine.	

Instruments*:	Aqueous phenolic solution at recommended use dilution.	30 minutes
Thermometers*:	Aqueous phenolic solution at recommended use dilution. Rinse thoroughly before use.	30 minutes

Environmental surfaces:
  Walls, floors, tables,
  machine panels, etc.
	Aqueous phenolic solution at recommended use dilution.	

Items contaminated by* Hepatitis virus:	Iodophor solution with minimum 0.5% available iodine.	30 minutes
Items entering skin** or mucous membranes:	Requires heat sterilization by steam under pressure.	30 minutes at 121°C (250°F)

* Must be cleansed with soap and water before disinfection.

** It is strongly recommended that all items which will be used to enter the skin or be in direct contact with mucous membranes (i.e., hypodermic needles, urinary catheters, suction catheters, etc.) be single-use, disposable items.

Handwashing

Washing hands often and thoroughly is one way to prevent the spread of disease.

It is important to wash hands:

• Before and after coming in contact with a patient.

• Before handling a patient's food or food tray.

• After handling a patient's articles, dressings, or any equipment or supplies used in his care.

• Before eating.

• After using the bathroom.

When washing hands, this procedure should be followed:

• Completely wet the hands and wrists under warm water.

• Apply soap (from a dispenser, if available, or a bar of soap). Spread the soap over the entire surface of the hands and wrists.

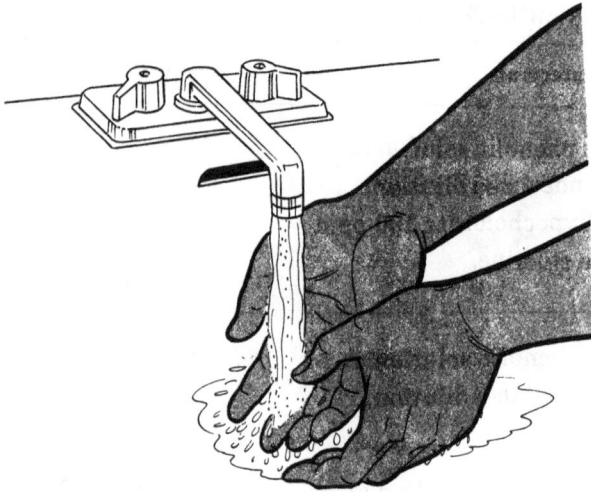

Fig. 7–15. Handwashing—Rinse with hands pointed downward.

• Work up a lather and spread it over hands and wrists. Work the lather in between the fingers and under the fingernails. Clean under the nails with an orangewood stick.

• Rinse thoroughly under warm running water with the hands down. (See Fig. 7–15.)

• Dry the hands with a paper towel. Use a paper towel to turn off the faucet.

Sterile Gloves

When putting on sterile gloves, it should be remembered that the hands only are surgically clean. Therefore, never touch the outside of the glove as this will render it unsterile.

When putting on sterile gloves, this procedure should be followed:

• Wash hands thoroughly and clean under the fingernails. Dry with a sterile towel.

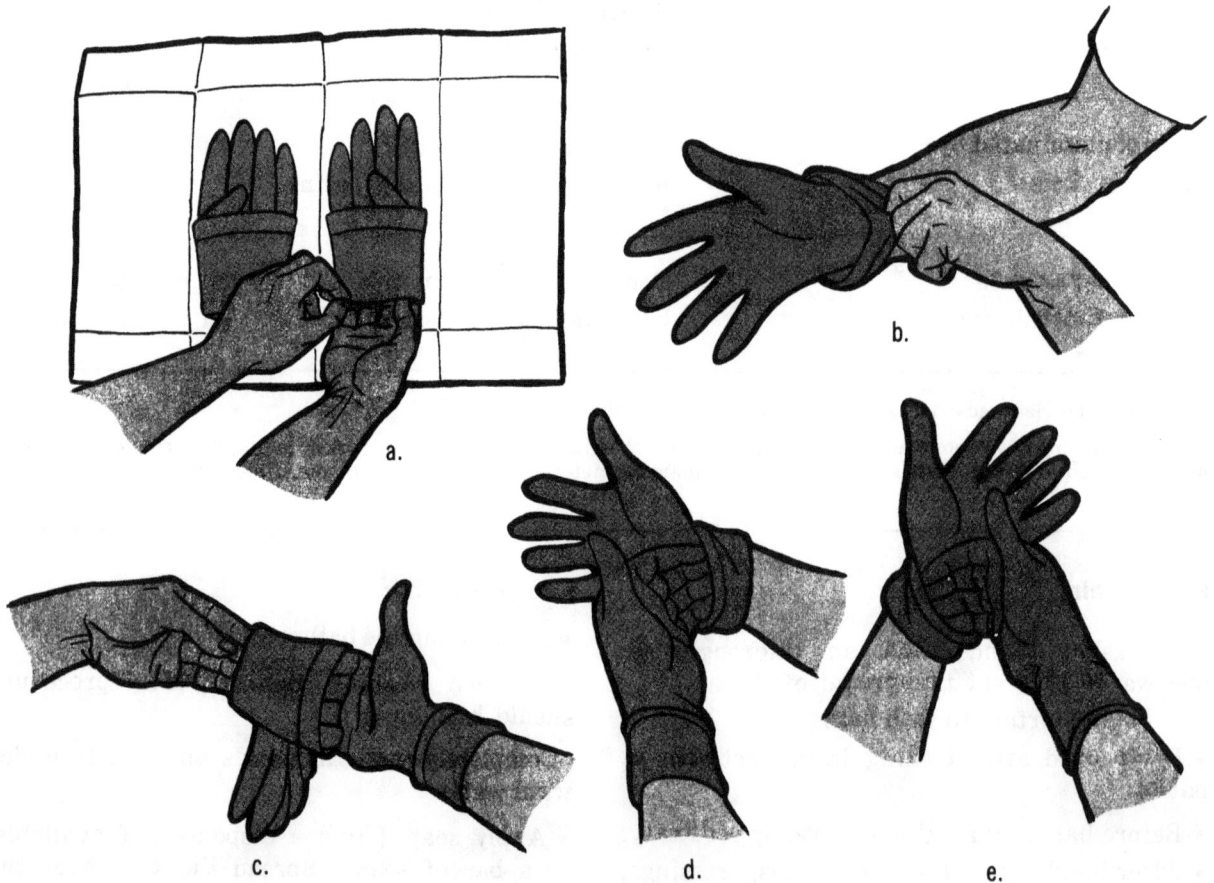

Fig. 7–16. Putting on sterile rubber gloves.

• Open the sterile glove package as directed on the disposable wrapper.

• With the left hand, pick up the right glove by the folded-down cuff (avoid touching the outside of the glove) and pull it onto the right hand, leaving the cuff intact. (See Figs. 7–16a and 7–16b.)

• Insert the gloved fingers of the right hand *under* the cuff of the left hand glove, and slip the left hand into the glove. (See Fig. 7–16c.)

• If it is necessary to pull up the cuffs, keep the gloved fingers on the outer side of the gloves (under the cuff). (See Figs. 7–16d and 7–16e.)

• The outside of the glove should not be touched by bare hands or any other unsterile material.

Isolation Techniques

Patient Care in Isolation

The nursing care of a patient with a communicable disease is identical to the nursing care provided for any patient with a disease of corresponding severity. However, certain precautions must be taken to prevent the spread of the disease from the patient to attendants or to other crew members.

A communicable disease usually spreads by direct contact with the individual having the disease or with articles that have been used by the patient. *Therefore, it is important to isolate the patient and the articles needed for his care.* If possible, the isolation room should have private toilet facilities.

Certain precautions must be observed. The patient should be instructed to cover his mouth and nose with a tissue wipe, when coughing or sneezing. The hands of the attendant must be washed each time after caring for the patient or handling articles that have been in contact with him.

Under the following circumstances, a protective gown and mask should be worn each time one enters the patient's room:

• If a person plans to remain in the room more than one minute.

• If anyone is going to give the patient personal care.

A gown and mask need not be worn when delivering or picking up material or equipment which does not involve any personal care or close contact with the patient.

Eating utensils should be cleaned of food scraps before they are removed from the sickroom. The solid portion of the patient's uneaten food should be discarded in a double-waxed paper bag that has been opened and put on preplaced newspapers outside the entrance to the patient's room. The liquid portion of the unused food should be discarded into the toilet.

The dishes and utensils can be placed in the large double paper bag located outside the entrance to the patient's room. Care should be taken not to contaminate the outside of the paper bag.

Dishes and utensils should be washed separately from those used by other members on shipboard, unless a dishwasher is available. Disposable items should be used when available.

Linens should be placed in a double cloth bag and labeled "isolated." They should be stored until they can be laundered. Linens from most patients can be decontaminated through normal procedures in a commercial laundry.

No visitors should be allowed. Only the person giving care should be permitted in the room.

Use of Gown and Mask

Hands should be washed before putting on a gown and mask. (See p. 319.) The gown should come together in the back and be long enough to cover to the knee or below. These should be donned outside the patient's room.

When putting on a gown and mask, this procedure should be followed:

• Slip the arms into the sleeves of the gown without touching the outer side.

• Fasten the gown at the top of the neck, at the waist, and tie in front.

• Put on a mask to cover the nose and mouth.

When removing a gown and mask, this procedure should be followed:

• Wash the hands thoroughly with soap and water and dry with paper toweling.

• Remove the face mask being careful to touch only the strings or elastic.

• Unfasten the gown at the neck and the waist.

• Remove the gown taking care not to contaminate the clothes underneath it.

• Fold the gown so that the contaminated portion is folded inside.

• Wash the hands again taking care to point them downward while rinsing. Dry with paper toweling.

TREATMENT AND PROCEDURES

Application of Cold

Exposure to cold slows down the work in the cells, and the blood supply to a body part is decreased because the blood vessels narrow. Therefore, cold applications should be applied to any part of the body which is injured and may bleed, in order to narrow the blood vessels and prevent hemorrhage.

Cold applications also are indicated in persons with certain infections (as an infected appendix or abscessed tooth) to prevent swelling and further damage that the swelling could cause. Thus, icecaps frequently are used when bleeding is highly possible, after an injury (as a blow to the lips or a sprained ankle) or in treating an infected area to prevent it from filling with blood and swelling.

Prolonged applications of cold, or exposure to excessive cold, may cause death of the body cells. Cold narrows the blood vessels so that the blood supply to the body part is cut off. Then, even though cellular activity is slowed down, the cells die because they are unable to take in food and oxygen or remove waste material. Signs of death of tissue include paleness, grayish-white appearance, or blueness (cyanosis) of the skin. Therefore the body part receiving a cold application must be watched as carefully as one receiving a hot application. The attendant should be on the alert for any signs that indicate tissue destruction.

Cold Eye Compresses

Cold, in the form of cold compresses, often is applied to an inflamed (reddened) eye to lower the blood flow to the eye. This reduces the bloodshot appearance of the eye and eases the pain caused by swelling.

When applying cold eye compresses, this procedure should be followed:

• Assemble equipment
  Sterile 4″ x 4″ compresses or eyepads
  Small round basin
  Bath towel
  Paper bag

• Place several large pieces of ice in the basin and add tap water.

• Drape the person with a bath towel.

• Dip a compress into the cold solution, wring it out and place it over the eye.

• Prepare the next compress. Remove the one on the eye and replace it with the fresh cold compress. Apply these cold compresses for a period of 15 to 30 minutes.

• If the eye is infected, use a fresh compress each time and discard the used one into a paper bag.

Cold Moist Compresses

With any compress, warm or cold, care must be taken to show that the patient does not have an adverse reaction to the treatment. Cold moist compresses should be discontinued if the patient complains of numbness, or if the body part shows signs of paleness (either grayish-white or blue).

When applying a cold moist compress, this procedure should be followed:

• Assemble equipment
  Basin with water
  Ice
  Compresses, 4″ x 4″ or 4″ x 6″ (suitable in size for the part of the body to be treated)
  Foil
  Waterproof sheet
  Bulb syringe

• Place the pieces of ice into a basin and add cold tap water.

• Place the compresses on top of a piece of foil, fold the edges of foil toward the material (try to avoid sharp edges).

• Wet the compresses with cold water drawn into a bulb syringe, and place over the affected part. (Water is drawn into the bulb syringe by first depressing the bulb with the fingers before placing it in the basin of water. Release the bulb when the tip of the syringe is under water.)

• Repeat the procedure when the compress is no longer cold.

• Remove the compresses after a 20 to 30 minute treatment.

• Dry the area after the treatment is completed.

Ice Cap (Dry Cold)

When applying an ice cap, this procedure should be followed:

• Fill the ice cap about one-half full of ice.

• Expel the air before closing the cap. (Air increases the rapidity with which the ice melts and decreases the flexibility of the cap.)

• Test the cap for leakage.

• Cover the ice cap with a soft absorbent material.

• Apply the ice cap to the affected part. If the ice cap has a metal top, keep it turned away from the patient's body.

• Apply for one-half hour and discontinue for one hour. Then reapply. Remove the ice cap if the patient complains of numbness, or if any sign of extreme whiteness or blueness of the part occurs.

• Refill as the ice melts.

Application of Heat

Heat should be applied to a patient's body when an infection is present, to increase circulation to a body part, help reduce congestion and inflammation, and relieve pain. In cases of abdominal pain or suspected appendicitis, NEVER APPLY HEAT—and contact a physician for directions.

When heat is applied to a patient's body, these safety measures should be carried out:

• Test the water solution to be sure it is the exact temperature required. The following temperatures are guides only:

    Hot bath: 110°F (43.3°C).

    Warm bath: 95°F (35°C).

    Foot Soak: 110°F (43.3°C).

    Hot wet dressing: 110°F (43.3°C).

    Hot water bottle: 115°F (46.1°C).

• Watch carefully for excessive redness on the patient's skin which may indicate that a burn is occurring.

• Apply the heat for the specified time.

• To prolong the effects of the treatment, keep the treated part warm, after the heat application is removed.

• To reheat the soak solution used on an arm or leg, *first remove the patient's limb from the container before adding the hot water* required to raise the solution to the desired temperature.

Dry Heat

Hot Water Bottle (110°F to 120°F or 43.3°C to 48.9°C)

When applying a hot water bottle, this procedure should be followed:

• Fill the hot water bottle (one-half or three-fourths full) with water at about 115°F (46.1°C).

• Expel the air until the water comes to the top. Test for leakage.

• Cover with a towel.

• Apply to the specified area of the body.

• Return to the patient in 15 minutes and check his skin for excessive redness or possible burning.

• Refill as necessary (at least every hour) to keep the water at the desired temperature.

Heating Pad

A heating pad also can be used to supply dry heat. However, care must be taken to insure that the temperature of the pad is not increased accidentally. Also, to avoid possible injury to the patient, electrical wiring and connections should be checked for flaws.

The area of application to the body should be checked at least every hour to offset possible burning of the patient's skin.

Warm Wet Soaks

When applying warm wet soaks (continuous dressings), this procedure should be followed:

• Assemble equipment

    4″ x 4″ sterile compresses, abdominal pads (ABDs) 8″ x 7½″, or bath towel. (Choose dressing that is suitable in size for the part of the body to be treated.

Basin of warm water 110°F (43.3°C).

Waterproof sheet.

Bath towel or bath blanket.

Gauze bandage strips.

Bulb syringe

• Place the bath towel or blanket over the waterproof sheet; then place it under the body part to be soaked.

• Place the compresses to be used in a basin of warm water, wring out well, and place them on the part in such a way that the area is covered completely.

• Wrap the waterproof sheet and bath blanket around the body part and tie them securely in position with strips of gauze bandages.

• Return to the person's bedside every two hours and dampen the compresses with warm water using a bulb syringe. Rewrap the part.

Continuous hot wet soaks to a flat surface of the body (as the chest or abdomen) can be applied and covered with a small piece of plastic and held in place with an elastic bandage. (*Do not have the plastic contact the skin.*) A hot water bottle one-third full, with the air expelled, can be placed on top of the soaks to maintain the heat for a longer period.

Cool or Tepid Sponge Bath

Usually this is done for fevers over 102°F (38.9°C). The patient must be watched for any adverse reaction to the cool sponge.

When giving a cool or tepid sponge bath, this procedure should be followed:

• Assemble equipment

Basin with cool water, temperature about 60°F (15.6°C)

Washcloths (2)

Large waterproof sheet

Cotton blankets (2)

Towels

• Keep the patient covered with a cotton blanket during the procedure. Remove pillows and pajamas.

• Place the waterproof sheet covered with a cotton blanket under the patient to protect the bedding.

• Check the patient's vital signs and record them on a sheet of paper, including the time.

• Sponge the body in orderly fashion, uncovering one part at a time. Proceed so that no part is missed, doing arms, chest, abdomen, front part of legs, back, buttocks, and back part of legs. Alternate the washcloths as necessary.

• Watch the patient's color and check his pulse. If the pulse becomes weak or the lips turn blue, discontinue the treatment.

• Continue the treatment for 20 minutes, if no complications occur.

• Using a towel, pat the skin dry (rubbing may increase body temperature) when the bath is completed.

• Cover the patient with a sheet folded in half. Leave his arms, chest, and legs exposed to promote heat loss.

• Remove the waterproof protection and the cotton blanket from under the patient.

• Make the patient comfortable and allow him to rest.

• Check the patient's temperature (rectally) every 15 minutes. *If tolerated,* give the patient a drink of ice water after his temperature is taken and recorded. Continue until the temperature is normal.

• If the procedure is not to be repeated, make the patient comfortable. Remove and clean the used equipment.

Surgical Dressings

Dressings serve several purposes. If used properly, dressings and the materials used to secure them help to prevent infection, absorb secretions, protect the area from trauma, and restrict motion that might disrupt the approximation (bringing tissue edges close together for suturing) of the wounded edges.

To change a dressing, a procedure should be used that will remove the old dressing without contaminating the wound or the fingers of the person removing it. Equipment will be needed to cleanse the wound, dress it adequately, and secure it. *Sterile instruments must be used to remove the dressings adhering to the wound and for treating it. In some instances, sterile gloves may be used.*

The size, number, and types of dressings used will depend on the nature of the wound. Packs with individual instruments and dressings should provide the ultimate in safety for the patient.

When applying a surgical dressing, this procedure should be followed:

• Assemble equipment.

Sterile disposable dressing set

Adhesive strips

Disposable gloves

Waxed paper bag for old dressing

• Wash hands thoroughly.

• Undo materials securing the dressing. Lift the dressing off by touching the outside portion only. If it is soiled, use an individual forceps or put on sterile disposable gloves.

• Drop the soiled dressing into a waxed paper bag. Later, staple shut and discard into trash.

• Open the gauze dressing packs.

• Using sterile forceps, remove the gauze dressing from its wrapper and place it on the wound. Take care not to touch the portion of the dressing that is going to be placed next to the wound.

• Apply tape to keep the dressing in place.

Catheterization of the Urinary Bladder

Catheterization is the insertion of a catheter (tube) through the urethra into the bladder to remove urine. When performed in a hospital by skilled persons, this procedure is relatively safe. *When improperly performed, there is danger of infection or perforation of the bladder. Therefore, catheterization should be done only by skilled persons.* In most instances aboard ship, when it is necessary to catheterize a patient, an indwelling catheter probably will be indicated.

A patient who has been consuming a normal amount of fluid but has not urinated in 24 hours, probably needs catheterization. Before performing it, try the following to induce a normal flow of urine:

• Provide privacy and the sound of running water.

• Let the patient stand, sit, or kneel.

• Apply a hot water bottle to the lower abdominal area.

If catheterization is considered necessary, get medical advice by radio and ask the physician if a Foley (indwelling) or a French catheter should be used. If the physician recommends an indwelling catheter, then go to p. 327 where the retention procedure is described. If a routine catherization will suffice, proceed as directed below.

Equipment Needed: The following should be obtained—

A sterile disposable catheterization tray which contains a 14 French straight catheter, sterile gloves, small forceps, cotton balls, lubricant, antiseptic solution, underpad and drape, specimen container, and label.

Catheterization (Male)

Explain the procedure to the patient and state that there will be only a slight discomfort. Fear and worry will stimulate the patient's muscles to tighten and it will be difficult to pass the catheter into the bladder.

Preparation of Male Patient: Assemble the equipment. Before opening the tray, the patient should be prepared for routine catheterization, as follows:

• Fanfold the top covers to the foot of the bed while covering the patient with a sheet or light blanket.

• Have the patient on his back with knees bent.

• Expose his penis, keeping the rest of the body covered. This can be done by pushing the bath blanket in from the side.

After the patient is prepared, the attendant's hands should be scrubbed thoroughly, especially under the fingernails.

Procedure (Male): For a routine catheterization of a male patient, the following procedure should be used—

• Follow the directions for opening the catheter and catheter tray, as written on the wrapper.

• Put on sterile gloves (see p. 320).

• Grasp the penis with the left hand and stand at the patient's right side. With the right hand scrub the end of the penis with povidone-iodine skin cleanser (or the cleanser provided in the disposable catheterization tray) and cotton balls.

• Pick up the catheter, holding it at least eight inches from the tip. Do not touch the part of the catheter which is to be inserted inside the patient.

• Apply the lubricant to at least seven inches of the catheter. *Thorough lubrication is essential.*

• Hold the penis straight with the left hand while inserting the catheter (see Fig. 7–17). This position straightens out the urethra.

• Use gentle but steady pressure to insert the catheter. A slight resistance may be felt upon approaching the bladder's sphincter muscle, but gentle pressure should push the catheter past it. If the catheter cannot be inserted with gentle pressure, and a firm resistance is felt— *then stop!* Get medical advice by radio. *Never force the catheter as it may seriously damage the bladder or urethra.*

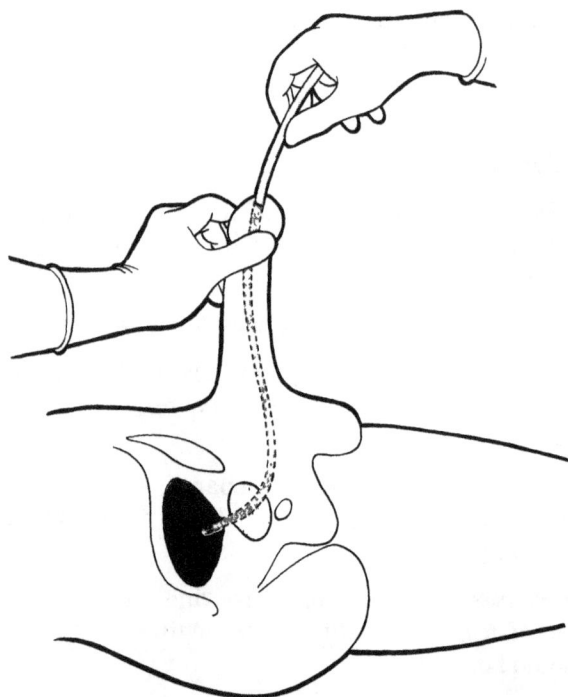

Fig. 7–17. Catheterization (male).

• Position the basin under the catheter.

• Insert the catheter (usually seven to eight inches) until urine begins to flow.

• Withdraw the catheter when the steady stream of urine starts to diminish. *Never empty the bladder completely.*

• Record the date and time of day for the procedure, and the amount and color of the urine obtained.

Catheterization (Female)

If catheterization is considered necessary, medical advice by radio should be obtained on the procedure, including whether a Foley (indwelling) or a French catheter should be used. If the physician recommends an indwelling catheter, then go to p. 327 where the retention procedure is described. If a routine catheterization will suffice, proceed as directed below.

Always explain to the patient the procedure and assure her that she may feel only slight discomfort. Try to keep her relaxed, because fear and worry will stimulate the muscles to tighten, and make it difficult to pass the catheter into the bladder.

Assemble the necessary equipment (see p. 325). A floor lamp will help the attendant to locate and see clearly the urinary meatus of the female.

Preparation of Female Patient

Before opening the tray, the female patient should be prepared for routine catheterization as follows:

• Fanfold the top covers to the foot of the bed, while covering her with a sheet or light blanket.

• Have the patient lie on her back with the knees bent, thighs separated, and feet flat on the mattress. Drape her thighs and legs with the right and left corners of the sheet and tuck the free edges under her feet.

• Do not fold back the bottom corner of the sheet to expose the vulva, until ready to start the catheterization.

• Place the lamp on the far side of the bed and adjust the light to shine on the perineal area.

• Scrub the hands. Maintaining aseptic technique, uncover the sterile tray.

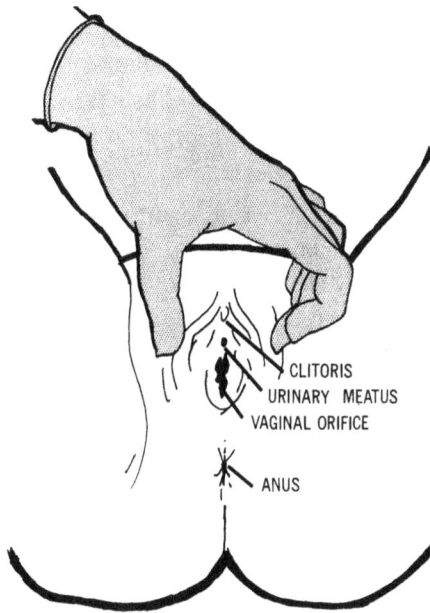

Fig. 7–18. Site for catheterization (female).

CLITORIS
URINARY MEATUS
VAGINAL ORIFICE
ANUS

• Fold back the drape sheet to expose the vulva. Encourage the patient to relax. Have her breathe regularly and slowly to lessen tension.

• Put on sterile gloves. (See p. 320.)

• Pour the prescribed solution over four cotton balls in the container provided.

• Squeeze the lubricant onto a gauze sponge.

• Place the sterile towel between the patient's thighs and pull the top edge just under the buttocks. Fold about three inches of the towel over the gloved hands to offset possible contamination of the gloves, while placing the towel under the buttocks. Use care to protect the exposed sterile surface. Do not contaminate the gloves.

• With the gloved left hand, separate the labia to expose the urinary meatus. (See Fig. 7–18.) The meatus should be visible as a small opening about one-fourth inch above the vagina.

• Keep the left hand in position, holding the labia apart until the catheter has been inserted. *Remember, the gloved left hand is no longer sterile.*

• With the gloved right hand, pick up one saturated cotton ball in the solution basin; with no retracing, cleanse the meatus and vestibule

from above downward. Repeat this procedure with the remaining cotton balls. Try to prevent the right hand from touching the meatus. Discard each cotton ball into the waste basin.

• With the gloved right hand, pick up the sterile basin and place it on the sterile towel, close to the buttocks and below the separated labia.

• With the gloved, sterile right hand, pick up the catheter, holding it about three inches from the tip. Lubricate it.

• Insert the catheter into the meatus about two inches, or until the urine starts to flow. Do not use force if there is resistance. Do not insert more than two inches.

• When the flow of urine decreases, pinch off the catheter and gently withdraw it.

• Leave the patient dry, covered, and comfortable.

• Record the date and time of day for the procedure, and the total amount and color of the urine obtained.

Retention Catheterization (Indwelling) and Urinary Bladder Drainage

A retention (indwelling) Foley catheter is used to permit continuous drainage of the urinary bladder without repeated catheterization. The catheter commonly used is a self-retaining urethral catheter (Foley type). This has a double lumen, with one opening for drainage and the other for inflation of the retention device, which is a small balloon at the tip of the catheter. The retention balloon is inflated with a measured amount of sterile water (or air) following its placement into the bladder. When a retention catheter is used, provision must be made for bladder drainage by tubing connected to a plastic drainage bag. Aseptic technique during urinary drainage is required because the indwelling catheter exposes the patient to a source of chronic irritation which increases susceptibility to infection.

An accurate record of the intake and output of fluid should be kept on patients having an indwelling catheter.

Equipment Needed: For a retention catheterization, the following should be obtained—

• A sterile disposable catheterization tray, which contains a Foley catheter, sterile gloves, small forceps, cotton balls, lubricant, antiseptic solution, a needle and syringe with sterile water, underpad and drape, specimen container and label.

- Sterile drainage tubing with plastic container.
- Safety pins.

Preparation of the patient: Before opening the tray, the patient should be prepared for indwelling catheterization the same as described for routine catheterization on p. 325 (male) or p. 326 (female).

Procedure for Placement of Retention Catheter
- To open the Foley catheter tray, follow the directions written on the wrapper.

- Put on sterile gloves and check the retention catheter for defects by injecting the specified amount of sterile water or air into the balloon lumen. The capacity of the balloon is written on the catheter. Then deflate the balloon before proceeding with the catheterization.

- Insert the catheter as for a routine catheterization.

- Inflate the catheter balloon after inserting the catheter. Inject the required amount of sterile water (or air) into the self-sealing balloon lumen. When properly positioned and inflated, the balloon will lie within the bladder at the bladder outlet. *The patient will experience severe pain if the balloon is inflated when in the urethra.*

- Clamp off the catheter and protect the open drainage lumen temporarily with a dry sterile gauze square.

- Use adhesive to secure the catheter in place. *For female patients,* anchor the catheter to the skin of the inner thigh, placing the adhesive toward the groin. *For male patients,* use the thigh also *unless medical advice by radio* specifies that the penis is to be positioned upward on the pubis, with the catheter anchored to the lower abdomen. This position helps prevent urethral edema.

- Connect the catheter to the urinary drainage tubing and drainage bottle, maintaining sterility of the drainage system.
(1) Connect the open end of the drainage tubing to the catheter.
(2) Unclamp the catheter.

(3) Adjust the tubing from the catheter to the drainage bottle *so that no kinks and no loops of tubing extend below the level of the entrance of the tubing into the bottle. This is necessary to provide effective gravity drainage.*

(4) Check the air-vent opening in the bottle or plastic bag closure. The vent must be open to insure drainage from the bladder.

(5) Loop an elastic band around the drainage tubing, and pin this loop to the bottom sheet. There should be no strain on the catheter and just enough length of tubing (about 40 inches) to enable the patient to turn and move freely.

(6) Place and secure the drainage container below the bedframe.

Followup Care: The retention catheter and drainage system may be continued for days or weeks, as directed over the radio. If the catheter stops draining, it should be changed as directed by a physician over the radio. Daily continuing care of the patient and the equipment includes the following essentials—

- Maintain an accurate record of the intake and output. Unless otherwise ordered, encourage the patient to drink daily at least 3000 ml of fluids to provide an effective internal irrigation system for the bladder, catheter, and the drainage tubing.

- Check the tubing and catheter connections frequently for kinks. Make sure the patient does not lie on the tubing because this will obstruct drainage and cause undue pressure on the skin.

- Maintain cleanliness and protect the urethral meatus. This requires direct observation and specific hygiene measures. For females, wash the perineal area carefully from front to back. Cleanse the urinary meatus around the catheter with sterile sponges moistened with povidone-iodine solution 1%. To help reduce irritation and possible infection, remove gently but thoroughly secretions of mucus and other discharges.

- Replace the drainage set (tubing, connector, and bottle) with a sterile set daily to reduce bacterial growth and odor.

• Measure and record the collected output of urine. Do not let the drainage bottle get more than three-fourths full, in order to prevent the tubing outlet from becoming immersed in the urine that is draining.

• Use aseptic technique to disconnect the catheter from the drainage tubing when the drainage set is replaced, a specimen is collected, or the catheter is irrigated:

(1) Wash the hands.

(2) Before disconnecting, clamp the catheter. A hemostat clamp may be used, with the tips covered with rubber tubing to prevent damage to the catheter. Be sure to unclamp the catheter after reconnecting it to the drainage tubing.

(3) As the catheter is disconnected, wipe the end of both catheter and connector with an individual germicide-saturated sponge. Cover the ends of the catheter and connector with a dry, sterile sponge, securing each with a rubber band. *Do not allow the drainage tubing to fall to the floor. If this should occur, the tubing will be contaminated and must be replaced.*

(4) Remove the sterile sponge before reconnecting the catheter to the drainage tubing.

The Ambulatory Patient

• To provide continuing gravity drainage for the ambulatory patient:

(1) The patient must carry the drainage bottle lower than his urinary bladder; and

(2) When standing upright, check to see that the tubing is not excessively long and not looped below the level of the bottle or above the urinary bladder.

Removal of a Retention Catheter

• Always deflate the balloon of a self-retaining catheter before removal.

• After the balloon is deflated, the catheter is removed in the same way as a French catheter.

Irrigation of the Bladder

Irrigation of the bladder is done primarily to wash out the catheter and prevent obstruction. This is a sterile procedure that must be done gently to prevent injury and spread of infection within the bladder.

The following equipment is needed:

Sterile bulb syringe, 30 ml
Sterile solution basin
Flask of prescribed sterile solution
Sterile towel
Sterile gauze sponges
Hemostat, rubber-shod
Elastic bands
Emesis basin

To irrigate the bladder proceed as follows:

• Scrub the hands thoroughly.

• Open the sterile packages. Pour the prescribed solution, which must be at room temperature, into the basin. Fill the bulb syringe.

• Open the sterile towel halfway and place to one side of the catheter-connector attachment.

• Clamp off the catheter, detach the connector, and place the end of the catheter on the sterile towel. Protect the open connector with the sterile gauze sponge and elastic band.

• Insert the tip of the bulb syringe into the catheter. Unclamp the catheter. Allow the solution to run in slowly with only gentle pressure on the syringe bulb. Pinch off the catheter while removing the bulb syringe. Keep the bulb of the syringe deflated when removing the syringe from the catheter. Allow 30 ml of solution to flow into the catheter at one time. Do not aspirate the irrigating fluid back. Pinch the catheter closed, remove the syringe and invert the end of the catheter over the emesis basin. Let the solution flow into the basin. Continue the irrigation until the return is clear.

• If the irrigating fluid flows in readily but fails to return, a clot may be obstructing the catheter opening. Do not add additional fluid, but try to dislodge the clot by gently squeezing or "milking" the tubing just below the connector.

• Reconnect the catheter to the tubing after terminating the procedure.

• Record the time of day and total amount of irrigation. If an input and output record is being maintained, measure and record the amount of return, if any, in the emesis basin. Subtract the total amount of irrigating fluid from the output total in the drainage bottle.

Enemas

An enema is an injection of fluid into the rectum. The two types of enemas are the *cleansing enema* and the *retention enema*.

In a *cleansing enema*, the fluid is expelled after five minutes. In the *retention enema*, the fluid should be retained in the rectum for four hours; then expelled.

Several pharmaceutical companies manufacture prepackaged, disposable, cleansing, and retention enema units. They come with directions for use. *It is recommended that disposable units be used whenever possible* because of the convenience of use, storage, and elimination of the need for cleaning and disinfecting. The disposable enema is stored at room temperature and can be given to the patient at that temperature.

Cleansing Enema

The procedure should be explained to the patient. A rubber sheet with covering should be placed under the patient. When giving an enema, this procedure should be followed:

- Assemble equipment.
  Disposable enema package
  Bedpan
  Toilet paper

- Instruct the patient to lie on the left side with the knees bent upward.

- Remove the cover from the rectal tube on the disposable enema.

- Insert the already lubricated rectal tube (three inches long) into the rectum.

- Inject the fluid by squeezing the plastic bottle until it is empty.

- Remove the rectal tube.

- If ambulatory, send the patient to the bathroom. If not ambulatory, place the patient on the bedpan.

- Raise the patient until he is in a sitting position on the bedpan. The patient usually has a bowel movement in five to ten minutes.

- Discard the disposable enema set.

Oil Retention Enema

An oil retention enema usually is given to soften a hard fecal mass that has formed in prolonged constipation.

Before giving the enema, the patient should be told that this fluid is to be retained and not expelled.

If an oil retention enema is to be given and a prepackaged disposable unit is available, no additional preparation will be required. The directions on the package should be followed. If no prepackaged unit is available, this procedure should be followed:

- Pour four ounces of olive oil or mineral oil into a container.

- Place the container of oil into a basin of warm water.

- Remove the container of oil from the water bath when a drop feels warm on the inner part of the wrist, and put it on a tray containing:
  a 14 French catheter
  small funnel
  toilet tissue

- Turn the patient onto his left side and keep the bed flat.

- Give the oil retention enema as follows:
  Lubricate the catheter by dipping it into the oil.

  Insert the catheter about three inches into the rectum.

  Attach the funnel to the other end of the catheter.

  Pour the oil onto the side of the elevated funnel and let it run into the rectum. This prevents air from being forced into the rectum.

  Continue until all the oil is given.

- Remove the catheter and at the same time apply pressure to the rectum with a large wad of toilet tissue as you squeeze the buttocks together.

- Place the patient into a back-lying position.

- Leave the waterproof sheet and drawsheet in place as there is usually seepage of oil from the rectum.

An oil retention enema usually is followed in four hours by a cleansing enema.

SPECIAL DIETS

Introduction

In many instances, the treatment of a patient's illness includes the type and quantity of food that the person eats. Special diets, as any other mode of treatment, should be used upon the advice and prescription of a physician. There are, of course, many different types of special diets. Some of the ship's company already may be on such a diet, which was prescribed by a physician to help control an existing condition. The following special diets include: (1) a *bland diet* that consists of easily digested, non-irritating foods; (2) a *mild salt (sodium)-restricted diet;* and (3) two frequently used *diabetic diets* that are designed for loss of weight or weight maintenance. These diets should not be considered as replacement diets for patients who already have been placed on a special diet by a physician. The diets are basic information, if a special diet is required.

Bland Diet

The *bland diet* is designed for those individuals who must avoid foods known to be irritating to the gastrointestinal tract. The diet that follows consists of approximately 2,300 calories —230 grams carbohydrate, 110 grams protein, and 110 grams fat. The *bland diet* meets the recommended daily allowance of the National Research Council (NRC), when foods are eaten in the amounts described hereafter, which consist of three meals and three intermediate feedings. Meals should be small and the patient should be urged to chew his food well.

Table 7–4: Bland Diet
RECOMMENDED DAILY FOOD ALLOWANCES

4 servings	Milk*
1 or 2	Egg*
6 oz	Meat*
3-6 slices	Bread
2 servings	Potato (or substitute)
1 serving	Cereal
2 servings	Vegetable (cooked)
3 servings (at least 1 citrus fruit)	Fruit
1-2 servings	Dessert*
3-6 servings	Fat*

*In cases of obesity and hyperlipidemia, modification of the diet should follow foods allowable within the caloric restrictions and the recommendations of the National Institutes of Health, respectively.

Table 7–5: Bland Diet
MEAL PATTERN SUGGESTED

Breakfast

Fruit or Fruit Juice
Cereal
Egg
Toast
Margarine
Milk
Sugar
Jelly
Salt

Midmorning

Meat or Substitute
Fruit

Lunch

Cream Soup
Meat or Substitute
Potato or Substitute
Vegetable
Dessert or Fruit
Bread
Margarine
Milk
Salt
Sugar

Midafternoon

Bread or Substitute
Meat or Substitute
Margarine

Dinner

Meat or Substitute
Potato or Substitute
Vegetable
Dessert or Fruit
Bread
Margarine
Milk
Salt
Sugar

Evening

Bread or Substitute
Milk

Table 7–6: Bland Diet

FOOD PATTERN SUGGESTED

Type of Food	Foods to Include	Foods to Avoid, if Intolerable
Meats, Eggs, Cheeses	Baked, broiled, roasted, or stewed: beef, lean pork, ham, veal, lamb, liver, poultry—Canned, fresh, frozen fish and other seafood—Soft, hard-cooked, poached, or scrambled eggs—Cottage cheese, cream cheese, mild processed cheese, cheddar cheese—Plain yogurt.	Fried or highly seasoned meats, fish, poultry, or eggs; smoked fish or meats; frankfurters or cold cuts of meat; other cheeses.
Potato or Substitute	White or sweet potatoes without skin, hominy grits, macaroni, noodles, spaghetti, refined rice.	Potato skins, fried potatoes, potato chips, whole grain rice, corn.
Soups	Cream soups and vegetables made from foods allowed.	Soups made from dried beans or peas, bouillon, broth, or consomme.
Sweets	Candy without fruit or nuts, honey, jelly, molasses, sugar, syrups (all in moderation).	Candy containing fruits or nuts; jams and preservatives with seeds and skins.
Vegetables	Vegetable juices—Canned or cooked: asparagus, beets, carrots, green or wax beans, spinach, pumpkin, squash, green peas, tomatoes, peeled eggplant, baby lima beans, leafy lettuce (chopped).	All raw and strongly flavored vegetables; broccoli, brussels sprouts, cabbage, cauliflower, cucumbers, onion, pepper, radish, turnips, dried beans, and legumes.
Miscellaneous	Salt, smooth peanut butter, cinnamon, and vanilla.	Catsup, horseradish, mustard, nuts, olives, pickles, popcorn, relishes, chili sauce, spices, pepper, chili powder, cloves, mustard seed, and nutmeg.

Mild Sodium-Restricted Diet
(2 to 3 grams of sodium)

The mild sodium-restricted diet is prepared using regular foods from the galley, with *no salt added* at the table. The following foods in Table 7–7 should be totally excluded from this special diet.

Diabetic Diets

The 1,800 and 2,200 calorie diets, recommended by the American Diabetes Association and the American Dietetic Association, are to be used in conjunction with the *food exchange lists*. Both the 1,800 and 2,200 calorie diets are designed to lower blood glucose levels. Also, the 1,800 calorie level is used for weight loss. (See Table 7–8.) And the 2,200 calorie diet is intended to maintain weight. (See Table 7–9.)

Table 7–7: Mild Sodium-Restricted Diet

FOOD TO BE TOTALLY EXCLUDED

Breads	Salted crackers, salted popcorn, salted potato chips, salted pretzels, salted cheese crackers
Fats	Bacon drippings, commercial salad dressings
Meats & Fish	Cured meats (ham, bacon, sausage, frankfurters, cornedbeef, cold cuts) and cheese
Soups	Salted soup, bouillon, broth, canned soup
Vegetables	Sauerkraut
Miscellaneous	Salt, celery salt, garlic salt, and onion salt—Gravies or stews made with gravy —Catsup, chili sauce, mustard, soy sauce, steak sauce, and other sauces— Pickles, olives, and salted nuts

Table 7–8*

1,800 CALORIES DIABETIC DIET—DESIGNED FOR WEIGHT LOSS
(Carbohydrates 180 grams, Protein 83 grams, Fat 80 grams)

Meals	Lists 1A & 1B Milk	Lists 2A & 2B Vegetables	List 3 Fruit	List 4 Bread	List 5 Meat	List 6 Fat
Breakfast	none	none	1 exchange	2 exchanges	2 exchanges	2 exchanges
Lunch	1 exchange	2A–2 exchanges	1 exchange	2 exchanges	2 exchanges	1 exchange
Supper	none	2A–1 exchange 2B–1 exchange	1 exchange	2 exchanges	2 exchanges	1 exchange
Evening	1 exchange	none	none	2 exchanges	1 exchange	1 exchange

* Recommended by the American Diabetes Association and the American Dietetic Association. See Table 7–10, for Food Exchange Lists.

Table 7–9*

2,200 CALORIES DIABETIC DIET—DESIGNED FOR WEIGHT MAINTENANCE
(Carbohydrates 220 grams, Protein 95 grams, Fat 100 grams)

Meals	Lists 1A & 1B Milk	Lists 2A & 2B Vegetables	List 3 Fruit	List 4 Bread	List 5 Meat	List 6 Fat
Breakfast	none	none	1 exchange	2 exchanges	2 exchanges	2 exchanges
Lunch	1 exchange	2A–2 exchanges	1 exchange	3 exchanges	2 exchanges	2 exchanges
Supper	none	2A–1 exchange 2B–1 exchange	1 exchange	3 exchanges	3 exchanges	3 exchanges
Evening	1 exchange	none	none	2 exchanges	2 exchanges	1 exchange

* Recommended by the American Diabetes Association and the American Dietetic Association. See Table 7–10, for Food Exchange Lists.

Table 7–10

FOOD EXCHANGE LISTS

List 1A
WHOLE MILK EXCHANGES
One exchange is 1 of the following:

1 cup	Whole milk
½ cup	Evaporated milk

List 1B
SKIM MILK EXCHANGES
One exchange is 1 of the following:

1 cup	Skim milk
⅓ cup	Powdered skim milk
1 cup	Buttermilk

List 2A
VEGETABLE EXCHANGES
One exchange is 1 cup cooked (raw as desired):

Asparagus	Lettuce
Broccoli	Mushrooms
Brussels sprouts	Okra
Cabbage	Peppers
Cauliflower	Radishes
Celery	Sauerkraut
Chicory	String beans
Cucumbers	Summer squash
Escarole	Tomatoes (1 whole)
Eggplant	or ½ cup
Greens (any kind)	Watercress

List 2B
VEGETABLE EXCHANGES
One exchange is ½ cup:

Beets	Pumpkin
Carrots	Rutabagas
Onions	Winter Squash
Green peas	Turnips

Table 7–10

Food Exchange Lists (continued)

List 3

FRUIT EXCHANGES

(Unsweetened)

One exchange is 1 of the following:

1 small (2" across)	Apple
⅓ cup	Apple juice
½ cup	Applesauce
2 medium	Apricots (fresh)
4 halves	Apricots (dried)
½ small	Banana
1 cup	Blackberries
⅔ cup	Blueberries
¼ small	Cantaloupe
10 large	Cherries
2	Dates
2 large	Figs (fresh)
1 small	Figs (dried)
½ cup	Fruit cocktail
½ small	Grapefruit
½ cup	Grapefruit juice
⅛ medium	Honeydew melon
1 small	Orange
½ cup	Orange juice
1 medium	Peach (fresh)
½ cup	Peaches (canned)
1 small	Pear (fresh)
½ cup	Pears (canned)
½ cup	Pineapple
⅓ cup	Pineapple juice
2 medium	Plums
2 medium	Prunes (dried)
¼ cup	Prune juice
2 tablespoonfuls	Raisins
1 cup	Raspberries
1 cup	Strawberries
1 large	Tangerine
1 cup	Tomato juice
1 cup	Watermelon

List 4

BREAD EXCHANGES

One exchange is 1 of the following:

1 slice	Bread or toast
1 medium	Roll or biscuit
1 medium (2" across)	Muffin
1 cube (1½")	Cornbread
½ cup	Cereals (cooked)
¾ cup	Cereals (dry)
½ cup	Cooked rice, grits, noodles, macaroni, spaghetti
2 (2½" square)	Graham crackers
20	Oyster crackers
5 (2" square)	Saltines
3 (2½" square)	Soda crackers
6	Crackers (round, thin)
2½ tablespoonfuls	Flour
¼ cup	Beans, baked (no pork)
½ cup	Beans, lima
½ cup	Beans, dried (cooked)
½ cup	Peas, dried (cooked)
⅔ cup	Parsnips
⅓ cup	Corn
1 cup	Popcorn
1 small	Potato, white
½ cup	Potato, white (mashed)
¼ cup	Potato, sweet (yam)
1 (1½" cube)	Sponge cake
½ cup	Ice cream (also omit 2 fat exchanges)
½ cup	Tomato soup (undiluted)
½ cup	Vegetable soup (undiluted)

List 5

MEAT EXCHANGES

One exchange is 1 of the following:

1	Egg
1 ounce	Meat, lean (beef, pork, lamb, liver, veal)
1 ounce	Fish
1 ounce	Poultry
1 (1-ounce slice)	Cold cuts
1	Frankfurter (8 or 9 per pound)
¼ cup	Fish, canned
¼ cup	Lobster or crab
5 small	Shrimp, clams, or oysters
3 medium	Sardines
1 ounce	Cheese (American or Swiss)
¼ cup	Cheese (cottage)
2 tablespoonfuls	Peanut butter (only once daily)

List 6

FAT EXCHANGES

One exchange is 1 of the following:

1 teaspoonful	Butter or margarine
1 slice	Bacon, crisp
2 tablespoonfuls	Cream for coffee
1 tablespoonful	French dressing
1 tablespoonful	Cream, whipping
1 tablespoonful	Cheese, cream
2 small	Olives
6 small	Nuts
⅛	Avocado
1 teaspoonful	Oil or other fats
1 teaspoonful	Mayonnaise

Recipes

Lemon Gelatin

(May be used in any amount)

1 teaspoonful—Unflavored gelatin
2 tablespoonfuls—Cold water
1 tablespoonful—Lemon juice
½ cup—Water

Put cold water in the top of a double boiler and add the gelatin. Let stand for 10 minutes at room temperature. Place over boiling water to dissolve the gelatin. *To flavor, an approved* substitute for sugar may be added.* Remove from the stove. Add lemon juice and ½ cup of water. Chill. To make COFFEE GELATIN, omit the

*Approved by the U.S. Food and Drug Administration.

lemon juice and use ½ cup of coffee instead of ½ cup of water.

Orange Gelatin

(1 serving equals 1 fruit exchange)

Proceed as directed above for *lemon gelatin*. However, omit the lemon juice and add ½ cup of orange juice to ½ cup of water.

Baked Custard

(1 serving equals ½ cup of milk and 1 meat exchange)

1—Egg
½ cup—Milk
A few grains—Table salt
⅛ teaspoonful—Vanilla
A sprinkle of—Nutmeg

Beat the egg slightly; stir in the milk, salt, and vanilla. *To flavor, an approved* substitute for sugar may be added.* Pour into a custard cup and sprinkle with nutmeg. Set in a pan of hot water and bake in a moderate oven, 350° F (176° C), about 45 minutes. The vanilla may be replaced by other flavors (as almond, lemon, orange, or maple).

Zero Salad Dressing

(May be used in any amount)

½ cup—Tomato juice
2 tablespoonfuls—Lemon juice or vinegar
1 tablespoonful—Onion, finely chopped
Salt and pepper

If desired, chopped parsley or green pepper, horseradish or mustard, among others, may be added. Combine all the ingredients and store in a jar with a tightly fitted top. Shake well before using. Refrigerate.

Suggestions for Patients on Special Diets

To *measure* foods, use a standard 8 oz measuring cup, a standard teaspoon, and a standard tablespoon. It is not necessary to buy special foods. Patients may eat the same foods bought for the galley: milk, vegetables, breads,

*Approved by the U.S. Food and Drug Administration.

meats, fats, and fruits (without added sugar). Food for patients may be prepared with the meals for the rest of the crew; however, portions for patients should be separated before extra fat or flour is added.

To *season* food for special diets, the following may be used: chopped parsley, cinnamon, pepper and other spices, lemon, lime, vinegar, or an *approved* sugar-substitute*. Other foods that do not have to be measured are: clear broth (without fat), bouillon, gelatin (without sugar), sour pickles, unsweetened dill pickles, cranberries, and rhubarb.

Fruits (fresh, frozen, or canned) may be eaten, as long as no sugar has been added. Labels on canned or packaged foods should be read to make sure there are statements as: *unsweetened* or *no sugar added*.

Vegetables should be cooked in plain salted water. Vegetables may be seasoned with part of the meat or fat allowed. Vegetables, meat, and milk exchanges in a patient's meal plan may be combined to make soups, stews, or other dishes. *If the vegetables are cooked, no more than 1 cupful should be eaten at a meal.* Raw vegetables as lettuce, radishes, celery, and other salad greens may be eaten as desired.

Meats should be cooked by broiling, baking, or roasting, instead of frying. If one wants to fry the meat, use only the amount of fat allowed for the meal. Measure meats after they are cooked. A 3-ounce serving of cooked meat is equivalent to 4 ounces of raw meat.

Foods to Avoid on Special Diets

Sugar	Marmalade	Cake
Candy	Syrup	Cookies
Honey	Preserves	Condensed milk
Jam	Molasses	Chewing gum
Jelly	Pie	Soft drinks

Wine, beer, and other alcoholic beverages usually are not allowed.

*Approved by the U.S. Food and Drug Administration.

Chapter VIII

Medical Care of Castaways and the Rescued

INTRODUCTION

THIS CHAPTER DEALS WITH SURVIVAL after abandonment of a vessel or aircraft at sea. It describes the medical treatment of survivors on the survival craft and aboard the rescue vessel. The need for prior training on these principles and continuing follow-up instruction cannot be overemphasized. During an abandonment, there will be little or no time to review a manual.

ABANDONMENT OF VESSEL (Ditching)*

Lifeboat drills must be conducted to prepare for possible disaster. Both crew and passengers must be instructed in the procedures to be followed. Reasons for the instructions should be given to all concerned because procedures will be remembered better when the necessity for them is understood.

Forced immersion is the primary hazard to life after surviving the initial impact of hitting the water. It should be kept in mind that no ocean or lake has a temperature equal to body temperature. Thus in all latitudes, anyone in open water will lose heat, and heat loss lowers the internal body temperature. As the

---

* The aviation term *ditching* as used here means the forcible abandonment of a vessel or aircraft in open water. The *ditch survivor* is one who immediately survives the abandonment, whether immersed or immediately evacuated to a survival craft. The terms *ditch survivor* and *castaway* are used interchangeably.

internal body (core) temperature (taken by rectum) falls below normal (*generalized hypothermia*), the heart increasingly becomes prone to develop ventricular fibrillation and cardiac arrest.

The extent to which generalized hypothermia threatens life is determined by the water temperature and time of exposure. The bodily effects of subnormal temperature will vary depending on geography, season of the year, duration and activity in the water, and body insulation (the amount of fatty tissue and clothing of the individual). (See Fig. 8–1 and Generalized (Immersion) Hypothermia p. 339.)

LIFE EXPECTANCY WITH NO EXPOSURE SUIT

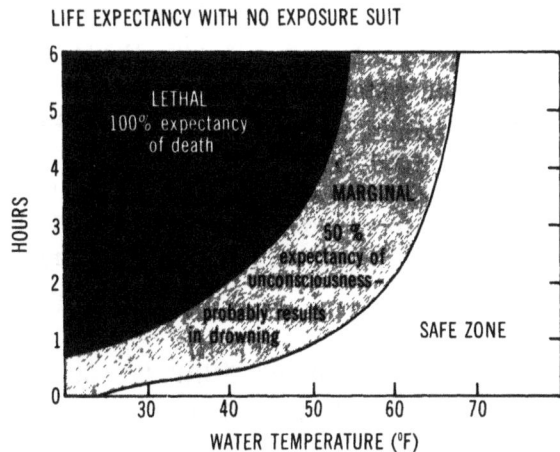

Fig. 8–1. Survival in cold water.

These practical suggestions should be followed prior to forced abandonment of a vessel:

• Dress as warmly as possible! Wear an exposure suit and waterproof gloves, if available. Even wet clothing insulates the body against cold.

• Wear a lifejacket. Bulky lifejackets will not interfere with a person's ability to float or swim.

• Bring any personal medicines taken regularly.

• Eat or drink nothing before entering the water because the colder temperature may cause stomach cramps. Alcohol especially is dangerous, because it causes rapid heat loss and impairs judgment.

• If it is necessary to jump into the water, jump feet first. Hold both arms over the head and try to make a vertical entry into the water.

Landing in a sitting position may result in fractures of the midspinal column or other internal injuries, especially to the kidneys. Landing in a horizontal position often will result in lung, kidney, or other internal injuries. Diving headfirst into the water may result in injury to the head and neck. (These facts are useful when diagnosing a survivor's injuries. If a castaway has been injured, try to find out how the person entered the water.)

• Do not thrash about or swim farther than is necessary. This wastes energy, and by increasing the flow of water around the body, activity may cause more rapid cooling.

• Remain as calm as possible. Panic when entering the water might result in holding one's breath. Then gasping will occur, causing an intake of water into the lungs.

• If time permits, put extra blankets, clothing, water, and food into survival crafts. Extra weight can be jettisoned later, if necessary.

SURVIVOR PICKUP BY SURVIVAL CRAFT
(Lifeboat or Raft)

Surviving in a lifeboat or liferaft (here after referred to as the survival craft) is one of the most strenuous ordeals an individual can face. It involves combat against all the ele-

mental forces at sea, one's own physical limitations, and—most of all—fear, hysteria, and despair. Thus, before picking up survivors, or as soon as immediate rescue operations have been completed, a firm chain of command, based on previous positions of authority must be established aboard the vessel. The individual in command of a survival craft (referred to in this chapter as the Captain) is responsible for the immediate welfare (physical safety, medical condition, and morale) of its crew, as well as the survivors.

Before deciding whether to continue searching for castaways, the Captain must consider the sea and weather, the condition of survivors already aboard, and if known, survivors' prior physical condition, age, length of time in the water, and how they entered the water. Spending excessive energy in search activities is physically harmful and demoralizing to the crew of the survival craft.

When injury to a survivor is suspected, the same methods outlined in general first aid instructions should be used in the transfer to lifeboat or raft. (See Chapter III.) Before hauling a castaway aboard, it would be wise to inquire about injuries.

The Captain of the survival craft must be the one to decide how long resuscitative efforts on unconscious victims should be continued; how food, water, and medical supplies are distributed; and when to signal for help.

IMMEDIATE MEDICAL PROBLEMS
ABOARD SURVIVAL CRAFT

Trauma

Injuries should be handled as outlined in Chapter III. However, it is possible that a prepared medical survival kit might not be available; so the rescuers will have to improvise. Under such conditions, the following principles are suggested.

The first objective in caring for any injured person is to provide lifesaving treatment. Without equipment this may be accomplished by:

• Controlling hemorrhage with direct pressure.

• Giving mouth-to-mouth resuscitation when needed.

• Treating absent pulse or cardiac stoppage by cardiopulmonary resuscitation (See p. 115.)

• Treating shock by placing a survivor's head lower than the rest of his body; and keeping him warm.

• Treating fractures by strapping the extremity to the opposite side, if nothing is available which can be used for splinting. For example, splint one leg to the other, one arm to the chest, or one forearm to the other (with hands touching elbows).

• Relieving pain by simple reassurance, if medicines are not available.

Drowning

Those rescued promptly from drowning usually recover spontaneously, if uncomplicated by an abnormally lowered body temperature (hypothermia).

Treatment

Treatment for victims who almost drowned should consist of immediate mouth-to-mouth resuscitation and external cardiac massage, if needed. It has been established that *nearly-drowning in fresh water* requires different follow-up care after initial emergency treatment, than from *nearly-drowning in saltwater.* However, on a survival craft, the emergency treatment will be about the same for those rescued from drowning in both salt and fresh water. The only difference would be to provide extra fresh water rations for the victim rescued from drowning in saltwater, as soon as he is able to drink.

If there is trouble breathing, mouth-to-mouth resuscitation may be helpful, even though the victim is breathing on his own. Efforts to drain water from the lungs of those rescued from drowning generally are not indicated or helpful, and should not be attempted. However, victims tend to swallow large volumes of water and their stomachs may become distended. This distention impairs ventilation and circulation, and should be alleviated as soon as possible. (See Cardiopulmonary Resuscitation, p. 115, and Drowning, p. 125.)

Generalized Hypothermia (Acute) Due to Immersion

As mentioned previously, generalized hypothermia is the leading cause of death among shipwrecked survivors. The ability to recognize and treat this condition is essential. Generalized hypothermia commonly occurs in most survivors extracted from cold water. These victims are strikingly pale, frequently have generalized muscular rigidity, are shivering, and exhibit varying levels of consciousness and shock.

Treatment

Victims aboard the survival craft who exhibit the above symptoms of generalized hypothermia should be assumed to have subnormal body temperatures. Treatment by rapid warming should be started promptly. The victims should be wrapped in blankets and warm clothing, if available, and warmed as fast as possible to reduce further heat loss. Lying close to others under covers may speed the warming process.

There will be a high risk of ventricular fibrillation and cardiac arrest as the body warms again. Should cardiac arrest occur, it should be treated immediately with a blow to the midchest and then if necessary with external massage and artificial respiration. (See p. 115+.)

Nothing should be given by mouth for 24 hours. Both alcoholic beverages and smoking should be avoided during this period.

Emotional Factors

Under ideal conditions the healthy uninjured person may be able to survive three days at sea in a lifeboat or raft. However, survival for longer than one month is not uncommon. The single most important factor in castaway survivorship is the poorly defined *WILL TO LIVE.* This has been proved time and again in sea disasters and ditchings. Often survivors made every mistake in the book, but were saved by their determination to live.

The actions and emotional stability of the castaways depend first upon the morale and psychologic strength of both the group and the individual. A group of experienced seamen, for instance, will be psychologically stronger to face ditching than a group of dependents. That individuals vary greatly, both mentally and physically, in their reactions to stress is self-evident and needs no discussion. Also, injuries sustained during ditching or aboard the liferaft may be new trauma for some castaways, while for others it may be an aggravation of preexisting medical or psychiatric conditions. Mental derangement may appear anytime, before or after the rescue.

As time is spent on the survival craft awaiting rescue, the group's morale may weaken seriously. Keeping survivors active is important. An assignment to various tasks—nursing care, supply tally, rescue watch, among other activities—will divert and occupy the mind and may help to keep hopes high. Lone survivors should make every effort to conserve energy and resources. They may imagine that they hear voices, or see things which are not really there. Keeping the mind active with mental exercises, may help to prevent this state.

Recognition and treatment of mental disturbances is the duty of all survivors, but the ultimate responsibility rests with the Captain of the survival craft. Anxiety is most contagious and can well destroy chances for survival on the open sea. Immediately after rescue, bewilderment and disbelief are to be expected, and some victims will be hysterical and agitated.

Treatment

The best treatment for anxiety is to reassure patients and assign small tasks to keep them occupied. Acute agitation should be treated promptly, as the situation demands. For some victims forcible restraint may need to be applied. Morphine sulfate 10 mg may be given intramuscularly and may be repeated every four hours as needed to calm the anxious person.

OTHER MEDICAL PROBLEMS ABOARD SURVIVAL CRAFT

1. Preexisting Medical Problems

Preexisting medical problems often call for a change in management on the survival craft. Unless withdrawal of prescribed medications is life-threatening, they should *not* be taken while awaiting rescue.

Prescribed medications which *should* be continued are digitalis preparations, medicines for the control of epilepsy (other than barbiturates), cortisone-like drugs, and nitroglycerin. Other medicines should be withheld unless there is danger of an immediate and serious medical problem.

2. Seasickness

Seasickness (motion sickness) is an acute illness characterized by loss of appetite, nausea, dizziness, and vomiting. Preventive measures often are effective. However, attacks of motion sickness are difficult to treat.

Treatment

Those known to be prone to seasickness should be given cyclizine hydrochloride 50 mg every four to six hours by mouth, if it can be retained.

3. Sunburn

Sunburn is one of the principal medical hazards of survival on the open sea, regardless of latitude. It may vary from a first to a third degree burn, depending upon the exposure and protection available to the victim. Initially, sunburn is generally characterized by redness, edema, and tenderness of the skin. It may be accompanied by local pain, fever, nausea, vomiting, diarrhea, weakness, or even prostration.

Sunburn is prevented by keeping fully clothed at all times, and if possible, staying under a canopy. Survivors should avoid looking directly into the sun or at the glare from the water. Those aboard the survival craft should wear sunglasses during all daylight hours. In addition to these obvious precautions, a sunscreening agent should be applied liberally to all exposed body parts, during periods of exposure to strong sunlight.

4. Injuries due to Marine Animals

Injuries from marine animals include not only direct trauma, but chemical poisoning and allergic reactions such as those caused by animals like the jellyfish, Portuguese man-of-war, and stingrays. Local symptoms may vary from hives to blisters to painful swellings, depending on the animal contacted. Generalized symptoms of headache, sneezing, difficult breathing, fever, and chills may be present.

Treatment

The body area affected should be cleansed thoroughly for conditions caused by marine animals. Acetaminophen 600 mg may be given for pain and fever or chills. The patient should be kept warm. For difficult breathing with wheezing, a 0.5 ml injection of epinephrine hydrochloride 1:1000 should be given subcutaneously.

5. Hydration and Nutrition

If rescue is delayed, maintaining both hydration and nutrition aboard the survival craft are likely to become progressively more serious problems. Food supplies are less essential than water. Lifeboat stores often are limited to hard candy, which provides a small amount of energy. Its main value is boosting the morale of hungry survivors.

Although survival craft (lifeboats and liferafts) carry a limited quantity of potable water, they may be equipped with desalting kits or a solar still which would provide additional drinking water. Each desalting kit provides about one pint of safe drinking water. Although the water is likely to be acrid and discolored, it is safe when prepared according to the instructions on the kit. The capacity of a solar still is limited; it will yield about eight pints of water per day in temperate climates with sunlight. This distilled water looks and smells better than the water produced by desalination. Efforts should be made to store rainwater.

If it is likely that more than one day will pass before rescue, minimal water should be issued during the first 24 hours. This will allow the body to activate water-saving mechanisms that later will reduce the need for water. Survivors who have spent some time in the water, or who have swallowed seawater, may have a demanding thirst; this should be satisfied partially. After the first day, one pint of water daily per person should be consumed. If stores are adequate while in tropical climates, the ration should be increased beyond one pint per day to compensate for excessive loss of water due to sweating.

6. Heat Exposure Injuries

Special problems are created aboard survival craft by exposure to tropical heat. In certain circumstances, fluid loss by sweating alone can be extremely high. The body will adjust to exceptional heat to some extent, but full acclimatization rarely occurs.

Dehydration

Dehydration can be prevented by minimizing activity during the daylight hours and by making best use of clothing or a canopy.

Treatment

Treatment for dehydration consists of increasing the water ration, as supplies permit. (See section 5, above.)

Heat Exhaustion

Heat exhaustion is caused by a loss of body water and salt. (For symptoms and treatment, see Chapter III, p. 49.)

Heat Cramps

Heat cramps are painful spasms of the muscles of the extremities, back, or abdomen due to salt depletion. The skin usually is moist and cool with muscle twitching frequently present. (For other information and treatment, see Chapter III, p. 105.)

Heatstroke (Sunstroke)

Heatstroke is a medical emergency. (For discussion and treatment, see Chapter III, p. 105.)

MEDICAL RESOURCES ABOARD LIFEBOAT

Lifeboats, liferafts, lifefloats, and buoyant apparatus are required by regulations * to be provided with certain provisions. This required equipment must be of good quality, efficient for the purpose they are intended to serve, and kept in good condition. The lifeboats for ocean and coastwise seagoing self-propelled vessels must be equipped with a *First Aid Kit (U.S. Coast Guard Approved)*. The provisions for approval and the contents of the *First Aid Kit* are stated in 46 CFR 160.041.

---

* Title 46, Code of Federal Regulations, Parts 33, 75, 94, and 192.

Table 8-1
Medical Survival Kit [1]
Suggested for Lifeboats Aboard Merchant Vessels

Description of Item	Unit	No. of Units	Comments
Medications			
Acetaminophen Tablets, 300 mg, 100s	bot.	1	Minor aches or pain, antipyretic
Cyclizine Hydrochloride Tablets, 50 mg, 100s	bot.	5	Seasickness, mild antihistamine
Diphenylhydantoin Sodium Capsules, 100 mg, 100s	bot.	1	Anticonvulsant antiepileptic
Diazepam Tablets, 5 mg, 100s [2]	bot.	3	Tranquilizer
Diphenoxylate Hydrochloride 2.5 mg and Atropine Sulfate 0.025 mg, Tablets, 100s [3]	bot.	1	Antidiarrheal
Epinephrine Hydrochloride Injection, 1:1000, 1 ml disposable cartridge, 10s	pkg.	1	Asthmatic attack, or difficulty in breathing after marine animal trauma
Morphine Sulfate Injection, 10 mg/ml, 1 ml Disposable Cartridge, 10s [4]	pkg.	1	Analgesic, sedative
Sodium Chloride, 1g Tablets, 100s	bot.	1	Heat cramps
Sunscreen Preparation	pkg.	40	Protection against sunburn
Tetracycline Hydrochloride Capsules, 250 mg, 100s	bot.	2	Broad spectrum antibiotic
Surgical Supplies			
Bandage, Elastic, 4 in, Roll, 12s	box	1	
Bandage, Gauze, Roll, Sterile 4 in x 10 yd 12s	box	1	
Bandage, Absorbent, Adhesive, 3/4 in x 3 in, 100s	box	1	
Insect Repellent	bot.	2	
Pad, Sterile, 4 in x 4 in, 100s	box	2	
Scissors, Bandage, Lister	each	1	
Soap, Surgical	cake	20	
Sunglasses	each	20	
Syringe, Hypodermic Cartridge Holder [5]	each	2	
Tape, Adhesive, Surgical, 2 in x 5 yd, Roll, 6s	box	1	
Thermometer, Clinical, Fever	each	2	

[1] To be available for forced abandonment of a vessel in cold water areas and infrequented waterways.
[2] Controlled Substance, Schedule III.
[3] Controlled Substance, Schedule V.
[4] Controlled Substance, Schedule II.
[5] Disposable cartridge for medication and syringe holder should be purchased from an identical supplier, to make sure that the cartridge will fit the syringe.

When ships travel infrequently-used waterways or in colder climates, it is advisable to have *in addition* a more comprehensive survival kit (in waterproof packaging) prepared and ready to be placed aboard lifeboats or liferafts, when needed. The proposed contents of such a kit are shown in Table 8–1. This list of medications and surgical supplies is planned for a complement of 20 to 30 survivors for a period of one week.

The Master should assign the individual in charge of the *Sickbay and Medicine Chest* to prepare *Medical Survival Kits,* or have them prepared ashore. The person designated by the Master to be responsible for these kits should store them in a compartment that can be maintained at temperatures above freezing, *but not above room temperature. On abandoning ship, it would be this individual's responsibility to see that the officer-in-charge of a lifeboat receives such a kit. Morphine sulfate injectable dosages may be stored in these kits. However, the ship's compartment in which morphine sulfate is stored should be locked securely at all times, and checked at frequent intervals by the Master. The Master and the officer concerned should be the only ones with the key or lock combination.*

SEARCH AND RESCUE PRIORITIES

1. Safety of Rescuers

Vessels responding to a distress call must consider the same problems that confront Captains of survival crafts: factors of sea and weather, the condition of survivors already picked up, probable condition of missing victims, and the condition of the rescue ship and crew. *The lives and safety of the rescue crew must be the first consideration.* The treatment of survivors will depend on the nature of the rescue facility, and the number and medical condition of the survivors.

2. Condition of Survivors (Triage Groups)

Personnel on the rescue vessel should sort rapidly all survivors according to their physical condition. The sorting or triage categories are:

(a) Those with minor injuries whose condition will not be worsened by delay in treatment.

Treat these last or as time permits. If their condition warrants, they may be put to work helping with the emergency or relieving others who can help.

(b) Those sick or injured but potentially treatable with facilities at hand.

This includes those who urgently require medical attention. Some in this group may be given first aid and relegated to triage group (a). For example, a broken arm could be splinted quickly and be set later, after other more critical problems are taken care of.

(c) The dead and the dying.

The dying are those who probably will not survive with the treatment available. They may be difficult to identify. This group should be treated after group (b) but before group (a). Within this group, try to pick those with the best chances for survival *before* the less hopeful cases.

MEDICAL PROBLEMS OF THE RESCUED CASTAWAY ABOARD RESCUE VESSEL

1. Drowning

Victims rescued from drowning must receive immediate treatment as previously discussed in this chapter on p. 339; and in more detail under Cardiopulmonary Resuscitation and Drowning, p. 115. Although there are different physiological variations from freshwater and seawater submersion in drowning, it is again emphasized that basic life support resuscitation procedures are the same for both. *Also, every submersion victim, even one requiring minimal treatment, should be evacuated to a hospital for follow-up care.*

2. Cold Exposure Injuries, Local

For discussion of the emergency treatment for local cold exposure injuries (Chilblain, Immersion Foot, Trench Foot, and Frostbite), see Chapter III, p. 45.

3. Generalized (Immersion) Hypothermia, Acute, Wet Cold, Aboard the Rescue Vessel

The following discussion on *generalized hypothermia,* plus material presented previously in this chapter, covers the various medical problems of patients with hypothermia. If this material is read it will be easier for the reader to understand the underlying causes of a patient's symptoms and carry out the treatment required.

In *generalized hypothermia, temperature* and *moisture* govern the level of body reaction; while *wind* and *length of exposure* govern the severity and speed of development.

At environmental temperatures less than 68 to 70°F (20 to 21°C), man's survival depends upon insulation (body fat, clothing), the ratio of body surface to volume, the basal metabolic rate (BMR), and *the will to survive.* Below 95°F (35°C) rectal temperature, hypothermia produces diminishing BMR, heart rate, blood pressure, and uncontrollable shivering. Hallucinations, apathy, and stupor or unconsciousness occur at 80°F to 86°F (27°C to 30°C); and death from ventricular fibrillation or cardiac arrest at 70°F to 82°F (21°C to 28°C).

Seawater freezes at 28.4°F (−2°C). It may be assumed that most polar water with ice is this cold. In polar water the body temperature falls very rapidly. Consciousness lasts 5 to 7 minutes, the ungloved hand is useless in 1 to 5 minutes, and death occurs in 10 to 20 minutes. It has been found that severe cold exposure to the head and neck can cause massive cerebral hemorrhage. This part of the anatomy should be specially protected for ditching.

Treatment

Treatment of generalized (immersion) hypothermia begins with resuscitation, using oxygen if available. An oral airway should be inserted. When respiration is absent or poor, or where there is *no detectable carotid pulse,* it may be difficult to tell if the patient is dead or alive. If there is uncertainty on the possibility of life, *always try to resuscitate.*

After carrying out lifesaving measures, wet clothing should be removed and plans for immediate and rapid warming made. If possible, immersion in a hot bath carefully maintained between 104°F to 107.6°F (40°C to 42°C) is desirable. If facilities are not available for maintaining a hot bath, hot water bottles or heating pads with layers of blankets can be

used on patients. Great care is needed to avoid burns, as the cold patient especially is vulnerable. Also, an airway must be maintained if the patient is unconscious.

It is recommended that heat only be applied to the central core of the body. It is of critical importance NOT to attempt to warm the victim's arms or legs since heating of the limbs causes cold blood to flow from them to the body core, causing further detrimental cooling of the core. Such incorrect treatment of hypothermia may induce a condition known as "after-drop."

The patient should be placed in the controlled temperature bath, or other methods of warming applied until the rectal temperature is above 95°F (35°C) and the patient has stopped shivering.

With a large number of cases, *treat first those not breathing (but alive) and the unconscious.* Continuous pouring of water at 104°F to 107.6°F (40°C to 42°C) over those waiting for treatment will increase the number of survivors.

The patient with hypothermia must be observed closely. Depression of breathing and cough reflexes may occur, and secretions may be retained. If a suction unit is available, catheter suction of the airway should be done frequently to remove secretions.

Nothing should be given by mouth because the patient may aspirate (inhale liquid into the lungs), or he may vomit due to a lack of bowel motility. Alcoholic beverages should not be given until 12 to 24 hours after recovery.

Intravenous fluids may be needed, but should be given after getting medical advice by radio. A 1000 ml solution of dextrose 5% and sodium chloride 0.45% injection should be allowed to run into the vein over the first hour, and more IV fluid should be given if the blood pressure remains low. This should be given at the rate of 1000 ml per hour as long as the systolic blood pressure is less than 100 mm of mercury and the patient is producing urine. It may be advisable to place an indwelling catheter into the bladder. (See p. 325.)

To combat metabolic acidosis, 50 ml of sodium bicarbonate (3.75 g) should be injected directly into the vein as soon as possible, after starting the intravenous dextrose and sodium chloride fluid. After tourniquet application, if there is any difficulty finding a suitable vein, the arm should be allowed to hang over the side of the bunk with the hand in warm water, with the tourniquet in place for a few minutes. Local heat frequently will make the veins apparent.

It is most important to control shivering because of the dangerous loss of heat and energy which accompanies it. Shivering usually occurs between the levels of 86°F to 98.6°F (30°C to 37°C). For shivering, morphine sulfate 10 mg should be given slowly, directly into the vein. It should be repeated in one to two hours, if needed, and the respiration is not slow and shallow. Approval to use morphine sulfate to control shivering should be sought by radio from a physician. If breathing becomes shallow or slow, mouth-to-mouth resuscitation should be used to support the patient's respiration. (See p. 115.)

In the unconscious patient with hypothermia, the pulse and blood pressure should be checked every 15 minutes and the rectal temperature every half hour. If the patient is comatose or appears to be in shock, a hydrocortisone sodium succinate 100 mg injection should be given intravenously immediately.

When the patient has been conscious for approximately 12 to 24 hours, tetracycline hydrochloride 500 mg should be given by mouth every six hours and continued for five days.

Plans should be made to evacuate the patient from the vessel to the nearest medical facility as soon as possible.

Chapter IX

Birth and Death at Sea

REGISTRATION OF DEATHS, MARRIAGES, AND BIRTHS AT SEA

Logbook Entries

Every vessel bound on any foreign voyage, or of the burden of 75 tons or greater on any intercoastal voyage, shall have an official logbook. The Master of such vessel shall make entries in the logbook on such matters as provided for in Title 46 United States Code, Section 201, which includes among other matters, the particulars regarding death, marriage, and birth.

Reports Required of Vessels Inbound to the United States from a Foreign Voyage

Immigration and Naturalization Service regulations require that the fact of death, marriage, or birth of an individual in the course of the voyage be entered in the passenger manifest or crew list which is turned over to that Service on port entry.

The laws of many States or cities of the United States require or permit the Master of an inbound vessel to file with the appropriate civil authorities a certificate of death, marriage, or birth for each such event occurring on a voyage, when the first port of entry is a U.S. port. Because requirements of law and forms vary from port to port, it may be necessary to seek assistance from the *local civil authorities*.

Reports to United States Consular Offices by Vessels Bound on any Foreign Voyage

The death, marriage, or birth of a U.S. citizen aboard any vessel on a foreign voyage is reported to the U.S. consular officer at the first port, where such officer is available, after the occurrence of such event. These reports are subsequently forwarded to the U.S. Department of State by the consular officer, where certified copies of their contents are made available upon request. This procedure has been followed for years as a service to U.S. citizens, although no statute requires that it be followed.

Report Required to the United States Coast Guard

Whenever there is a loss of life on any merchant vessel, whether in foreign-going or domestic service, the Master, agent, or person in charge shall, as soon as possible, give notice to the nearest marine inspection office of the Coast Guard. When the deceased is a seaman, the Master shall within 48 hours after arrival at his port of destination in the United States give an account of moneys, clothes, and effects to the Coast Guard official to whom the duties of shipping commissioner have been delegated, in accordance with the provisions contained in Title 46, United States Code, Sections 621, 622, 623, 624, 625, 626, 627, 628, and 706.

CHILDBIRTH

Introduction

Occasionally, a person without medical or nursing education has to deliver a baby on board ship. A baby normally is born without any manipulation. The attendant should receive the baby, tie and cut the cord, receive the placenta (afterbirth), and provide proper care for the mother and baby following delivery. A very important function is to reassure the mother and make her feel that there is someone close at hand upon whom she can rely. This feeling of confidence by the mother will increase in proportion to the calmness and efficiency that the attendant exhibits.

When confronted with a woman in labor, the attendant should be able to evaluate the mother properly and if delivery is imminent, prepare to assist her in giving birth. If possible, the mother should be transported to a hospital where a well trained staff is available with the appropriate equipment, supplies, and drugs.

In order to decide whether or not to transport the mother to the hospital, certain information should be obtained by questioning and examination. Ask the mother:

- How many children she has delivered previously?

- How long she has been in labor?

- Whether the "bag of waters" has broken?

- If she feels as though she has to strain to move her bowels?

Also:

- Examine the mother for *crowning* (top of the baby's head appears).

- Determine if time is available to evacuate her to the nearest hospital.

The average time of labor for the mother of a first child is 15 hours, but labor is considerably shorter for subsequent babies. Thus, if the mother says that she is having her first baby and that she has not been in labor long, there may be time to transport her to a hospital. However, the decision should not be based on this information alone without finishing the evaluation.

The mother's indication that she feels she must strain or move her bowels means that the baby has moved from the uterus into the birth canal, a reliable sign that birth is imminent. This sensation is caused by the baby pressing the wall of the vagina against the rectum.

The attendant also should examine the vaginal opening for crowning before making a final decision about transporting the patient. This procedure may be embarrassing to the mother and it is important that the attendant fully explain what is being done and why. Every effort should be made to protect the mother from embarrassment during both the examination and delivery.

In many cases a hasty decision to transport the mother means that the delivery could take place in a helicopter or ambulance, under the worst possible circumstances. Therefore, it is very important to weigh this information before deciding to evacuate the mother from the ship.

As the mother's contractions increase in intensity and frequency, she may become restless, moan, and cry out. As labor progresses, the contractions will cause the mother to "bear down," as she would if straining to have a bowel movement. She should be encouraged to relax and rest between contractions.

To give intelligent assistance to the woman in labor, the attendant should know something about what is happening to the body as labor progresses, as well as the symptoms which will occur.

Stages of Labor

Labor, which is the process of childbirth, consists of contractions of the wall of the uterus (womb). These contractions force the expulsion of the baby into the outside world. (See Fig. 9–1.) Labor is divided into three general stages. *The first stage* usually lasts several hours (up to 18 hours or more for a first baby), from the first contraction to full dilation of the cervix. The small opening at the lower end of the uterus (the cervix) gradually stretches until it is large enough to let the baby pass through. The contractions usually begin as an acutely aching sensation in the small of the back; in a short time, they turn into cramplike pains recurring regularly in the lower abdomen. At first, these

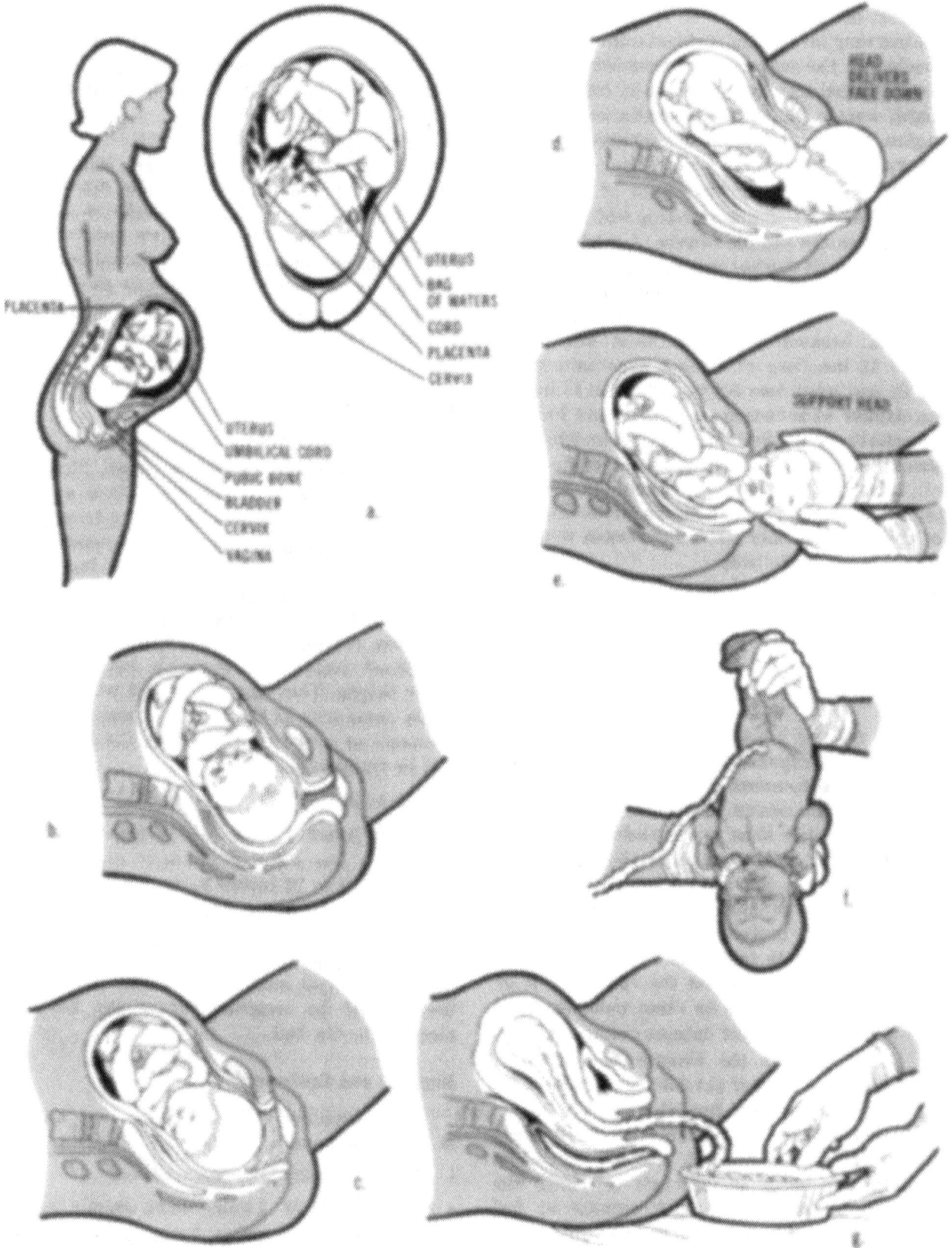

Fig. 9-1. Anatomy of pregnancy and normal stages in labor.

contractions are from 10 to 15 minutes apart, are not very severe, and last but a few moments. Gradually, the intervals between contractions grow shorter and they increase in intensity. A slight, watery, bloodstained discharge from the vagina may accompany contractions or occur before the labor begins.

At the end of the *first stage* of labor, the "bag of waters" (amniotic sac), which encases the baby in the uterus, breaks. A pint or more of watery fluid discharges. Sometimes the "bag of waters" breaks during the first stage of labor. This should not cause the attendant any concern, because it usually does not affect labor. If the "bag of waters" breaks prematurely and labor does not begin within 12 hours, the danger of infection to mother and baby is potentially great. Seek medical advice by radio about possible evacuation of the mother.

The *second stage* lasts about 30 minutes to two hours or more. It begins when the neck of the cervix is fully open, and it ends with the actual birth of the baby.

During the *third stage,* lasting about 15 minutes or more, the afterbirth (placenta) is expelled.

Preparing the Patient

As soon as labor begins, if the birth does not seem to be imminent, the patient should be given an enema, unless she is able to administer it herself. The enema should be expelled into a bedpan rather than a commode. She should take a shower or sponge bath, unless the birth seems imminent. She should be advised to use a heavy lather to clean the inner sides of the thighs and the rectal area, during which she must be careful to prevent soap or water from entering the vagina. After the sponge bath or shower she should put on clean clothing.

The patient should urinate frequently during labor to keep the bladder as empty as possible at the time of the delivery of the baby. As labor progresses, her diet should be restricted to soft, easily digested foods and liquids. She need not get into bed until the contractions occur at intervals of about five minutes. In fact, she ought to remain up and active during the early stages of labor, unless the rolling of the ship makes this dangerous.

At the onset of the first contractions, usually there is plenty of time to get ready for the delivery. The expectant mother should be asked to tell the attendant when contractions first start, so that all preparations for the birth can be completed.

An assistant should be chosen from among the crew or passengers. If possible, this should be someone who has had previous experience with childbirth, or with medical affairs in general. Also, one or two other crew members or passengers (preferably women) should be asked to stand-by to assist. They should be shown how to maintain supplies of clean towels and linen, and instructed how to care for the newborn baby.

Beds for Mother and Baby

For the delivery, a single bed or a bunk with an open foot should be used. The bed should be made up as follows: Place a wide board under the mattress to keep it from sagging. Cover the mattress with a rubber sheet or piece of canvas about three or four feet square, and spread a cloth sheet over this. Draw both sheets tight, and tuck them under the mattress. A pad, made of a folded sheet, should be placed under the woman's buttocks and upper thighs. Then the bed should be made up in the usual way. If the room has been properly warmed, no covering other than the top sheet will be required.

The Baby's Bed

A satisfactory bed can be improvised by building a box about the size of an ordinary pillow and 8 to 12 inches high. A pillow placed in the box can serve as a mattress. If in a temperate climate, wrap a hot water bottle in the baby's blanket and put it into the bed to warm both bed and blanket. The hot water bottle must be removed before the baby is placed into the bed.

Supplies and Equipment

The supplies and equipment that should be assembled are as follows:

• A dozen freshly laundered towels.

• Four pieces of 1-inch wide sterile gauze bandage, about 9 inches long, to be used in tying the baby's cord. Usually only two are used; the other two are extra.

• Sterile gauze dressings, 4 inches square, to wrap around the stump of the cord.

• Sterile scissors for cutting the cord. If sterile scissors are not available, scissors can be cleaned with soap and water and boiled for five minutes in a clean container.

• A dropper bottle of polymyxin B-neomycin-gramicidin eye drops.

• A soft warm blanket to wrap around the baby.

• A basin with a cover to receive the placenta.

• Sterile gloves.

• Sterile or clean gown.

• Rubbing alcohol (isopropyl alcohol, 70% or equivalent) for the cord dressing.

• A roll of 3-inch gauze bandage.

• A sanitary belt.

• Sanitary pads (uncontaminated) from an unopened package, to catch the vaginal discharge, which will continue for several weeks after delivery.

If the patient does not have an unopened package of sanitary pads, cut sterile cotton into pads 10 inches long, 4 inches wide, and 1 inch thick, using sterile scissors. Work on a surface covered with a freshly laundered towel and use a sterile forceps to handle the cotton and gauze. Then cut sterile gauze or freshly ironed cloth into pieces large enough to wrap around each pad and leave two or three inches at each end. Grasp the ends when doing the wrapping. The padded part should not be touched. The towel should be folded over the pads for storage until they are used.

Delivery of Baby and Placenta

When the labor contractions occur regularly every five minutes, the patient should get into bed. *No anesthetic or sedative of any kind should be given to relieve the discomfort without medical advice by radio.*

The attendant should lay out the supplies in a convenient place ready for use. Then the attendant's hands should be scrubbed thoroughly with soap and water.

Because of the danger of introducing infection into the vagina, one never should attempt to clean or disinfect the area between the patient's thighs or around the openings of the vagina, either before or after delivery. Any gross contamination such as feces should be wiped away. However, care must be taken not to introduce any additional bacteria into the vagina. The patient should remain covered with a sheet until just before the baby is born.

It is important to keep calm. It should be remembered that most babies are born without undue difficulty. If there is any marked divergence from the following description of the baby's birth, or if for any reason there seems to be cause for alarm, *medical advice by radio should be sought.*

The "bag of waters" probably will break shortly before the child is born; this may go unnoticed, or a pint or more of clear or blood-stained fluid may come from the vagina.

At this time, the attendant should scrub his hands thoroughly, open the sterile supplies, put on a clean surgical gown and sterile gloves. (See p. 320+.)

The patient should lie on her back with her knees bent and spread apart. If possible, the bed should be well lighted. Normally, the baby's head comes out first, with the face downward. The attendant should place one hand under the baby's forehead and have the other ready to receive the body. As soon as the head is born, the body and limbs usually follow quickly.

If the umbilical cord is wrapped around the neck when the head and neck appear during delivery, try to slip the cord over the baby's head so that it will not be strangled. (See Fig. 9-2.) If this cannot be done, tie the cord in

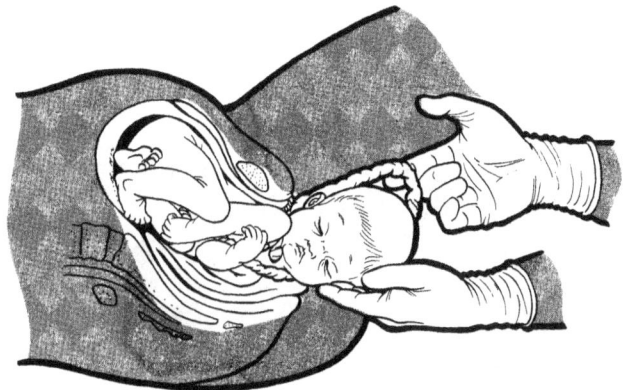

Fig. 9–2. Umbilical cord wrapped around baby's neck.

two places, two inches apart, and cut between the ties. Then, unwind the cord from around the baby's neck.

After the baby is born, a fold of towel should be wrapped around its ankles to prevent slipping. With one hand the baby should be held up by the heels, taking care that the umbilical cord is slack. To get a good grip, insert one finger between the baby's ankles. *Don't spank the baby.* If breathing does not start spontaneously, snap the forefinger of your hand on the sole of the baby's foot. The baby will be very slippery, and should be held over the bed in case it slips from the attendant's grasp. The attendant's other hand should be placed under the baby's forehead with its head bent back slightly, so that fluid and mucus can run out of its mouth. A small rubber ear syringe may be used to remove excess mucus from the mouth, if necessary. Remember—always squeeze the bulb before inserting the tip of the syringe into the baby's nose or mouth, and gently release the bulb to remove the mucus. When the baby begins to cry, lay it on its side on the bed close enough to its mother to keep the cord slack. Note the time of delivery. Later, in the patient's record and the official ship's logbook, record the date, time of delivery, the baby's sex, and the names of the parents.

Tie a strip of sterile gauze around the cord about three inches from the baby's body, and another piece of sterile gauze tied about two inches farther along toward the mother. Do not use any material so thin that it will cut through the cord when tightened. Make square knots and *be sure the ties are tight.* Using sterile scissors, cut the cord between the two knots. (See Fig. 9–3.)

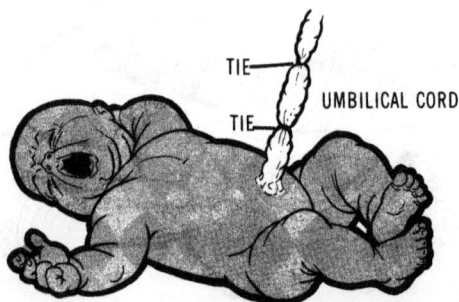

Fig. 9–3. Tying and cutting the umbilical cord.

A pad of sterile gauze, moistened with rubbing alcohol, should be placed under and over the stump. Shortly after cutting the cord, examine the cut end attached to the baby for signs of continued bleeding. If there is evidence of bleeding from the cord, do not attempt to adjust or tighten the existing knot or clamp. Tie or clamp the cord again a short distance from the original closure. It is very important that the cord be closed off completely. The baby should be wrapped in a warmed blanket and placed on its left side in its bed where an assistant can watch it. The baby should be observed carefully during the first 24 hours.

The Placenta

Continue to observe the mother. Contractions usually stop after the birth of the baby, but will begin again to expel the placenta. This usually occurs in 15 to 30 minutes, and is accompanied by a gush of blood. *Do not pull on the cord.* When the placenta is delivered, it should be wrapped in a towel, placed in a plastic bag and refrigerated until transported with the mother and baby to the hospital. The physician will want to examine the placenta for completeness because any portion of the placenta that was not delivered must be removed. Any tissue remaining in the mother's uterus could cause prolonged, excessive bleeding. *If excessive bleeding occurs, seek medical advice by radio.*

Care of Mother After Delivery

After the placenta has been delivered, the attendant's hand should be placed on the mother's abdomen, just below the navel. The contracted uterus feels like a hard lump about as big as a grapefruit. If a hard lump is not felt, the abdomen should be massaged firmly and gently until one forms under the hand. Gentle massage will stimulate a relaxed uterus, causing it to contract. If the uterus does not contract, there is danger of hemorrhaging. Therefore, the uterus should be felt every 15 minutes for hardness to assure that it is contracted. *If the uterus does not become hard, continue the massage and seek medical advice by radio.*

The mother's blood pressure should be taken every 15 minutes after delivery for two hours, or until stabilized. When one knows that the uterus has contracted, the patient's thighs and buttocks should be bathed with soap and water and dried. *Do not bathe the area between the thighs or around the vagina.* A sanitary pad should be applied, the soiled pad and towels removed, and the bunk made up with fresh linen.

The attendant should not try to suture any lacerations in the vaginal opening. The mother should lie on her back with a pillow beneath her knees, and her legs together. She may have a slight chill, so she should be kept warm with blankets. A warm (not hot) drink of sweetened tea, milk, or boullion may be given to her, and her face and hands wiped with a damp towel. She may drop off to sleep. If she remains awake and is restless due to pain, codeine sulfate 30 mg and aspirin 600 mg may be administered by mouth. If aspirin is not well tolerated by the patient, acetaminophen may be given at the same dosage and frequency, along with the codeine sulfate. This dosage may be repeated for discomfort, every four hours for the first 24 to 48 hours after delivery. *The medication should not be continued for more than 48 hours without advice from a physician.*

The mother's diet after delivery may include all foods, except onions and cabbage. She should be encouraged to drink plenty of fluids, particularly milk. If fresh milk is not available, canned milk can be made more palatable by diluting it with equal parts of water, and adding sugar, eggs, chocolate, or other flavoring.

The mother's elimination of wastes should be checked carefully. If her bowels have not moved within three days after delivery, an enema should be given. The enema should be repeated every other day, if the bowels do not move naturally. Her output of urine should be measured carefully and should be at least 1500 ml during the first 24 hours. After each voiding, the perineal area should be cleansed with warm water poured from a sterile container. A sufficient fluid intake must be maintained to assure an adequate output of urine.

The mother's bed should be made up with clean linen daily. Every morning she should be provided with the necessary articles for mouth care and for a sponge bath.

Normally, the mother should rest and be restricted to limited activities for three days following the birth. If her temperature rises above 100°F (37.7°C) for more than 12 hours, an initial dose of penicillin V 500 mg should be given by mouth followed by 250 mg every six hours. If the patient is suspected of being allergic to penicillin, use oral erythromycin in the same dosage and frequency. The patient should be kept on the antibiotic until at least four days after she becomes afebrile (without fever). *If fever persists, seek medical advice by radio.*

Care of Baby After Delivery

Within 30 minutes after the baby is born, two drops of polymyxin B-neomycin-gramicidin eye drops must be placed in each eye to prevent infection, in case any bacteria have entered the eyes during birth.

The baby should be observed every half hour for the first three hours and then every hour for the next 24 hours. Skin color and breathing rate should be noted.

A fresh alcohol dressing should be applied to the stump of the umbilical cord each time it becomes soiled. This may have to be done several times daily. The stump will fall off within seven to ten days. The small area remaining should be redressed until it is healed.

Resuscitating the Newborn Baby

If the baby is not breathing spontaneously within 30 seconds after delivery (about the time it takes to clear the blood and mucus from his nose and mouth), or if he is born limp and apparently lifeless, resuscitative measures must be initiated without delay. The following procedure should be used.

Again, quickly suction the infant's mouth and nose to assure that there is no blockage due to blood or mucus. Replace the baby on its side, with the head lower than the body. Grasp the baby's feet between the second, third, and fourth fingers of one hand, and snap the forefinger of your other hand sharply against the soles of its feet. This stimulation should cause the infant to gasp and breathe, and perhaps to cry lustily. If not, go on to the next step.

Begin mouth-to-mouth resuscitation. (See p. 119.) Quickly blow several small puffs of air from your cheeks into the baby's mouth and nose, and then check for signs of breathing. If the baby has started to breathe spontaneously at this point, administer oxygen until it is pink and breathing well. Do not place the oxygen mask directly over the face; instead, hold it in front of the child's face a slight distance away.

If mouth-to-mouth efforts are still unsuccesful after two minutes, and if at that time you cannot locate a pulse, start cardiopulmonary resuscitation. (See p. 122.) Remember to use only one or two fingers on the sternum and to apply very little pressure. *Caution: Mechanical resuscitation devices never should be used on a newborn infant.*

Feeding the Newborn Baby

The baby should be put to the mother's breast twice the first day and every three hours thereafter, even though the milk does not come into the breast for two or three days. Until the mother has milk, the baby should be given about one ounce of boiled water every two or three hours. The water should be about body temperature. It may be given from a medicine dropper or teaspoon which has been sterilized by boiling; or from a sterile baby bottle with nipple, if available.

Abnormal Conditions of Pregnancy

The majority of births are normal and uncomplicated and pose no particular threat to either the mother or baby. There are, however, numerous complications that can occur. Some of these can be alleviated by the attendant but others require the skill of trained professionals in a hospital with the necessary equipment and supplies.

If a woman goes into labor at sea, medical advice by radio should be sought as soon as possible, instead of waiting until the delivery actually begins.

This book does not provide information on all possible complications of pregnancy and delivery because the possibility of delivering a baby aboard ship at sea is slight. Also, there are possible complications that would require

immediate care by a physician. The following complications are examples of some of the abnormal conditions that might occur. The use of the radio to obtain medical advice provides the best approach in dealing with these problems:

• Vaginal bleeding at anytime during the last three months of pregnancy usually constitutes an emergency. The mother should be placed in bed and taken to port as soon as possible for evaluation by a physician. The mother also should be placed in bed if vaginal bleeding occurs during the first trimester of pregnancy.

• Rupture of the "bag of waters" without labor and with no labor within 12 hours also is considered an emergency. The danger of infection to mother and baby is potentially great. *Seek medical advice by radio.*

• The breech presentation is the most common of abnormal deliveries. This is when the buttocks is delivered first rather than the head-first presentation as in a normal delivery. In a breech presentation, the same procedures should be followed as in a normal delivery. Let the baby deliver with as little interference as possible.

• A prolapsed umbilical cord occurs when the cord comes out of the vagina before the baby is born. Because the cord is already in the birth canal and the uterine contractions are pushing the baby into the canal, the cord will be squeezed between the baby's head and the wall of the vagina and the underlying pelvic structure. Because the baby still is dependent on the blood circulating through the cord for its oxygen supply, the danger of suffocation develops very quickly. Without facilities to perform an emergency Caesarian section, there is virtually nothing that can be done to save the baby. The delivery should be handled in the usual manner.

Baptizing a Newborn Baby

A baby born at sea might exhibit signs that it is not going to survive. In such circumstances attendees at the birth or the Master should ask the mother if she wants the child baptized in conformance with her religious beliefs. If the mother is not conscious, the Master should use his own discretion on the matter.

Nothing is quite so sad as a baby born dead or dying shortly after birth. It is a tragic moment for all concerned—the parents, who have waited so long for their child, and the attendants, who have shared the experience of childbirth.

A simple act of kindness may provide the distraught parents with spiritual comfort. When a baby is stillborn or death appears imminent, any person regardless of religious belief, may baptize the newborn of Christian parents. The attendant should sprinkle drops of water on the baby's bare skin, preferably the head, and say, *I baptize thee in the name of the Father, and of the Son, and of the Holy Spirit.* This exact form should be used. Naturally, resuscitation efforts should be continued during and after the baptism.

Emergency Baptism of Fetus or Embryo

A miscarried fetus or embryo, no matter how small, also can be baptized. Putrefaction or advanced general decomposition is the only certain sign of real death. Break the membranes or open the blood clot surrounding the embryo. Immerse it in a pan of water making sure the water contacts the fetus itself. Then, while moving it about in the water so that there will be a washing or flowing or "baptizing," say the words of conditional baptism: *"If you are capable, I baptize you in the name of the Father, and of the Son, and of the Holy Spirit."* Finally, remove it from the water. The fetus should be immersed in a preservative within a container that has a tight-fitting lid, for examination upon arrival at the first port.

DEATH AT SEA

Because cargo ships usually do not have a physician or lawyer aboard, the Master must assume certain responsibilities concerned with death. These include taking the dying declaration (antemortem statement) of a patient and pronouncing the person dead.

Antemortem Statement

When it appears that a person at sea is about to die, he should be advised that he can make a legally valid statement, if he so desires. The Master, other officer, or crew member may be called upon to record the statement. This is an extremely serious matter, because such a statement may be of vital importance in connection with the cause or circumstances of a person's impending death; the disposition of property, money, or personal effects; or with some incident in his past life. The welfare of many individuals can be influenced by the statement. For instance, a statement may affect the well-being and future security of the patient's family; or the liberty of a person who might be accused of causing the patient's death and thus be subject possibly to criminal prosecution. Whoever receives the declaration must make very effort to understand clearly and completely what is said, *and to take it down in writing—exactly as given.* The recorder must ascertain the patient's attitude, and determine to the best of his ability that the patient is in his right mind, is thinking clearly, rationally, and is fully conscious.

The importance of any statement a patient is about to make should be fully explained to him. The statement must be voluntary; that is, no coercion, threat, or force can be used to obtain it. The statement should be written exactly in the patient's own words without any deletions, additions, or changes. Extraordinary care should be taken not to attempt to interpret what the patient might seem to mean, but to confine the statement to the exact words as spoken by the patient.

The written statement should be read back to the patient. Every effort should be made to obtain his signature on the statement, together with signatures of the witnesses. Any writing intended to serve as the patient's last will and testament *should be signed by him and by three witnesses, whenever possible.*

If a statement made by a dying person cannot be recorded verbatim, the person to whom it is made should make adequate notes at the earliest opportunity, so that he may be able to refresh his memory on the contents of such statement, if he is required to testify in court at a later date. Any declarations, exclamations, acts, or gestures of the dying person, which might in any way indicate his intentions or desires, should be noted and described in writing. It should be remembered that the legal competency or admissibility of a dying person's statement (written or oral) will be affected by the character of the statement, the circumstances under which it is made, the type of proceeding (civil, criminal, or probate) to occur, and the laws of the particular court (Federal, State, or foreign) in which it might be desired to introduce such statement in evidence. Attendants and others concerned should be careful, thorough, and accurate whenever they must record statements of a dying person.

Signs of Death

A merchant marine officer may have to declare a person dead. This is a heavy responsibility. Ship's officers should be equipped with a working knowledge of how to recognize death. The signs of death may be divided into two classes, depending upon whether they arise *shortly after death* or *some time later*.

Early signs of death are absence of heartbeat and breathing for at least 20 minutes. It is difficult for a layman without skill in the use of diagnostic instruments to determine with certainty when the heart stops beating. Besides feeling for the pulse, the heart sounds should be sought by listening with an ear or stethoscope applied directly to the chest, just to the left of the breastbone.

The following is considered a time-honored test, if breathing is not superficially apparent: obtain a clean mirror, make sure it is cooler than body temperature, and hold it before the patient's mouth and nostrils. If the patient is breathing, even shallowly, the mirror will fog; that is, moisture from the breath will condense on its cool surface. If a polished mirror is not available, a wisp of cotton placed on the slightly opened lips of the patient, or before a nostril opening should indicate any air current, if there is life and breathing.

It never should be forgotten that a person may appear to be dead when he still is alive. *Death* is the cessation of life beyond the possibility of resuscitation. *Suspended animation (or death trance),* which imitates death, is total unconsciousness with scarcely any respiration, heartbeat, or other obvious sign of life. Suspended animation may occur as a part of such things as neuropsychiatric disorders (hys-

teria for instance), debilitating disease, submersion, gas poisoning, electric shock, or any major injury followed by shock, whether or not there are large wounds or massive hemorrhage or extensive tissue damage. Breathing may be so shallow that it cannot be distinguished by ordinary methods; or breathing may stop before the heart stops beating. Heart sounds may be so faint that they cannot be heard by ordinary means. The pulse may be so feeble that it cannot be detected by touch. The pupils of the eyes may be dilated and fail to react to light. The eyelids may be half-closed and the cornea (the transparent covering of the front of the eyeball) insensitive to touch.

Therefore, if the circumstances suggest suspended animation, resuscitation efforts should not be stopped until the fact of death is definitely established—although one or more of the early signs of apparent death are present. Unless the patient unquestionably is dead, time should not be wasted in looking for the early, minute signs of death. Instead, every effort should be centered on resuscitation.

In most cases, death is unmistakable when it occurs. It will not be necessary to wait for the later signs to confirm death. Nevertheless, the body rarely, if ever, is buried at sea before the late signs of death have occurred. From a medicolegal and other points of view, the record of the case should include a description of those later signs of death that were observed. *The later conclusive signs of death include:*

• *Changes in the appearance of the eye*—The cornea loses its transparency, turns milky or cloudy, and becomes wrinkled.

• *Drop in body temperature*—In doubtful cases, a clinical thermometer should be placed in the rectum. Occasionally, the temperature remains stationary or rises for a short time after death. However, cooling soon occurs and usually the body temperature drops several degrees Fahrenheit each hour for the first 8 or 10 hours after death, except in the tropics or under circumstances where the room temperature approaches body temperature (98.6°F or 37°C). The rate of fall depends upon the temperature at the time of death, the amount of fatty tissue under the skin, the amount of clothing worn, and weather conditions.

• *Rigor mortis*—A stiffening of the muscles and rigidity of the body, usually appears within two to eight hours after death, and lasts 16 to 24 hours. However, the onset of rigor mortis and its duration are subject to wide variation. Rigor mortis, usually begins in the facial muscles, extends gradually to the legs, and disappears in the same order.

Care must be taken not to confuse rigor mortis with the muscular spasm and rigidity that sometimes occurs almost immediately after an electric shock or in some cases of poisoning. Early rigidity is not a reason for discontinuing artificial respiration or other attempts at resuscitation.

• *Postmortem lividity*—The skin upon which the body rests—usually at the buttocks, back, and shoulders—gradually becomes discolored several hours after death. This discoloration is due to the settling of blood into the lowest parts of the body as it lies in one position. These purplish or reddish-violet spots are known as "death spots," corpse lividity, postmortem lividity, or cadaveric lividity.

These spots, sometimes mistaken for bruises, usually can be distinguished from bruises in two ways: (1) *lividity spots* would not have been present before death and (2) *bruises* will show considerable blood or perhaps a clot, while the lividity spots will not. Lividity spots provide a sure sign of death.

• *Putrefaction* (rotting, decomposition)—This is absolute proof of death. Putrefaction occurs after rigor mortis has disappeared. Ordinarily its onset is not apparent for at least one day after death; and it may be delayed for several days, depending upon such circumstances as the cause of death, and whether in a cold or in a hot moist climate.

Care of the Body After Death

Ship's officers are not expected to embalm a body. The following outline is not concerned with the preservation of a body after death; only its general care.

In the presence of a corpse, everyone should be respectful, quiet, orderly, and subdued. There should be no attempt at humor; such efforts usually indicate an embarrassed covering up of kinder emotions which would be better to express. The behavior of the medical attendant can do much to preserve a proper atmosphere in the death room. It should be remembered that the death of a member of the crew may be very depressing to the rest of the ship's company. They should not see the body until it is properly laid-out and prepared for burial.

When rigor mortis occurs within a few hours after death, it becomes difficult to make adjustments to the positions of the limbs. As soon as death has been pronounced, it is essential that the body be placed in the conventional position for burial. The body should be placed on its back, with the legs straightened and the knees held together with a loosely knotted bandage. The arms should be positioned along the sides, with the elbows bent and the forearms carried across the abdomen so that the hands will meet. The wrists should be secured in this position by a loosely knotted bandage.

The head should be elevated slightly by means of a pad. The eyelids should be closed. At times they will not stay closed, and it will be necessary to place a piece of damp cotton on top of the lids. If this will not keep them closed, the lids should be lifted up, and a very small wisp of cotton inserted under the upper eyelids. Then the lid should be closed over the cotton. One should be sure that the cotton is not thick enough to disfigure the eyelids' appearance and that none of the white cotton is visible after the lids are closed.

The mouth must be closed. If the deceased wore false teeth, they should be carefully placed in position so that the facial appearance is as normal as possible. The lower jaw usually sags before rigor mortis sets in; it should be supported by a folded towel or a broad bandage knotted over the top of the head. After a few hours, this bandage may be removed (before any of the crew members view the body).

Discharges may appear from body openings; the nostrils, mouth, penis, and anus; these openings should be plugged with cotton. Care must be taken to assure that the cotton plugs in the nostrils are not visible from the outside.

The face should be washed carefully and dried. The hair should be combed in the fashion used by the deceased when he was alive.

Usually, there is no question about the identification of a crewman's body, because members of the crew presumably were identified properly at the time of signing-on. However, for some legal reason, absolutely certain identification may be needed. Therefore, it is recommended that (1) fingerprints be taken; and (2) a careful, written description be made of the location, and exactly measured size of other peculiarities, as scars, tatto marks, moles, and birthmarks. Fingerprints are made by pressing the palmar (front) side of the last joint of each finger, one after the other, on an inking stamp pad, and making the impression of the finger markings by pressing the inked surface of each finger onto a piece of paper. Each imprint should be identified by noting under it "left thumb," "left index finger," "left middle finger," and so on for all the fingers.

If the patient died of a contagious disease, the body (except for the face and head) should be carefully and completely wrapped in a sheet which has been previously dampened with phenolic disinfectant solution.

Disposition of the Body

If a decision is made *not* to bury at sea, the remains should be put into a *leakproof mortuary body transfer bag* and kept in a refrigerated area aboard ship. *The remains must not be frozen,* in order to keep it in good condition for possible viewing by relatives of the deceased, or for possible later medical-legal investigation.

Burial Arrangements

The Master will get in touch with the shipping company, which in turn will contact the next-of-kin for instructions on disposition of the remains. The company will relay these instructions back to the Master. It could be decided (1) to retain the remains aboard ship until arrival at a U.S. port; (2) send the remains to a mortuary in a foreign port; or (3) burial could be at sea. United States law is silent as to when there *must* be a burial at sea, or when the remains *must* be returned to port.

In some circumstances the laws of the country at the next port of entry will determine the disposition of the remains. Before entering a foreign port, the Master should *contact local health officials in advance.*

There may be occasions when the remains would be transported by air to the United States. This could happen when requested by next of kin, the vessel's owner, the deceased person's labor union, or any number of other possibilities that could influence the Master to decide on such a move.

Burial at Sea

Today burial at sea is the exception. If it is decided to conduct a burial at sea, the body should be encased from head to foot carefully and completely in a sheet, and then sewed tightly in canvas. A heavy weight should be enclosed in the canvas at the feet.

If the body is to be kept on board ship for a day or two, it should be washed and petroleum jelly applied to the face and hands. If possible, the body should be placed in cold storage.

All available information about the deceased, his family, his friends, and a complete history of his illness, a careful record of his words, such as messages, expressed wishes, and last statement, should be gathered together in a file for delivery to the proper shore authorities. His personal belongings should be gathered together, listed, placed in a sealed package, and stored in a safe place.

Burial Service for Ships Without a Chaplain

At the spot on the afterdeck where the burial is to be held, two sawhorses or similar supports should be placed about the height of the ship's railing. All the ship's company who are available for the ceremony should assemble at the place of burial. The flag-draped body of the deceased is then brought forth on a stretcher (or other similarly shaped flat surface) by four or six attendants (pallbearers), two or three on each side. The stretcher is placed on the supports, feet outboard. The attendants step back slightly but retain their relative position with regard to the stretcher. All uncover.

The ship's Master, or someone representing him, shall step forward and slowly and solemnly read a suitable prayer, as the following—*

---

* Because the following prayer has been highly regarded in past editions, it is presented again in this revised edition.

PRAYER

Out of the depth have I cried unto Thee, O Lord: Lord hear my voice.

Let Thine ears be attentive to the voice of my supplication.

If Thou, O Lord, wilt mark iniquities, Lord who shall stand it?

For with Thee there is merciful forgiveness; and by reason of Thy law, have I waited for Thee, O Lord,

My soul hath hoped in the Lord.

From the morning watch even until night; let Israel hope in the Lord,

Because with the Lord there is mercy; and with Him plenteous redemption.

And He shall redeem Israel from all his iniquities.

Eternal rest grant unto him. O Lord, And Let perpetual light shine upon him.

Come to his assistance, ye Saints of God. Meet him, ye Angels of the Lord. Receive his soul, and present it to the Most High.

May Christ who called thee, receive thee; and may the Angels lead thee into the bosom of Abraham.

Eternal rest grant to him, O Lord, and let perpetual light shine upon him.

The Master, or his representative, may talk about the deceased for 3 to 5 minutes, highlighting things that made him an honorable man among men.

The Master or his representative then nods to the attendants at the bier; they grasp the flag with one hand and lift it slightly above the corpse. If necessary, the two attendants at the foot-end of the stretcher will lift that end so that it rests on the rail.

The two attendants at the head-end of the stretcher will tilt it up and permit the body to slide, feet foremost, into the sea. As the body is consigned to the deep, attendees stand in reverence.

When someone who is next of kin is present at the burial service, the flag can be folded neatly and presented to that person. If no next of kin are present, the flag may be placed temporarily with the effects of the deceased.

Family Notified

When the family is notified that the remains were committed to the deep, the Master should indicate the longitude and latitude where the event occurred. Also, the Master should find out if the next of kin wants the flag sent to the family with the personal effects of the deceased.

Chapter X

Prevention and Control of Communicable Diseases

THE PRACTICE OF MEDICINE includes not only the treatment of diseased individuals but also the prevention and control of disease and injury. Prevention always has been considered the most desirable way to attain good health. Aboard ship, maintenance of the highest possible levels of health should be the aim of all. Specific measures can be taken to prevent, control, or remove threats to health and efficiency. These measures include quarantine, immunization, proper sanitation, vector control, chemophylaxis (use of medication or other chemicals to prevent disease), and presentation of educational talks or audiovisual aids. Those in command of the vessel are responsible for provision or enforcement of these and other measures.

COMMUNICABLE DISEASES

Communicable diseases are those which can be transmitted from one host to another. Transmission may be direct or indirect to a well person from an infected person or animal; at times through an intermediate animal host, a vector; or the inanimate environment. Illnesses result when an infectious agent invades and multiplies in the host.

The occurrence and spread of disease are determined by an interplay of factors specific to the causative agent, the environment, and the individuals or groups to whom the disease occurs. Epidemics may endanger the operation and safety of the ship. If many fall ill, medical facilities, supplies, and personnel may be utilized so heavily that the sick will not receive adequate care. Thus, it is important to know how various diseases are spread and what measures should be taken to assure their prevention and control.

Environmental Sanitation

Environmental sanitation, which is very important in the control of communicable diseases, seeks to prevent the spread of pathogens by eliminating both sources and modes of transmitting the agents. Among examples are sanitary treatment, handling, distribution, and dispensing of water, milk, and food; treatment and disposal of sewage to avoid contamination of water and food supplies; air hygiene and sanitation to prevent airborne infection; and the control of vectors of disease agents. Due to programs of environmental sanitation, malaria and many of the enteric diseases, such as typhoid fever and cholera, have either been eradicated or significantly reduced in the United States and other countries.

Infectious Agents

Organisms that produce disease in man range in size from the submicroscopic viruses to the fish tapeworm, which may attain a length of over 30 feet. Microorganisms are found in both plants and animals, as single cell and many-celled types.

Several groups of infectious agents (and representative diseases which they cause) may be classified as follows:

Bacteria: (sore throat, pneumonia, tuberculosis, syphilis, bacillary dysentery, cholera).

Viruses: (common cold, influenza, poliomyelitis, smallpox, measles, and viral pneumonia).

Rickettsiae: (typhus fever and Rocky Mountain spotted fever).

Protozoa: (malaria, amebic dysentery, African sleeping sickness).

Metazoa: (filariasis, trichinosis, hookworm, and tapeworm diseases).

Fungi: (ringworm and athlete's foot).

Infectious agents usually are specific in their disease-producing capabilities. Several different organisms can produce diseases which resemble each other clinically (symptoms and course of the disease) and pathologically (anatomical changes caused by a disease). For example, the meningococci, tubercle bacilli, and the mumps virus can produce meningitis, which is an inflammation of the membrane that envelops the brain and spinal cord. However, a specific disease, such as tuberculosis, only can be caused by a specific agent—in this case the tubercle bacillus.

Disease Incidence (Occurrence)

After infection, the number of cases of a disease that will occur is determined by many factors, some of which are:

Number of infective organisms entering into the exposure; that is, whether the exposure was minimal or massive.

Virulence (disease-producing power) of the organism; that is, the degree of change it can produce in the host. *Pathogenicity* means the ability of the microorganism to produce disease. Some strains of a pathogenic species may be more virulent than others.

Susceptibility of the host, or its ability to resist infection. Immunities may be acquired through vaccination or by inheritance. In addition, the natural resistance of the body and a state of good health constitute strong defenses against infections. Infection by a disease-producing organism, therefore, does not result necessarily in clinically detectable disease. In the control of communicable disease, infected but apparently healthy people are as significant as those with all the symptoms and signs of the disease.

Chain of Infection

The chain of infection spreading through a host population has five links:

• A reservoir of infection or source of the agent.

• A portal of exit or mode of escape of the agent from the reservoir.

• A method of transmission of the agent from the source to the new host.

• A portal of entry into the new host.

• A susceptible new host.

Knowledge of the infection chain is required for the development of effective measures to prevent or control the spread, because the interruption or absence of any single link will prevent transmission of the disease. Thus, communicable diseases often are classified on the basis of their method of passing from the source to the host.

Sources of Infection

A reservoir of infection is the habitat of the infecting organisms, the sum of all sources of infection. Sources or reservoirs of infection may be human, animal, or environmental.

Most of the infectious diseases harmful to man have a *human source* or reservoir. Manifestations of the presence of the infective agent in the human reservoir range in degree from an asymptomatic (symptom-free) healthy carrier to frank (unmistakable) disease. The obvious cases of a disease vary downward in severity from fatal, through severe to moderate, to mild. The disease may be *atypical* or *abortive:* that is, the usual manifestations of the disease may not develop (atypical); or the patient may recover before all signs or symptoms occur (abortive). *Missed cases* are those which are not recognized either by the patient or the physician.

Carriers of infection may be transient or chronic. *Incubationary carriers* are those who harbor the infection during the incubation period prior to the onset of the disease. *Convalescent carriers* are those who continue to harbor the organism after recovering from the disease. Carriers of disease can be as important a source of infection as those who are ill with the disease. The relative importance of a carrier category differs with each specific disease. In meningococcal meningitis, for example, the number of asymptomatic (without symptoms) or transient carriers may far outnumber those who are ill with the disease. On the other hand, in measles the human is the source of infection only from the beginning of the catarrhal stage, until about five days after the rash appears. There are no asymptomatic carriers of measles as far as is known.

In general, *diseases of animals* (zoonoses) affect man only accidentally. In most cases, man is not a natural host for the infective agent. However, in certain diseases both man and another animal or animals are essential to the normal life cycle of the infecting agent. In these instances, the infective agents have differentiated stages in their life cycle that require two or more hosts for their development. Malarial mosquitoes, most tapeworms, the blood flukes of schistosomiasis, and the round worms causing filariasis are examples. In other instances, either man or another animal can serve as reservoirs of infection.

Animal species which can serve as reservoirs of infectious diseases that affect man include:

Gastropods
slugs, snails, mussels, oysters, clams;

Arthropods
(a) *insects* (lice, fleas, flies, bees),

(b) *arachnids* (spiders, mites, ticks),

(c) *crustaceans* (lobsters, shrimp, crabs, water fleas);

Fish; Birds; and such Mammals as
(rats, bats, cattle, horses, swine, dogs, cats, monkeys).

Some infectious agents live in the soil; thus the inanimate environment is the reservoir of infection in these illnesses. *Fungi* (such as those causing coccidioidomycosis, histoplasmosis, and blastomycosis) and *molds* are found in soil and dust or on vegetation grown in endemic areas (places where the disease is common). Certain species of bacteria which form spores also are found in the soil, but only if the soil has been contaminated previously with the spore. Tetanus (lockjaw) and anthrax are examples of diseases that may be acquired in this manner.

Portals of Exit

The ease with which an organism can escape from its infected host partly determines the ease with which it is transmitted to another host. Some agents never leave their hosts under ordinary circumstances. The larvae of the pork worm (*trichina*) that cause trichinosis, for instance, cannot escape from the tissues unless the host is eaten by another animal. In some diseases, the infecting organism cannot leave its host during certain stages of its development; for example, there is no spread of the *Treponema* that cause syphilis from a patient with the late stages of syphilis. From an epidemiologic (occurrence and distribution of a disease) standpoint, the important fraction of the reservoir of infection is that portion from which the agent *can* escape.

Usually there is only a single portal of exit for each species of infectious agent, but there can be more; for example, the respiratory tract and skin lesions in smallpox. Usually, the portal of exit is the same as the portal of entry. However, there are many exceptions to this rule.

Modes of Transmission

The spread of disease also depends upon the ability of the infecting organism to survive outside its reservoir (source). Transmission of the agent may be either direct or indirect.

Direct transmission methods include:

• *Direct contact* with the infected person, as in kissing or sexual intercourse.

• *Droplet spread*, in which an infected person, through sneezing, coughing, or talking, sprays the face of a noninfected person with droplets containing the disease-causing agent.

• *Fecal-oral spread,* in which fecal material from an infected person is transferred to the mouth of a noninfected person, usually by the hands. Usually the hands are contaminated by touching such things as soiled clothing, bedding, towels, and then touching the mouth where transmission occurs.

Indirect transmission of infectious organisms involves *vehicles* and *vectors* which carry disease agents from the source to the host.

Vehicles are inanimate or non-living means of transmission of infectious organisms. They include:

Water—If polluted specifically by contaminated sewage, it is the vehicle for such enteric (intestinal) diseases as typhoid fever, cholera, amebic and bacillary dysentery.

Milk—The vehicle for diseases of cattle transmissible to man, including bovine tuberculosis, undulant fever, and streptococcal infections from infected udders. Diseases in which milk serves as the link between man and man include typhoid fever, scarlet fever, and diphtheria. Milk also serves as a growth medium for some agents of bacterial diseases.

Food—It is the vehicle for typhoid and paratyphoid fevers, amebic dysentery, food infections, and poisoning. To serve as a vehicle, food must be moist, bland (not too acid or alkaline), raw or inadequately cooked, or improperly refrigerated after cooking, as well as having been in intimate contact with an infected source. Virtually any food meeting these requirements may be a vehicle for transmitting organisms that cause disease.

Air—It is the vehicle for the common cold, pneumonia, tuberculosis, influenza, whooping cough, measles, and chickenpox. Discharges from the mouth, nose, throat, or lungs take the form of droplets which remain suspended in the air from which they may be inhaled. When the moisture in these droplets evaporates, bacteria and viruses form "droplet nuclei" which remain for a long time to contaminate air, dust, and clothing. The nuclei thus suspended are sometime called aerosols. Although disease agents entering their hosts by way of the respiratory tract usually are airborne, direct contact by kissing, eating contaminated food, or using con-

taminated drinking glasses also provide entrance through the gastrointestinal tract.

Soil—It can be the vehicle for tetanus, anthrax, hookworm, and some wound infections. In general, however, the soil does not carry human pathogens that are spread from one person to another.

Fomites—This term embraces all inanimate objects other than water, milk, food, air, or soil which might play a role in the transmission of disease. Fomites include bedding, clothing, books, even doorknobs and drinking fountains. In the past, great importance was placed on the role of fomites in transmitting disease. It was the reason for the emphasis on fumigation. Today it is generally believed that most pathogenic organisms do not live very long away from the host and are readily destroyed by drying and sunlight. Thus, the amount of disease spread by fomites is relatively small and does not warrant undue emphasis, especially if these precautions lead to the neglect of more important measures that will limit the spread of infection.

Vectors are animate or living vehicles which transmit infections in the following ways:

Mechanical transfer — Contaminated mouthparts or feet of some insect vectors mechanically transfer the infectious organisms to the bite-wound or to food. For example, flies may transmit bacillary dysentery, typhoid fever, or other intestinal infections by walking over feces of the typhoid or dysentery host, and later leaving the disease-producing germs on food over which it walks.

Intestinal harborage—Certain insects harbor pathogenic (cause disease) organisms in their intestinal tracts. The organisms are passed in the feces or are regurgitated by the vector, and the bite wounds or food are contaminated. For example, in the transmission of the rickettsiae causing typhus fever, the organism is passed in the feces of the body louse and is rubbed into the bite-wound or other skin abrasion by the human host. In bubonic plague, the plague bacillus multiplies in the stomach of the flea, causing an obstruction. When the flea bites a rodent or man, the blood obtained is regurgitated into the wound and carries the plague bacilli with it.

Biologic transmission—This term refers to a vital change in the infectious agent during its stay in the body of the vector. The vector takes in the organism along with a blood meal but is not able to transmit infection until after a definite period, during which the pathogen changes. These biologic changes may be sexual reproduction, maturation, or multiplication; the time required for these biologic changes is referred to as the "extrinsic incubation period."

The parasite which causes malaria is an example of an organism which completes the sexual stages of its life cycle within its vector, the mosquito. The larvae of filarial worms undergo part of their development and mature in various flies and mosquitoes. The virus of yellow fever multiplies in the bodies of mosquitoes; and the microorganisms of the rickettsiae family multiply in the bodies of mites, ticks, fleas, and lice. Such environmental factors as temperature and humidity may affect the vector and the extrinsic incubation period.

Portals of Entry

The portal of entry is the anatomic route by which the infectious agent gains entrance into the body of the host. Often the portal of entry is the same as the portal of exit. Portals of entry and exit may be found in the following systems of the human body:

Respiratory system, including the nose, mouth, pharynx, larynx, trachea, bronchi, and lungs.

Gastrointestinal system, including the mouth, pharynx, esophagus, stomach, small and large intestines, rectum and anus, as well as the accessory organs of digestion that include the salivary glands, liver, gallbladder, and pancreas.

Skin, including special membranes such as mucous membranes, of which the conjunctiva is a type. However, unbroken skin is a barrier to infectious agents.

Genitourinary system, including the urethra, bladder, ureters, and kidneys in both sexes; the prostate, seminal vesicles, spermatic duct, epididymis, and testes in the male; and the vagina, uterus, fallopian tubes, and ovaries in the female.

In some cases the organ-system primarily involved in the disease process is also the portal of entry and exit of the causative organism. This is true, for example, of most of the respiratory and gastrointestinal diseases. On the other hand, the portal of entry frequently bears no relation to the organ-system involved in the disease. In rabies, for instance, the virus enters the host through a wound in the skin, produces a disease process in the central nervous system, and leaves the host through the saliva. Disease agents transmitted by arthropod vectors, for such diseases as malaria and yellow fever, enter and leave the host through the skin, but involve other tissues in the disease process.

Susceptible Host

A host is a living organism which harbors or nourishes another organism. This kind of relationship is called *symbiosis,* from a Greek word that means "living together." If the relationship is mutually beneficial to the two partners, it is called *mutualism.* In contrast, when one organism may injure, destroy, or live at the expense of the other, the relationship is called *parasitism.* Communicable diseases are manifestations of parasitism.

The occurrence of infection and disease, stated previously, is determined by a complex interplay of factors that pertain to the host and the infecting agent (parasite). In the host, these factors determine the host's *susceptibility* or resistance to infection. Susceptibility and *immunity* may be thought of as opposite ends of a scale, or range, with varying degrees in between of susceptibility or resistance. Both are relative expressions. Much depends upon the *virulence* (disease-producing power) of the infective agent and whether the dose is minimal or massive.

Immunity and Resistance

Immunity and resistance are the result of several processes, many of which are not yet fully understood, and no doubt there are other factors as yet unsuspected. Some factors are known to be inherent to living organisms, while others are known to be acquired. *Inherent host factors* which contribute to a human being's *resistance to infection* include:

Mechanical barriers, such as the skin and mucous membranes of the respiratory, gastrointestinal, and genitourinary tracts.

Body secretions which either destroy, trap, or wash away infecting organisms, such as tears, the urine, the digestive juices, perspiration, and the mucus of the respiratory tracts.

Certain cells of the blood (leukocytes), and cells of the reticuloendothelial system (macrophages) found in the liver, spleen, bone marrow, and lymph nodes. These remove infecting organisms and foreign particles from the body by engulfing and destroying them, in a process known as *phagocytosis.*

Acquired immunity is developed by the host after previous experiences with infecting organisms or their products. It is specific, that is, limited to those particular organisms. The immune process may be explained in this way:

When foreign protein is injected into the body, formation of an opposing substance is stimulated. The substance injected is called an *antigen (anti*body *gen*erator), and the opposing substance is called an *antibody* (bodies that are antagonistic). After entering the tissues, foreign substances such as bacteria and their toxins act as antigens and stimulate the tissues to form specific antibodies. Even though the immunity is specific for each antigen, a phenomenon of cross-immunity does exist. This is due to a similarity of reactive groups to different antigens. Thus, immune bodies formed in response to one disease frequently help protect against another. Antibodies react in many ways with the antigen which stimulated their production.

Antitoxins neutralize toxins (poisons) which are produced by snakes, insects, and plants as well as by bacteria. Some bacteria do not themselves enter the blood but pour their toxins into it, as in the case of tetanus, diphtheria, and botulism. Because such toxins are antigens that excite antibody formation, these antibodies are known as antitoxins. Because the toxin is prepared to act upon cells when it enters the blood, the progress of the disease is likely to be extremely rapid; death may occur before the body can make sufficient antitoxin

to combat the poison. This is true of the toxins (venoms) of certain snakes. Unless treated promptly with immune serum (antivenin), the snakebite victim may succumb within a few hours.

Acquired immunity may develop either *actively* or *passively.*

Active immunity results when the host is stimulated by an antigen to produce its own antibodies. This occurs naturally as a result of infection, or artificially after injection of antigens, which are known as vaccines and are developed in laboratories.

Passive immunity occurs when the host receives antibodies obtained from another human being, or from another animal which has been immunized actively against the antigen. Passive immunity occurs naturally in the newborn infant who receives antibodies from its mother through the placenta. In passive immunity, the injected foreign immune bodies usually circulate in the recipient's blood until they are destroyed by the reticuloendothelial system after three to five weeks.

Passive immunity is preferable to active immunity in treatment of acute illnesses, for it can be instituted within minutes. A good example of lifesaving passive immunity is that resulting from injection of antivenin for snakebite. Those who have been actively immunized, either naturally or through injection of vaccine, will produce antibodies more vigorously when exposed to the antigen of a particular disease than those lacking previous experience with the antigen. This is the so-called "booster" effect. The booster effect does not occur following passive immunization.

Other factors affect host resistance to infection and disease. These factors, which are imperfectly understood, are related to the environment, to conditions intrinsic to the host, and to the interactions of the two. Such environmental factors as temperature and humidity seem to influence the host's receptivity and reactions to infection.

Ionizing radiation, such as X-rays and gamma rays from nuclear reactions, is known to depress host resistance to infection. The physiologic status of the host—as determined by nutrition, fatigue, age, or the presence of pathologic conditions—is significant in the development of infectious diseases. Resistance may be sex-linked. Communicable disease death rates are generally higher in males than females, with the exception of whooping cough. Some authorties believe that race also influences resistance or susceptibility to communicable diseases, but this has not been established conclusively.

CONTROL OF COMMUNICABLE DISEASES

Measures for the prevention or control of communicable diseases are intended to break the chain of infection at its weakest link. In general, control measures attempt to prevent exposure to infection. These measures are strengthened by increasing the resistance of the susceptible host. This can be achieved by active or passive immunization or by the prophylactic use of drugs.

Reservoir Eradication

Exposure to infection can be prevented by eradicating the reservoir of infection, closing the portals of exit from the sources, and eliminating the modes of transmission. For example, in the United States, human tuberculosis caused by the bovine (infecting cattle) strain of the tubercle bacillus has been virtually eradicated by searching for and destroying infected cattle. Outbreaks of bubonic plague long have been controlled—that is, prevented from reaching epidemic proportions—by destroying rats and other rodents.

Isolation

Isolation of the infected persons and quarantine of susceptible contacts are among the oldest public health procedures. They have many shortcomings if attendants neglect other sources such as missed cases, atypical cases, and healthy carriers of infection.

Immunization

Every seagoing person, if only for self-protection and convenience, should be immunized against smallpox, diphtheria, tetanus, and poliomyelitis. In some ports, shore liberty should be contingent upon valid evidence of recent successful immunizations. "Booster" immunizations for smallpox *every three years* and diphtheria-tetanus *every ten years* should be kept current.

Protection against smallpox by vaccination has been observed for many years. Although it is no longer required in most areas of the United States, vaccination will be essential for international travel as long as smallpox continues to exist anywhere in the world. Protection against tetanus (lockjaw) by injection of a toxoid is recommended universally as part of good preventive medical practice. Regular "booster" immunization at *10-year intervals* is advisable for everyone regardless of occupation. Tetanus exposure is especially high on ships carrying cattle, hides, or similar cargoes and is common on land throughout the world.

A second category of special immunizations is the use of vaccines for yellow fever, cholera, and typhoid fever, depending on the route and destination of the vessel. Yellow fever vaccine is required at *ten-year intervals* for disembarkation in many tropical American and African countries. Cholera vaccine may be required at *six-month* intervals for travel to certain parts of the world. Avoiding food and water, which may be contaminated, is the most effective means of protection against typhoid fever and cholera. Typhoid vaccine may be a helpful adjunct when traveling in countries where typhoid commonly occurs, and food and water control cannot be effected.

A third category of protective agents includes those considered elective for special situations. For instance, plague vaccine might be considered for seamen anticipating frequent or prolonged travel in Southeast Asia, currently one of the few areas reporting much plague. *Immune serum globulin (ISG)* protection against hepatitis might be considered for those traveling in hepatitis-endemic areas of the world. Booster doses of ISG *every six months* might be useful for *perhaps three or four years,* if prolonged exposure cannot be avoided.

Malaria prophylaxis, with weekly doses of 500 mg of chloroquine phosphate (equivalent to 300 mg of chloroquine) is a necessity for all seamen working or stopping over in most tropical areas of the world. Routine immunization against typhus is not indicated today, as louse control remains the most effective method of control.

Seaman's Immunization Record

Every seaman should have immediately at hand, written evidence of the immunizations and prophylaxis that he has received. Having these records immediately available is more than a convenience for going ashore. It will prevent repeated and unnecessary immunizations when signing-on, or entering an infected port, or a port that requires immunization documents.

Over-immunization usually can be recognized by a severe local reaction following a routine booster, as for example, diphtheria-tetanus toxoid. *This should be noted in the seaman's record.* Generally no specific treatment for such a reaction is required.

Although some immunizations can be completed by a single procedure that will require only a few minutes, others require two or three doses over a two to eight week period. This can present a problem to merchant seamen. It is recommended that they arrange for multi-dose immunizations during layovers ashore, if no staff officer in the crew is qualified to administer them. (See p. 450+.) Seamen should contact the Public Health Service hospital or outpatient clinic to receive the appropriate immunizations. These facilities also have the current regulations concerning the immunizations required for various parts of the world.

Chapter XI

Environmental Control Aboard Ship

A BACKGROUND TO ENVIRONMENTAL SANITATION

ENVIRONMENTAL CONTROLS deal with the complex of climatic, family, physical, and biological factors that act on an individual, his community, and his natural or man-made surroundings. These controls ultimately determine his health and survival.

The seaman's health and survival depend mainly on three related controls:

(1) His own efforts to maintain his physical and mental efficiency at an optimum level;

(2) The organization of the physical facilities and the supplies necessary to maintain him in a state of maximum efficiency, and

(3) The efforts of other personnel, ashore and afloat, to create and maintain conditions intended to promote the seaman's good health.

The seaman should expect and find certain facilities, supplies, and healthful conditions in his shipboard environment. In turn, he and his fellow crew members have a major responsibility for the state of that environment. Individual and group health are totally dependent on a proper give-and-take attitude among the crew.

A give-and-take attitude is particularly important in maintaining good environmental sanitation aboard ship. Proper sanitation is impossible unless each crew member cooperates. At the same time, the Master should ensure the good sanitary conditions of the vessel through periodic inspections by appropriate persons to whom he delegates this responsibility.

Proper ventilation, lighting, food sanitation, liquid transport, waste disposal, personal hygiene, ship inspection, and the management of disease vectors (carriers) will be discussed in this chapter.

VENTILATION

Ships are compartmentalized to keep them buoyant and watertight. This makes proper ventilation difficult. Various methods of air conditioning, exhausting, and forced ventilation have been tried. Modern vessels use ventilation and forced air to create conditions most suitable for working in ships' compartments.

For effective ventilation there must be an adequate flow of clean air with sufficient oxygen content; controlled humidity to prevent "sweating," mold, and allergic reactions; and controlled temperatures to make the air comfortable.

The design and operation of the ventilation system should assure that air is provided to all living spaces as required for personnel and equipment safety. Air should not be recirculated from any exhaust system without adequate filtration to remove bacteria, foreign bodies, toxic gases, odors, smoke, and other hazards or annoyances. All ducts should be located where they are accessible to inspection, maintenance and repair, and filters should be placed properly, cleaned, and inspected on a regular basis. Ventilation rates and temperature criteria should conform to the directives issued by the Naval Sea Systems Command, U.S. Department of the Navy.

Microorganisms

One of the dangers of a faulty ventilation system is the transmission of diseases caused by microorganisms, although airborne infections usually are of minor importance except for certain respiratory diseases of bacterial and viral origin.

Because of the limited living space aboard some vessels and the possibility of the ventilation system recycling air through the vessel, the entire crew can be infected with virulent organisms. To prevent this, controls should be used. Two control methods are disinfection of the air by ultraviolet light and filtration of the air by mechanical or electrostatic means. Each method has its drawbacks. It is the responsibility of the Chief Engineer to use one or more of these mechanisms when there is a danger of airborne infections being circulated through the ventilation system of the ship.

Gases

Besides bacterial contamination of air, a common hazard aboard ship is the accumulation of gases in holds, bunkers, paint lockers, tanks and other confined areas. Such gases may be toxic (poisonous) or they may displace oxygen. Seamen entering such an enclosed space may become ill or die of asphyxia (suffocation).

Among commonly found toxic gases are carbon monoxide, carbon dioxide, ammonia, chlorine, nitrogen, and petroleum gases. These gases and others are found in varying combinations in shipboard fires; in empty oil, chemical, and storage tanks; and in the bilges, skin tanks, and certain cargo holds. Certain classes of cargo absorb oxygen or give off toxic gases. This is particularly true of products of plant origin such as linseed cakes, resin, and tobacco.

Poisonous gases or fumes may be formed in chemical, petroleum or whale-oil tanks as a result of decomposition of residues remaining after the tanks are emptied. Fumes can develop from cargoes of hides that have become moist and have fermented. Enclosed freshly-painted compartments can be lethal if not properly ventilated. Also dangerous are ships' tanks which have been painted.

Mechanical refrigeration systems are potentially dangerous due to leakage of ammonia, Freon,® or other refrigerants into enclosed spaces. Cyanide or other gases that are used to fumigate ships present a serious hazard, during and after fumigation until properly aired.

In all cases, safety rests with proper ventilation and proper individual precautions. It is the responsibility of the Deck Officer and/or Chief Engineer to assure that when compartments or tanks must be entered or cleaned that the area has been ventilated thoroughly, all explosive gases have been vented, and the oxygen supply is adequate. Also, the responsible officer should make sure that the first person entering the area wears a lifeline so that he can be retrieved if he becomes faint or ill. The work crew should be checked continuously during the first half hour of work. Proper oxygen canister-type gas masks and someone who knows how to use them should be available, if a rescue becomes necessary.

These precautions should be reinforced by frequent training demonstrations and emergency drills for all ship's personnel on the use of rescue and mask equipment. For reference, every ship's officer should have in his possession a copy of "Gas Hazards on Shipboard," by Alan Osbourne, *Modern Marine Engineer's Manual*, Vol. 1. A Bayne Meild, Jr., editor. Cambridge, Maryland: Cornell Maritime Press, Inc., 1965.

LIGHTING

Adequate lighting aboard ship is essential for efficiency and safety. Fatigue and eyestrain develop rapidly in poor illumination. Work performance is reduced, accidents increase, and consciously or unconsciously the individual's morale deteriorates.

The amount of light needed varies with the type of work or activity being performed. For instance, less light is needed for eating, resting, or general recreation than for reading, plotting charts, or carrying out other detailed work.

Good lighting is important especially in the engine room, galley, chartroom, and companion ways. In the engine room, high illumination free from glare is desirable. Lights should be located so that crew members will cast the fewest possible body shadows upon their work, and equipment will not create pools of darkness.

The light focused on a work surface is *local light,* as distinguished from the *general illumination* of a compartment. The amount of general illumination should be at least one-tenth that of the local light because it is difficult for the eyes to adjust back and forth from a brightly lighted work surface to a dimly lighted compartment.

The relationship of lighting to safety in the engine room, companion ways, and ladder wells is obvious. Good visibility in the galley, pantry, scullery, and head also is necessary. Adequate illumination in the food service and preparation areas is essential to proper food handling and to maintain adequate sanitation standards.

Proper lighting depends on such factors as brightness, location, and color of the light sources; size, shape, color, and contents of the area being lighted; and texture of the surfaces. The most important and readily adjusted of these factors are brightness and location of the source. The amount of light can be controlled by varying the distance to the source, its brightness (by wattage, shape, size, color, clarity, or frosting), and the use of shades, mirrors and reflectors. The surface on which the light falls can be changed to improve visibility.

The energy source should be located so that adequate light hits the work area, but does not shine into the eyes or create glare. Glare pro-

duces temporary blindness and fatigue, which might lead to accidents.

The Chief Engineer must see that lighting is adequate for the work to be done and that dangerous reflection, glare, and shadows are eliminated. To further eliminate danger to seamen, he must see that light sources are shielded and are immediately replaced when they fail.

FOOD SANITATION

Food procurement, preparation, and services aboard most vessels are the primary responsibility of the Steward's department. The galley crew and others in the department are responsible for the cleanliness of food preparation and storage areas, as well as for the sanitary manner in which food is served in the mess areas and dining saloons.

It is the responsibility of the Master and the Chief Steward to monitor the health of the food handlers; and to make regular and unscheduled inspections of areas used for the storage, preparation, and service of food, as well as self-dispensing food service units aboard ship.

The proper care of a ship's food services and supplies involves the handlers of food; the conditions of purchase; surroundings in which food is stored, prepared, and served; the care of the utensils and utilities; the disposal of food wastes; and the control of vectors of disease, as insects and rodents.

The Food Handler

Aboard a merchant vessel, the food handler should be a member of the Steward's department and directly responsible to the Chief Steward for overall direction.

Requirements for the examination of the food handler are listed in current publications of the U.S. Coast Guard, U.S. Public Health Service, State and local health agencies, and many ship companies.

A food handler should have a thorough physical examination at least once a year, and inspections for communicable diseases at more frequent intervals. Physical examinations for food service personnel are provided in major ports by the medical departments of the operating company; the U.S. Public Health Service;

city health departments; and other facilities designated by the company, the union, or the country.

A carrier of typhoid or other communicable disease should not be permitted to prepare or handle food. Crew members with skin infections or open wounds should not handle food, eating utensils, or dishes that will be used by others.

It is the responsibility of the Purser, Chief Steward, and Chief Cook to assure that any food handler signed aboard has proper health certification. Pierhead jumpers and others who may sign on without proper examinations should never be assigned duty in the Steward's department until each has passed a complete and thorough medical examination.

The food handler should be trained for his job and impressed with the critical importance of helping to reduce the potential for communicable diseases among the crew. He must be scrupulous in the cleanliness of his body and clothing. The food handler must wear clothing designed for food service areas, and this clothing should be laundered regularly and worn only during working hours.

To encourage high standards of personal hygiene among food service workers, the "head," with its toilet and lavatory facilities, must be readily accessible to the food preparation area. Hand washing facilities, with sanitary soap dispensers and individual towels, should be available in the food preparation area. It is the Chief Cook's responsibility to see that the facilities are utilized.

Food Service Facilities

All food service facilities aboard ship should conform to the minimum requirements in the U.S. Public Health Service's publications: *Handbook on Sanitation of Vessel Construction*,* Public Health Service Publication No. 393, 1967; and *Handbook on Sanitation of Vessels in Operation*, Public Health Service Publication No. 68, 1963.

In general, surfaces of all decks, bulkheads, and deckheads in the food processing, serving, and storage areas should be corrosion-free, smooth, and easy to clean. All surface materials

---

* Published by the Interstate Travel Sanitation Branch, Food and Drug Administration, U.S. Department of Health, Education, and Welfare, 200 C Street, S.W., Washington, D.C. 20204.

coming into contact with foods should be corrosion-resistant, non-toxic, nonabsorbent, smooth, durable, and easy to clean.

Utensils and Equipment

Cooking utensils and equipment must be made of materials that are non-toxic; that is, they should not be made of metals such as cadmium, lead, zinc, or antimony. The positioning of this equipment and storage of utensils should be planned for safe, efficient use. Each item should be designed, constructed, and installed to permit ease of cleaning, disassembling, and maintenance. All permanently installed or stationary equipment should be constructed so that flashing or closing strips will exclude openings to adjacent structures or other equipment, unless adequate clearance for proper cleaning is provided.

Commissary equipment to be purchased on the open market, such as dishwashing machines, food mixers, ranges, and other food handling, preparation or storage equipment, should be procured only if judged acceptable by the U.S. Public Health Service. Such acceptance is based on a careful review and evaluation of the equipment and its component parts and materials, to assure freedom from undesirable sanitation features, ability to perform its sanitary function satisfactorily, and its ease of cleaning.

Proper plumbing equipment in the food service areas is mandatory. Potable water only should be piped into food service spaces, except that non-potable water may be piped to garbage grinder eductors. Food service equipment and spaces should be adequately drained, and the drains should be protected from backflow of wastes.

The Chief Steward and the Chief Engineer must assure that the foregoing recommendations are implemented, and make regular sanitary inspections to see that no health hazards develop.

Food Storage

Non-refrigerated Items

The non-refrigerated foods can be divided into *bulk items* and *broken or lot items*. The bulk items are boxed, bagged, or canned. While each has specific storage needs, all have certain common requirements such as a storage area that can be locked and separated from non-food items. Bulk items must be kept free of dampness, condensation or waste waters, and free of poisons and contaminants. They should be stored in a protected, cool, dry area; rotated regularly, and kept free of rodent and insect contamination. If such food becomes infected or outdated, it must be destroyed.

Once foods are removed from the dry stores storeroom and dispensed to the day stores, they must be protected from contamination after the original protective packaging is removed.

Bulk foods must be stored so that access for inspection is provided. They also must be stored to be readily accessible for use and secured so the ship's roll will not allow rupture, shift, or drift. The foods must be kept clear of all cleaning or chemical agents. Supplies should not be stored directly on the deck but should be elevated at least six inches to facilitate cleaning and to reduce insect and rodent harborage.

After loading aboard ship, storage requirements for *boxed foods* demand that they be utilized quickly to minimize vermin infestation. They must be dated for proper utilization and never left in storage in an opened state.

Non-refrigerated *bulk items* such as cereals, beans and sugar, as well as vegetables such as potatoes and onions, are extremely susceptible to external contamination, insect and rodent infestation, and rupture. They must be protected by storage in easily-cleaned vermin-proof containers or bins.

Non-refrigerated *canned or bottled items* usually are stored in boxes or crates. They are best protected by maintaining a rotating inventory, keeping the units dry and preferably cool, and eliminating damaged or distorted cans or tins. Corrugated paper boxes should be emptied and removed from the ship as soon as possible, as they are apt to harbor insects. Some items, such as pickled goods, are stored in barrels or hogsheads, casks or kegs and are best kept in cool areas.

By observing these controls, non-refrigerated foodstuffs can be stored so that the health of the crew and passengers is protected.

The Chief Steward must assure the quality and safety of stored non-refrigerated food stuffs.

Refrigerated Items

The same basic requirements apply to the storage of refrigerated items. However, refrigerated storage is more confined, and specified temperatures must be maintained.

Refrigerated foods fall into two general groups—*frozen foods* and *cooled foods*.

Frozen foods must be kept at $0°F$ to $-10°F$ ($-18°C$ to $-23.2°C$) from time of freezing until time of preparation. Under these conditions, food retains normal taste and appearance and has a shelf life from one to six months. Once thawed, however, such food must be used immediately and not refrozen under any circumstances. Once food is thawed, it rapidly deteriorates and may become toxic due to bacterial action. For best utilization, frozen food is stored in packaged units. Once a package is opened, the contents must be wrapped, kept frozen in the day stores, and used at the earliest opportunity.

Cooled food items kept in storage most often are fresh fruits and vegetables, processed and cooked meat products, and foods prepared for rapid utilization. These, as well as leftovers, should be kept covered and stored at from $32°F$ to $45°F$ ($0°C$ to $7.2°C$) depending on the product.

Both the freezer and cooler compartments should have highly accurate, adjustable thermostats for temperature control. Thermometers should be easily visible to persons working in passageways serving the refrigerated spaces and on the Engineer's control panel.

In cooled food storage areas, humidity ranges from moderate to high. Cooled foods, properly handled, have a storage life of from one day to four months, depending on the item. Leftover food should be assumed to have a shelf life of not more than 48 hours because of the possibility of contamination. At $40°F$ ($4.4°C$) and below, this danger is minimized.

Both frozen and cooled foods keep better when the refrigeration unit is properly drained, kept clean, and free of ice, frost, food spillage or residue, fungus, and slime. For freezer efficiency, remove frost or ice before it reaches one-quarter inch in thickness.

When defrosting, wash the freezer with steam or heavily chlorinated warm soapy water to remove slime, dirt, grease and fungus growth. Shelves, hooks and grids should be removed and washed with a warm detergent solution, then steamed down, rinsed in hot water and, if possible, sun dried or heat dried. The refrigerator decks should be cleaned and scrubbed with a hot detergent solution and then rinsed. The drains should discharge preferably into a separate drainage system or into a separate vented tank— *never into the plumbing system or open bilge.* When the refrigerator empties into a sewerage or drainage system, there must be an air gap between the refrigerator drain and the system.

After cleaning, the refrigerator should be loaded so that stores are placed neatly, with no physical overloading and separated to allow free circulation or air. Foods to be refrigerated should be stored in shallow metal pans or plastic containers covered with wax paper, plastic, or aluminum foil.

The Chief Steward must assure the cleanliness of the storage areas and food storage equipment; and the Chief Engineer must assure the effective functioning of these units.

The Galley

It is most important that the general galley be constructed so that work spaces are clear and the decks are covered with waterproof, non-slipping surfaces. Also, the galley should be equipped, illuminated, and maintained to assure good sanitation. Equipment should be made of corrosion-resistant, non-toxic materials that are easy to clean. All galley areas, especially the cooking areas, should be fire-protected, easy to clean, and capable of being rapidly vented of smoke, steam, odors, and gases. (See Fig. 11-1.) Proper ventilation will keep the galley dry and pleasant.

All galley water must be potable, except nonpotable water may be piped to the garbage grinder eductor. Back-siphonage must be prevented. All drains must be trapped and should have easily accessible "clean outs."

Waste, particularly food scraps, should be kept in tightly covered sturdy garbage cans.

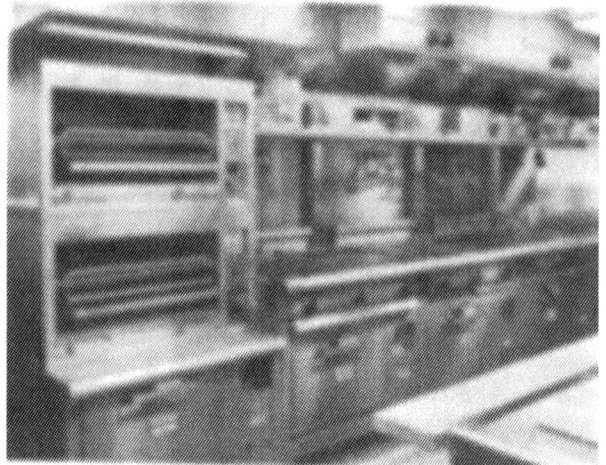

Fig. 11-1. Cooking area of main galley.

Where possible, these should be stored in refrigerated areas until the garbage can be disposed of properly.

Pipes carrying nonpotable liquids, as drains and overboard water, should be kept to a minimum in the areas used for the storage, preparation, and serving of food.

It is the Master's duty to work with the Chief Steward to ensure the sanitary and safety conditions of the galley areas.

Where possible, all galley equipment and utensils should be fixed in place. Non-fixed utensils should be hung or stored to avoid loss, damage, or injury to seamen when the ship rolls.

Foodstuffs, supplies, cookware, crockery and utensils should be thoroughly cleaned after each use and stored in containers that can be secured when the items are not in use.

LIQUID TRANSPORT

Ship's Liquid Transport Systems

Specialized piping systems on ships include the *bilge system* which collects drainage that must be pumped overboard; the *clean ballast system* which maintains the proper trim, stability, and immersion of the vessel; and the *fuel oil and oily ballast* which stores and transfers clean oil to the ship's fuel system, and secondarily replaces the oil with sea water as part of the ballast system.

Other specialized piping systems are the *fire system* which supplies water under pressure to the ship's fire stations and to the deck and anchor wash areas; the *sanitary system* which supplies water to the heads and other sanitary fixtures; and the *wash water system* which supplies fresh water from skin and/or peak tanks. *The wash water system must be independent of all other piping systems and labeled: not fit to drink.*

An important specialized piping system is the *drinking water system* that supplies potable water to fountains, washing, and culinary units. The drinking water system must be protected as well as isolated from all other systems, and its water must conform to the *National Interim Primary Drinking Water Regulations,* effective June 24, 1977. These regulations are under the jurisdiction of the Office of Water Supply, U.S. Environmental Protection Agency (EPA), 401 M Street, S.W., Washington, D.C. 20460. For further information, contact the EPA.

Miscellaneous systems aboard ships include transport steam, compressed air, foam, and numerous other specialized liquid and gaseous agents.

Potable Water Sources

The handling of water must be rigidly controlled from source to consumer to avoid contamination.

Potable water on shipboard is derived either from distillation or from natural sources. Distilled water is either fresh or salt water that has been converted to steam and back to water. It is relatively free of impurities but has a flat taste. Natural water, or "shore water," usually is obtained from wells, springs, or fresh water bodies ashore. Usually it must be treated, either ashore or afloat, to protect the health of the seaman.

Potable Water Transport Systems

The water system of a port city is the usual source of potable water. It is made available to the ship either through watering points at dockside or from water boats.

The Master must determine if a water source is safe by consulting either his local company agent or the local public health department. In the United States, this can be determined from the current OFFICIAL CLASSIFICATION OF VESSEL WATERING POINTS,* (unnumbered publication), 1976.

Each vessel currently is required to carry sufficient potable water hose to load its potable water. This special hose is kept in a storage cabinet labeled *"Potable Water Hose Only,"* and it is not to be used for any other purpose. (See Fig 11-2.)

A Deck Officer is responsible for the cleanliness and safety of his ship's filling hose and its ends, as well as the connections of dockside, water boat, or shipside filling lines. These connections—outlet and inlet—must be at least 18 inches above the dock, water boat deck, and ship's deck, and housed with a proper fitting. Each such watering point connection must be labeled *"Potable Water Filling."*

Potable Water Storage

To avoid contamination, potable water tanks should have no common partition with

---

* Published by the Interstate Travel Sanitation Branch, Food and Drug Administration, U.S. Department of Health, Education, and Welfare, 200 C Street, S.W., Washington, D.C. 20204. Available from 10 regional offices of the U.S. Department of Health, Education, and Welfare. The publication is revised annually.

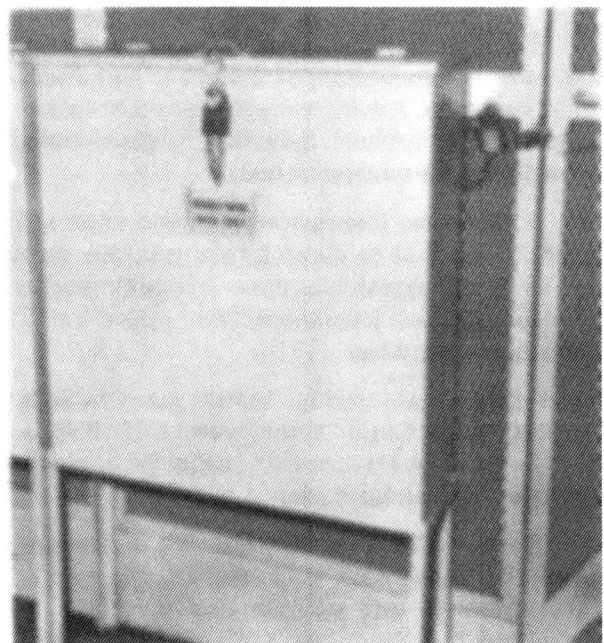

Fig. 11-2. Storage cabinet clearly marked for special hose used only for potable water.

tanks containing nonpotable liquids—including skin tanks—unless the water is to receive additional treatment by a method approved by the U.S. Public Health Service, the World Health Organization, or the government registering the vessel. No "head" may be constructed over that part of the deck which forms the top of the water storage tank, and no non-gravity tunnel may pass through it. The tank must be labeled *"Potable Water"* and be accessible through a watertight, preferably side-mounted, manhole. It must have an overflow and relief valve or vent, be drainable completely from a bottom drain, able to withstand pressure, and have water level gauges or petcocks.

Potable Water Pipelines and Service Units

Potable water should be transported from the storage areas to dispensing units through identified (i.e., color-coded non-cross-connected pipes made of safe metals or plastic). All potable water outlets must be protected from back-siphonage by an air-gap or approved vacuum breaker. Drinking fountains should be constructed so the mouth of the seaman does not have to touch the spout, and the fountains should be fitted with splash guards.

Disinfection of Potable Water Systems

Historically, waterborne diseases have been the most common cause of disability and death among seamen. Among such diseases are dysentery, cholera, typhoid, hepatitis, poliomyelitis, amebiasis, and schistosomiasis.

Waterborne diseases would be a constant threat if not held in check by the sanitary control of fresh water supplies. Drinking water must be obtained, transported, and stored under protected conditions.

Potable water tanks, which must have a suitable inner lining that meets U.S. Public Health Service standards, should be cleaned and sanitized at least once a year.

The system should be filled with water and superchlorinated with hypochlorite (50 ppm). To be effective this solution should remain in the system for four hours, after which the tank should be flushed and refilled with potable water.

LIQUID AND SOLID WASTE DISPOSAL

Liquid wastes are organic materials that can be moved in a liquid. These include body excretions such as feces, urine, sputum, and vomitus; sink, laundry and washroom wastes; food, tank, bilge, and engine room wastes; and other degradable materials. Aided by flushing from the sanitary water system, these wastes are mixed with water and carried out of the vessel by its waste pipes and/or scuppers.

Solid wastes are any discarded materials which are not readily degradable without heat or pressure. Aboard ship, these include discarded items such as surgical dressings, disposable unit containers, and refuse.

Both liquid and solid wastes are health hazards. Contamination by these wastes can cause outbreaks of typhoid fever, paratyphoid fever, cholera, or dysentery. Rats, flies and other vectors of disease thrive on solid wastes. Consequently, waste disposal from vessels must be accomplished without endangering the lives of persons aboard the vessel or in off-ship areas.

Throughout the developed world and much of the developing world, it is illegal to discharge sewage, bilge water, ballast, or solid waste near public water supply intakes; or in any other areas restricted by national, State or local laws, regulations or codes. In the United States these restrictions can be obtained from any Regional Office of the U.S. Department of Health, Education, and Welfare, the U.S. Coast Guard, the U.S. Environmental Protection Agency, and the U.S. National Oceanic and Atmospheric Administration.

As a further safeguard, the Master should consult with local authorities before the vessel discharges wastes in possibly restricted areas, because each locality and country has regulations which are highly individual.

CONTROL OF DISEASE VECTORS

Throughout maritime history, ships' crews and inhabitants of ports have been decimated and incapacitated by vector-borne diseases. Rats, mice, and monkeys carry disease. Parrots and parakeets are common bird vectors, and common insect disease carriers include mosquitoes, flies, bedbugs, lice, ticks, and cockroaches.

Control of vectors aboard ship is the responsibility of the Master and those persons he designates. Control of vector entry into, and exit from the port is primarly the responsibility of U.S. Public Health Service and port authorities.

The shipping company, through the Master, also has a major responsibility for the cleanliness of the ship. Hospitalization or return home of sick seamen is a major cost under the "maintenance and cure" clause of maritime law. In extreme circumstances, quarantine of an infected or infested vessel has been known to have caused a loss to the company of a quarter of a year's income, while acquiring new clearance papers.

While it is the Master's responsibility to keep his ship clean and free of vectors of disease, he also must see that an officer, such as the First Mate or Marine Physician Assistant, maintains a ship's medical log of: (1) all diseases and illnesses of the crew and passengers; (2) quarantine declarations, deratinization or exemption certificates, and passenger and crew lists (with their immigration, vaccination, and inoculation histories), and (3) other special declarations required by the country, port, or agency.

Control of Rodents

Rats on a ship are a health menace and a nuisance. They cause extensive damage to cargo and food, and rat droppings contain organisms which produce intestinal diseases. Because rats usually attempt to forage in the galley and provision storeroom areas, these organisms are likely to be introduced into the food supplies. Rats carry fleas which may transmit plague and murine typhus. Because of these dangers, ships heavily infested with rats must be fumigated, and fumigation is a laborious, expensive, and dangerous procedure. It can be avoided through adequate rat-control measures.

Despite reasonable precautions by the ship's personnel and port authorities, some rats may be aboard. However, infestation can be avoided by *not* providing food and nesting places for rats, and by trapping or otherwise

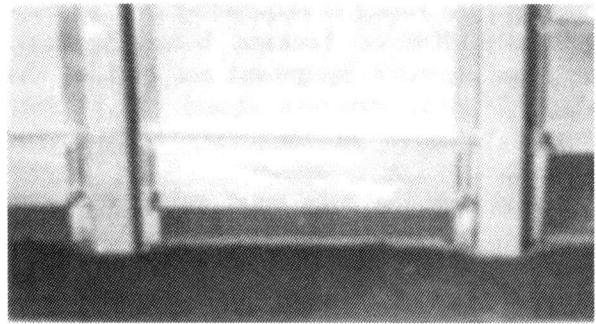

Fig. 11–3. Ratproofing of bulkhead.

destroying them before they breed and develop colonies.

Frequent inspection of a ship for signs of rat life (trails or runs marked by dirt or droppings) will indicate the kind of measures that should be taken to prevent rat infestation. There are four general measures available:

(1) keeping the rats from getting aboard;

(2) ratproofing the ship, thus "building out" the rats by elimination of their living places or harborages (see Fig. 11–3);

(3) keeping all food protected and avoiding accumulation of food scraps, thus "starving out" the rodents; and

(4) killing them by trapping, poisoning, or expert fumigation by personnel from authorized agencies.

All chemicals (rodenticides and insecticides), that are used to control vectors, should be kept in their original containers, properly labeled and securely stored away from food (stores and cargo).

To prevent rats from coming aboard, every available precaution should be taken. This includes proper placement and maintenance of rat guards on all mooring lines and keeping the gangplank well illuminated.

Ratproof construction is built into most modern ships. The increased construction cost of ratproofing is more than repaid by preventing damage to cargo and avoiding excessive fumigation and other quarantine delays.

Ratproofing includes the elimination of hidden spaces and dead spaces for rat harborages. If such spaces cannot be eliminated, they should be constructed in a manner that makes the entry of rats impossible. The ship must be kept in good repair if ratproofing is to be continuously effective. Lockers, boxes, dunnage, or other movable equipment not part of the ship's original structure should not be permitted to serve as temporary shelters for rodents.

Starving the rats must accompany ratproofing. All food and garbage should be stored in metal containers with tightly fitting metal covers. Nothing edible should be left exposed. Food or edible waste spilled accidently in any part of the ship should be cleaned up promptly. These measures will help to control flies and cockroaches as well as rats and mice.

Trapping is a good method of keeping down the rat population. Snap traps, which are more effective and practicable than the cage type, should be set along ledges, bulkheads, and other places used as rat runs. Meat, bacon rind, or cheese may be used as bait for the traps if the rats cannot get at these foods in any other place. Apples, pears, dates, potatoes, and turnips also make good bait. The bait trigger should be pointed toward the bulkhead or rat run. The rat should be given the chance to nibble at the bait for the first few days before the trap is set. After a rat is caught, the trap should *not* be flamed or scalded; the odor of the rat will help in catching others. One should vary the kind of bait. Precautions should be taken to avoid touching the dead rat because of the danger of infected fleas.

Red squill, zinc phosphide, and the anticoagulants are the rodenticides (rat poisons) generally recommended by health departments for use by the public. These rodenticides are available commercially and are ones which the untrained individual is least likely to experience difficulties in handling.

The anticoagulant rodenticides, such as warfarin and diphacinone, kill in a radically different manner from the older acute (single dose) poisons such as zinc phosphide. They must be ingested for several consecutive days before they become effective.

Although it is extremely costly, a badly infested ship may be treated best by fumigation. The decision to fumigate a ship will depend upon the estimated number of rats aboard, the type of cargo, and the history of the voyage. For example, fumigation may be necessary, if a ship recently has touched a plague port.

The gases most commonly used for ship fumigation are hydrogen cyanide and methyl bromide. *These are extremely poisonous to human beings as well as to insects and rodents. Therefore, fumigation must be carried out by experts.*

Before fumigation is begun, the ship must be tied up at a distance from other vessels. It is absolutely necessary to make sure there is *no one on board* except those authorized to do the fumigating.

The ship to be fumigated must be cleared of all excess gear and dunnage. Drawers and lockers must be open for proper penetration and action of the gas. Ports, ventilators, and other openings must be secured to prevent the escape of gas.

After fumigation, the holds and superstructures must be aired. Tests must be made for the gas, after about an hour of airing. Beds and clothing must be thoroughly aired on deck for at least two hours because the gas has a strong tendency to remain in clothing and bedding. *Men have died as a result of returning too soon to compartments not completely aired and free of gas. A fumigated ship should not be boarded until released by the fumigating officer.* Also, any food that had been exposed to the gaseous fumigant must be discarded.

Control of Insects

Even with present control measures it is impossible to keep a ship completely free of insects. This is because of the variety of insects, their many methods of gaining access to the ship, and their ability to survive despite efforts to destroy them. Flies and mosquitoes may board the vessel at wharves or in harbors. Bedbugs, fleas, lice, and ticks may be brought aboard on the bodies, clothing, or personal gear of crew or passengers. Fleas also may be carried aboard by rats. Cockroaches and weevils may be present in provisions or cargo brought aboard the ship.

Insects transmit disease when germs on their bodies come in contact with food or other articles. Insects also may pick up and pass on disease by biting. For example, *Anopheles* mosquitoes transmit malaria, lice transmit epidemic typhus, and fleas transmit plague.

Suppression of insect infestation aboard ship demands coordination by ship and shore personnel. Unless control is continued at sea, the most thorough campaign to destroy insects and rodents on a ship in port will not pay off. It is easier and less costly to maintain controls constantly, rather than to apply sporadic intensive measures only in port. Furthermore, living and working conditions will be better at all times.

To fight insects successfully, one must first know the habits of each type and apply this knowledge. For example, *body lice* live on the human body and clothing; therefore, personal cleanliness will go a long way toward preventing louse infestation. *Bedbugs* are most likely to seek shelter in mattresses and cracks around beds; thus cleanliness and frequent inspection are valuable control measures. *Cockroaches* breed prolifically in areas where food is available; therefore, strict cleanliness in areas where food is stored, prepared, or eaten is of great importance. *Flies* are attracted by unprotected food and refuse; hence, they can be curbed if exposure of food is kept at a minimum, and if refuse is placed in clean, tightly covered cans for prompt disposal.

Personal and environmental cleanliness are the most satisfactory elements of long-range insect control. Insecticides are useful in providing immediate, although temporary, relief from a heavy insect infestation. The sporadic or casual use of insecticides is of little value if the underlying conditions persist, because the insecticide's effects wear off, and the surviving insects, new generations and newly-introduced insects rapidly recreate the infestation. For best results, insecticides should be used only as a supplement to cleanliness and other permanent control measures.

Insect control operations present hazards through contact with poisons, machinery, and flammable materials. The safest effective pesticide should be used, and personnel should be aware constantly of the special hazards. Only properly trained, responsible personnel should be allowed to do insect control work. *Personnel should work in pairs, never alone.* Bystanders should be kept away, and chemicals and equipment should be under constant control to prevent their being stolen or picked up by accident. Regular maintenance and careful use of equipment are imperative.

Following are the insects most commonly found aboard ship, some of their characteristics, and suggested methods of control:

Flies

Domestic flies, some of which bite, may transmit enteric (intestinal) diseases to man. Their larvae and eggs may infest human flesh and intestines as well as stored foods.

Environmental Controls: Store all refuse in durable cans with tight lids and maintain insect screening.

Chemical Controls: Use residual and space sprays indoors and residual sprays outdoors.

Mosquitoes

Several species of mosquitoes suck blood and may transmit encephalitis, malaria, yellow fever, filariasis, and other diseases.

Environmental Controls: Eliminate standing water and maintain insect screening.

Chemical Controls: Use same measures as above for domestic flies.

Cockroaches

Roaches produce unpleasant odors, transmit diarrhea and dysentery, and damage food stores.

Environmental Controls: Eliminate cracks, crevices and dead spaces; store food and garbage properly; keep entire area scrupulously clean; watch for, and destroy, all cockroaches and their egg cases, particularly those introduced with luggage, food stores and furniture; remove corrugated cardboard boxes and cartons from provision storerooms as soon as feasible.

Chemical Controls: Spray cracks, crevices, baseboards, furniture, fixtures and cabinets with a pinstream spray of an appropriate insecticide, and dust an insecticide into dead spaces and on items which sprays might damage, such as power panels. Special precautions are required in food service areas.

Lice, Bedbugs, and Fleas

These ectoparasites which live on the outside of the body cause discomfort and may transmit disease.

Environmental Controls: Maintain personal hygiene by bathing and by laundering clothing and bedding frequently; keep cabins clean by vacuuming floors, rugs, and upholstered furniture weekly; watch for, and eliminate, ectoparasites introduced with luggage, clothing, bedding or furniture; eliminate cracks and crevices where they hide; avoid furniture with wood-to-wood joints and pillows or mattresses with rolled seams; eliminate rodents.

Chemical Controls: For *lice*, dust infested individuals and contacts with insecticide powders or materials prescribed by a physician. For *bedbugs*, spray cracks, crevices and furniture in infested dwellings with appropriate insecticides. Special attention should be given to the tufts and seams of mattresses. For *fleas*, dust infected areas and infested pets with an appropriate insecticide powder.

Pests in Stored Products

These pests (cockroaches, beetles, moths, ants, mites, silverfish, springtails) damage clothing and rugs and ruin many millions of dollars worth of stored foods annually. Also they produce or transmit human diseases.

Environmental Controls: Store foods and products in an orderly, sanitary manner in a cool, dry room on racks up off the floor; use old stocks first; inspect stocks regularly and dispose of any found to be infested.

Chemical Control: Spray storerooms with insecticide approved for use in food service areas, making sure none gets in or on stored food.

SANITARY INSPECTION OF A SHIP

The U.S. Public Health Service recommends that ships registered under the American flag carry a *Sanitary Log* (Form No. 9452), which can be obtained from any U.S. quarantine station. The purpose of this log is ". . . *to provide quarantine officers, sanitary inspectors, ship's officers, agents, owners, and others with information regarding the sanitary history of vessels through systematically recorded reports of previous inspections* . ."

In wartime and under various peacetime circumstances, a ship unexpectedly may change its itinerary. It is difficult for government agencies to obtain a complete, accurate sanitary record of the vessel without such a log. If properly kept, the *Sanitary Log* should speed quarantine procedures.

All vessels arriving in the United States in ports of entry are subject to quarantine inspection by the Public Health Service of the U.S. Department of Health, Education, and Welfare. For detailed information see Appendix C, entitled *Regulations Governing Foreign Quarantine*, p. 436.

Regular inspections are necessary to maintain a vessel in good sanitary condition. The persons making the inspections should be on the alert for signs of vermin and rodent infestation. Areas which should be inspected thoroughly include:

Forepeak	Sewage disposal
Provision storeroom	Washroom and head
Galley	Cold storage space
Pantry	Refrigeration space
Issue room	Mess space
Sickbay	Living spaces
Scullery	Shelter deck
Garbage disposal	Holds
Brig spaces	

PERSONAL HYGIENE

Hygienic living protects the health of the individual. The health of a seaman depends in part, on his own efforts to maintain habits of cleanliness and neatness.

Personal cleanliness includes good care of the skin, hair, nails, mouth and teeth, and proper maintenance of clothing, towels, and other personal gear. A daily bath or shower, particularly in hot weather or after working in hot compartments, is conducive to good health and lessens the possibility for infection of cuts or scratches. Brisk rubbing with a rough towel after a bath or shower stimulates circulation, promotes good skin tone, and gives a feeling of well being. Clean clothing should be put on following a bath or shower.

Care of the mouth and teeth by regular use of a toothbrush after meals and daily use of dental floss are essential to assist in the prevention of gum disease, infection, and tooth decay. Before brushing natural teeth, any partial dentures should be removed and carefully cleaned with a brush and mild soap or special denture cleanser. Unclean removable dentures are particularly harmful to remaining natural teeth. Full artificial dentures should be cleaned regularly after meals, and particularly at bedtime, to remove food residue which can cause mouth odor and encourage infection.

The importance of washing hands at appropriate times cannot be overemphasized. Crew members should wash their hands before eating. Also, it is of vital importance, if cleanliness is to be maintained and the spread of infection reduced, that hands be washed immediately after urinating or defecating.

In cold weather, hands are less likely to chap if the skin is dried thoroughly. A little petroleum jelly, cold cream, or hand lotion rubbed into the skin after washing may help to prevent chapping and to keep the skin in good condition.

Adequate sleep is necessary for the health, well-being, and efficiency of the individual. Sleep requirements may vary considerably, and the sleeping habits of crew members may be quite dissimilar. However, unbroken periods of rest for everyone are desirable.

Hair should be shampooed frequently, cut at regular intervals, and preferably kept short.

Cleanliness aboard ship can be encouraged by providing sufficient hot water in convenient wash places to facilitate cleansing. Installation of a laundry and drying room for washing clothes also helps to maintain a high standard of cleanliness.

Each member of the crew should use only his own towels and be responsible for their cleanliness. Wet towels should not be folded and stowed; dirty towels should be laundered as soon as possible and not allowed to accumulate. Single-use paper towels are satisfactory only if waste receptacles are provided and used.

Chapter XII

Radio in Medical Emergencies

*Part 1—*DH MEDICO
Medical Advice by Radio

EXCEPT IN WARTIME when radio silence is imposed on ships at sea the Master can and should radio for medical advice when it is needed. Although United States merchant vessels may be hundreds of miles from land, they can obtain medical advice in a quick and efficient manner through the DH MEDICO program. If the request is not handled directly by the hospital involved, medical advice in most cases is received within the hour by radio message through one of the public coast stations or by phone patch.

DH MEDICO is a service that furnishes *medical advice by radio* 24 hours every day. Medical officers of the U.S. Public Health Service receive requests for medical advice through the U.S. Coast Guard, U.S. Navy, or commercial radio stations along the coast of the United States. Because the service is free, the term DEADHEAD* MEDICO or DH MEDICO is used. The DH MEDICO radio service which began in 1921 has provided medical advice for thousands of cases and saved the lives of many merchant seamen.

The system of furnishing medical advice to ships at sea was adopted by other nations and now is international in scope. The U.S. Public Health Service will provide medical in-

formation to foreign vessels. U.S. vessels can obtain similar assistance from foreign countries.

So that language difficulties can be avoided when a ship requests information from a foreign country, an *International Code of Signals*† that contains a medical section was developed and adopted for worldwide use. Although this code always is available for use, medical advice should be sought and given in plain language (English) whenever possible. However, when language difficulties are met, the code should be used.

For the sake of uniformity and to avoid confusion and delay, even when the message is in English, the text of the code and instructions should be followed *in sequence*, as far as possible. In part 2 of this chapter, pp. 386 to 419, the MEDICAL SIGNAL CODE with instructions (Chapter 3 of the International Code of Signals†) is reproduced from the publication listed in the footnote below.

Each U.S. Coast Guard station has pre-arranged direct communication to a U.S. Public Health Service hospital for rapid handling of

---

* *Deadhead* is an old railroad term that generally refers to a free rider or a free passage.

† Publication No. H.O. 102. INTERNATIONAL CODE OF SIGNALS, UNITED STATES EDITION, 1969. Chapter 3, pp. 97–130. Published by the U.S. Naval Oceanographic Office, U.S. Government Printing Office, Washington, D.C. 20402.

DH MEDICO messages. The calls should be made to the nearest station when its call sign is known. If the call sign is not known, the general Coast Guard call NCG (any Coast Guard radio station) should be used. *The use of CQ [call for unknown station(s) or general call to all stations] is discouraged for medical messages.*

DH MEDICO Frequencies To Be Used

The frequencies to be used for DH MEDICO in calling the U.S. Coast Guard and other radio stations are 500 kHz (A1 A2) and the various HF calling bands listed in the table that follows. For those vessels equipped with a radio telephone, 2182 kHz or 156.8 MHz (F3) (Channel 16) in the VHF band is used. If a vessel is unable to establish communications on 500 kHz due to extreme range, the HF

calling band providing the required propagation for the time of day should be utilized.

Urgent Medical Advice

In American waters, requests for medical advice of an urgent nature should be preceded by the urgent signal (XXX XXX XXX), in order to give them priority over other radio traffic except distress communications. If the request is sent to a United States station, the message also should be prefixed by **DH MEDICO.**

Unless specifically addressed, Coast Guard Stations will deliver all DH MEDICO messages to the nearest U.S. Public Health Service facility. (See Appendix A, p. 428.)

NOTE

The locations of the U.S. Coast Guard Radio Stations and Communication Stations are listed on the next page. Since this information changes periodically, it is recommended that the publication LIST OF RADIO DETERMINATION AND SPECIAL SERVICE STATIONS be used. This publication is available from:

General Secretariat
International Telecommunications Union
Place Des Nations CH-1211
Geneva 20, Switzerland

The medical information is listed in Volume 2 of the 1976 edition. All ships licensed by the FCC should have a copy on board.

Table 12–1

U.S. Coast Guard—Radio Stations and Communication Stations

Call Sign	Location and Type of Station	Working Frequency	HF Band Guarded			
			Day*		Night*	
		kHz	kHz	MHz	kHz	MHz
NMF	Communication Station Boston, Mass.	472. 8728. 12834.5 22487.5	500.	8. 12. 22.	500.	8. 12.
NMN	Communication Station Portsmouth, Va.	466. 8465. 12718.5 17151.2	500.	8. 12. 16.	500.	8. 12.
NMA	Radio Station Miami, Fla.	440.	500.		500.	
NMG	Communication Station New Orleans, La.	428.	500.		500.	
NMR	Radio Station San Juan, Puerto Rico	466. 8471. 12700. 17002.4	500.	8. 12. 16.	500.	8. 12.
NMC	Communication Station San Francisco, Calif.	420. 8574. 12743. 17218.4 22476.	500.	8. 12. 16. 22.	500.	8. 12.
NMJ	Radio Station Ketchikan, Alaska	416.	500.		500.	
NOJ	Communication Station Kodiak, Alaska	470.	500.		500.	
NOX	Radio Station Adak, Alaska	450.	500.		500.	
NRV	Radio Station Guam, Marianas Islands	466.	500.		500.	
NMO	Communication Station Honolulu, Hawaii	400. 8650. 12889.5 17247.2	500.	8. 12. 16.	500.	8. 12.
NMW	Radio Station Astoria, Oregon	448.	500.		500.	
4YH	38.00N 71.00W	500.	500.		500.	

Ships—Calling Bands

4178.–4187. kHz	8356.– 8374. kHz	16712. –16748. kHz
6267.–6280.5 kHz	12534.–12561. kHz	22222.5–22267.5 kHz

*Note: Day: 2 hours after sunrise until 2 hours before sunset (local time).
Night: 2 hours before sunset until 2 hours after sunrise (local time).

Chapter XII—Part 2

Medical Signal Code of the International Code of Signals

(See p. 419 for a *Special Index* that relates to the *Medical Signal Code*.)

Part 2 of Chapter XII, which begins on this page, reproduces the *Medical Signal Code* of the INTERNATIONAL CODE OF SIGNALS.* THE INTERNATIONAL CODE OF SIGNALS was developed to provide a means of communication when language difficulties occur in situations related essentially to safety of navigation and persons.

Generally, medical advice should be sought and given in plain language (English). However, when language difficulties are met, the code should be used to get medical advice by radio. See p. 419 for a *Special Index* that relates to the *Medical Signal Code*.

* The *medical section* of the *International Code of Signals* is reproduced on pages 386 to 419. Its source is Publication No. H.O. 102, INTERNATIONAL CODE OF SIGNALS, UNITED STATES EDITION, 1969. Chapter 3, pp. 97–130. Published by the U.S. Naval Oceanographic Office. U.S. Government Printing Office, Washington, D.C. 20402.

Chapter XII—Part 2
MEDICAL SIGNAL CODE

Section 2— **Request for Medical Assistance** (Continued)

Part 2—Section 1
EXPLANATION AND INSTRUCTIONS

General

1. Medical advice should be sought and given in plain language whenever it is possible but, if language difficulties are encountered, this Code should be used.

2. Even when plain language is used, the text of the Code and the instructions should be followed as far as possible.

3. Reference is made to the procedure signals "C", "N", or "NO" and "RQ" which, when used after the main signal, change its meaning into affirmative, negative, and interrogative, respectively.

Example:
"MFE N" = "Bleeding is not severe."
"MFE RQ" = "Is bleeding severe?"

---

* The signal "C" should be used to indicate an affirmative statement or an affirmative reply to an interrogative signal; the signal "RQ" should be used to indicate a question. For a negative reply to an interrogative signal or for a negative statement, the signal "N" should be used in visual or sound signaling and the signal "NO" should be used for voice or radio transmission.

When the signals "N" or "NO", and "RQ" are used to change an affirmative signal into a negative statement or into a question, respectively, they should be transmitted after the main signal.

Examples:
"CY N" (or "NO" as appropriate) = "Boat(s) is(are) not coming to you."
"CW RQ" = "Is boat/raft on board?" The signals "C", "N", or "NO", and "RQ" cannot be used in conjunction with single-letter signals.

---

* *Source:* The three paragraphs in the box are reprinted from Chapter 1, Section 6 on *Flashing Light Signaling*, paragraph 3(j), p. 12, Pub. No. H.O. 102, INTERNATIONAL CODE OF SIGNALS, UNITED STATES EDITION, 1969. U.S. Government Printing Office, Washington, D.C. 20402. The rest of this chapter reproduces Chapter 3, *The Medical Signal Code*, from the same source.

INSTRUCTIONS TO MASTERS

Standard method of case description

1. The master should make a careful examination of the patient and should try to collect, as far as possible, information covering the following subjects:

(*a*) Description of the patient (Section 2B, Pages 390 and 391);

(*b*) Previous health (Section 2C, Page 391);

(*c*) Localization of symptoms, diseases or injuries (Section 2D, Page 391);

(*d*) General symptoms (Section 2E, Pages 391 through 394);

(*e*) Particular symptoms (Section 2F, Pages 394 through 404);

†(*f*) Diagnosis (Section 3B, Pages 404 and 405).

2. Such information should be coded by choosing the appropriate groups from the corresponding sections of this chapter. It would help the recipients of the signal if the information is transmitted in the order stated in Paragraph 1.

3. Section 2A, Page 390, contains signals which can be used independently, i.e., with or without the description of the case.

4. After a reply from the doctor has been received and the instructions therein followed, the master can give a progress report by using signals from Section 2G, Pages 403–404.

INSTRUCTIONS TO DOCTORS

1. Additional information can be requested by using Section 3A, Page 404.

Example:
"MQB" = "I cannot understand your signal, please use standard method of case description."

---

† Part 2, Section 3B, Pages 404 and 405, "Diagnosis," can be used by both the master ("request for medical assistance") and the doctor ("medical advice").

2. For diagnosis,† Section 3B, Pages 404 and 405, should be used.

Example:

"MQE 26" = "My probable diagnosis is cystitis."

3. Prescribing should be limited to the "List of Medicaments" ‡, which comprises Table M–3 in Section 4, Pages 413 through 418 of the Code.

4. For special treatment, signals from Section 3C, Pages 405 and 406, should be used.

Example:

"MRP 4" = "Apply ice-cold compress and renew every 4 hours."

5. When prescribing a medicament (Section 3D, Pages 406 and 407) *three signals should be used* as follows:

(a) *the first* (Section 3D–1, Page 406 and Table M–3 in Section 4, Pages 413 through 418) to signify the medicament itself.

Example:

"MTD 32" = "You should give aspirin tablets."

(b) *the second* (Section 3D–2, Page 406) to signify the method of administration and dose.

Example:

"MTI 2" = "You should give by mouth 2 tablets/capsules."

(c) *the third* (Section 3D–3, Page 407) to signify the frequency of the dose.

"MTQ 8" = "You should repeat every 8 hours."

6. The frequency of external applications is Coded in Section 3D–4, Page 407.

Example:

"MTU 4" = "You should apply every 4 hours."

7. Advice concerning diet can be given by using signals from Section 3E, Page 407.

Example:

"MUC" = "Give water only in small quantities."

---

† Part 2, Section 3B, Pages 404 and 405, "Diagnosis," can be used by both the master ("request for medical assistance") and the doctor ("medical advice").

‡ Table M–3 has been modified to include an *Equivalent List of Medications* in a right-hand column. The *name* and *number* of each medication is the same as shown in Table 6–1, Chapter VI, pp. 257 to 262. Masters of American vessels are urged to stock aboard ship the recommended *Equivalent List of Medications*.

EXAMPLES

As an example, two cases of request for assistance and the corresponding replies are drafted below:

Case One

Request for medical assistance

"I have a male age (44) years. Patient has been ill for (2) days. Patient has suffered from (bronchitis acute). Onset was sudden. Patient is delirious. Patient has fits of shivering. Temperature taken in mouth is (40). Pulse rate per minute is (110). The rate of breathing per minute is (30). Patient is in pain (chest). Part of the body affected is right (chest). Pain is increased on breathing. Patient has severe cough. Patient has bloodstained sputum. Patient has been given (penicillin injection) without effect. Patient has received treatment by medicaments in last (18) hours. My probable diagnosis is (pneumonia)."

Medical advice

"Your diagnosis is probably right. You should continue giving (penicillin injection). You should repeat every (12) hours. Put patient to bed lying down at absolute rest. Keep patient warm. Give fluid diet, milk, fruit juice, tea, mineral water. Give water very freely. Refer back to me in (24) hours or before if patient worsens."

Case Two

Request for medical assistance

"I have a male aged (31) years. Patient has been ill for (3) hours. Patient has had no serious previous illness. Pulse rate per minute is (95). Pulse is weak. Patient is sweating. Patient is in pain in lumbar (kidney) region. The part affected is left lumbar (kidney) region. Pain is severe. Pain is increased by hand pressure. Bowels are regular."

Request for additional information

"I cannot make a diagnosis. Please answer the following question(s). Temperature taken in the mouth is (number). Pain radiates to groin and testicle. Patient has pain on passing water. Urinary functions normal. Vomiting is present."

Additional information

"Temperature taken in mouth is (37). Pain radiates to groin and testicle. Patient has pain on passing water. Patient is passing small quantities of urine frequently. Vomiting is absent. Patient has nausea."

Medical advice

"My probable diagnosis is kidney stone (renal colic). You should give morphine injection. You should give by subcutaneous injection (10) milligrams. Give water freely. Apply hot water bottle to lumbar (kidney) region. Patient should be seen by doctor when next in port."

Part 2—Section 2
REQUEST FOR MEDICAL ASSISTANCE

Code	*Meaning*	*Cross Reference*

A. REQUEST—GENERAL INFORMATION

Code	Meaning	Cross Reference
MAA	I request urgent medical advice.	
MAB	I request you to make rendezvous in position indicated.	
MAC	I request you to arrange hospital admission.	
MAD	I am . . . (indicate number) hours from nearest port.	
MAE	I am converging on nearest port.	
MAF	I am moving away from nearest port.	
	I require medical assistance	**W**
	I have a doctor on board	**AL**
	Have you a doctor?	**AM**
	I need a doctor	**AN**
	I need a doctor; I have severe burns	**AN 1**
	I need a doctor; I have radiation casualties	**AN 2**
	I require a helicopter urgently with a doctor	**BR 2**
	I require a helicopter urgently to pick up injured/sick person	**BR 3**
	Helicopter is coming to you now (or at time indicated) with a doctor	**BT 2**
	Helicopter is coming to you now (or at time indicated) to pick up injured/sick person	**BT 3**
	I have injured/sick person (or number of persons indicated) to be taken off urgently	**AQ**
	You should send a helicopter/boat with a stretcher	**BS**
	A helicopter/boat is coming to take injured/sick	**BU**
	You should send injured/sick persons to me	**AT**

B. DESCRIPTION OF PATIENT

Code	Meaning	Cross Reference
MAJ	I have a male aged . . . (number) years.	
MAK	I have a female aged . . . (number) years.	

Code	*Meaning*	*Cross Reference*

MAL	I have a female . . . (number) months pregnant.	
MAM	Patient has been ill for . . . (number) days.	
MAN	Patient has been ill for . . . (number) hours.	
MAO	General condition of the patient is good.	
MAP	General condition of the patient is serious.	
MAQ	General condition of the patient is unchanged.	
MAR	General condition of the patient has worsened.	
MAS	Patient has been given . . . (Table M–3 in Section 4, Pages 413 through 418) with effect.	
MAT	Patient has been given . . . (Table M–3 in Section 4, Pages 413 through 418) without effect.	
MAU	Patient has received treatment by medicaments in last . . . (indicate number) hours.	

C. PREVIOUS HEALTH

MBA	Patient has suffered from . . . (Table M–2 in Section 4, Page 412).	
MBB	Patient has had previous operation . . . (Table M–2 in Section 4, Page 412).	
MBC	Patient has had no serious previous illness.	
MBD	Patient has had no relevant previous injury.	

D. LOCALIZATION OF SYMPTOMS, DISEASES, OR INJURIES

MBE	The whole body is affected.	
MBF	The part of the body affected is . . . (Table M–1 in Section 4, Page 409).	
*MBG	The part of the body affected is right . . . (Table M–1 in Section 4, Page 409).	
*MBH	The part of the body affected is left . . . (Table M–1 in Section 4, Page 409).	

---

* To be used when right and left side of the body or limb need to be differentiated.

E. GENERAL SYMPTOMS

| MBP | Onset was sudden. | |
| MBQ | Onset was gradual. | |

Temperature

| MBR | Temperature taken in mouth is . . . (number). | |
| MBS | Temperature taken in rectum is . . . (number). | |

Code	*Meaning*
MBT	Temperature in morning is . . . (number).
MBU	Temperature in the evening is . . . (number).
MBV	Temperature is rising.
MBW	Temperature is falling.

Pulse

MBX	The pulse rate per minute is . . . (number).
MBY	The pulse rate is irregular.
MBZ	The pulse rate is rising.
MCA	The pulse rate is falling.
MCB	The pulse is weak.
MCC	The pulse is too weak to count.
MCD	The pulse is too rapid to count.

Breathing

MCE	The rate of breathing per minute is . . . (number) (in and out being counted as one breath).
MCF	The breathing is weak.
MCG	The breathing is wheezing.
MCH	The breathing is regular.
MCI	The breathing is irregular.
MCJ	The breathing is strenuous (noisy).

Sweating

MCL	Patient is sweating.
MCM	Patient has fits of shivering (chills).
MCN	Patient has night sweats.
MCO	Patient's skin is hot and dry.
MCP	Patient is cold and clammy.

Mental State and Consciousness

MCR	Patient is conscious.
MCT	Patient is semiconscious but can be roused.
MCU	Patient is unconscious.
MCV	Patient found unconscious.

Code	Meaning	*Cross Reference*
MCW	Patient appears to be in a state of shock.	
MCX	Patient is delirious.	
MCY	Patient has mental symptoms.	
MCZ	Patient is paralyzed . . . (Table M–1 in Section 4, Page 409).	
MDC	Patient is restless.	
MDD	Patient is unable to sleep.	

Pain

MDF	Patient is in pain . . . (Table M–1 in Section 4, Page 409).	
MDG	Pain is a dull ache.	
MDJ	Pain is slight.	
MDL	Pain is severe.	
MDM	Pain is intermittent.	
MDN	Pain is continuous.	
MDO	Pain is increased by hand pressure.	
MDP	Pain radiates to . . . (Table M–1 in Section 4, Page 409).	
MDQ	Pain is increased on breathing.	
MDR	Pain is increased by action of bowels.	
MDT	Pain is increased on passing water.	
MDU	Pain occurs after taking food.	
MDV	Pain is relieved by taking food.	
MDW	Pain has no relation to taking food.	
MDX	Pain is relieved by heat.	
MDY	Pain has ceased.	

Cough

Code	Meaning	
MED	Cough is present.	
MEF	Cough is absent.	

Bowels

Code	Meaning	
MEG	Bowels are regular.	
MEJ	Patient is constipated and bowels last opened . . . (indicate number of days).	
MEL	Patient has diarrhea . . . (indicate number of times daily).	

| | | *Cross* |
| *Code* | *Meaning* | *Reference* |

Vomiting

MEM   Vomiting is present.

MEN   Vomiting is absent.

MEO   Patient has nausea.

Urine

MEP   Urinary functions normal.

MEQ   Urinary functions abnormal.

Bleeding

MER   Bleeding is present . . . (Table M–1 in Section 4, Page 409).

MET   Bleeding is absent.

Rash

MEU   A rash is present . . . (Table M–1 in Section 4, Page 409).

MEV   A rash is absent.

Swelling

MEW   Patient has a swelling . . . (Table M–1 in Section 4, Page 409).

MEX   Swelling is hard.

MEY   Swelling is soft.

MEZ   Swelling is hot and red.

MFA   Swelling is painful on hand pressure.

MFB   Swelling is discharging.

MFC   Patient has an abscess . . . (Table M–1 in Section 4, Page 409).

MFD   Patient has a carbuncle . . . (Table M–1 in Section 4, Page 409).

F. PARTICULAR SYMPTOMS

F–1. Accidents, Injuries, Fractures, Suicide, and Poisons

Bleeding is present . . . (Table M–1 in Section 4, Page 409 _____ **MER**

MFE   Bleeding is severe.

MFF   Bleeding is slight.

MFG   Bleeding has been stopped by pad(s) and bandaging.

MFH   Bleeding has been stopped by tourniquet.

MFI   Bleeding has stopped.

MFJ   Bleeding cannot be stopped.

Code	Meaning	Cross Reference
MFK	Patient has a superficial wound . . . (Table M–1 in Section 4, Page 409).	
MFL	Patient has a deep wound . . . (Table M–1 in Section 4, Page 409).	
MFM	Patient has penetrating wound . . . (Table M–1 in Section 4, Page 409).	
MFN	Patient has a clean-cut wound . . . (Table M–1 in Section 4, Page 409).	
MFO	Patient has a wound with ragged edges . . . (Table M–1 in Section 4, Page 409).	
MFP	Patient has a wound discharging . . . (Table M–1 in Section 4, Page 409).	
MFQ	Patient has contusion (bruising) . . . (Table M–1 in Section 4, Page 409).	
MFR	Wound is due to blow.	
MFS	Wound is due to crushing.	
MFT	Wound is due to explosion.	
MFU	Wound is due to fall.	
MFV	Wound is due to gunshot.	
MFW	Patient has a foreign body in wound.	
MFX	Patient is suffering from concussion.	
MFY	Patient cannot move the arm . . . (Table M–1 in Section 4, Page 409).	
MFZ	Patient cannot move the leg . . . (Table M–1 in Section 4, Page 409).	
MGA	Patient has dislocation . . . (Table M–1 in Section 4, Page 409).	
MGB	Patient has simple fracture . . . (Table M–1 in Section 4, Page 409).	
MGC	Patient has compound fracture . . . (Table M–1 in Section 4).	
MGD	Patient has comminuted fracture . . . (Table M–1 in Section 4, Page 409).	
MGE	Patient has attempted suicide.	
MGF	Patient has cut throat.	
MGG	Patient has superficial burn . . . (Table M–1 in Section 4, Page 409).	
MGH	Patient has severe burn . . . (Table M–1 in Section 4, Page 409).	
MGI	Patient is suffering from noncorrosive poisoning (no staining and burning of mouth and lips).	
MGJ	Patient has swallowed corrosive (staining and burning of mouth and lips).	
MGK	Patient has swallowed unknown poison.	

Code	Meaning	Cross Reference
MGL	Patient has swallowed a foreign body.	
MGM	Emetic has been given with good results.	
MGN	Emetic has been given without good results.	
MGO	No emetic has been given.	
MGP	Patient has had corrosive thrown on him . . . (Table M–1 in Section 4, Page 409).	
MGQ	Patient has inhaled poisonous gases, vapors, dust.	
MGR	Patient is suffering from animal bite . . . (Table M–1 in Section 4, Page 409).	
MGS	Patient is suffering from snakebite . . . (Table M–1 in Section 4, Page 409).	
MGT	Patient is suffering from gangrene . . . (Table M–1 in Section 4, Page 409).	

F–2. Diseases of Nose and Throat

Code	Meaning	Cross Reference
MGU	Patient has nasal discharge.	
MGV	Patient has foreign body in nose.	
MHA	Lips are swollen.	
MHB	Tongue is dry.	
MHC	Tongue is coated.	
MHD	Tongue is glazed and red.	
MHF	Tongue is swollen.	
MHG	Patient has ulcer on tongue.	
MHJ	Patient has ulcer in mouth.	
MHK	Gums are sore and bleeding.	
MHL	Throat is sore and red.	
MHM	Throat has pinpoint white spots on tonsils.	
MHN	Throat has gray white patches on tonsils.	
MHO	Throat hurts and is swollen on one side.	
MHP	Throat hurts and is swollen on both sides.	
MHQ	Swallowing is painful.	
MHR	Patient cannot swallow.	
MHT	Patient has hoarseness of voice.	
	Patient has swallowed a foreign body _____	MGL
MHV	Patient has severe toothache.	

Code	Meaning	Cross Reference

F—3. Diseases of Respiratory System

MHY Patient has pain in chest on breathing . . . (Table M–1 in Section 4, Page 409).

Breathing is wheezing _____ **MCG**

MHZ Breathing is deep.

MIA Patient has severe shortness of breath.

MIB Patient has asthmatical attack.

Cough is absent _____ **MEF**

MIC Patient has severe cough.

MID Cough is longstanding.

MIF Patient is coughing up blood.

MIG Patient has no sputum.

MIJ Patient has abundant sputum.

MIK Sputum is offensive.

MIL Patient has bloodstained sputum.

MIM Patient has blueness of face.

F—4. Diseases of the Digestive System

MIN Patient has tarry stool.

MIO Patient has clay-colored stool.

Patient has diarrhea . . . (indicate number of times daily) _____ **MEL**

MIP Patient has diarrhea with frequent stools like rice water.

MIQ Patient is passing blood with stools.

MIR Patient is passing mucus with stools.

Patient has nausea _____ **MEO**

MIT Patient has persistent hiccough.

MIU Patient has cramp pains and vomiting.

Vomiting is present _____ **MEM**

Vomiting is absent _____ **MEN**

MIV Vomiting has stopped.

MIW Vomiting is persistent.

MIX Vomit is streaked with blood.

MIY Patient vomiting much blood.

MIZ Vomit is dark (like coffee grounds).

Code	*Meaning*	*Cross Reference*
MJA	Patient vomits any food and liquid given.	
MJB	Amount of vomit is . . . (indicate in deciliters: 1 deciliter equals one-sixth of a pint).	
MJC	Frequency of vomiting is . . . (indicate number) daily.	
MJD	Patient has flatulence.	
MJE	Wind has not been passed per anus for . . . (indicate number of hours).	
MJF	Wind is being passed per anus.	
MJG	Abdomen is distended.	
MJH	Abdominal wall is soft (normal).	
MJI	Abdominal wall is hard and rigid.	
MJJ	Abdominal wall is tender . . . (Table M–1 in Section 4, Page 409).	
	Patient is in pain . . . (Table M–1 in Section 4, Page 409) _____	**MDF**
	Patient has a swelling . . . (Table M–1 in Section 4, Page 409) _____	**MEW**
MJK	Hernia is present.	
MJM	Hernia cannot be replaced.	
MJN	Hernia is painful and tender.	
MJO	Patient has bleeding hemorrhoids.	
MJP	Hemorrhoids cannot be reduced (put back in place).	

F–5. Diseases of the Genitourinary System

Code	*Meaning*	*Cross Reference*
	Patient is in pain . . . (Table M–1 in Section 4, Page 409) _____	**MDF**
MJS	Patient has pain on passing water.	
MJT	Patient has pain in penis at end of passing water.	
MJU	Patient has pain spreading from abdomen to penis, testicles, or thigh.	
MJV	Patient is unable to hold urine (incontinent).	
MJW	Patient is unable to pass urine.	
MJX	Patient is passing small quantities of urine frequently.	
MJY	Amount of urine passed in 24 hours . . . (indicate number in deciliters: 1 deciliter equals one-sixth of a pint).	
	Urinary functions normal _____	**MEP**
MKA	Urine contains albumen.	
MKB	Urine contains sugar.	
MKC	Urine contains blood.	
MKD	Urine is very dark brown.	

| | | *Cross* |
| *Code* | *Meaning* | *Reference* |

MKE	Urine is offensive and may contain pus.
MKF	Penis is swollen.
MKH	Foreskin will not go back to normal position.
MKI	Patient has swelling of testicles.
MKJ	Shall I pass a catheter?
MKK	I have passed a catheter.
MKL	I am unable to pass a catheter.

F–6. Diseases of the Nervous System and Mental Diseases

MKP	Patient has headache . . . (Table M–1 in Section 4, Page 409).	
MKQ	Headache is throbbing.	
MKR	Headache is very severe.	
MKS	Head cannot be moved forward to touch chest.	
MKT	Patient cannot feel pinprick . . . (Table M–1 in Section 4, Page 409).	
MKU	Patient is unable to speak properly.	
MKV	Giddiness (vertigo) is present.	
	Patient is paralyzed . . . (Table M–1 in Section 4, Page 409)	**MCZ**
	Patient is conscious	**MCR**
	Patient is semiconscious but can be roused	**MCT**
	Patient is unconscious	**MCU**
MKW	Pupils are equal in size.	
MKX	Pupils are unequal in size.	
MKY	Pupils do not contract in a bright light.	
MKZ	Patient has no control over his bowels.	
MLA	Patient has fits associated with rigidity of muscles and jerking of limbs—indicate number of fits per 24 hours.	
	Patient has mental symptoms	**MCY**
MLB	Patient has delusions.	
MLC	Patient is depressed.	
	Patient is delirious	**MCX**
MLD	Patient is uncontrollable.	
	Patient has attempted suicide	**MGE**
MLE	Patient has had much alcohol.	

Code	Meaning	Cross Reference

MLF   Patient has delirium tremens.

MLG   Patient has bedsores . . . (Tables M–1 in Section 4, Page 409).

F–7. Diseases of the Heart and Circulatory System

Patient is in pain . . . (Table M–1 in Section 4, Page 409) _____ MDF

MLH   Pain has been present for . . . (indicate number of minutes).

MLI   Pain in chest is constricting in character.

MLJ   Pain is behind the breastbone.

Pain radiates to . . . (Table M–1 in Section 4, Page 409) _____ MDP

Patient has blueness of face _____ MIM

MLK   Patient has pallor.

The rate of breathing per minute is . . . (number) (in and out being counted as one breath) _____ MCE

The pulse is weak _____ MCB

The pulse rate is irregular _____ MBY

The pulse is too weak to count _____ MCC

The pulse is too rapid to count _____ MCD

MLL   Breathing is difficult when lying down.

MLM   Swelling of legs that pits on pressure.

MLN   Patient has varicose ulcer.

F–8. Infectious and Parasitic Diseases

MLR   Rash has been present for . . . (indicate number of hours).

MLS   Rash first appeared on . . . (Table M–1 in Section 4, Page 409).

MLT   Rash is spreading to . . . (Table M–1 in Section 4, Page 409).

MLU   Rash is fading.

MLV   Rash is itchy.

MLW   Rash is not itchy.

MLX   Rash looks like general redness.

MLY   Rash looks like blotches.

MLZ   Rash looks like small blisters containing clear fluid.

MMA   Rash looks like larger blisters containing pus.

MMB   Rash is weeping (oozing).

MMC   Rash looks like wheals.

Code	*Meaning*	*Cross Reference*

MMD Rash consists of rose-colored spots that do not blanch on pressure.

MME Skin is yellow.

Patient has an abscess . . . (Table M–1 in Section 4, Page 409) ____ **MFC**

MMF Patient has buboes . . . (Table M–1 Section 4, Page 409).

MMJ Patient has been isolated.

MMK Should patient be isolated?

MML I have had (indicate number) similar cases.

Patient has diarrhea with frequent stools like rice water _____ **MIP**

Patient has never been successfully vaccinated against smallpox ____ **MUT**

Patient was last vaccinated . . . (date indicated) _____ **MUU**

Patient has vaccination marks _____ **MUV**

F–9. Venereal Diseases

(See also Diseases of Genitourinary System.)

MMP Patient has discharge from penis.

MMQ Patient has previous history of gonorrhea.

MMR Patient has single hard sore on penis.

MMS Patient has multiple sores on penis.

Patient has buboes . . . (Table M–1 in Section 4, Page 409) _____ **MMF**

MMT Patient has swollen glands in the groin.

MMU End of penis is inflamed and swollen. ___ ___ ___ ___ ___ ___ _____

F–10. Diseases of the Ear

Patient is in pain . . . (Table M–1 in Section 4, Page 409) _____ **MDF**

MMW Patient has boil in ear(s).

MMX Patient has discharge of blood from ear(s).

MMY Patient has discharge of clear fluid from ear(s).

MMZ Patient has discharge of pus from ear(s).

MNA Patient has hearing impaired.

MNB Patient has foreign body in ear.

Giddiness (vertigo) is present _____ **MKV**

MNC Patient has constant noises in ear(s).

Code	*Meaning*	*Cross Reference*

F–11. Diseases of the Eye

Patient is in pain . . . (Table M–1 in Section 4, Page 409) _____ **MDF**

MNG — Patient has inflammation of eye(s).

MNH — Patient has discharge from eye(s).

MNI — Patient has foreign body embedded in the pupil area of the eye.

MNJ — Eyelids are swollen.

MNK — Patient cannot open eyes (raise eyelids).

MNL — Patient has foreign body embedded in the white of the eye.

MNM — Patient has double vision when looking at objects with both eyes open.

MNN — Patient has sudden blindness in one eye.

MNO — Patient has sudden blindness in both eyes.

Pupils are equal in size _____ **MKW**

Pupils are unequal in size _____ **MKX**

Pupils do not contract in a bright light _____ **MKY**

Patient has a penetrating wound . . . (Table M–1 in Section 4, Page 409) _____ **MFM**

MNP — Eyeball is yellow in color.

F–12. Diseases of the Skin

See Infectious and Parasitic Diseases in Paragraph F–8 of Section 2, Pages 400 and 401.

F–13. Diseases of Muscles and Joints

MNT — Patient has pain in muscles of . . . (Table M–1 in Section 4, Page 409).

MNU — Patient has pain in joint(s) . . . (Table M–1 in Section 4, Page 409).

MNV — Patient has redness and swelling of joint(s) . . . (Table M–1 in Section 4, Page 409).

MNW — There is history of recent injury.

MNX — There is no history of injury.

F–14. Miscellaneous Illnesses

Patient has had much alcohol _____ **MLE**

MOA — Patient is suffering from heat exhaustion.

MOB — Patient is suffering from heat stroke.

MOC — Patient is suffering from seasickness.

Code	Meaning	Cross Reference
MOD	Patient is suffering from exposure in lifeboat—indicate length of exposure (number) hours.	
MOE	Patient is suffering from frostbite . . . (Table M–1 in Section 4, Page 409).	
MOF	Patient has been exposed to radioactive hazard.	

F–15. Childbirth

Code	Meaning	
MOK	I have a patient in childbirth aged . . . (number) years.	
MOL	Patient states she has had . . . (number) children.	
MOM	Patient states child is due in . . . (number) weeks.	
MON	Pains began . . . (number) hours ago.	
MOO	Pains are feeble and produce no effect.	
MOP	Pains are strong and effective.	
MOQ	Pains are occurring every . . . (number) minutes.	
MOR	The bag of membranes broke . . . (number) hours ago.	
MOS	There is severe bleeding from the womb.	
MOT	The head is coming first.	
MOU	The buttocks are coming first.	
MOV	A foot has appeared first.	
MOW	An arm has appeared first.	
MOX	The child has been born.	
MOY	The child will not breathe.	
MOZ	The placenta has been passed.	
MPA	The placenta has not been passed.	
MPB	I have a nonpregnant woman who is bleeding from the womb.	

G. PROGRESS REPORT

Code	Meaning	
MPE	I am carrying out prescribed instructions.	
MPF	Patient is improving.	
MPG	Patient is not improving.	
MPH	Patient is relieved of pain.	
MPI	Patient still has pain.	
MPJ	Patient is restless.	
MPK	Patient is calm.	

Code	*Meaning*	*Cross Reference*
MPL	Symptoms have cleared.	
MPM	Symptoms have not cleared.	
MPN	Symptoms have increased.	
MPO	Symptoms have decreased.	
MPP	Treatment has been effective.	
MPQ	Treatment has been ineffective.	
MPR	Patient has died.	

Part 2—Section 3
MEDICAL ADVICE

A. REQUEST FOR ADDITIONAL INFORMATION

MQB   I cannot understand your signal; please use standard method of case description.

MQC   Please answer the following question(s).

B. DIAGNOSIS

MQE   My probable diagnosis is . . . (Table M–2 in Section 4, Page 412).

MQF   My alternative diagnosis is . . . (Table M–2 in Section 4, Page 412).

MQG   My probable diagnosis is infection or inflammation . . . (Table M–1 in Section 4, Page 409).

MQH   My probable diagnosis is perforation of . . . (Table M–1 in Section 4, Page 409).

MQI   My probable diagnosis is tumor of . . . (Table M–1 in Section 4, Page 409).

MQJ   My probable diagnosis is obstruction of . . . (Table M–1 in Section 4, Page 409).

MQK   My probable diagnosis is hemorrhage of . . . (Table M–1 in Section 4, Page 409).

MQL   My probable diagnosis is foreign body in . . . (Table M–1 in Section 4, Page 409).

MQM   My probable diagnosis is fracture of . . . (Table M–1 in Section 4, Page 409).

MQN   My probable diagnosis is dislocation of . . . (Table M–1 in Section 4, Page 409).

MQO   My probable diagnosis is sprain of . . . (Table M–1 in Section 4, Page 409).

		Cross
Code	*Meaning*	*Reference*

MQP	I cannot make a diagnosis.
MQT	Your diagnosis is probably right.
MQU	I am not sure about your diagnosis.

C. SPECIAL TREATMENT

MRI	You should refer to your International Ship's Medical Guide if available or its equivalent.
MRJ	You should follow treatment in your own medical guide.
MRK	You should follow the instructions for this procedure outlined in your own medical guide.
MRL	Commence artificial respiration immediately.
MRM	Pass catheter into bladder.
MRN	Pass catheter again after . . . (number) hours.
MRO	Pass catheter and retain it in bladder.
MRP	Apply ice-cold compress and renew every . . . (number) hours.
MRQ	Apply hot compress and renew every . . . (number) hours.
MRR	Apply hot-water bottle to . . . (Table M–1 in Section 4, Page 409).
MRS	Insert ear drops . . . (number) times daily.
MRT	Insert antiseptic eye drops . . . (number) times daily.
MRU	Insert anaesthetic eye drops . . . (number) times daily.
MRV	Bathe eye frequently with hot water.
MRW	Give frequent gargles one teaspoonful of salt in a tumblerful of water.
MRX	Give enema.
MRY	Do not give enema or laxative.
MRZ	Was the result of the enema satisfactory?
MSA	Give rectal saline slowly to replace fluid loss.
MSB	Give subcutaneous saline to replace fluid loss.
MSC	Apply well-padded splint(s) to immobilize limb. Watch circulation by inspection of color of fingers or toes.
MSD	Apply cotton wool to armpit and bandage arm to side.
MSF	Apply a sling and/or rest the part.
MSG	Give light movements and massage daily.
MSJ	Place patient in hot bath.
MSK	To induce sleep give two sedative tablets.

Code	Meaning	Cross Reference

MSL   Reduce temperature of patient as indicated in general nursing chapter of Medical Guide.

MSM   The swelling should be incised and drained.

MSN   Dress wound with sterile gauze, cotton wool, and bandage.

MSO   Dress wound with sterile gauze, cotton wool, and apply well-padded splint.

MSP   Apply burn and wound dressing and bandage lightly.

MSQ   Dress wound and bring edges together with adhesive plaster.

MSR   The wound should be stitched.

MST   The wound should not be stitched.

MSU   Stop bleeding by applying more cotton wool, firm bandaging, and elevation of the limb.

MSV   Stop bleeding by manual pressure.

MSW   Apply tourniquet for not more than fifteen minutes.

MSX   Induce vomiting by giving an emetic.

MSY   You should pass a stomach tube.

MSZ   Do not try to empty stomach by any method.

D. TREATMENT BY MEDICAMENTS

D–1. Prescribing

MTD   You should give ... (Table M–3 in Section 4, Pages 413 through 418).

MTE   You must not give ... (Table M–3, in Section 4, Pages 413 through 418).

D–2. Method of Administration and Dose

MTF   You should give one tablespoonful (15 ml or ½ oz).

MTG   You should give one dessertspoonful (7.5 ml or ¼ oz).

MTH   You should give one teaspoonful (4 ml or 1 drachm).

MTI   You should give by mouth ... (number) tablets/capsules.

MTJ   You should give a tumblerful of water with each dose.

MTK   You should give by intramuscular injection ... (number) milligrams.

MTL   You should give by subcutaneous injection ... (number) milligrams.

MTM   You should give by intramuscular injection ... (number) ampoule(s).

MTN   You should give by subcutaneous injection ... (number) ampoule(s).

Code	*Meaning*	*Cross Reference*

D–3. Frequency of Dose

MTO	You should give once only.	
MTP	You should repeat after . . . (number) hours.	
MTQ	You should repeat every . . . (number) hours.	
MTR	You should continue for . . . (number) hours.	

D–4. Frequency of External Application

MTT	You should apply once only.	
MTU	You should apply every . . . (number) hours.	
MTV	You should cease to apply.	
MTW	You should apply for . . . (number) minutes.	

E. DIET

MUA	Give nothing by mouth.	
MUB	Give water very freely.	
MUC	Give water only in small quantities.	
MUD	Give water only as much as possible without causing the patient to vomit.	
MUE	Give ice to suck.	
MUF	Give fluid diet, milk, fruit, juices, tea, mineral water.	
MUG	Give light diet such as vegetable soup, steamed fish, stewed fruit, milk puddings, or equivalent.	
MUH	Give normal diet as tolerated.	

F. CHILDBIRTH

MUI	Has she had previous children?	
MUJ	How many months pregnant is she?	
MUK	When did labor pains start?	
	Give enema _____	MRX
MUL	Encourage her to rest between pains.	
MUM	Encourage her to strain down during pains.	
MUN	What is the frequency of pains (indicate in minutes).	
	To induce sleep give two sedative tablets _____	MSK
MUO	Patient should strain down and you exert steady but gentle pressure on lower part of the abdomen but not on the womb to help expulsion of the placenta.	

Code	Meaning	Cross Reference
MUP	You should apply tight wide binder around lower part of abdomen and hips.	
MUQ	You should apply artificial respiration gently by mouth technique on infant.	

G. VACCINATION AGAINST SMALLPOX

MUR	Has the patient been successfully vaccinated?	
MUS	Has the patient been vaccinated during the past three years?	
MUT	Patient has never been successfully vaccinated against smallpox.	
MUU	Patient was last vaccinated . . . (indicate date).	
MUV	Patient has vaccination marks.	

H. GENERAL INSTRUCTIONS

MVA	I consider the case serious and urgent.	
MVB	I do not consider the case serious or urgent.	
MVC	Put patient to bed lying down at absolute rest.	
MVD	Put patient to bed sitting up.	
MVE	Raise head of bed.	
MVF	Raise foot of bed.	
MVG	Keep patient warm.	
MVH	Keep patient cool.	
MVI	You should continue your local treatment.	
MVJ	You should continue your special treatment.	
MVK	You should continue giving . . . (Table M–3 in Section 4, Pages 413 through 418).	
MVL	You should suspend your local treatment.	
MVM	You should suspend your special treatment.	
MVN	You should cease giving . . . (Table M–3 in Section 4, Pages 413 through 418).	
MVO	You should isolate the patient and disinfect his cabin.	
MVP	You should land your patient at the earliest opportunity.	
MVQ	Patient should be seen by a doctor when next in port.	
MVR	I will arrange for hospital admission.	
MVS	I think I should come on board and examine the case.	
MVT	No treatment advised.	
MVU	Refer back to me in . . . (number) hours or before if patient worsens.	

Part 2—Section 4
TABLES OF COMPLEMENTS
(See illustrations pp. 410–411)

Table M–1

REGIONS OF THE BODY

Side of body or limb affected should be clearly indicated—right, left

Figure 1 (Front)

1. Frontal region of head
2. Side of head
3. Top of head
4. Face
5. Jaw
6. Neck front
7. Shoulder
8. Clavicle
*9. Chest
10. Chest mid
11. Heart
12. Armpit

13. Arm upper
14. Forearm
15. Wrist
16. Palm of hand
17. Fingers
18. Thumb
19. Central upper abdomen
20. Central lower abdomen
*21. Upper abdomen
*22. Lower abdomen
*23. Lateral abdomen
*24. Groin

25. Scrotum
26. Testicles
27. Penis
28. Upper thigh
29. Middle thigh
30. Lower thigh
31. Knee
32. Patella
33. Front of leg
34. Ankle
35. Foot
36. Toes

Figure 2 (Back)

37. Back of head
38. Back of neck
39. Back of shoulder
40. Scapula region
41. Elbow
42. Back upper arm
43. Back lower arm

44. Back of hand
*45. Lower chest region
46. Spinal column upper
47. Spinal column middle
48. Spinal column lower
*49. Lumbar (kidney) region
50. Sacral region

51. Buttock
52. Anus
53. Back of thigh
54. Back of knee
55. Calf
56. Heel

Other Organs of the Body

57. Artery
58. Bladder
59. Brain
60. Breast
61. Ear(s)
62. Eye(s)
63. Eyelid(s)
64. Gall bladder
65. Gullet (esophagus)
66. Gums
67. Intestine
68. Kidney

69. Lip lower
70. Lip upper
71. Liver
72. Lungs
73. Mouth
74. Nose
75. Pancreas
76. Prostate
77. Rib(s)
78. Spleen
79. Stomach
80. Throat

81. Tongue
82. Tonsils
83. Tooth, teeth
84. Urethra
85. Uterus, womb
86. Vein
87. Voice box (larynx)
88. Whole abdomen
89. Whole arm
90. Whole back
91. Whole chest
92. Whole leg

---

* Indicate side as required.

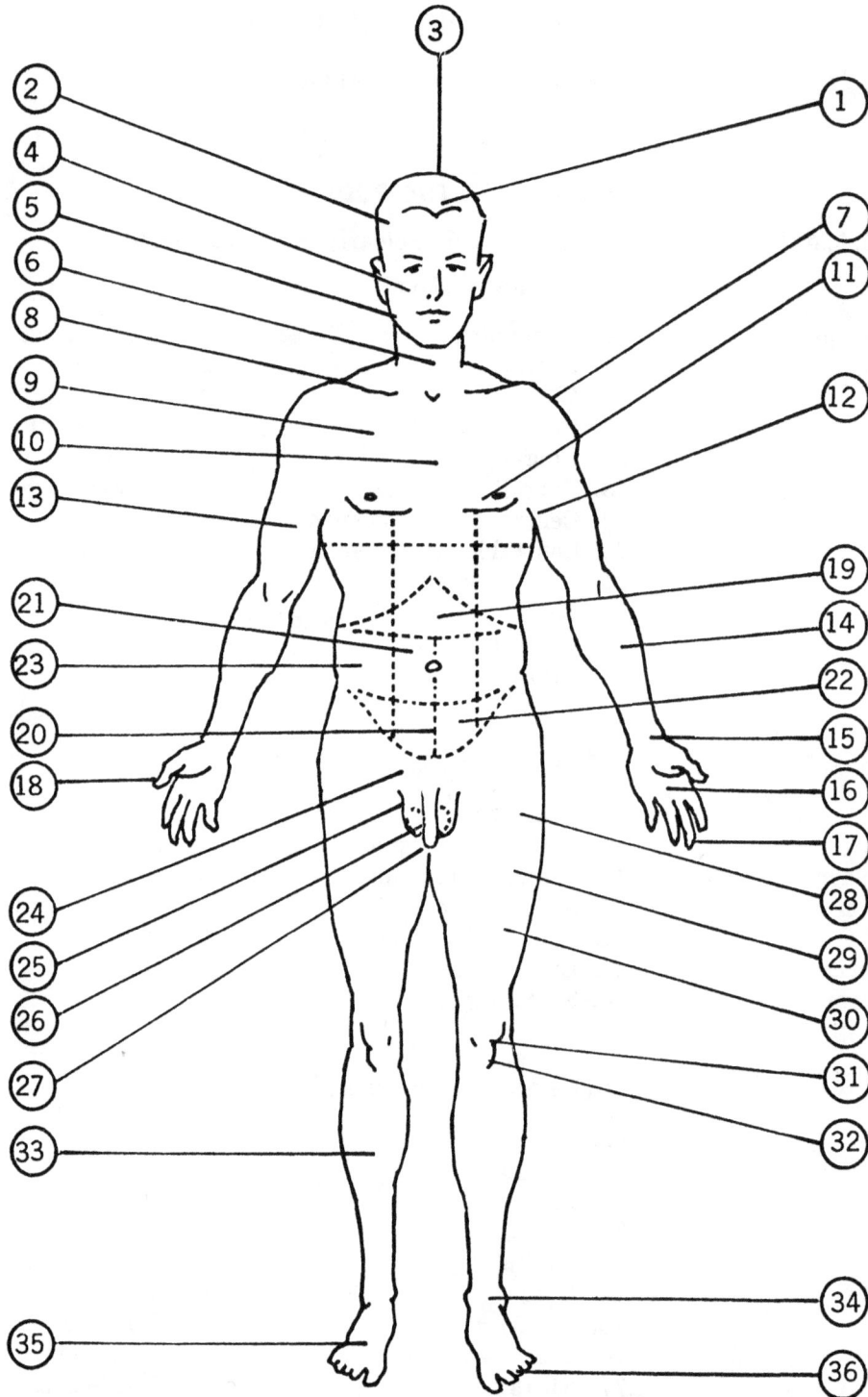

Fig. 12-1. To get MEDICAL ADVICE BY RADIO, use the numbers shown in this figure or those in Figure 12-2. This is a *front view* (diagrammatic) of the human body. Each body part or body area is assigned a specific number. In the radio message, the *side* of the body or *limb* affected should be clearly indicated as *right side* or *left side* (see p. 391.) Refer to Table M-1 to identify the body parts associated with the numbers.

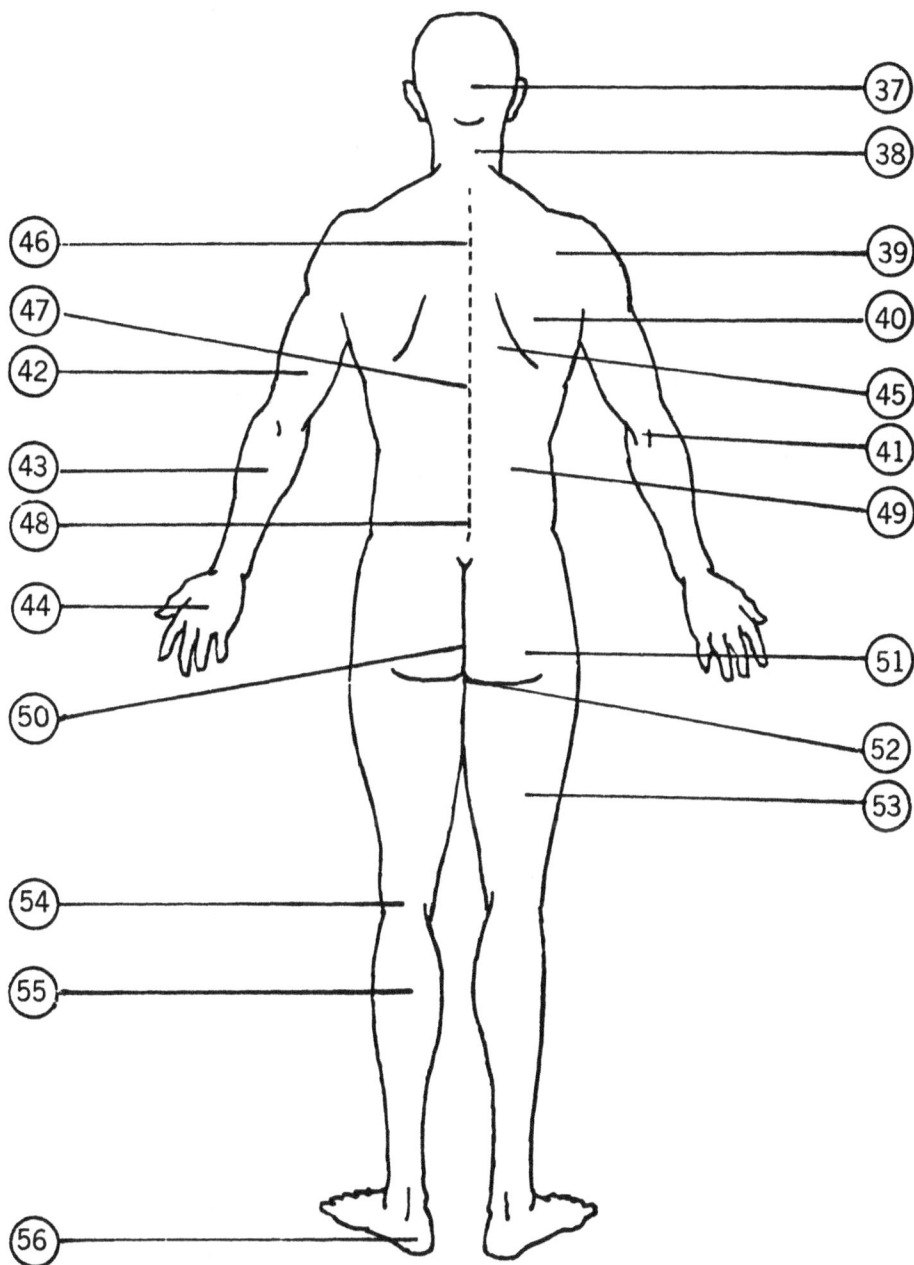

Fig. 12–2. To get MEDICAL ADVICE BY RADIO, use the numbers shown in this figure or those in Figure 12–1. This is a *back view* (diagrammatic) of the human body. Each body part or body area is assigned a specific number. In the radio message, the *side* of the body or *limb* affected should be clearly indicated as *right side* or *left side*. (See p. 391.) Refer to Table M–1 to identify the body parts associated with the numbers.

Table M—2

LIST OF COMMON DISEASES

1. Abscess	33. Eczema	65. Piles
2. Alcoholism	34. Erysipelas	66. Plague
3. Allergic reaction	35. Fits	67. Pleurisy
4. Amoebic dysentery	36. Gangrene	68. Pneumonia
5. Angina pectoris	37. Gastric ulcer	69. Poisoning (corrosive)
6. Anthrax	38. Gastroenteritis	70. Poisoning (noncorrosive)
7. Apoplexy (stroke)	39. Gonorrhea	71. Poisoning (barbiturates)
8. Appendicitis	40. Gout	72. Poisoning (methyl alcohol)
9. Asthma	41. Heat cramps	73. Poisoning (gases)
10. Bacillary dysentery	42. Heat exhaustion	74. Poliomyelitis
11. Boils	43. Heat stroke	75. Prolapsed intervertebral disc (slipped disc)
12. Bronchitis (acute)	44. Hepatitis	76. Pulmonary tuberculosis
13. Bronchitis (chronic)	45. Hernia	77. Quinsy
14. Brucellosis	46. Hernia (irreducible)	78. Rheumatism
15. Carbuncle	47. Hernia (strangulated)	79. Rheumatic fever
16. Cellulitis	48. Immersion foot	80. Scarlet fever
17. Chancroid	49. Impetigo	81. Sciatica
18. Chickenpox	50. Insulin overdose	82. Shingles (herpes zoster)
19. Cholera	51. Indigestion	83. Sinusitis
20. Cirrhosis of the liver	52. Influenza	84. Shock
21. Concussion	53. Intestinal obstruction	85. Smallpox
22. Compression of brain	54. Kidney stone (renal colic)	86. Syphilis
23. Congestive heart failure	55. Laryngitis	87. Tetanus
24. Constipation	56. Malaria	88. Tonsillitis
25. Coronary thrombosis	57. Measles	89. Typhoid
26. Cystitis (bladder inflammation)	58. Meningitis	90. Typhus
27. Dengue	59. Mental illness	91. Urethritis
28. Diabetes	60. Migraine	92. Urticaria (nettle rash)
29. Diabetic coma	61. Mumps	93. Whooping cough
30. Diphtheria	62. Orchitis	94. Yellow fever
31. Drug reaction	63. Peritonitis	
32. Duodenal ulcer	64. Phlebitis	

Table M–3

*LIST OF MEDICAMENTS

*List of Medicaments

(Identified by *number* and *name*) from the medical section of the *International Code of Signals**

† List of Equivalent Medications

(Identified by *number* and *name*) recommended in Chapter VI, pp. 257 to 262 of this publication, THE SHIP'S MEDICINE CHEST AND MEDICAL AID AT SEA

A. FOR EXTERNAL USE

1. Auristillae Glyceris
   Glycerin eardrops
   EARDROPS

≡ No equivalent. Obtain further medical advice.

2. Guttae Sulfacetamidi
   Sulfacetamide eye drops
   ANTISEPTIC EYE DROPS

82. Polymyxin B-Neomycin-Gramicidin
    Eye Drops
    (See page 261.)

3. Guttae Tetracainae
   Tetracaine eye drops
   ANESTHETIC EYE DROPS

87. Proparacaine Hydrochloride
    Eye Drops
    (See page 261.)

4. Linimentum Methylis Salicylatis
   Methyl salicylate liniment
   SALICYLATE LINIMENT

61. Menthol Ointment, Compound
    (See page 260.)

5. Lotio Calaminae
   Calamine Lotion
   CALAMINE LOTION

18. Calamine Lotion
    (See page 257.)

6. Lotio Cetrimidi
   Cetrimide lotion
   ANTISEPTIC LOTION

84. Povidone-Iodine Solution
    (See page 261.)

7. Naristillae Ephedrine
   Norephedrine hydrochloride drops
   NASAL DROPS

78. Phenylephrine Hydrochloride
    Nasal Spray, 0.25%
    (See page 260.)

8. Paraffinum Molle Flavum
   Yellow soft paraffin
   SOFT PARAFFIN

≡ No equivalent. Obtain further medical advice.

---

† Masters of American vessels are urged to stock aboard ship the EQUIVALENT MEDICATIONS listed in the above right-hand column. Each EQUIVALENT MEDICATION has a number which may be used to identify it in Table 6–1, p. 257 and pp. 271 to 293 of Chapter VI.

Each medication listed in the left-hand column has its *equivalent* listed directly opposite in the right-hand column.

IN ALL CASES, BE SURE TO VERIFY THE CORRECT DOSAGE OF THE MEDICATION TO BE USED. Where no similar medication is stocked aboard ship, medical advice must be sought by radio.

---

* Preparations listed above in the left-hand column are reproduced from Publication No. H.O. 102, INTERNATIONAL CODE OF SIGNALS, UNITED STATES EDITION, 1969. Chapter 3, pp. 97 to 130. For the sake of uniformity, medicaments are indicated in the first place by their Latin denomination so that a correct translation can be found in each language.

Table M–3(Continued)

*LIST OF MEDICAMENTS

*List of Medicaments	† List of Equivalent Medications
(Identified by *number* and *name*) from the medical section of the *International Code of Signals**	(Identified by *number* and *name)* recommended in Chapter VI, pp. 257 to 262 of THE SHIP'S MEDICINE CHEST AND MEDICAL AID AT SEA

9. Paraffinum Molle Flavum Carbasi
     Absorbentis
   Tulle gras dressing (Paraffin gauze)
   BURN/WOUND DRESSING

≡ No equivalent. Obtain further medical advice.

10. Unguentum Bacitracini
    Bacitracin ointment
    ANTIBIOTIC OINTMENT

14. Bacitracin Ointment
    (See page 257.)

11. Unguentum Benzocaini Compositum
    Compound benzocaine ointment
    PILE OINTMENT

47. Hemorrhoidal Suppository
    (See page 259. Note different dosage form.)

12. Unguentum Xylocaini Hydrochloridi
    Mylocaine ointment
    LOCAL ANESTHETIC OINTMENT

≡ No equivalent. Obtain further medical advice.

B. FOR INTERNAL USE

Allergic Conditions

13. Compressi Promethazini Hydrochloridi
    Promethazine hydrochloride tablets
    ANTIHISTAMINE TABLETS
    (25 mgs per tablet)

33. Diphenhydramine Hydrochloride Capsules, 25 mg
    (See page 258.)

14. Injectic Adrenalini
    Adrenaline injection
    ADRENALINE
    (1 mg in "Ampins")

38. Epinephrine Hydrochloride Injection, 1:1000, 1 ml cartridge
    (See page 258.)

Caution: USE ABOVE INJECTION NO. 14 ONLY ON MEDICAL ADVICE BY RADIO—EXCEPT IN CASE OF ANAPHYLACTIC SHOCK DUE TO PENICILLIN INJECTION

Caution: USE ABOVE INJECTION NO. 38 ONLY ON MEDICAL ADVICE BY RADIO—EXCEPT IN CASE OF ANAPHYLACTIC SHOCK DUE TO PENCILLIN INJECTION.

Antibiotics

15. Capsulae Tetracyclini Hydrochloridi
    Tetracycline hydrochloride capsules
    TETRACYCLINE CAPSULES
    (250 mgs per capsule)

101. Tetracycline Hydrochloride Capsules 250 mg
     (See page 262.)

---

* See footnote, p. 413, left-hand column.   † See footnote, p. 413, right-hand column.

Table M–3 (Continued)

*LIST OF MEDICAMENTS

List of Medicaments	† *List of Equivalent Medications*
(Identified by *number* and *name*) from the medical section of the *International Code of Signals**	(Identified by *number* and *name)* recommended in Chapter VI, pp. 257 to 262 of THE SHIP'S MEDICINE CHEST AND MEDICAL AID AT SEA

16. Compressi Phenoxymethylpenicillini
Phenoxymethylpenicillin
PENICILLIN TABLETS
(125 mgs per tablet)

73. Penicillin V Potassium Tablets, 250 mg
(See page 260. Note: Compensation is required for difference in tablet strength.)

17. Compressi Sulfadimidini
Sulfadimidine tablets
SULFONAMIDE TABLETS
(500 mgs per tablet)

96. Sulfisoxazole Tablets, 500 mg
(See page 261.)

18. Injectio Benzylpenicillini
Procaine penicillin G
PENICILLIN INJECTION
(600,000 units per ampoule)

71. Penicillin G Procaine, Sterile Suspension, 600,000 units/ml
(See page 260.)

19. Injectio Streptomycini Sulfatis
Streptomycin sulfate injection
STREPTOMYCIN INJECTION
(1,000 mgs per ampoule)

≡ No equivalent. Obtain further medical advice.

20. Injectio Tetracyclini Hydrochloridi
Tetracycline hydrochloride
TETRACYCLINE INJECTION
(100 mgs per ampoule)

≡ No equivalent. Obtain further medical advice.

Asthma

21. Compressi Aminophyllini
Aminophylline tablets
ASTHMA RELIEF TABLETS
(300 mgs per tablet)

8. Aminophylline Suppository Rectal, 500 mg
(See page 257. Note different dosage form and route of administration.)

Caution: THIS TABLET NO. 21 TO BE USED ONLY ON MEDICAL ADVICE BY RADIO

22. Compressi Ephedrini Hydrochloridi
Ephedrine Hydrochloride tablets
EPHEDRINE TABLETS
(30 mgs per tablet)

37. Ephedrine Sulfate Capsules, 25 mg
(See page 258.)

* See footnote, p. 413, left-hand column.   † See footnote, p. 413, right-hand column.

Table M–3 (Continued)

*LIST OF MEDICAMENTS

*List of Medicaments	*† List of Equivalent Medications*
(Identified by *number* and *name*) from the medical section of the *International Code of Signals**	(Identified by *number* and *name*) recommended in Chapter VI, pp. 257 to 262 of THE SHIP'S MEDICINE CHEST AND MEDICAL AID AT SEA

23. Tinctura Benzoini Composita
    Tincture of benzoin compound
    INHALATION MIXTURE

≡ No equivalent. Obtain further medical advice.

Cough

24. Compressi Codeini Phosphatis
    Codeine phosphate tablets
    CODEINE TABLETS
    (15 mgs per tablet)

24. Codeine Sulfate Tablets, 30 mg
    (See page 258. Note: Compensation is required for difference in tablet strength.)

25. Linctus Scillae Opiata
    Linctus of squill, opiate
    COUGH LINCTUS

27. Dextromethorphan Hydrobromide Syrup with Glyceryl Guaiacolate
    (See page 258.)

Diarrhea

26. Mistura Kaolini et Morphinae
    Kaolin and morphine mixture
    DIARRHEA MIXTURE

56. Kaolin Mixture with Pectin
    (See page 259.)

Heart

27. Compressi Glycerylis Trinitratis
    Glycerin Trinitrate tablets
    HEART TABLETS
    (0.5 mg per tablet)

68. Nitroglycerin Tablets, 0.4 mg
    (See page 260.)

NOTE: For congestive heart failure, the following preparations are available on board ship, but they should be used only on medical advice transmitted in plain language and not by code:

Compressi Chlorothiazidi
(Chlorothiazide) or equivalent
(500 mgs per tablet)

43. Furosemide Tablets, 40 mg
    (See page 259.)

Compressi Digoxin (Digoxin tablets) or
    equivalent
(0.25 mg per tablet)

32. Digoxin Tablets, 0.25 mg
    (See page 258).

---

* See footnote, p. 413, left-hand column.   † See footnote, p. 413, right-hand column.

Table M–3 (Continued)

*LIST OF MEDICAMENTS

List of Medicaments	† *List of Equivalent Medications*
(Identified by *number* and *name*) from the medical section of the *International Code of Signals**	(Identified by *number* and *name)* recommended in Chapter VI, pp. 257 to 262 of THE SHIP'S MEDICINE CHEST AND MEDICAL AID AT SEA

Indigestion

28. Compressi Magnesii Trisilicas
Magnesium trisilicate
STOMACH TABLETS

7. Aluminum Hydroxide, with Magnesium Hydroxide or Magnesium Trisilicate, Chewable Tablets
(See page 257.)

Laxatives

29. Compressi Colocynthidis et Jalapae Compositae
Compound Colocynth and Jalap tablets
VEGETABLE LAXATIVE TABLETS

≡ No equivalent. Obtain further medical advice.

30. Magnesii Hydroxidum
Magnesium hydroxide mixture
LIQUID LAXATIVE—"Milk of Magnesia"

64. Milk of Magnesia
(See page 260.)

Malaria

31. Compressi Chloroquini Sulfatis
Chloroquine sulfate tablets
MALARIA TABLETS
(200 mgs per tablet)

22. Chloroquine Phosphate Tablets, 250 mg
(See page 257).

Pain

32. Compressi Acidi Acetylasalicylici
Acetylsalicylic acid tablets
ASPIRIN TABLETS
(300 mgs per tablet)

12. Aspirin Tablets, 300 mg
(See page 257).

33. Injectio Morphini
Morphine sulfate injection
MORPHINE INJECTION
(15 mgs per ampoule)

66. Morphine Sulfate Injection, 10 mg/ml
(See page 260. Note: Compensation is required for difference in strength.)

---

* See footnote, p. 413, left-hand column.

† See footnote, p. 413, right-hand column.

Table M–3 (Continued)

*LIST OF MEDICAMENTS

*List of Medicaments

(Identified by *number* and *name*) from the medical section of the *International Code of Signals**

† List of Equivalent Medications

(Identified by *number* and *name*) recommended in Chapter VI, pp. 257 to 262 of THE SHIP'S MEDICINE CHEST AND MEDICAL AID AT SEA

Sedation

34. Compressi Butobarbitali
Butobarbitone tablets
SEDATIVE TABLETS
(100 mgs per tablet)

35. Compressi Phenobarbitali
Phenobarbitone tablets
PHENOBARBITONE TABLETS
(30 mgs per tablet)

36. Compressi Chlorpromazini
Hydrochloridi
Chlorpromazine hydrochloride tablets
TRANQUILLIZER TABLETS
(LARGACTIL)
(50 mgs per tablet)

Caution: THIS TABLET NO. 36 TO BE USED ONLY ON MEDICAL ADVICE BY RADIO.

74. Pentobarbital Sodium Capsules, 50 mg
(See page 260. Note: Compensation is required for difference in strength.)

77. Phenobarbital, Tablets, 30 mg
(See page 260.)

31. Diazepam Tablets, 5 mg
(See page 258.)

Salt Depletion or Heat Cramps

37. Compressi Natrii Chloridi Solv
Sodium chloride tablets
SALT TABLETS
(500 mgs per tablet)

94. Sodium Chloride Tablets, 1 g
(See page 261. Note: Compensation is is required for difference in strength.)

Seasickness

38. Compressi Hyoscini Hydrobromidi
Hysocine Hydrobromide tablets
SEASICKNESS TABLETS
(0.3 mg per tablet)

25. Cyclizine Hydrochloride Tablets, 50 mg
(See page 258.)

---

* See footnote, p. 413, left-hand column.

† See footnote, p. 413, right-hand column.

INDEX
MEDICAL SIGNAL CODE
(Numbers Refer to Pages)

Part 3—AMVER System
Automated Mutual-assistance VEssel Rescue System

The AMVER (Automated Mutual-assistance VEssel Rescue) system operated by the United States Coast Guard, is an international program designed to assist the safety of merchant vessels on the high seas. Merchant vessels of all nations on offshore passages throughout the world are encouraged to send sail plans upon departure from port, and periodic position reports enroute, to cooperating radio stations who will forward them to the AMVER Center on Governors Island in lower New York Harbor. There, the information is entered into a computer which calculates positions by dead reckoning for the ships throughout their voyages, based upon most recent information. When a recognized *Rescue Coordination Center (RCC)* of any nation learns of an emergency at sea, it is encouraged to obtain a computer-predicted listing of ships in the vicinity of the emergency to see which, if any, might be well-suited to provide help. Valuable search and rescue data, such as each ship's radio watch schedule and whether she carries a doctor, are kept on file in the computer and also printed for each ship listed. The location of an individual vessel, if participating, may be obtained by rescue authorities if her safety is in question.

DH MEDICO

DH MEDICO messages and responses thereto may be coordinated, or at least monitored, by a Rescue Coordination Center (RCC) of some nation. Most DH MEDICO messages sent via U.S. Coast Guard radio stations are handled by a Coast Guard RCC. The RCC will assist in the determination of the necessary action, if treatment by ship's personnel until arrival in port is insufficient for the well-being of the patient. The necessary action is determined by such things as seriousness of the case, position of the ship, and the location of nearby assisting facilities. The recommended action simply may be treatment by the ship's person-

nel, evacuation of the patient by helicopter, diversion of the ship to port to put the patient ashore, or a rendezvous at sea with another ship which is carrying a doctor on board. If such a rendezvous is necessary, arrangements can be faciliated by use of information from the U.S. Coast Guard's AMVER system.

Rendezvous at Sea

To arrange for a rendezvous at sea for a vessel with a medical case, a Rescue Coordination Center (RCC) may ask the AMVER Center in New York for a surface picture (SURPIC) listing vessels in the vicinity with a doctor on board. For example, the computer may be asked for all such ships within a radius of 500 miles from the position of the vessel with a medical case, or all such ships along the trackline from its present position to its destination. If such vessels show up on the SURPIC, the RCC may provide the patient's vessel with information on the most appropriate one so that a rendezvous can be arranged. Communications between the patient-vessel and the doctor-ship should be established as soon as practicable. Any rendezvous and subsequent transfer of personnel must be mutually agreeable to the Masters of the vessels involved.

It should be pointed out there is no guarantee that another ship with a doctor on board will be in a position to help the vessel with the medical problem. However, AMVER information often has been used to arrange MEDICO rendezvous with mutual benefit to all concerned.

The current list of radio stations cooperating in the AMVER program is printed in the AMVER Bulletin, published every two months by the AMVER Center. Masters may request their vessels to be placed on the mailing list for the AMVER Bulletin by writing to:

AMVER Center

U.S. Coast Guard

Governors Island, N.Y. 10004

Chapter XIII

Helicopter Evacuation At Sea *

A GUIDE FOR MERCHANT VESSELS

WHEN A MERCHANT VESSEL is faced with a medical evacuation at sea, lives depend on knowing the right procedures and on planning well in advance. Obviously, getting a patient to a doctor is foremost in everyone's mind. However, the patient is not the only one in danger. An oversight or poor planning on the ship can imperil the helicopter, its crew, and even the patient's shipmates helping on deck. Knowing the correct evacuation procedure makes it safer for everyone. Most procedures used by U. S. Coast Guard helicopters are identical to those practiced throughout the world.

First, distance will determine whether an evacuation is even possible. The maximum range of the types of helicopters now used by the U. S. Coast Guard, the HH–52A amphibious single-turbine powered and the HH–3F amphibious twin-turbine-powered, is 150 and 300 nautical miles respectively. This is in *ideal* weather with *ideal* weight aboard, and includes going out, hovering for 10 minutes, and returning. Bad weather or extra weight shorten these distances.

Obviously, if a merchant vessel is 500 miles at sea and needs a helicopter evacuation, she will have to divert and head for a point where a helicopter can reach her. Normally, the *Rescue Coordination Center* working on the case will tell the ship if a diversion is necessary, and a rendezvous point will be established.

The sooner the Captain acknowledges by message that the ship will be diverted to the designated rendezvous point and gives its estimated time of arrival, the sooner the helicopter can be launched. If the vessel already is within helicopter range, a diversion in the direction of the helicopter's base may be beneficial to speed the removal of the patient.

For planning the evacuation and discussing the patient's condition, good ship-helicopter communication is crucial. A fixed-wing aircraft often escorts a helicopter during an offshore evacuation, both to locate the ship in order to guide the helicopter to the scene, and to help with communications. Therefore, it is not unusual for a fixed-wing aircraft to circle the vessel and communicate with it before the helicopter arrives, relaying information until the helicopter is within communication range.

Voice communications between ship and aircraft normally are conducted on international distress and/or calling frequencies such as 2182 kHz and 156.8 MHz. Other frequencies common to both helicopter and vessel may be used, but once good communications have been established, frequency changes should be avoided. If necessary, helicopters can transmit and receive voice—Double Side Band or Single Side Band—on high frequencies between 2,000 kHz and 30,000 kHz. Homing capabilities for the

* Source: AMVER BULLETIN (*A*utomated *M*utual-assistance *VE*ssel *R*escue System). Issue Number 11/12:73, pp. 5–9. Published bimonthly by the Commander, Atlantic Area United States Coast Guard, Governor's Island, New York, N.Y. 10004.

helicopter often are available on many frequencies.

If voice communications cannot be established when it arrives on the scene, the helicopter will attempt to set up communications through other means. These consist of: lowering a portable radio, using a portable loud hailer, dropping message blocks, lowering a handset connected to the helicopter's intercommunications equipment, using a chalk board, or using hand signals. If there is no practical way of communicating, the helicopter may move right into position and begin the hoist.

Whatever the communication method on scene, the vessel earlier should have provided the *Rescue Coordination Center* with as accurate a position as possible, including course, speed, weather and sea conditions, and wind direction and velocity. *Medical information on the patient should include whether or not he is ambulatory. Coast Guard helicopters normally do not carry a stretcher, so if one is needed, the crew must know before takeoff so it can be put aboard.*

After the helicopter has taken off, the vessel will be told its estimated time of arrival (ETA). Most probably, communications will be established first with the fixed-wing aircraft, and later with the helicopter as it gets closer. Frequent transmissions may be requested from the ship for homing purposes, so she should stand a continuous watch on the assigned frequency.

With or without ship-to-aircraft communication, the Captain can prepare for the hoist prior to the helicopter's arrival. Most merchant vessels have a clear area from which the hoist can be made safely, usually on the fantail. The more space made available, the easier and less hazardous is the hoist. A horizontal distance of 50 feet in all directions from the helicopter body is a minimum safe clearance. Although Coast Guard helicopters can hoist from substantial heights, the higher the hoist, the more difficult and dangerous it is.

If the hoist is to be from the fantail and an awning covers it, this should be removed and tied up securely, along with any other items that may be blown about by the rotor downwash of the helicopter. Booms extending aft near the fantail should be raised as vertically as possible alongside the king posts. Aft flagstaffs should be taken down and antenna wires or cables extending to the stern removed, if possible. Any reduction of obstruction on the stern, or wherever the hoist is made, will mean a lower and easier hoist.

Shortly before the helicopter arrives, and if the weather and the patient's condition permit, the patient should be brought up from below and placed under cover near, but not in, the hoist area. Blankets should be wrapped securely around the patient so the rotor downwash does not blow them away.

As the helicopter arrives, change the vessel's course into the wind, ideally with it about 20 degrees on the port bow. It is not only unnecessary for the vessel to slow or stop, but actually preferable to maintain normal speed because the helicopter can make the hoist with better control at a forward speed of 10 to 15 knots.

Final instructions for the hoist will be given by the pilot after seeing the ship and its obstructions. The pilot may not want to use the planned position, but will lower the basket or stretcher to another section of the vessel, if that appears safer. *The helicopter is equipped with a rescue basket for patients able to sit in it. However, if a stretcher is needed, it should have been requested so that a specially-equipped one with a hoisting bridle can be used. It is difficult to adapt quickly a ship's stretcher to this type of suspension.*

During its flight, the aircraft builds up a static electricity charge. Anyone who reaches up to take hold of the basket or stretcher will most certainly get a shock. *Therefore, always let the basket or stretcher touch the deck before handling it.* If a high hoist is involved, or if the hoist is from a confined space, the helicopter may lower a trail line. Deck personnel can guide the basket to the deck with this line, as long as they do not touch the basket itself.

Instinctively, the patient will grasp the side of the basket. The patient should be warned of the possibility of injuring his fingers if the basket hits the side of the helicopter as it is being brought aboard. When the patient is ready for the hoist he should nod his head. Then deck personnel will signal the hoist operator in the helicopter by indicating thumbs up, and the hoist begins. The basket or stretcher should be steadied to minimize swinging, and steadying lines used if the hoist is so equipped. For safety, nobody should stand under the basket.

If the patient is so ill that the stretcher must be brought to him, it will have to be unhooked from the hoist cable. *Don't try to take the stretcher away from the hoist point without unhooking and letting it go free.* Normally, the pilot will retrieve the cable, then pull away from the ship until he sees the patient aboard the stretcher and ready to be hoisted. *Never hook the cable to any part of the ship! Never secure the litter or the rescue basket to the vessel, while the hoist cable still is attached to the litter or basket!*

Special lighting precautions will be necessary if the hoist takes place at night. Because of visibility and depth perception problems and the pilot's inability to judge his height above the water, he probably will have to make an instrument approach to the vessel. Lighting of the ship and the hoist area is necessary, but it is important not to shine any lights into the cockpit of the aircraft, nor to have any deck lights pointing up toward the helicopter. Such lights can disorient or blind the pilot. If a searchlight is used to help the aircraft locate the ship, it should point vertically and be secured, once the helicopter has reached the area. Any boom lights used to light the deck should be directed downward.

Hoists can be made from the deck of ocean-going vessels 99 percent of the time. Although using a small boat from which to hoist the patient has been done successfully, it is the exception rather than the rule. If a small boat must be used, the sea should be relatively calm, with the boat underway during the hoist to maintain steerageway and to keep from foundering in the rotor wash of the helicopter. Again, the wind should be dead ahead or on the port bow.

Every helicopter medical evacuation at sea is different, and each presents its own problems. Communications between pilot and ship may be impossible. Operations at night, or under poor weather conditions, require the utmost caution and capability of the pilot. But in each case, knowing what to expect and how to prepare, and what the accepted procedure is, can save time, effort—and a life.

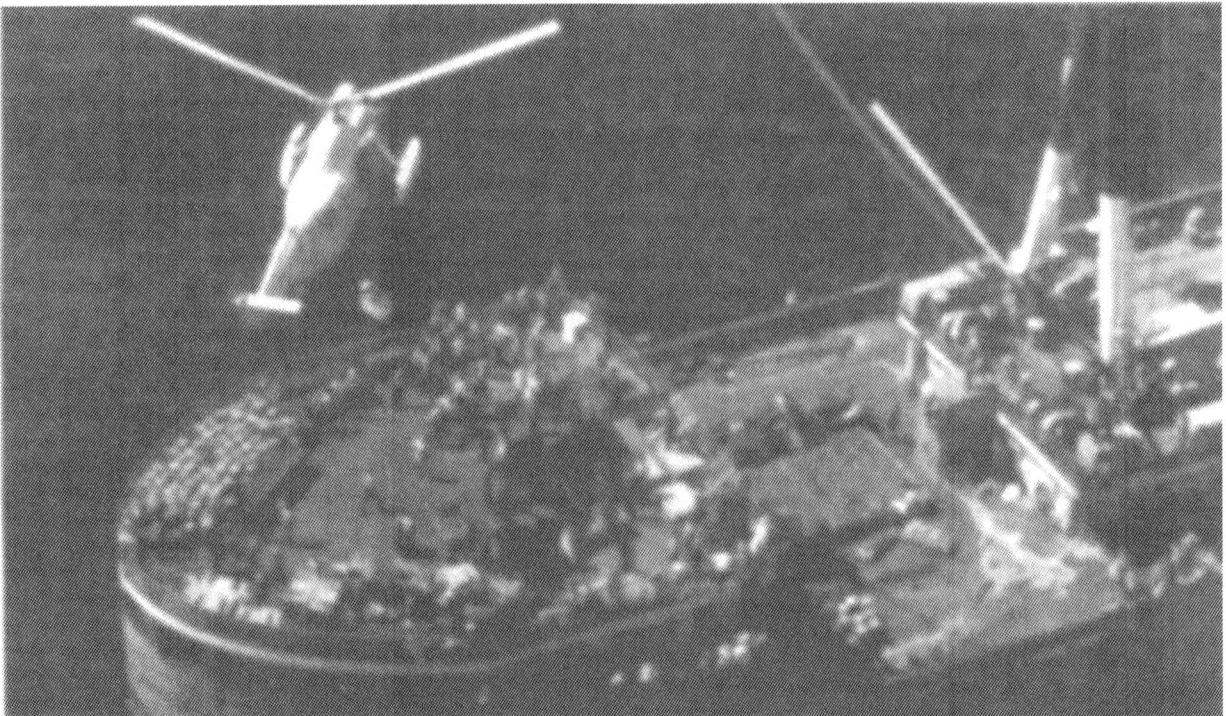

Fig. 13–1. During a medical evacuation at sea, a basket is lowered from helicopter to vessel to pick up the patient.

HELICOPTER EVACUATION CHECKOFF LIST

This checkoff list was prepared for use in evacuations carried out by U.S. Coast Guard helicopters. In general, these procedures are applicable to helicopter operations conducted by other rescue agencies.

Remember:

Helicopter evacuation is a hazardous operation to the patient *and* the plane crew, and it should be attempted only when the life of the patient is gravely threatened. Provide the doctor with all the information you can about the patient so that an intelligent evaluation can be made on the need for evacuation.

When requesting helicopter assistance:

1. Give an accurate position, speed and course of the vessel; time; weather conditions; wind direction and velocity; voice and CW frequencies.

2. If not already provided, give *complete* medical information including whether or not the patient is ambulatory.

3. If your vessel is beyond helicopter range, advise on your diversion intentions so that a rendezvous point may be selected.

4. If there are any changes, advise immediately. Should the patient expire prior to arrival of the helicopter, be sure to advise. Remember, the flight crew are risking their lives attempting to help you.

Preparations prior to arrival of the helicopter:

1. Provide continuous radio guard on 2182 kHz, or specified *voice* frequency if possible. The helicopter cannot operate CW.

2. Select and clear the most suitable hoist area, preferably aft, with a minimum 50-foot radius. This must include the securing of loose gear, awnings, and antenna wires. Trice up running rigging and booms. If the hoist is aft, lower the flagstaff.

3. If the hoist is at night, light the pickup area as well as possible. *Be sure you do not shine any lights on the helicopter,* so the pilot is not blinded. If there are obstructions in the vicinity, put a light on them so the pilot will be aware of their positions.

4. Point searchlights vertically to aid in locating the ship, and secure them when the helicopter is on scene.

5. Advise on the location of the pickup area *before* the helicopter arrives, so that an approach may be made aft, amidships, or forward, as required.

6. There will be a high noise level under the helicopter, making voice communication almost impossible. Arrange a set of hand signals among the crew who will assist.

HELICOPTER EVACUATION CHECKOFF LIST (Continued)

Hoist operations:

1. If possible, move the patient to a position as close to the hoist area as his condition permits—*time is important.*

2. Normally, if a litter is required, it will be necessary to move the patient to the special litter which will be lowered by the helicopter. Be prepared to do this as quickly as possible. Be sure the patient is strapped in, face up, *with a life jacket, if his condition permits.*

3. Be sure the patient is tagged to indicate what medication, if any, was administered, and when.

4. Have the patient's medical record and necessary papers in an envelope or package ready for transfer *with* him.

5. Change course so the ship rides as easily as possible with the wind on the bow, preferably on the port bow. Try to choose a course to keep stack gases clear of the hoist area.

6. Reduce speed if necessary to ease the ship's motion, but maintain steerageway.

7. If you do not have radio contact with the helicopter, when you are in all respects ready for the hoist, signal the helicopter to come in with a "come-on" by hand, or at night by flashlight.

8. **To avoid static shock, allow the basket or stretcher to touch the deck prior to handling.**

9. If a trail line is dropped by the helicopter, guide the basket or stretcher to the deck with the line. Keep the line clear at all times.

10. Place the patient in the basket, sitting with both hands clear of the sides, or in the litter as described above. Signal the helicopter hoist operator when ready for the hoist. The patient should signal by nodding his head, if he is able. Deck personnel should give thumbs up.

11. If it is necessary to take the litter away from the hoist point, unhook the hoist cable and keep it free for the helicopter to haul in. *Do not secure the cable to the vessel or attempt to move the stretcher without unhooking.*

12. When the patient is strapped in the stretcher, signal the helicopter to lower the cable, hook up, and signal the hoist operator when ready to hoist. Steady the stretcher from swinging or turning.

13. If the trail line is attached to the basket or stretcher, use to steady. Keep feet clear of the line.

Appendices

Appendix A

HOSPITALS AND OUTPATIENT CLINICS
CONTRACT PHYSICIANS
U.S. Public Health Service

Hospitals and Outpatient Clinics

Since 1798, the Federal Government has furnished medical care to sick and disabled American merchant seamen. Table A–1 that follows lists eight hospitals and 30 outpatient clinics of the U.S. Public Health Service which provide emergency and followup general medical care for eligible merchant seamen.

Contract Physicians

Many of the PHS facilities have contracted with private physicians to provide medical care to seamen. These *contract physicians* generally are located in geographic areas where there are no PHS facilities. If merchant seamen require medical care, and no PHS hospital or outpatient clinic is nearby, they should check the local telephone directory to determine whether a local physician may be listed as a *contract physician* for the U.S. Public Health Service. In the local telephone directory, turn to the section on the UNITED STATES GOVERNMENT—Health, Education, and Welfare, Department of.

Also seamen may phone or write to the nearest PHS facility (see Table A–1) to inquire where there is a conveniently located *contract physician* to whom they might go for eligible medical care.

Table A–1

HOSPITALS AND OUTPATIENT CLINICS
U.S. Public Health Service

Location	Street Address	Area Code	Telephone Number
HOSPITALS			
Baltimore, Maryland 21211	3100 Wyman Park Drive	301	338–3000
Boston, Mass. 02135	77 Warren Street	617	782–3400
Nassau Bay, Texas 77058	2050 Space Park Drive		
New Orleans, La. 70118	210 State Street	504	899–3441
Norfolk, Virginia 23508	6500 Hampton Blvd.	804	423–5800
San Francisco, Calif. 94118	15th Ave. and Lake St.	415	752–1400
Seattle, Washington 98144	1131 14th Ave. So.	206	324–7650
Staten Island, N.Y. 10304	Bay St. and Vanderbilt Ave.	212	447–3010
OUTPATIENT CLINICS			
Atlanta, Georgia 30333	1600 Clifton Road, N.E.	404	633–3311
Balboa Heights, Canal Zone	------------------	---	52–7968
Buffalo, New York 14203	50 High Street, Rm. 609	716	846–4721

Table A–1 (Continued)

HOSPITALS AND OUTPATIENT CLINICS
U.S. Public Health Service

Location	Street Address	Area Code	Telephone Number
OUTPATIENT CLINICS ((Continued)			
Charleston, S.C. 29403	214 Fed. Bldg., 334 Meeting St.	803	577–4171 (Ext 256)
Charlotte Amalie Virgin Islands 00801	U.S. Federal Office Bldg. Veterans Blvd.	809	774–2301
Chicago, Illinois 60605	1439 S. Michigan Avenue	312	353–5900
Cincinnati, Ohio 45202	P.O. and Courthouse Bldg. 5th and Walnut Sts.	513	684–2115
Cleveland, Ohio 44113	New P.O. Bldg., West 3rd St. and Prospect Ave.	216	522–4524
Detroit, Michigan 48215	14700 Riverside Drive	313	822–9300
Galveston, Texas 77550	4400 Avenue N	713	763–1211
Honolulu, Hawaii 96807	591 Ala Moana Boulevard	808	546–5670
Houston, Texas 77002	204 U.S. Customs Building 701 San Jacinto St.	713	226–4871
Jacksonville, Fla. 32201	P.O. Bldg., Suite 118 311 W. Monroe St.	904	791–3541
Juneau, Alaska 99801	Bartlett Mem. Hosp. 419-6th Street	---	--------
Memphis, Tennessee 38104	969 Madison Ave.	901	725–9550
Miami, Florida 33130	51 S.W. 1st Ave., Rm. 712	305	350–5385
Mobile, Alabama 36602	125 Federal Bldg.	205	690–2261
New York, N.Y. 10014	245 West Houston St.	212	620–3217
Philadelphia, Pa. 19106	U.S. Custom House, Rm. 700 2nd and Chestnut Streets	215	597–4099
Pittsburgh, Pa. 15219	U.S. Post Office and Courthouse 7th Ave. and Grant St.	412	644–3376
Port Arthur, Texas 77640	Fed. Office Building, Rm 209 5th St. and Austin Ave.	713	982–2732
Portland, Maine 04103	331 Veranda St.	207	775–3131
Portland, Oregon 97205	220 Courthouse Broadway and Main St.	503	221–2147
St. Louis, Missouri 63103	1520 Market St.	314	425–4851
San Diego, Calif. 92101	2105 Fifth Ave.	714	293–5020
San Juan, Puerto Rico 00904	8½ Fernandez Juncos Ave.	809	723–5200
San Pedro, Calif. 90731	825 S. Beacon St.	213	548–2611
Savannah, Georgia 31401	1602 Drayton Street	912	232–4321 (Ext 308)
Tampa, Florida 33601	601 Florida Ave.	813	228–2674
Washington, D.C. 20201	Switzer Bldg. 4th and C Sts., S.W.	202	245–1638

Appendix B

REGULATIONS GOVERNING MEDICAL CARE
FOR SEAMEN AND CERTAIN OTHER PERSONS

U.S. Public Health Service

The following excerpt from the Code of Federal Regulations states the requirements which must be met by American seamen in order to be provided medical services by the United States Public Health Service (PHS).

For further information on PHS medical care for American seamen, contact the director of any PHS hospital or PHS outpatient clinic in the United States. (See Directory, Appendix A, pp. 428–9.)

Title 42—Public Health

Chapter 1—Public Health Service, U.S. Department of Health, Education, and Welfare

AUTHORITY: Sec. 2, 321, 322, 58 Stat. 682, 695, 696 as amended; 42 U.S.C. 2, 248, 249. Sec. 32.86 to 32.90 issued under sec. 331 and 332, 58 Stat. 696, 698 as amended; 42 U.S.C. 255, 256.

SOURCE: 40 FR 25816, June 19, 1975, unless otherwise noted.

Definitions

§32.1   *Meaning of terms.*

All terms not defined herein shall have the same meaning as given them in the Act.

(a) "Act" means the Public Health Service Act, approved July 1, 1944, 58 Stat. 682, as amended;

(b) "Service" means the Public Health Service;

(c) "Secretary" means the Secretary of Health, Education, and Welfare and any other officer or employee of the Department of

Health, Education, and Welfare to whom the authority involved may have been delegated.

(d) "Seamen" includes any person employed on board in the care, preservation, or navigation of any vessel, or in the service on board, of those engaged in such care, preservation, or navigation, but does not include the owner or joint owners of a vessel or the spouse of any such owner, except owner-operators as described in §32.6(a)(12);

(e) "Vessel" includes every description of watercraft or other artificial contrivance used, or capable of being used, as a means of transportation on water, exclusive of aircraft and amphibious contrivances;

(f) "Authorizing Official" means Service officers or employees duly designated by the Director, Division of Hospitals and Clinics to authorize and provide care and treatment to beneficiaries at Service expense;

(g) "Active Duty," with respect to an enrollee of the United States Maritime Service, means that the enrollee is on the active list of that service, as distinguished from being on inactive status, and includes absence on authorized leave or liberty;

(h) "Commercial fishing operations" means the gathering of any form of either fresh water or marine animal life for sale on a commercial basis through available markets.

Beneficiaries

§32.6 *Persons eligible.*

(a) Under this part the following persons are entitled to care and treatment by the Service as hereinafter prescribed:

1. Seamen employed on vessels of the United States registered, enrolled, or licensed under the maritime laws thereof, other than canal boats engaged in the coasting trade, hereinafter designated as American seamen;

2. Seamen employed on United States or foreign flag vessels as employees of the United States;

3. Seamen, not enlisted or commissioned in the military or naval establishments, who are employed on State school ships or on vessels of the United States Government of more than five tons burden;

4. Seamen on vessels of the Mississippi River Commission;

5. Officers and crew members of vessels of the Fish and Wildlife Service;

6. Enrollees in the United States Maritime Service on active duty and members of the Merchant Marine Cadet Corps;

7. Cadets at State maritime academies or on State training ships;

8. Seamen-trainees while participating in maritime training programs to develop or enhance their employability in the maritime industry;

9. Persons afflicted with Hansen's disease;

10. Seamen on foreign flag vessels other than those seamen employed on foreign flag vessels specified in subparagraph (2) of this paragraph;

11. Non-beneficiaries for temporary treatment and care in case of emergency;

12. Persons who own vessels registered, enrolled, or licensed under the maritime laws of the United States, who are engaged in commercial fishing operations, and who accompany such vessels on such fishing operations, and a substantial part of whose services in connection with such fishing operations are comparable to services performed by seamen employed on such vessel or on vessels engaged in similar operations.

(b) Separate regulations govern:

1. The medical care of certain personnel and their dependents, of the Coast Guard, National Oceanic and Atmospheric Administration and Public Health Service (see Part 31 of this chapter);

2. physical and mental examinations of aliens (see Part 34 of this chapter);

3. care and treatment of narcotic addicts (see Part 33 of this chapter); and (4) Medical Care for Indians. (See Part 36 of this chapter.)

(c) While regulations of the Public Health Service are not required with respect thereto, circular instructions by the Service cover the care and treatment or physical examination of the following;

1. Persons not otherwise eligible for treatment for purposes of study;

2. Persons detained in accordance with quarantine laws;

3. Persons detained by the Immigration and Naturalization Service, for treatment at the request of that Service;

4. Persons entitled to treatment under the Federal Employees' Compensation Act and extensions thereof;

5. Beneficiaries of other Federal agencies on a reimbursable basis;

6. Medical examinations of;

i Employees of the Alaska Railroad and employees of the Federal Government for retirement purposes;

ii Employees in the Federal classified service, and applicants for appointment, as requested by the Civil Service Commission for the purpose of promoting health and efficiency;

iii Seamen for purposes of qualifying for certificates of service; and

iv Employees eligible for benefits under the Longshoremen's and Harbor Workers' Compensation Act, as amended as requested by any deputy commissioner thereunder.

American Seamen

§32.11 Scope of benefits.

(a) American seamen (hereinafter referred to in §§32.11 to 32.23, inclusive, as seamen) shall, on presenting evidence of eligibility, be entitled to medical, surgical, and dental treatment or hospitalization at medical care facilities operated by the Service or, in accordance with these regulations, at Service contract medical facilities at the expense of the Service.

(b) Where medical facilities of the Service are not available, medical care and services may be obtained from contract medical providers designated by the Service. Expenses for medical care and services obtained from non-Service providers or in non-Service facilities not arranged for by the Service in behalf of seamen is not an obligation of the Service and will not be paid.

§32.12 Provision of services.

(a) When a seaman requires medical, surgical and dental treatment or hospitalization which the Service is unable to provide in the local Service operated facility, or in the case of an emergency, arrangements for such medical, surgical, and dental treatment or hospitalization at the expense of the Service shall be made by an authorizing official.

(b) If eligibility cannot be established at the time of application by the seaman or by the person who applies in his behalf, the applicant shall be notified that the authorization for treatment is conditional and that the payment of reasonable expenses by the Service for such treatment shall be subject to proof of eligibility.

(c) The authorizing official shall keep himself informed regarding the progress of the case in order that treatment or hospitalization shall not be unnecessarily prolonged.

§32.13 Application for treatment.

(a) In nonemergency cases, a sick or disabled seaman, in order to obtain the benefits of the Service, must apply in person, or by proxy if too sick to do so, to an authorizing official as specified in §32.12, and must furnish satisfactory evidence of his eligibility for such benefits.

(b) In emergency cases, a sick or disabled seaman shall, upon admission for such condition or as soon thereafter as is practicable under the circumstances, either personally or by proxy, notify the nearest authorizing official of the fact of such admission and treatment and shall furnish appropriate identification and satisfactory evidence of eligibility for such benefits.

§32.14 Evidence of eligibility.

(a) As evidence of his eligibility a seaman must present a properly executed MASTER'S CERTIFICATE, or a continuous discharge book, or a certificate of discharge, showing that he has been employed on a registered, enrolled, or licensed vessel of the United States. The certificate of the owner or accredited commercial agent of a vessel as to the facts of the employment of any seaman on said vessel may be accepted in lieu of the MASTER'S CERTIFICATE where the latter is not procurable. When an applicant cannot furnish any of the foregoing documents, his certification as to the facts of his most recent (including his last) employment as a seaman, stating names of vessels and dates of service, may be accepted as evidence in support of his eligibility. Documentary evidence of eligibility, excepting continuous discharge books and certificates of discharge, shall be filed at the medical care facility of the Service where application is made. Where continuous discharge books and certificates of discharge are submitted as evidence of eligibility, the pertinent information shall be abstracted therefrom, certified by the officer accepting the application, and filed at the station.

(b) Except as otherwise provided in §§32.11 to 32.23, inclusive, documentary evidence of eligibility must show that the applicant has been employed for 60 days of continuous service on a registered, enrolled, or licensed vessel of the United States, a part of which time must have been during the 180 days immediately preceding application for relief. There may be included as a part of such 60 days of continuous service as a seaman time spent in training as:

1. an active duty enrollee in the United Maritime Service;

2. a member of the Merchant Marine Cadet Corps;
member of the Merchant Marine Cadet Corps;

3. a cadet at a State maritime academy; or

4. a cadet on a State training ship. The phrase "60 days of continuous service" shall not be held to exclude seamen whose papers show brief intermissions between short services that aggregate the required 60 days: Provided, that any such intermission does not exceed 60 days. The time during which a seaman has been treated as a patient of the Service shall not be considered as absence from the vessel in determining eligibility. When the seamen's service on his last vessel is less than 60 days, his oath or affirmation as to previous service may be accepted.

§3215. Sickness or injury while employed.

A seaman taken sick or injured on board or ashore when actually employed on a vessel shall be entitled to care and treatment without regard to length of service.

§32.16 Seamen from wrecked vessels.

Seamen taken from wrecked vessels of the United States and returned to the United States, if sick or disabled at the time of their arrival in the United States, shall be entitled to care and treatment without regard to length of service.

§32.17 Lapse of more than 180 days since last service.

(a) Where more than 180 days have elapsed since an applicant's last service as a seaman, he will no longer be eligible for benefits from the Service: Provided, That if he can show that he has not definitely changed his occupation, such period of time shall not exclude him from receiving care and treatment (1) if due in whole or in part to closure of navigation or economic conditions resulting in decreased shipping with consequent lack of opportunity to ship; or (2) if he provides satisfactory evidence that he has been under continuous medical supervision and treatment at other than Service expense for a condition which occurred or arose during any period of treatment at a Service facility or at Service expense.

(b) Where a seaman receives care and treatment by the Service or at Service expense during a period of eligibility for a condition or illness which requires, in the opinion of the attending physician, continuing and recurring care and treatment on a regular and frequent basis, such periods of continuing and recurring care and treatment whether obtained privately by the seaman or at Service facilities or Service expense shall not be included in the computation of the 180 day period above.

§32.18 Procedure in case of doubtful eligibility.

When a reasonable doubt exists as to the eligibility of an applicant for service, the matter shall be referred immediately to the appropriate authorizing official or Hospital Director for decision. If, in the opinion of such person the applicant's condition is such that immediate care and treatment is necessary, temporary care and treatment shall be given pending the decision as to eligibility.

§32.19 False document evidencing service.

The issue or presentation of a false document as evidence of service with intent to procure the treatment of a person as a seaman shall be immediately reported to the Headquarters of the Service.

§32.20 Treatment during voyage.

The Service shall not be liable for expenses incurred during a voyage for the care of sick and disabled seamen.

§32.21 Care while in custody.

Seamen shall not be provided treatment at the expense of the Service while in police custody.

§32.22 *Reconsideration of eligibility denial.*

A decision of the authorizing official or Hospital Director denying eligibility shall be communicated to the seaman in writing, shall set forth the reasons therefor, and shall state that such decision may be reconsidered by the Secretary upon written request setting forth the facts in support of such request.

§32.23 *Certificate of discharge from treatment.*

A certificate of discharge from treatment may, at the discretion of the officer in charge, be given to a hospital patient, but such certificate, when presented at another medical care facility shall not be taken as establishing the seaman's eligibility for further care and treatment, but may be considered in connection with other documentary evidence of eligibility submitted by the seaman.

Seamen; State School Ships and Vessels of the United States Government

§32.46 *Conditions and extent of treatment.*

Seamen, not enlisted or commissioned in the military naval establishments, who are employed on State school ships, on vessels of the United States Government of more than five tons burden, or on vessels of the Mississippi River Commission or of the Fish and Wildlife Service, shall be entitled to care and treatment by the Service under the same conditions, where applicable, and to the same extent as is provided for American seamen.

Owner-Operators of Commercial Fishing Vessels

§32.57 *Conditions and extent of treatment.*

Persons who own vessels registered, enrolled, or licensed under the maritime laws of the United States, who are engaged in commercial fishing operations, and who accompany such vessels on such fishing operations, and a substantial part of whose services in connection with such fishing operations are comparable to services performed by seamen employed on such vessel or on vessels engaged in similar operations shall be entitled to care and treatment by the Service under the same conditions, where applicable, and to the same extent as is provided for American seamen.

Maritime Service Enrollees and Merchant Marine Cadets

§32.61 *Use of Service facilities.*

(a) Enrollees in the United States Maritime Service on active duty and members of the Merchant Cadet Corps shall, upon written request of the responsible officer of the station or training ship to which such enrollees or cadets are attached, identifying the applicant, be entitled to medical, surgical, and dental treatment or hospitalization at medical care facilities of the Service or at Service expense. Whenever an enrollee or cadet applies for care without the above-mentioned written request and in the opinion of the responsible Service officer the applicant's condition is such that immediate care and treatment is necessary, temporary care and treatment shall be given pending verification of the applicant's status as an enrollee or cadet.

(b) If eligibility cannot be established at the time of application by the enrollee or cadet or by the person who applies in his behalf, the applicant shall be notified that the authorization for treatment is conditional and that the payment of reasonable expenses by the Service for such treatment shall be subject to proof of eligibility.

(c) The authorizing official shall keep himself informed regarding the progress of the case in order that treatment or hospitalization shall not be unnecessarily prolonged.

§32.62 *Injury while in custody.*

Enrollees on active duty or cadets shall not be provided treatment at the expense of the Service while in police custody.

§32.63 *Absence without leave.*

Enrollees on active duty or cadets shall not be entitled, when absent without leave, to receive medical care except at a medical care facility of the Service or under contract to the Service.

Cadets at State Maritime Academies or on State Training Ships

§32.76 *Conditions and extent of treatment.*

Cadets at State maritime academies or on State training ships shall be entitled to care and treatment by the Service under the same conditions and to the same extent as is provided for American seamen. Provided, however, that the written request of the superintendent or other responsible officer of an academy, including the Master of a training ship, shall be accepted in lieu of the documentary evidence of eligibility required of American seamen.

Persons with Hansen's Disease

§32.86 *Admissions to Service facilities.*

Any person with Hansen's disease who presents himself for care or treatment or who is referred to the Service by the proper health authority of any State, Territory, or the District of Columbia shall be received into the Service hospital at Carville, Louisiana, or into any other hospital of the Service which has been designated by the Secretary as being suitable for the accommodation of persons with Hansen's disease.

§32.87 *Confirmation of diagnosis.*

At the earliest practicable date, after the arrival of a patient at the Service hospital at Carville, Louisiana, or at another hospital of the Service the medical staff shall confirm or disprove the diagnosis of Hansen's disease. If the diagnosis of Hansen's disease is confirmed, the patient shall be provided appropriate inpatient or outpatient treatment. If the diagnosis is not confirmed, the patient shall be discharged. [40 FR 25816, June 19, 1975; 49 FR 36774, Aug. 22, 1975]

§32.88 *Examinations and treatment.*

Patients will be provided necessary clinical examinations which may be required for the diagnosis of primary or secondary conditions, and such treatment as may be prescribed.

§32.89 *Discharge.*

Patients with Hansen's disease will be discharged when, in the opinion of the medical staff of the hospital, optimum hospital benefits have been received.

§32.90 *Notification to health authorities regarding discharged patients.*

Upon the discharge of a patient the medical officer in charge shall give notification of such discharge to the appropriate health officer of the State, Territory, or other jurisdiction in which the discharged patient is to reside. The notification shall also set forth the clinical findings and other essential facts necessary to be known by the health officer relative to such discharged patient.

Seamen on Foreign Flag Vessels

§32.106 *Conditions and extent of treatment; rates; burial.*

(a) Seamen on foreign flag vessels may, when suitable accommodations are available and on application of the Master, owner, or agent of the vessel, be provided treatment at medical care facilities of the Service at rates prescribed by the Secretary.

(b) Upon application, the Service may assist in arranging for private hospitalization of such seamen or private services in connection with their treatment at the expense of the Master, owner, or agent of the vessel.

(c) If any such seaman dies while receiving treatment by the Service, the expenses of burial shall be paid directly to the vendors by the Master, owner, or agent.

Nonbeneficiaries: Temporary Treatment in Emergency

§32.111 *Conditions and extent of treatment; charges.*

(a) Persons not entitled to treatment by the Service may be provided temporary care and treatment at medical care facilities of the Service in case of emergency as an act of humanity.

(b) Persons referred to in paragraph (a) of this section who, as determined by the officer in charge of the Service facility, are able to defray the cost of their care and treatment shall be charged for such care and treatment at the following rates (which shall be deemed to constitute the entire charge in each instance): In the case of hospitalization, at the current interdepartmental reciprocal per diem rate; and, in the case of outpatient treatment, at rates established by the Secretary.

Appendix C

REGULATIONS GOVERNING FOREIGN QUARANTINE
U.S. Public Health Service

Introduction

The U.S. Public Health Service administers foreign quarantine procedures at ports of entry under the control of the United States.

All vessels arriving at ports under the control of the United States are subject to public health inspection. Only the following vessels upon arrival are subject to *routine boarding* for quarantine inspection:

(1) vessels which have been in a smallpox-infected country in the 15 days prior to arrival;

(2) vessels which have been in a plague-infected country within 60 days prior to arrival; and

(3) vessels which have had on board *any of the following signs of illness* during the 15 days preceeding arrival—

(a) A temperature of 100° F (38° C) or greater, which was accompanied or followed by any one or all of the following; rash, jaundice, glandular swelling; OR

(b) Diarrhea severe enough to interfere with work or normal activity; and

(c) Death, regardless of foregoing criteria.

Masters of vessels having illness aboard compatible with the above criteria must provide notification of the illness by radio through their agent to the quarantine station at the intended U.S. port of arrival.

Vessels arriving at ports under control of the United States are subject to sanitary inspection to determine whether measures should be applied to prevent the introduction, transmission, or spread of communicable diseases.

Specific public health laws, regulations, policies, and procedures may be obtained by contacting United States Quarantine Stations, United States Consulates, or the

> Director, Quarantine Division
> Bureau of Epidemiology
> Center for Disease Control
> U.S. Public Health Service
> Atlanta, Georgia 30333

International Health Regulations (1969)*

THE UNITED STATES GOVERNMENT is a member of the World Health Organization (WHO) of the United Nations and is a signatory of the international health regulations, without reservations. Following are some of the pertinent articles that deal with quarantine requirements. See pp. 445–62 for copies of important forms that include: (1) a DERATTING CERTIFICATE and/or DERATTING EXEMPTION CERTIFICATE; (2) a MARITIME PUBLIC HEALTH DECLARATION; and (3) INTERNATIONAL CERTIFICATES OF VACCINATION (available as a booklet).

Article 54†

1. Every ship shall be either:
   (a) permanently kept in such a condition that it is free of rodents and the plaque vector; or
   (b) periodically deratted.

2. A Deratting Certificate or a Deratting Exemption Certificate shall be issued only by the health authority for a port approved for that

---

*Adopted by the Twenty-second World Health Assembly in 1969 and amended by the Twenty-sixth World Health Assembly in 1973. (Source: INTERNATIONAL HEALTH REGULATIONS—1969, Second Annotated Edition. Published by the World Health Organization, Geneva. 1974.)

† (a) Deratting Certificates and Deratting Exemption Certificates are valid for a maximum of six months but, under certain conditions, the validity of such certificates may be extended only once by a period of one month. (*Off. Rec. Wld Hlth Org., 79,* 502; *87,* 404; *95,* 482)

(b) If inspection of a ship, carried out at the end of the period of validity of its Deratting Exemption Certificate, proves that the ship is still entitled to a Deratting Exemption Certificate, a new certificate should be issued. Periodic deratting of ships is not necessary if inspection proves that the ship is entitled to a Deratting Exemption Certificate. (*Off. Rec. Wld Hlth Org., 87,* 405)

(c) There is no provision in the Regulations for endorsement by a port health authority of a valid Deratting Certificate or Deratting Exemption Certificate to the effect that inspection of the ship has confirmed the accuracy of the information given on the certificate. (*Off. Rec. Wld Hlth Org., 79,* 502) purpose under Article 17. Every such certificate shall be valid for six months, but this period may be extended by one month for a ship proceeding to such a port if the deratting or inspection, as the case may be, would be facilitated by the operations due to take place there.

3. Deratting Certificates and Deratting Exemption Certificates shall conform with the model shown on pp. 446–7.

4. If a valid certificate is not produced, the health authority for a port approved under Article 17, after inquiry and inspection, may proceed in the following manner:

(a) If the port has been designated under paragraph 2 of Article 17, the health authority may derat the ship or cause the deratting to be done under its direction and control. It shall decide in each case the technique which should be employed to secure the extermination of rodents on the ship. Deratting shall be carried out so as to avoid as far as possible damage to the ship and to any cargo and shall not take longer than is absolutely necessary. Wherever possible deratting shall be done when the holds are empty. In the case of a ship in ballast, it shall be done before loading. When deratting has been satisfactorily completed, the health authority shall issue a Deratting Certificate.

(b) At any port approved under Article 17, the health authority may issue a Deratting Exemption Certificate if it is satisfied that the ship is free of rodents. Such a certificate shall be issued only if the inspection of the ship has been carried out when the holds are empty or when they contain only ballast or other material, unattractive to rodents, of such a nature or so disposed as to make a thorough inspection of the holds possible. A Deratting Exemption Certificate may be issued for an oil tanker with full holds.

5. If the conditions under which a deratting is carried out are such that, in the opinion of the health authority for the port where the operation was performed, a satisfactory result cannot be obtained, the health authority shall make a note to that effect on the existing Deratting Certificate.

Article 84

1. The Master of a seagoing vessel making an international voyage, before arrival at its first port of call in a territory, shall ascertain the state of health on board, and, except when a health administration does not require it, he shall, on arrival, complete and deliver to the health authority for that port a Maritime Declaration of Health which shall be countersigned by the ship's surgeon if one is carried.

2. The Master, and the ship's surgeon if one is carried, shall supply any information required by the health authority as to health conditions on board during the voyage.

3. A Maritime Public Health Declaration shall conform with the model shown on pp. 448–9.

4. A health administration may decide:
(a) either to dispense with the submission of the Maritime Declaration of Health by all arriving ships; or
(b) to require it only if the ship arrives from certain stated areas, or if there is positive information to report.

In either case, the health administration shall inform shipping operators.

Article 92

1. Special treaties or arrangements may be concluded between two or more States having certain interests in common owing to their health, geographical, social or economic conditions, in order to facilitate the application of these Regulations, and in particular with regard to:

(a) the direct and rapid exchange of epidemiological information between neighboring territories;

(b) the health measures to be applied to international coastal traffic and to international traffic on inland waterways, including lakes;

(c) the health measures to be applied in contiguous territories at their common frontier;

(d) the combination of two or more territories into one territory for the purposes of any of the health measures to be applied in accordance with these Regulations;

(e) arrangements for carrying infected persons by means of transport specially adapted for the purpose.

2. The treaties or arrangements referred to in paragraph 1 of this Article shall not be in conflict with the provisions of these Regulations.

3. States shall inform the Organization of any such treaty or arrangement which they may conclude. The Organization shall send immediately to all health administrations information concerning any such treaty or arrangement.

Article 93

1. These Regulations, subject to the provisions of Article 95 and the exceptions hereinafter provided, replace, as between the States bound by these Regulations and as between these States and the Organization, the provisions of the following existing International Sanitary Conventions, Regulations and similar agreements:

(a) International Sanitary Convention, signed in Paris, 3 December 1903;

(b) Pan American Sanitary Convention, signed in Washington, 14 October 1905;

(c) International Sanitary Convention, signed in Paris, 17 January 1912;

(d) International Sanitary Convention, signed in Paris, 21 June 1926;

(e) International Sanitary Convention for Aerial Navigation, signed at The Hague, 12 April 1933;

(f) International Agreement for dispensing with Bills of Health, signed in Paris, 22 December 1934;

(g) International Agreement for dispensing with Consular Visas on Bills of Health, signed in Paris, 22 December 1934;

(h) Convention modifying the International Sanitary Convention of 21 June 1926, signed in Paris, 31 October 1938;

(i) International Sanitary Convention, 1944, modifying the International Sanitary Convention of 21 June 1926, opened for signature in Washington, 15 December 1944;

(j) International Sanitary Convention for Aerial Navigation, 1944; modifying the International Sanitary Convention of 12 April 1933, opened for signature in Washington, 15 December 1944;

(k) Protocol of 23 April 1946 to prolong the International Sanitary Convention, 1944, signed in Washington;

(l) Protocol of 23 April 1946 to prolong the International Sanitary Convention for Aerial Navigation, 1944, signed in Washington;

(m) International Sanitary Regulations, 1951, and the Additional Regulations of 1955, 1956, 1960, 1963, and 1965.

2. The Pan American Sanitary Code, signed at Habana, 14 November 1924, remains in force with the exception of Articles 2, 9, 10, 11, 16 to 53 inclusive, 61, and 62, to which the relevant part of paragraph 1 of this Article shall apply.

Appendix D

MERCHANT VESSELS AND CONTROLLED SUBSTANCES
(Narcotics, Depressants, and Stimulants)

- **Introduction to Federal Regulations**
- **Controlled Substances Act of 1970**
  Schedules I, II, III, IV, V
  Regulations Relating to Merchant Vessels
- **Controlled Substances for Vessels**
  Procurement
  Recordkeeping
  Security
  Forms
- **U.S. Department of Justice**
  Drug Enforcement Administration (DEA)
  DEA Regional Offices (Domestic and Foreign)

Introduction

Congress has enacted legislation over the years to assist in preventing abuse and illicit traffic in substances causing addiction or habituation. The major legislation included the Harrison Narcotic Act of 1914, with amendments, and the Drug Abuse Control Amendments of 1965 to the Federal Food, Drug, and Cosmetic Act. The latter legislation was needed to meet the problems of the growing abuse and illicit traffic in stimulant, depressant, and hallucinogenic substances. The Harrison Narcotic Act was enforced by the Federal Bureau of Narcotics of the Treasury Department and the Drug Abuse Control Amendments were enforced by the Bureau of Drug Abuse Control of the Food and Drug Administration.

Controlled Substances Act of 1970

In 1970, Congress passed the Comprehensive Drug Abuse Prevention and Control Act of 1970 (P. L. 91–513) which repealed the previous Federal legislation. The enforcement of this Act, which may be referred to as the Controlled Substances Act of 1970 (CSA), is the sole responsibility of the Drug Enforcement Administration (DEA) of the United States Department of Justice.

The drugs that come under jurisdiction of the Controlled Substances Act are placed into one of five schedules, depending on the degree of drug abuse potential. A brief description of each schedule, with examples of drugs included, follows:

Schedule I (C–1)

Drugs in Schedule I are those that have no accepted medical use in the United States and have high abuse potential. Some examples are heroin, marihuana, LSD, peyote, and mescaline.

Schedule II (C–II)

The drugs in Schedule II have a high abuse potential with high psychic or physical dependence liability. Schedule II controlled substances consist of the former Class A narcotic drugs, and drugs containing certain stimulants or depressants as the single active ingredient or in combination with each other. Examples of Schedule II controlled substances are: opium, morphine, codeine, hydromorphone (Dilaudid®), methadone (Dolophine®), meperidine (Demerol®), cocaine, oxycodone (one component of Percodan®), oxymorphone (Numorphan®), straight amphetamines and methamphetamines, and combination forms such as: Dexamyl®, Obedrin®, and Bamadex®. Also in Schedule II are phenmetrazine (Preludin®) and methylphenidate (Ritalin®). Barbiturates in Schedule II include amobarbital (Amytal®), pentobarital (Nembutal®), and secobarbital (Seconal®).*

Schedule III (C–III)

The drugs in Schedule III have an abuse potential less than those in Schedules I and II, and include many of the drugs formerly known as Class B Narcotics. Members of this schedule include nalorphine and paregoric, and non-narcotic drugs such as: glutethimide (Doriden®), methyprylon (Noludar®), and most barbitu-

---

*Registered trade names of selected controlled substances are provided for general information only. These drugs also may be commercially available generically or under other trade names.

rates (except phenobarbital, amobarbital, pentobarbital and secobarbital).*

Schedule IV (C–IV)

The drugs in Schedule IV have an abuse potential less than that of those listed in Schedule III and include drugs such as: phenobarbital, chlordiazepoxide (Librium®), diazepam (Valium®), chloral hydrate, ethchlorvynol (Placidyl®), meprobamate (Equanil®, Miltown®), and paraldehyde.*

Schedule V (C–V)

The drugs in Schedule V have a relatively low abuse potential and consist of those preparations formerly known as *Exempt Narcotics*, with the exception of paregoric (camphorated tincture of opium), which is in Schedule III. Several codeine-containing cough preparations and diphenoxylate-atropine sulfate (Lomotil®) are in this schedule.*

In order to be in conformance with this law, it is of the utmost importance that ships' owners, operators, medical officers, and Masters be fully aware of their responsibilities under Federal regulations relating to controlled substances aboard a vessel. The specific mention of ocean vessels (merchant vessels) in the Federal regulations is contained in the Code of Federal Regulations (CFR) Title 21, Part 1301.28. This Part, as amended through April 1, 1976, is reproduced in the next several paragraphs.

Code of Federal Regulations
Title 21—Food and Drugs

Chapter II—Drug Enforcement Admin., U.S. Department of Justice

§*1301.28 Registration regarding ocean vessels.*

(a) If acquired by and dispensed under the general supervision of a medical officer described in paragraph (b) of this section, or the Master of the vessel under the circumstances described in paragraph (d) of this section, controlled substances may be held for stocking, be maintained in, and dispensed from medicine chests, first aid packets, or dispensaries:

---

*Registered trade names of selected controlled substances are provided for general information only. These drugs also may be commercially available generically or under other trade names.

1. On board any vessel engaged in international trade or in trade between ports of the United States and any merchant vessel belonging to the U.S. Government;

2. On board any aircraft operated by an air carrier under a certificate of permit issued pursuant to the Federal Aviation Act of 1958 (49 U.S.C. 1301); and

3. In any other entity of fixed or transient location approved by the Administrator as appropriate for application of this section (e.g., emergency kits at field sites of an industrial firm).

(b) A medical officer shall be:

1. Licensed in a State as a physician;

2. Employed by the owner or operator of the vessel, aircraft or other entity; and

3. Registered under the Act at the location of the principal office of the owner or operator of the vessel, aircraft or other entity.

(c) A registered medical officer may serve as medical officer for more than one vessel, aircraft, or other entity under a single registration, unless he serves as medical officer for more than one owner or operator, in which case he shall attain a separate registration at the location of the principal office of each such owner or operator.

(d) If no medical officer is employed by the owner or operator of a vessel, or in the event such medical officer is not accessible and the acquisition of controlled substances is required, the Master of the vessel, who shall not be registered under the Act, may purchase controlled substances only with the approval of and upon special order form (HSA–590, Authorization to Purchase Controlled Substances for Vessels, formerly HSM–590) provided by a medical officer of the United States Public Health Service. Upon issuance, a copy of each Form HSA–590 will be immediately submitted by the USPHS facility where issued to the Drug Enforcement Administration Regional Office covering the area in which the facility is located. Blank or presigned Form HSA–590 may not be furnished to ships or shipping companies by USPHS.

(e) Any medical officer described in paragraph (b) of this section shall, in addition to complying with all requirements and duties prescribed for registrants generally, prepare an annual report as of the date on which his registration expires, which shall give in detail an accounting for each vessel, aircraft, or other entity, and a summary accounting for all vessels, aircraft, or other entities under his supervision for all controlled substances purchased, dispensed or disposed of during the year. The medical officer shall maintain this report with other records required to be kept under the Act and, upon request, deliver a copy of the report to the Administration. The medical officer need not be present when controlled substances are dispensed, if the person who actually dispensed the controlled substances is responsible to the medical officer to justify his actions.

(f) [Reserved]

(g) Owners or operators of vessels, aircraft, or other entities described in this section shall not be deemed to possess or dispense any controlled substance acquired, stored and dispensed in accordance with this section.

(h) The Master of a vessel shall prepare a report for each calendar year which shall give in detail an accounting for all controlled substances purchased, dispensed, or disposed of during the year. The Master shall file this report with the medical officer employed by the owner or operator of his vessel, if any, or, if not, he shall maintain this report with other records required to be kept under the Act and, upon request, deliver a copy of the report to the Administration.

(i) Controlled substances acquired and possessed in accordance with this section shall not be distributed to persons not under the general supervision of the medical officer employed by the owner or operator of the vessel, aircraft, or other entity, except in accordance with § 1307.21 of this chapter.

[37 F.R. 15918, Aug. 8, 1972, as amended at 38 F.R. 756, Jan. 4, 1973; 41 FR 9546, Mar. 5, 1976]

Procurement of Controlled Substances for Vessels

Federal regulations (21 CFR 1301.28) provide that controlled substances coming within the purview of the Controlled Substances Act of 1970 and used for stocking medicine chests, first aid packets, and dispensaries maintained on board any vessel engaged in international trade or in trade between ports of the United States, and any merchant vessel belonging to the Government, may be acquired in only two ways:

(1) They may be acquired by a medical officer (physician), employed by the owner or operator of such vessel, licensed in a State as a physician and registered under the Act at the location of the principal office of the owner or operator of the vessel. Such medical officer will procure the controlled substances direct from a vendor and, when procuring a controlled substance in Schedule II, will use an official Schedule II controlled substances order form issued to him by the DEA.

(2) If no such medical officer is employed by the owner or operator of a vessel, or in the event such medical officer is not accessible and the acquisition of controlled substances is required, the Master of the vessel, who shall not be registered under the Act, may procure controlled substances only with the approval of, and upon special order form HSA–590 (formerly PHS–2341), *Authorization to Purchase Controlled Substances for Vessels,* provided by a medical officer at a United States Public Health Service facility. (See Appendix A, p. 428 for a listing of U.S. Public Health Service Hospitals and Outpatient Clinics.) A sample of form HSA–590 is shown on pages 456–7.

When it is necessary for the Master to acquire controlled substances (narcotics, depressants or stimulants) he will present himself at a United States Public Health Service facility (see p. 428) to request approval for the purchase of the controlled substances needed. The medical officer of the U.S. Public Health Service will consider the reasonableness, adequacy, and propriety of the kinds and quantities of drug products requested in relation to the ship's itinerary, ship's crew and passengers, usage requirements, stock on board, and other pertinent factors.

If the USPHS Medical Officer approves the Master's request, the Medical Officer will prepare and sign Form HSA–590, and the Master will sign this form in the Officer's presence. (See p. 456.) The Master then will receive two copies: a *vendor's copy* and a *Master's copy.* He will use the vendor's copy to make a direct purchase of the controlled substances and will retain his copy for at least two years in the controlled substances file aboard his vessel.

A Master of a vessel under a foreign flag or registry may obtain controlled substances in the same manner as described above.

Recordkeeping of Controlled Substances

Complete records must be maintained aboard a merchant vessel for all transactions that relate to *controlled substances*. Two forms (A and B) recommended for this purpose, are shown at the end of this appendix. *Form A—Appendix D* is entitled, *Controlled Substance, Acquisition, Use, and Perpetual Inventory Record* (see p. 458); and *Form B—Appendix D* (see p. 462) relates to the *Transfer of Custody of Controlled Substances*. Both forms should be used to keep records of *all* controlled substance medications stocked aboard the vessel. A sample of a completed Form A (see p. 459) has been prepared to show the kinds of transactions that should be recorded.

Each controlled substance medication should be entered on a separate sheet of Form A, *Controlled Substance Acquisition, Use, and Perpetual Inventory Record*. For example, morphine sulfate injection 10 mg should be recorded on one copy of Form A; and codeine sulfate tablets 30 mg should be recorded on a second form. Each copy of Form A should list the name of only one medication for inventory purposes.

If the ownership or agency of a vessel changes, or if the person responsible for the keeping of controlled substances is changed, this should be noted in two ways:

(1) As a statement on each Form A—Appendix D, *Controlled Substances Acquisition, Use, and Perpetual Inventory Record,* which includes the signature of the person accepting responsibility for controlled substances at the time of changing agents or personnel; and

(2) As a separate transfer statement Form B—Appendix D, covering all controlled substances, which should be prepared and signed by both the person formerly responsible and the person assuming responsibility for controlled substances (see p. 462).

The original copy of these forms (A and B) shall remain aboard the vessel and be available for at least two years from the date of last required entry for inspection by agents of the Drug Enforcement Administration (DEA) of the U.S. Department of Justice or the Bureau of Customs of the U.S. Treasury Department. A new copy of Form A, *Controlled Substances Acquisition, Use, and Perpetual Inventory Record* should *not* be started for each voyage—*it should be continued in use until filled,* irrespective of the number of voyages.

Federal regulations, 21 CFR 1301.28(h), state that the Master of a vessel shall prepare a report for each calendar year, which will give in detail an accounting for all controlled substances purchased, dispensed, or disposed of during the year. The Master shall file this report with the Medical Officer employed by the owner or operator of his vessel or, if none, he shall maintain this report with other records required to be kept under the Act and upon request deliver a copy of the report to the Drug Enforcement Administration of the U.S. Department of Justice. This summary report should be prepared annually, using data from the file of Form A, *Controlled Substances Acquisition, Use, and Perpetual Inventory Record,* for each Controlled Substance carried aboard ship.

Security for Controlled Substances

Masters, medical officers, owners or operators are advised that the loss or theft of controlled substances should be reported to appropriate local authorities. In addition, registrants under the Controlled Substances Act must report any theft or significant loss of any controlled substances to the nearest Regional Office of the Drug Enforcement Administration of the U.S. Department of Justice in accordance with Parts 1301.74(c) and 1301.76(b) of the Drug Enforcement Administration (DEA) regulations. Because an immediate report to DEA will not always be possible in the case of merchant vessels at sea, the Master shall make an investigation to determine the reason or cause for any loss, theft, or inaccuracy in the records of the controlled substances. The Master shall include his findings and any remedial steps proposed or taken to prevent recurrence, when he subsequently reports the loss or theft to DEA. (Addresses of DEA Regional Offices are shown at the end of this appendix, p. 444.) DEA Form 106 (available from DEA Regional Offices) must be completed for any theft or loss. (Sample DEA Form 106 is shown on pp. 460–1.)

The requirements for physical security of controlled substances aboard a vessel are recommended to be as follows:

Schedule I: All controlled substances in Schedule C–I cannot be bought for use aboard ship.

Schedule II: All controlled substances in Schedule C–II shall be maintained in the Master's safe.

Schedules III, IV, V: All controlled substances in Schedules C–III, C–IV, and C–V shall be maintained either in the Master's safe or under lock in the ship's sick bay or dispensary.

The Master of a vessel has the primary responsibility for safeguarding these substances through the control and supervision of their receipt, storage, issue, use, and recordkeeping. Details concerned with the responsibility of safeguarding controlled substances may be delegated, subject to the Master's primary responsibility, to a senior officer aboard (marine physician assistant, first mate, or similar designee).

The Master shall make periodic inspections of the records for controlled substances and stocks on hand to insure that security and recordkeeping requirements for all controlled substances are fulfilled aboard the vessel. Such inspections should be made at least every six months.

U.S. DEPARTMENT OF JUSTICE
Drug Enforcement Administration (DEA)

DEA Regional Offices (Domestic)

Region 1—BOSTON
JFK Federal Bldg.
Room G–64
Boston, Mass. 02203
(617) 223–2170

Region 2—NEW YORK
555 West 57th St.
New York, N.Y. 10019
(212) 399–5151

Region 3—PHILADELPHIA
Wm. J. Green, Jr., Fed. Bldg.
Room 10224
600 Arch St.
Philadelphia, Pa. 19106
(212) 597–9530

Region 4—BALTIMORE
31 Hopkins Plaza
Room 955
Baltimore, Md. 21201
(301) 962–4800

Region 5—MIAMI
8400 N.W. 53rd St.
Miami, Fla. 33166
(305) 591–4870

Region 6—DETROIT
357 Federal Bldg.
231 W. Lafayette St.
Detroit, Mich. 48226
(313) 226-7290

Region 7—CHICAGO
Everett Dirksen Federal Bldg.
219 S. Dearborn St.
Suite 1800
Chicago, Ill. 60604
(312) 353–7875

Region 8—NEW ORLEANS
Plaza Tower
1001 Howard Ave.
Suite 1800
New Orleans, La. 70113
(504) 589–6841

(There is no Region 9.)

Region 10—KANSAS CITY
U.S. Courthouse
811 Grand Ave.
Suite 231
Kansas City, Mo. 64106
(816) 374–2631

Region 11—DALLAS
1100 Commerce St.
Room 4A5
Dallas, Tex. 75202
(214) 749–3631

Region 12—DENVER
U.S. Customs Office
Room 336
P.O. Box 1860
Denver, Colo. 80202
(303) 837–3951

Region 13—SEATTLE
221 First Avenue, West
Room 200
Seattle, Wash. 98119
(206) 442–5443

Region 14—LOS ANGELES
350 S. Figueroa St.
Los Angeles, Calif. 90071
(213) 688–3432

DEA Regional Offices (Foreign)

Region 15—MEXICO CITY
DEA/Justice
American Embassy
Apartado Postal 88–BIS
Mexico, D.F., Mexico

Region 16—BANGKOK
DEA/Justice
American Embassy
APO San Francisco 96346

Region 17—PARIS
DEA/Justice
American Embassy
APO New York 09777

Region 18—CARACAS
DEA/Justice
American Embassy
APO New York 09893

Region 19—ANKARA
DEA/Justice
American Embassy
APO New York 09254

Region 20—MANILA
DEA/Justice
American Embassy
APO San Francisco 96528

FORMS
Discussed in Appendices C and D
(For sources of all forms, refer to page numbers shown below)

CDC 4.452
8-75

**DEPARTMENT OF
HEALTH, EDUCATION, AND WELFARE**
PUBLIC HEALTH SERVICE

**DERATTING CERTIFICATE (¹) — CERTIFICAT DE DERATISATION (¹)
DERATTING EXEMPTION CERTIFICATE (¹) — CERTIFICAT D'EXEMPTION DE LA DERATISATION (¹)**

issued in accordance with Article 54 of the International Health Regulations
Délivré conformément à l'article 54 du Règlement Sanitaire International (1969)

(Not to be taken away by Port Authorities.)—(Ce certificat ne doit pas être retiré pas les autorités portuaires.)

PORT OF _____ Date _____
PORT DE _____ Date _____

THIS CERTIFICATE records the inspections and { derating / exemption } (a) *at this port and on the above date*

LE PRESENT CERTIFICAT atteste l'inspection et { la dératisation / l'exemption } (a) en ce port et à date ci-dessus

of the { ship / inland navigation vessel } (a) _____
du navire

of { net tonnage for a sea-going vessel / tonnage net dans le cas d'un navire de haute mer
de { tonnage for an inland navigation vessel / tonnage dans le cas d'un navire de navigation interieure } (a) (f)

At the time of { inspection / derating } (a) ____ *the holds were laden with* ____ tons of ____ cargo
Au moment de { l'inspection / la dératisation } (a) les cales étaient chargées de ____ tonnes de ____ cargaison

COMPARTMENTS(b)	RAT INDICATIONS / TRACES DE RATS (c)	RAT HARBORAGE / REFUGES A RATS		DERATTING — DERATISATION					
		discovered / trouvés (d)	treated / supprimés	by fumigation — par fumigation / Fumigant — Gaz utilisé / Hours exposure — Exposition (heures)		by catching, trapping, or poisoning / par capture ou poison			COMPARTIMENTS(b)
				Space (cubic feet) / Espaces (mètres cubes)	Quantity used / Quantités employées (e)	Rats found dead / Rats trouvés morts	Traps set or poisons put out / Pièges ou poisons mis	Rats caught or killed / Rats pris ou tués	
Holds 1.									Cales 1.
— 2.									— 2.

		English	French			
	3.		3.			
	4.		4.			
	5.		5.			
	6.		6.			
	7.		7.			
		Shelter deck space.	Entrepont			
		Bunker space.	Soute à charbon			
		Engine room and shaft alley	Chaufferies, tunnel de l'arbre			
		Forepeak and storeroom	Peak avant et magasin			
		Afterpeak and storeroom	Peak arrière et magasin			
		Lifeboats	Canots de sauvetage			
		Charts and wireless rooms	Chambre des cartes, T. S. F.			
		Galley	Cuisines			
		Pantry	Cambuses			
		Provision storerooms	Soute à vivres			
		Quarters (crew)	Postes (équipage)			
		Quarters (officers)	Chambres (officiers)			
		Quarters (cabin passengers)	Cabines (passagers)			
		Quarters (steerage)	Postes (émigrants)			
		Saloon	Salon			
		Messrooms	Salle à manger de l'équipage			
		Refrigerated storerooms	Soute à vivres réfrigérées			
		TOTAL	**TOTAL**			

For copies of this form, write to:
Quarantine Division,
Center for Disease Control,
U.S. Public Health Service,
Atlanta, Georgia 30333

(a) *Strike out the unnecessary indications.* — Rayer les mentions inutiles.
(b) *In case any of the compartments enumerated do not exist on the ship or inland navigation vessel, this fact must be mentioned.* — Lorsqu'un des compartiments énumérés n'existe pas sur le navire, on devra le mentionner expressément.
(c) *Old or recent evidence of excreta, runs, or gnawing.* — Traces anciennes ou récentes d'excréments, de passages ou de rongements.

RECOMMENDATIONS MADE. — OBSERVATIONS. — *In the case of exemption, state here the measures taken for maintaining the ship or inland navigation vessel in such a condition that it is free of rodents and the plague vector.* — Dans le cas d'exemption, indiquer ici les mesures prises pour que le navire soit maintenu dans des conditions telles qu'il n'y ait à bord ni rongeurs, ni vecteurs de la peste.

(d) *None, small, moderate, or large.* — Néant, peu, passablement ou beaucoup.
(e) *State the weight of sulphur or of cyanide salts or quantity of HCN acid used.* — Indiquer les poids de soufre ou de cyanure ou la proportion d'acide cyanhydrique.
(f) *Specify whether applies to metric displacement or any other method of determining the tonnage.* — Spécifier s'il s'agit de déplacement métrique ou, sinon, de quel autre tonnage il s'agit.

Seal, name, qualification, and signature of the inspector. — Cachet, nom, qualité et signature de l'inspecteur.

Forms Discussed in Appendices C and D

DEPARTMENT OF HEALTH, EDUCATION, AND WELFARE
PUBLIC HEALTH SERVICE
CENTER FOR DISEASE CONTROL
ATLANTA, GEORGIA 30333

MARITIME PUBLIC HEALTH DECLARATION
(SEE INSTRUCTIONS ON REVERSE SIDE)

FORM APPROVED
OMB NO. 68-R0439

RADIO CALL SIGN	NAME OF VESSEL

I. ALL VESSELS REQUESTING RADIO PRATIQUE INCLUDE THIS INFORMATION IN RADIO REQUEST

A. Itinerary for past 15 days or since last port under control of the U.S., whichever is shorter. Enter last port first.

Port City/Country	Date of Departure	Port City/Country	Date of Departure

For copies of this form, write to:
Quarantine Division,
Center for Disease Control,
U.S. Public Health Service,
Atlanta, Georgia 30333

NO   YES

B. Were any persons ill during past 15 days or since last U.S. Port (whichever is shorter)? ☐ ☐
   Illness to be reported:

   1. Temperature of 100°F (38°C) or greater (a) which persisted for 2 days or more;
      or (b) which was accompanied or followed by any one or all of the following:
      rash, jaundice, glandular swelling.

   2. Diarrhea severe enough to interfere with work or normal activity.

C. Was this vessel in a plague infected country since its last U.S. Port? ☐ ☐

D. If answer to C is yes, was vessel precleared for plague purposes when last in plague country? ☐ ☐

II. COMPLETE THIS SECTION BUT DO NOT INCLUDE IN RADIO REQUEST FOR PRATIQUE

Crew		Passengers		I certify the foregoing statements are true and to the best of my knowledge and belief, the vessel, passengers, officers, crew, and cargo conform, except as indicated above, to the applicable Quarantine Regulations and Laws of the United States.
No. of U.S. Citizens	No. of Aliens	No. of U.S. Citizens	No. of Aliens	
				Signature of Master · Date

III. THIS SECTION NOT FOR VESSEL USE

I   D   B   C   T/S   TV
M D Y   H M   H M   H M

CDC 4.573 (F.HSM 13.19)
3-78

INSTRUCTIONS

MARITIME PUBLIC HEALTH DECLARATION A vessel subject to routine public health inspection entering a port under the control of the United States is required to complete Sections I and II on Page 1 prior to arrival Upon arrival, the completed form (and a copy of the radio message, if radio pratique was requested) will be given to the public health inspector or the vessel's agent

RADIO PRATIQUE Radio pratique is public health clearance by radio, based upon information received from the vessel prior to its arrival in port Radio pratique is available at all U S ports A vessel granted radio free or provisional pratique for public health may proceed directly to berth and begin normal business activities The granting of radio pratique does not exempt a vessel from control measures or public health inspection subsequently deemed necessary or from the requirements of other government agencies

A vessel which does not request radio pratique will undergo complete inspection in accordance with normal port procedures

To request radio pratique, a vessel will transmit to its agent a brief message containing answers to Items A, B, C, and if applicable, D in Section I and the agent will inform the designated public health office during normal business hours, between 4 and 72 hours prior to the vessel's arrival For circumstances in which illnesses occur aboard a vessel subsequent to the vessel's radio pratique request, the vessel master must notify the agent immediately The agent will notify the designated public health office at once

The radio pratique request should include
1   Vessel's radio call sign
2   Vessel's itinerary for the 15 days prior to arrival
3   **One** of two codes
    a   RPR-AIN (for Radio Pratique Requested — All Items Negative) — if items B and C on the Declaration are negative, or
    b   RPR-AINX (for Radio Pratique Requested — All Items Negative Except) — if Item B and/or C on the Declaration is yes, give Item letter(s)

Example of request "KXYN Pto La Cruz 7/1/72 RPR-AIN"
The vessel is identified by the radio call sign KXYN The vessel has been in Pto La Cruz only (departure date July 1, 1972) during the last 15 days Radio pratique is requested — Items B and C are negative

Example of request "KXYN Pto La Cruz 7/1/72 RPR-AINX-B"
The vessel is identified by the radio call sign KXYN The vessel has been in Pto La Cruz only (departure date July 1, 1972) during the last 15 days Radio pratique is requested — Item C is negative — Item B is entered because there is illness on board The ill person(s) should be readily available for inspection upon arrival

Any illness which occurs after radio pratique is requested must be reported immediately through the agent to the public health office having jurisdiction at the U S port of entry where the vessel is first destined

A vessel diverted to another U S port after requesting radio pratique should resubmit the request through its agent to the public health office responsible for the port to which it is diverted

The Master should insure that the vessel is maintained in a rat-free and sanitary condition

SECTION I

Item A   Include last U S port if within 15 days

Item B   Enter "X" in appropriate box to indicate yes or no
Illness to be reported crew members and passengers (including those who have disembarked) who have, or have had, any of the following during the past 15 days or since the last U S port (whichever is shorter)
    1   Temperature of 100°F (38°C) or greater
        (a) which was accompanied or followed by any one or all of the following rash, jaundice, glandular swelling, OR
        (b) which persisted for two days or more
    2   Diarrhea severe enough to interfere with work or normal activity

Item C   Enter "X" in appropriate box to indicate yes or no

Item D   Enter "X" in appropriate box to indicate yes or no

SECTION II

Enter the number of crew members and passengers according to whether they are U S citizens or aliens

The Declaration must be signed by the Master

All cats, dogs, monkeys, and psittacine birds must remain on board until released for entry by an authorized official Contact a public health inspector for rodent inspection if Deratting/Deratting Exemption Certificate is expired or if renewal is required before the next port

HSM 13 19 (CDC) REV 5-72 **(BACK)**

FOLD HERE TO PLACE WITH PASSPORT

INTERNATIONAL CERTIFICATES OF VACCINATION
AS APPROVED BY
THE WORLD HEALTH ORGANIZATION
(EXCEPT FOR ADDRESS OF VACCINATOR)

CERTIFICATS INTERNATIONAUX DE VACCINATION
APPROUVÉS PAR
L'ORGANISATION MONDIALE DE LA SANTÉ
(SAUF L'ADRESSE DU VACCINATEUR)

TRAVELER'S NAME—NOM DU VOYAGEUR

ADDRESS—ADRESSE   (Number—Numéro)   (Street—Rue)

(City—Ville)

(County—Département)   (State—État)

U.S. DEPARTMENT OF HEALTH, EDUCATION, AND WELFARE

PUBLIC HEALTH SERVICE

PHS–731 (REV. 9-77)

For sale by the Superintendent of Documents,
U.S. Government Printing Office, Washington, D.C. 20402
Stock No. 017–001–00399–9

Booklet: Part 1 of six related pages (450–455)

A free single copy of the material on pp. 450–455 is available as a booklet (PHS–731) from the quarantine epidemiologists of State health departments.

Sales copies are available from the Superintendent of Documents, U.S. Government Printing Office, Washington, D.C.   20402

INSTRUCTIONS TO TRAVELERS

International Certificates of Vaccination or Revaccination are official statements verifying that proper procedures have been followed to immunize you against a quarantinable disease which could be a threat to the United States and other countries. The Certificates are essential in permitting uninterrupted international travel. THEY MUST BE COMPLETE AND ACCURATE IN EVERY DETAIL, or you may be detained at international ports of entry

Certain immunizations are required by the countries, other immunizations and preventive measures are sometimes advisable, depending upon the traveler's age, previous immunization status, and the nature and duration of travel. Yellow fever immunization may be given only by a designated Yellow Fever Vaccination Center. Other immunizations may be given by any licensed physician

When your itinerary is complete, your local or State Health Department, private physician, travel agency, or international air line can furnish you information on immunizations or prophylaxis required or recommended for your trip. Your local or State Health Department can inform you where in your area you may be vaccinated against yellow fever and have your Certificates validated

There is a risk of acquiring *MALARIA* when traveling to parts of the Caribbean, Central and South America, Africa, the Middle East, the Indian subcontinent, and the Far East. You are strongly advised to seek information from your local or State Health Department or private physician concerning the need for protection against malaria and for instructions on how the prophylactic drugs should be taken

If you need medications regularly, take an adequate supply with you. Because of possible serious consequences to your health, do NOT buy medications "over the counter" unless you are familiar with the product. Should you need medical assistance, the American Embassy or Consulate usually can provide names of physicians or hospitals

How to Complete Your International Certificates of Vaccination

1 Enter your name and address on the cover of the booklet before presenting it to your physician

2 On the Certificates required for your travel, print your name on the first line, sign your name on the second line, indicate your sex, and indicate your date of birth in the following sequence: day, month, year. Example: 5 June 1956

3 It is your responsibility to have the Certificates validated with an "approved stamp." THE CERTIFICATES ARE NOT VALID WITHOUT AN "APPROVED STAMP."

INSTRUCTIONS TO PHYSICIANS

INFORMATION REQUESTED ON EACH CERTIFICATE MUST BE COMPLETE FOR THE CERTIFICATE TO BE VALID

1 The space for primary vaccination against smallpox is to be used only when a person receives his vaccination against smallpox for the first time. If unsuccessful, a new Certificate must be used for a repeat primary vaccination

2 The dates on each Certificate are to be written with the day in arabic numerals, followed by the month in letters and the year in arabic numerals. Example: 2 Jan 1978

3 Vaccinations may be given by nurses and medical technicians if under the direct supervision of a qualified medical practitioner. The WRITTEN signature of the physician or other person authorized by the physician must appear on the Certificate. A signature stamp is not acceptable

4 If smallpox, yellow fever, or cholera immunization is required for your patient but is contraindicated on medical grounds, you should complete the "Medical Contraindication to Vaccination" statement in the "Personal Health History" section of the Certificates indicating the nature of the contraindication

5 There is a risk of acquiring *MALARIA* when traveling to parts of the Caribbean, Central and South America, Africa, the Middle East, the Indian subcontinent, and the Far East

6 Information on malaria prophylaxis, for areas where malaria transmission occurs, for the recommended prophylactic drug regimens, and on preparing patients for international travel may be obtained from your local or State Health Department.

SAVE THIS BOOKLET. YOU MAY HAVE OCCASION TO USE IT FOR FUTURE TRAVEL AND AS A RECORD OF YOUR VACCINATION HISTORY.

INTERNATIONAL CERTIFICATE OF VACCINATION OR REVACCINATION AGAINST SMALLPOX
CERTIFICAT INTERNATIONAL DE VACCINATION OU DE REVACCINATION CONTRE LA VARIOLE

This is to certify that
Je soussigné(e) certifie que_____ sex
                                                              sexe _____
whose signature follows   date of birth
dont la signature suit _____ né(e) le _____

has on the date indicated been vaccinated or revaccinated against smallpox with a freeze-dried or liquid vaccine certified to fulfill the recommended requirements of the World Health Organization
a été vacciné(e) ou revacciné(e) contre la variole à la date indiquée ci-dessous, avec un vaccin lyophilisé ou liquide certifié conforme aux normes recommandées par l'Organisation mondiale de la Santé

Date	Show by "X" whether / Indiquer par "X" s'il s'agit de	Signature, professional status, and address of vaccinator / Signature, titre, et adresse du vaccinateur	Manufacturer and batch no. of vaccine / Fabricant du vaccin et numéro du lot	Approved stamp / Cachet autorisé
1a	Primary vaccination performed / Primovaccination effectuée ☐			
1b	Read as successful Prise ☐ / Unsuccessful Pas de prise ☐			
2	☐ Revaccination			
3	☐ Revaccination			
4	☐ Revaccination			
5	☐ Revaccination			

This form is available as part of a booklet (PHS–731). INTERNATIONAL CERTIFICATES OF VACCINATION. (See p. 450 on availability of a free copy and/or sales stock.)

THE VALIDITY OF THIS CERTIFICATE shall extend for a period of 3 years, beginning 8 days after the date of a successful primary vaccination* or, in the event of a revaccination, on the date of that revaccination

The approved stamp mentioned above must be in a form prescribed by the health administration of the country in which the vaccination is performed

This certificate must be signed in his own hand by a medical practitioner or other person authorized by the national health administration, his official stamp is not an accepted substitute for his signature

Any amendment of this certificate, or erasure, or failure to complete any part of it, may render it invalid.

LA VALIDITÉ DE CE CERTIFICAT couvre une période de trois ans commençant huit jours après la date de la primovaccination effectuée avec succès (prise) ou, dans le cas d'une revaccination, le jour de cette revaccination

Le cachet autorisé doit être conforme au modèle prescrit par l'administration sanitaire du territoire où la vaccination est effectuée.

Ce certificat doit être signé de sa propre main par un médecin ou une autre personne habilitée par l'administration sanitaire nationale, un cachet officiel ne pouvant être considéré comme tenant lieu de signature

Toute correction ou rature sur le certificat ou l'omission d'une quelconque des mentions qu'il comporte peut affecter sa validité.

*See item 1, Instructions to Physicians.

Booklet: Part 3 of six related pages (450–455)

**INTERNATIONAL CERTIFICATE OF VACCINATION OR REVACCINATION
AGAINST YELLOW FEVER
CERTIFICAT INTERNATIONAL DE VACCINATION OU DE REVACCINATION
CONTRE LA FIÈVRE JAUNE**

This is to certify that
Je soussigné(e) certifie que _____

sex
sexe _____

whose signature follows
dont la signature suit _____

date of birth
né(e) le _____

has on the date indicated been vaccinated or revaccinated against yellow fever.
a été vacciné(e) ou revacciné(e) contre la fièvre jaune à la date indiquée.

Date	Signature and professional status of vaccinator / Signature et titre du vaccinateur	Manufacturer & batch number of vaccine / Fabricant du vaccin et numéro du lot	Official stamp of vaccinating center / Cachet officiel du centre de vaccination
1.			
2.			

This form is available as part of a booklet (PHS–731). INTERNATIONAL CERTIFICATES OF VACCINATION. (See p. 450 on availability of a free copy and/or sales stock.)

THIS CERTIFICATE IS VALID only if the vaccine used has been approved by the World Health Organization and if the vaccinating center has been designated by the health administration for the country in which that center is situated

THE VALIDITY OF THIS CERTIFICATE shall extend for a period of 10 years, beginning 10 days after the date of vaccination or, in the event of a revaccination, within such period of 10 years, from the date of that revaccination.

This certificate must be signed in his own hand by a medical practitioner or other person authorized by the national health administration, his official stamp is not an accepted substitute for his signature.

Any amendment of this certificate, or erasure, or failure to complete any part of it, may render it invalid.

CE CERTIFICAT N'EST VALABLE que si le vaccin employé a été approuvé par l'Organisation mondiale de la Santé et si le centre de vaccination a été habilité par l'administration sanitaire du territoire dans lequel ce centre est situé.

LA VALIDITÉ DE CE CERTIFICAT couvre une période de dix ans commençant dix jours après la date de la vaccination ou, dans le cas d'une revaccination au cours de cette période de dix ans, le jour de cette revaccination.

Ce certificat doit être signé de sa propre main par un médecin ou une autre personne habilitée par l'administration sanitaire nationale, un cachet officiel ne pouvant être considéré comme tenant lieu de signature.

Toute correction ou rature sur le certificat ou l'omission d'une quelconque des mentions qu'il comporte peut affecter sa validité.

Booklet: Part 4 of six related pages (450–455)

INTERNATIONAL CERTIFICATE OF VACCINATION OR REVACCINATION
AGAINST CHOLERA
CERTIFICAT INTERNATIONAL DE VACCINATION OU DE REVACCINATION
CONTRE LE CHOLÉRA

This is to certify that
Je soussigné(e) certifie que _____

sex
sexe _____

whose signature follows
dont la signature suit _____

date of birth
né(e) le _____

has on the date indicated been vaccinated or revaccinated against cholera.
a été vacciné(e) ou revacciné(e) contre le choléra à la date indiquée.

Date	Signature, professional status, and address of vaccinator / Signature, titre, et adresse du vaccinateur	Approved stamp / Cachet autorisé
1.		1.
2.		2.
3.		3.
11		11.
12.		12.

This form is available as part of a booklet (PHS–731). INTERNATIONAL CERTIFICATES OF VACCINATION. (See p. 450 on availability of a free copy and/or sales stock.)

The vaccine used shall meet the requirements laid down by the World Health Organization.
THE VALIDITY OF THIS CERTIFICATE shall extend for a period of 6 months, beginning 6 days after one injection of the vaccine or, in the event of a revaccination, within such period of 6 months, on the date of that revaccination.
The approved stamp mentioned above must be in a form prescribed by the health administration of the country in which the vaccination is performed.
This certificate must be signed in his own hand by a medical practitioner or other person authorized by the national health administration; his official stamp is not an accepted substitute for his signature.
Any amendment of this certificate, or erasure, or failure to complete any part of it, may render it invalid.
Le vaccin utilisé doit satisfaire aux normes formulées par l'Organisation mondiale de la Santé.
LA VALIDITÉ DE CE CERTIFICAT couvre une période de six mois commençant six jours après une injection de vaccin ou, dans le cas d'une revaccination au cours de cette période de six mois, le jour de cette revaccination.
Le cachet autorisé doit être conforme au modèle prescrit par l'administration sanitaire du territoire où la vaccination est effectuée.
Ce certificat doit être signé de sa propre main par un médecin ou une autre personne habilitée par l'administration sanitaire nationale, un cachet officiel ne pouvant être considéré comme tenant lieu de signature.
Toute correction ou rature sur le certificat ou l'omission d'une quelconque des mentions qu'il comporte peut affecter sa validité.

PERSONAL HEALTH HISTORY

This section is provided to include a record of the personal health history of the international traveler and to assist any physician called upon to provide treatment in case of illness or accident. Space is also provided to record immunizations that are not required for entrance into any country but have been obtained by the traveler for additional health protection.

OTHER IMMUNIZATIONS/PROPHYLAXIS RECEIVED
Autres immunisations/prophylaxies reçues
(Immunoglobulin, MALARIA, plague, poliomyelitis, rabies, tetanus/diphtheria, typhoid, typhus, etc. — Immunoglobuline, PALUDISME, peste, poliomyélite, rage, tétanos/diphtérie, typhoïde, typhus, et caetera)

Date	Vaccine/prophylactic drug Vaccin/drogue prophylactique	Dose	Physician's signature Signature du médecin

MEDICAL CONTRAINDICATION TO VACCINATION
Contre-indication médicale à la vaccination

This is to certify that immunization against
C'est pour certifier que l'immunisation contre

_____ for
(Name of disease — Nom de la maladie)   pour
                                          is medically
_____ est médicament
(Name of traveler — Nom du vogageur)

contraindicated because of the following conditions:
contra-indiquer à cause des conditions suivantes.

This form is available as part of a booklet (PHS–731). INTERNATIONAL CERTIFICATES OF VACCINATION. (See p. 450 on availability of a free copy and/or sales stock.)

(Signature and address of physician)
(Signature et adresse du médecin)

MEDICATIONS TAKEN REGULARLY (e.g., insulin, digitalis)
Médications pris regulièrement (e.g., insuline, digitale)

Health problem — Problème de santé	Generic and trade names of medication — Noms génériques et commerciaux de la médication	Medication dosage — Dose de médication	Physician's remarks — Remarques du médecin	Physician's signature — Signature du médecin

OPHTHALMIC INFORMATION (prescription glasses)
Information ophtalmique (lunnettes prescription)

	Sphere Sphere	Cylinder Cylindre	Axis Axe	Prism Prisme	Base Courbe
(OD) Ocular dexter Oculaire droit					
(OS) Ocular sinister Oculaire gauche					

Add _____   Base curve _____

Addition _____   Courbe base _____

Other _____

Autre _____

AUTHORIZATION TO PURCHASE CONTROLLED SUBSTANCES FOR VESSELS

Federal Regulations (21 CFR 1301.28) provide that controlled substances, coming within the purview of the Controlled Substances Act of 1970, for stocking medicine chests, first aid packets, and dispensaries maintained on board any vessel engaged in international trade, or in trade between ports of the United States, and any merchant vessel belonging to the Government may be acquired only in two ways. (1) By a medical officer, employed by the owner or operator of such vessel, licensed in a state as a physician and registered under the Act at the location of the principal office of the owner or operator of the vessel. (2) If no such medical officer is employed by the owner or operator of a vessel, or in the event such medical officer is not accessible and the acquisition of controlled substances is required, the master of the vessel, who shall not be registered under the Act, may purchase controlled substances only with the approval of, and upon this form HSA-590 (formerly HSM-590) provided by, a medical officer of the United States Public Health Service. Blank or presigned Form HSA-590 may not be furnished to ships or shipping companies by USPHS.

TO: *(Name and Address of Vendor)*	DATE

In accordance with the regulations noted above, you are authorized to furnish to the Master of the vessel identified below, the following controlled substances, which are to be used exclusively in stocking the medicine chest, dispensary, or first aid packets maintained on board said vessel.

ITEM	TO BE COMPLETED BY USPHS MEDICAL OFFICER			TO BE COMPLETED BY VENDOR	
	MEDICATION *(Include the controlled substance component(s) if not a part of the preparation's name)*	DESCRIPTION OF MEDICATION *(State dosage form, strength, and number or volume per container)*	NO. OF CONTAINERS REQUESTED	DATE FILLED	NO. OF CONTAINERS FURNISHED
A	B	C	D	E	F
1.					
2.					
3.					
4.					
5.					
6.					
7.					
8.					

Available only from medical officers of the United States Public Health Service. (See Appendix A, p. 428)

This authorization is for exactly _____ items.

NAME OF VESSEL, OFFICIAL NO., & COUNTRY OF REGISTRY	STATION NAME AND ADDRESS
OWNER OR OPERATOR OF VESSEL	NAME OF AUTHORIZING USPHS MEDICAL OFFICER *(Type or print)*
NAME OF MASTER OF VESSEL *(Type or print)*	TITLE
SIGNATURE OF MASTER OF VESSEL	SIGNATURE OF AUTHORIZING USPHS MEDICAL OFFICER

HSA-590 (FORMERLY HSM-590)
REV. 11-75

(See Instructions on Reverse)

MASTER'S COPY
(Retain aboard vessel)

INSTRUCTIONS FOR COMPLETION OF THIS FORM

1. The total number of items ordered on the form must be stated in the space provided for that purpose.

2. Only one item is to be entered on each numbered line. An item may consist of one or more containers of the same size, but must not be counted on the form as more than one item.

3. The purchaser must include in column B, "Medication", the controlled substance's component(s) if not a part of the preparation's name, e.g., Paregoric (Opium).

4. Column C, "Description of Medication", shall include the dosage form, e.g., tablets, capsules, or ampuls, etc., or if a liquid, the volume in the container, e.g., 240 ml. (8 fl. oz.) or 480 ml. (1 pt.), and the strength.

5. In column D, "Number of Containers Requested", enter the number of containers.

6. The vendor shall enter in columns E and F of both the original and the Master's copy of the form presented to him the date this order is filled and the number of containers furnished for each line item. If an item is not filled in its entirety, the vendor shall place in column F only the number of containers actually furnished.

DISPOSITION OF COPIES

VENDOR'S COPY (white)	Filed with the controlled substances records of the vendor filling the order.
MASTER'S COPY (blue)	Retained aboard the vessel.
REGIONAL OFFICE DIRECTOR'S COPY (yellow)	Mailed immediately by the USPHS facility where issued to the Drug Enforcement Administration Regional Office covering the area where the facility is located.
MEDICAL OFFICER'S COPY (pink)	Retained for USPHS issuing facility's files.

HSA-590 (BACK)
REV. 11-75

Form A – Appendix D

Name of Drug _____

Form _____

Strength _____

Unit _____
(Tablet, Ampul, Other)

CONTROLLED SUBSTANCE
Acquisition, Use, and Perpetual Inventory Record

Owner/Agent _____ Average Complement _____

Name of Vessel _____

Voyage Number	Date Voyage Begun	Date Voyage Ended	Date Received or Administered	No. of Units (tablet, ampul, etc.) acquired	No. of Units Administered	Total Number of Units Remaining on Hand	Patient's Name or Source of New Stock	Reason for Administering	Initials of Person Administering the Medications or Receiving New Stock

SUGGESTED FORMAT

Form A -- Appendix D

CONTROLLED SUBSTANCE
Acquisition, Use, and Perpetual Inventory Record

Name of Drug **Codeine Sulfate**

Form **Tablet**

Strength **30 mg**

Unit **Tablet**

(Tablet, Ampul, Other)

Name of Vessel **Seven Seas** Owner/Agent **Thomas & Co., Inc.** Average Complement **35**

SUGGESTED FORMAT THAT SHOWS HOW ENTRIES MAY BE MADE

Voyage Number	Date Voyage Begun	Date Voyage Ended	Date Received or Administered	No. of Units (tablet, ampul, etc.) acquired	No. of Units Administered	Total Number of Units Remaining on Hand	Patient's Name or Source of New Stock	Reason for Administering	Initials of Person Administering the Medications or Receiving New Stock
In port of Norfolk, Va.			Inventory		6-8-74	11			John E. Jones
In port of Norfolk, Va.			6-9-74			114	...york Wholesale Drug Co., Inc.		J.E.J.
15	6-10-74	6-15-74	6-15-74		1	113	Henry Jackson	Toothache pain	J.E.J.
16	7-30-74	9-15-74	Inventory		9-15-74	113	No Transactions		J.E.J.
17	11-15-74	12-27-74	11-21-74		1	112	Richard Hall	Sprained left foot-pain	J.E.J.
"	"	"	11-22-74		2	110	Richard Hall	pain	J.B.
In port of New York			Inventory		2/11/75	110	Custody assumed by		Robert E. Baker

459

Forms Discussed in Appendices C and D

U.S DEPARTMENT OF JUSTICE / DRUG ENFORCEMENT ADMINISTRATION	OMB APPROVAL
REPORT OF THEFT OR LOSS OF CONTROLLED SUBSTANCES	No 43 - RO464

Federal Regulations require registrants to submit a detailed report of any theft or loss of Controlled Substances to the Drug Enforcement Administration.
Complete this form in triplicate. Forward the original and duplicate copies to the nearest DEA Regional Office. Retain the triplicate copy for your records.

1 NAME AND ADDRESS OF REGISTRANT (Include ZIP Code)

ZIP Code ☐☐☐☐☐

2 PRINCIPAL BUSINESS OF REGISTRANT *(Check one)*

1 ☐ Pharmacy   3 ☐ Manufacturer/Distributor

2 ☐ Practitioner   4 ☐ Other _____

3 DEA REGISTRATION NUMBER
2 ltr prefix ☐☐   7 digit suffix ☐☐☐☐☐☐☐

4 COUNTY IN WHICH REGISTRANT IS LOCATED

5. DATE OF THEFT OR LOSS

6 NUMBER OF THEFTS OR LOSSES REGISTRANT EXPERIENCED IN LAST 12 MONTHS

7 WAS THEFT OR LOSS REPORTED TO POLICE
☐ YES   ☐ NO

8. NAME AND ADDRESS OF POLICE DEPARTMENT

9 TYPE OF THEFT OR LOSS (Check one)

1 ☐ Night Break-In (complete Item 10 below)   4 ☐ Customer Pilferage

2 ☐ Armed Robbery (complete Item 11 below)   5 ☐ Other (specify) _____

3 ☐ Employee Theft   6 ☐ Lost in Transit (complete Item 12 below)

10 IF NIGHT BREAK-IN, WHAT WAS THE POINT OF ENTRY ?

11 IF ARMED ROBBERY, WAS ANYONE INJURED ?
☐ NO   ☐ YES (If Yes, HOW ?)

12 IF LOST IN TRANSIT, COMPLETE THE FOLLOWING

A Name of Common Carrier	B Name of Consignee	C Consignee's DEA Registration Number

13 IF OFFICIAL CONTROLLED SUBSTANCES ORDER FORMS WERE STOLEN, GIVE NUMBERS

14 WHAT IDENTIFYING MARKS, SYMBOLS OR PRICE CODES WERE ON THE LABELS OF THESE CONTAINERS ? (Insert your pricing codes)

15 a IF CASH WAS TAKEN, WHAT AMOUNT ?

15b IF MERCHANDISE WAS TAKEN, VALUE ?

16 WHAT SECURITY MEASURES HAVE BEEN TAKEN TO PREVENT FUTURE THEFTS OR LOSSES ?

PRIVACY ACT INFORMATION

AUTHORITY: Section 301 of the Controlled Substances Act of 1970 (PL 91-513)

PURPOSE: Report theft or loss of Controlled Substances

ROUTINE USES: The Controlled Substances Act Registration Records produces special reports as required for statistical analytical purposes. Disclosures of information from this system are made to the following categories of users for the purposes stated:

A. Other Federal law enforcement and regulatory agencies for law enforcement and regulatory purposes

B. State and local law enforcement and regulatory agencies for law enforcement and regulatory purposes

C. Persons registered under the Controlled Substances Act (Public Law 91-513) for the purpose of verifying the registration of customers and practitioners

EFFECT: Failure to report theft or loss of controlled substances may result in penalties under Section 402 and 403 of the Controlled Substances Act.

DEA Form (Apr 1976) — **106**   Previous edition dated 9/75 is Obsolete

LIST OF CONTROLLED SUBSTANCES LOST

	NAME OF SUBSTANCE OR PREPARATION (Include Manufacturer)	NAME OF CONTROLLED SUBSTANCE IN PREP	DOSAGE FORM AND STRENGTH	QUANTITY	TOTAL NET WT (Gms.) OF CONTROLLED INGREDIENT
EX	EMPIRIN ++ 3	CODEINE	½ GR TAB.	100	3,200
1					
2					
3					
4.					
5.					
6					
7					
8.					
9.					
10.					
11					
12					
13					
14.					
15					
16					
17.					
18					
19					
20.					
21.					
22.					
23.					
24					
25					
26					
27					
28.					
29					
30.					
31.					
32					
33.					
34.					
35.					
36.					
37					

Reverse side of DEA Form 106: Report of Theft or Loss of Controlled Substances. Form available from DEA Regional Offices, U.S. Department of Justice.

FOR DEA REGIONAL USE ONLY	GRAMS
AMPHETAMINES	
BARBITURATES	
COCAINE	
CODEINE	
DIHYDROCODEINONE	
DILAUDID	
METHADONE	
METHAMPHETAMINE	
MORPHINE	
NUMORPHAN	
OPIUM	
OXYCODONE	
PETHIDINE	
OTHERS (List)	

I certify that the foregoing information is correct to the best of my knowledge and belief.

Signature _____

Title _____

Date _____

GPO 1976 O - 204-310

Form B — Appendix D

TRANSFER OF CUSTODY OF CONTROLLED SUBSTANCES
(Narcotics and Other Controlled Medications)

I, _____, Master of _____
attest that the physical inventory and perpetual inventory records of
the narcotics and other controlled substances listed below are in
balance, and that such records are complete and accurate records of all
activities relating to the medication listed below.

A transfer of these medications is made as of this date to
_____, my successor.

Date _____ Signature _____

	Drug	Form	Strength	Unit (Capsule, Tablet, etc.)
1.				
2.				
3.				
4.				
5.				
6.				
7.				
8.				
9.				
10.				
11.				
12.				

SUGGESTED FORMAT for keeping records on the transfer of custody of controlled substances. Shipping companies and/or owners of vessels may have this format printed in quantities that will meet their needs.
Copies of the form are NOT available from the U.S. Public Health Service.

ACCEPTANCE
I certify that I have received from _____ the
quantities listed in the perpetual inventory records as of this date.
I accept responsibility for the custody and issuances of these medications,
as well as for any additional received while I am Master of _____
_____.

Date _____ Signature _____

Index

A

Abandonment of vessel, 337–338
Abdominal
  cavity, 22
  distention, 163–164
  injuries, 94
  pain (stomachache), 148–149
Abrasion, 51
Abscess
  boils, 235–236
  dental, 152–153
Abuse
  alcohol definition, 201
  drug, 206–212
  marihuana, 211–212
  solvent, 212
Acetylsalicylic acid
  see Aspirin
Acetaminophen, 257, 262, 271
Acetazolamide, 257, 262–263, 271
Acids, poisoning, 111
Acne, 234
Acquired immunity, 366
Adam's apple, 20
Adenoids, 19
Adhesions, 22
Addiction
  alcohol, 200–206
  drug, 206–212
Administration of medicines
  see Medications
Administration set, intravenous, 296
Admission to sickbay, 303
Adrenal glands, 32–33
Agitated depression, 216–217
Ague, 178–180
Air conditioning
  see Ventilation
Air embolism, prevention in veni-
  puncture, 315
Air splints, inflatable, 81
Airway
  inserting an, 71
  open, in CPR, 116–117
  pharyngeal, 295
Alcohol, 111
  abuse, addiction, definition, body
    reaction, metabolism, 201
  poisoning, 111–112
  rubbing, 257, 271
Alcohols, 200–201
  ethyl, 200
  methyl, 200
  isopropyl, 200, 319
  denatured, 200
  grain, 200

Alcoholism, 200–206
  chronic, 24, 204
  convulsive state, 204
  definition, 201
  management of patients, 202
Alimentary canal, 22–23
Alkalies, poisoning, 111
Alkaline aromatic solution, 257, 271
Allergy
  acute, 223
  bacterial, 223
  bronchitis, 223–225
  chronic, 223
  irritation, due to, 223
  reactions, 220–221
  viral, 223
Aluminum acetate, 257, 263, 271
Aluminum hydroxide with magne-
  sium hydroxide or magnesium tri-
  silicate, 257, 263, 272
American Medical Association,
  address, 47
American Society of Hospital Phar-
  macists (ASHP), 262
Aminophylline suppository, rectal,
  257, 272
Ammonia
  inhalant, 257, 272
  poisoning, 111
Amoebic dysentery, 151
Amphetamine, 112, 210
Ampicillin, 257, 263, 272–273
AMVER system, 420
Amylnitrite inhalant, 257, 273
Anaphylactic shock, 221
Anatomical regions, 2
Anatomy, definition, 1
Angina pectoris, 136
Angio edema, 240
Animal bites, 59
Ankle
  bones, 13–14
  fracture, 92–93
Anopheles mosquito, 179
Antemortem statement, 355–356
Anthrax, 173
Antibodies, disease, immunity, 366
Antidote, general, poisoning, 109–110
Antihistamine poisoning, 112
Antitoxins, 366
Antivenin serum, 61
Anuria, urine retention, 172
Anus, 22–24
Anxiety attacks, 227
Apoplexy
  see Stroke
Apothecary system, 301
Appendices, 427–462
Appendicitis, 24, 149
Appendicular skeleton, 3, 4, 11

Appendix, 22, 24, 149
Arm
  bones of, 4
  fractures, 81–84
  structure, 11–12
Armpits, ringworm, 244
Arsenic poisoning, 114
Arteries
  names, 18
  pressure points, 55
Arthritis, 196–197
Artificial circulation, pressure point,
  122, 130–131
  see CPR
Artificial ventilation, alternate meth-
  od, 130–131
  see CPR
Ascending colon, 24
Asepsis, 317–318
Asiatic cholera, 174–175
Asphyxia, 115, 123
Aspirin, 257, 273
  poisoning, 114
Asthma, 221–222, 226
Athlete's foot, 244–245
Atopic dermatitis, 237
Atropine sulfate, 257, 273
Auditory nerves, 30
Autoclaving, 318
Autonomic nervous system, 28, 30, 31
Avoirdupois system, 301
Avulsions, 52
Axial skeleton, 3–4
Axillary thermometer, 305
Axon, 27

B

Baby, newborn
  baptizing, 354–355
  care after delivery, 353
  feeding, 354
  resuscitating, 353–354
Bacillary dysentery
  see Dysentery
Bacitracin ointment, 257, 273
Back
  bandage, 63–65
  injuries, 95
  pressure—arm lift technique, 130-
    131
Backache, 197–198
Backbone, fracture, 85, 88
Backrub, 259, 280
Bacterial bronchitis, 223
Bacterial food poisoning, 157–160
Bag, mortuary, 296–297, 357–358
Baking soda
  see Sodium bicarbonate

T